Rheumatology
IN PRIMARY CARE

JUAN J. CANOSO, M.D., F.A.C.P.

Adjunct Professor of Medicine
Tufts University School of Medicine
Private practice
American British Cowdray Hospital
Mexico City, Mexico

SOUTH COLLEGE
709 Mall Blvd.
Savannah, GA 31406

W.B. SAUNDERS COMPANY
A Division of Harcourt Brace & Company
Philadelphia   London   Toronto   Montreal   Sydney   Tokyo

W.B. SAUNDERS COMPANY
A Division of Harcourt Brace & Company

The Curtis Center
Independence Square West
Philadelphia, Pennsylvania 19106

Library of Congress Cataloging-in-Publication Data

Canoso, Juan J.

Rheumatology in primary care / Juan J. Canoso.

p. cm.

ISBN 0–7216–6080–0

1. Rheumatology. 2. Primary Care (Medicine) 3. Connective tissue—Diseases. 4. Musculo-skeletal system—Diseases. I. Title.

[DNLM: 1. Rheumatic Diseases. 2. Bone Diseases. 3. Primary Health Care. WE 544 C227r 1997]

RC927.C323 1997   616.7'23—dc21

DNLM/DLC   96-40174

RHEUMATOLOGY IN PRIMARY CARE   ISBN 0–7216–6080–0

Copyright © 1997 by W.B. Saunders Company.

All rights reserved. No part of this publication may be reproduced or transmitted in any form or by any means, electronic or mechanical, including photocopy, recording, or any information storage and retrieval system, without permission in writing from the publisher.

Printed in the United States of America.

Last digit is the print number: 9   8   7   6   5   4   3   2   1

In Memoriam

Professor Pablo Purriel, Montevideo
Sheldon M. Wolff, M.D., Boston

To

Mary-Carmen, and Adrian, Diego, Luis, and Mary

PREFACE

As its title suggests, the aim of *Rheumatology in Primary Care* is to provide primary care physicians, family practitioners, and internists with concise, practical information on the care and management of one particular group of patients: those afflicted with rheumatologic disorders.

The initial chapters on rheumatologic history, physical examination, pattern recognition, imaging studies, laboratory utilization, and general therapy should be read first. These concise chapters serve as a road map to the lengthier disease-specific chapters, as well as providing an introduction to good rheumatologic technique. Next, you should familiarize yourself with the various guidelines on rheumatic diseases presented at the end of the appendix. These have been put together by thoughtful and knowledgeable committees, most of them under the aegis of the American College of Rheumatology. The wealth of sound advice in the guidelines may then be applied in the appropriate clinical situations. Upon this foundation, read the disease-oriented chapters as you encounter rheumatic disease patients in your daily practice. These chapters are supplemented by relevant sections in the appendix—i.e., the guidelines, physical therapy instructions, and information on community and other resources. The material presented in the exercise instruction pages should be passed on to your patients, to serve as reminders after you have given them practical instruction on the correct performance of these exercises. (Without question, it would be ideal to have the help of physical therapists, occupational therapists, and physiatrists; but this is not always possible in the real world.) Finally, some actual case summaries are included in the text. These cases have taught me a lot. I hope you will find them enjoyable to read as well as instructive.

Two important areas are not included in the book. One is a description of rheumatic diseases in children; the other is a discussion of basic disease mechanisms. For information on these fascinating and complex topics, reference should be made to textbooks dealing specifically with them.

I wish you a rewarding reading experience and encourage any suggestions or criticisms you may have.

Acknowledgments

I thank Ray Kersey of the W.B. Saunders Company for his trust, guidance, and patience; Mary-Carmen Amigo, M.D., for helpful suggestions on the manuscript; Ma. Cristina Lara M., M.D., Radiologist at Centro Médico Nacional Siglo XXI, Mexico D.F., for radiographic material; Leonardo Zamudio, M.D., for his generosity in opening his library to all interested; Françoise Bartlett for invaluable help during the editorial process; Christina Viera for the attractive page layouts; and Nora Souza for her excellent drawings.

Mexico City
November 1996

Juan J. Canoso, M.D.

NOTICE

Medicine is an ever-changing field. Standard safety precautions must be followed, but as new research and clinical experience broaden our knowledge, changes in treatment and drug therapy become necessary or appropriate. The editors of this work have carefully checked the generic and trade drug names and verified drug dosages to ensure that the dosage information in this work is accurate and in accord with the standards accepted at the time of publication. Readers are advised, however, to check the product information currently provided by the manufacturer of each drug to be administered to be certain that changes have not been made in the recommended dose or in the contraindications for administration. This is of particular importance in regard to new or infrequently used drugs. It is the responsibility of the treating physician, relying on experience and knowledge of the patient, to determine dosages and the best treatment for the patient. The editors cannot be responsible for misuse or misapplication of the material in this work.

The Publisher

CONTENTS

Part I	**Introduction**	**1**
1	Introduction	3
2	Physical Examination	5
3	Pattern Recognition in Rheumatology	12
4	Imaging Studies	21
5	Laboratory Studies	27
6	Immunologic Studies	32
7	Questionnaires and Other Assessment Intruments; Criteria	37
8	Methods of Treatment	41
9	Special Situations in Rheumatic Disease Therapy	50
10	Rheumatic Manifestations of Endocrine, Hematologic, and Malignant Disease	52
11	Disability Issues	55
Part II	**Connective Tissue Disorders**	**57**
12	Rheumatoid Arthritis	59
13	Systemic Lupus Erythematosus (SLE), Primary Antiphospholipid Syndrome, and Sjögren's Syndrome	74
14	Inflammatory Conditions of Muscle	97
15	Systemic Sclerosis (Scleroderma) and Related Syndromes	104
16	The Vasculitides	115
17	The Spondyloarthropathies	133
18	Crystal-Induced Arthritis	150
19	Infectious Arthritis	162
20	Osteoarthritis	176
21	Infiltrative Conditions	183

Part III		**Bone Diseases**	**187**
	22	Bone Diseases	*189*
Part IV		**Musculoskeletal Conditions (Regional Rheumatic Diseases)**	**209**
	23	Hand and Wrist Pain	*211*
	24	Elbow Pain	*227*
	25	Shoulder Pain	*238*
	26	Neck, Dorsal, and Low Back Pain	*254*
	27	Hip Pain	*270*
	28	Knee Pain	*274*
	29	Foot Pain	*285*
Part V		**Pain Amplification Syndromes, Related Conditions, and Miscellanea**	**297**
	30	Pain Amplification Syndromes, Related Conditions, and Miscellanea	*299*
		Appendix	*317*
		Index	*355*

PART I

INTRODUCTION

CHAPTER 1

Introduction

A current listing by the American College of Rheumatology includes over 150 conditions that fall within the field of rheumatology. For most, etiology is unknown. Many of these conditions have been rather artificially delimited with a tendency to be overinclusive. Lack of a known cause and inclusiveness have resulted in wide disease spectra. From a clinician's viewpoint, patients present with complaints such as a painful knee or shoulder, abnormal findings such as a knobby hand, or clinical clusters or syndromes of varying complexity. Examples include inflammation in multiple joints (polyarthritis); a painful, swollen joint of a few days duration (acute arthritis); arthritis and inflammation at tendon insertions (reactive arthritis); arthritis, facial rash, and a pericardial rub (usually systemic lupus erythematosus); proximal weakness and dermatitis (dermatomyositis); and a history of recurrent fetal loss, livedo reticularis, and stroke in a young woman (primary antiphospholipid syndrome).

Seasoned clinicians place great emphasis on the history and physical examination because the clearer the observation, the narrower the differential diagnosis. Once at this point, after listening, looking, touching, and thinking, laboratory determinations and imaging procedures can be extremely helpful. Used earlier in the diagnostic process, however, they not only add unnecessary expense, but more likely positive findings will represent so-called false positives, resulting in confusion rather than enlightenment.

In addition, a thoughtful process of diagnostic reduction enables the clinician to initiate treatment in instances in which a definite diagnosis is wanting. For example, it may not be possible to tell whether an older patient with recent complaints has early late-onset rheumatoid arthritis or polymyalgia rheumatica with peripheral joint involvement. Nonspecific medications may be used, however, that help both conditions. The diagnostic dilemma may be solved when medications are reduced and discontinued after the expected duration of polymyalgia rheumatica, a self-limited disease, has elapsed. Relapse will be virtually diagnostic of rheumatoid arthritis.

Musculoskeletal History

Patients should be given an opportunity to describe in their own words, and with the only recommendation that they use descriptive words rather than labels, the *chief complaint* and the *very onset of symptoms*. Since pain is the main symptom in rheumatic disease, physicians should become conversant with leading pain patterns. Pain that originates in superficial structures such as the skin and superficial bursae is sharply localized to the diseased area. When deeper structures are involved such as joints, ligaments, tendons, and periosteum, pain may be experienced about the involved structure or at a more distant site. In general, superficial joints, ligaments, and tendons hurt locally whereas pain originating in deep-seated structures such as the shoulder and hip radiates distally in the limb along muscles derived from the same embryologic segment. It becomes quite important to differentiate deep pain radiation from dermatomic pain. Dermatomic pain arises from root irritation and is superficially experienced, sharply localized, and associates with pins and needles sensation. Deep pain is dull, boring, poorly localized, and may associate with muscle spasm and tender points within the painful area.

After obtaining this essential information I favor a guided interview. The initial task is to determine if one is dealing with regional or systemic disease. To this end, in all patients I use an initial set of questions or *systemic disease module:* "How well do you feel on waking up in the morning as compared with later in the day?", "Would you describe your early morning symptoms?", "How long does it take you to be at your best?" are questions used to sort out regional from systemic disease. People with mechanical/structural regional syndromes wake up well or with minimal symptoms and become achy with activities. People with systemic conditions from fibromyalgia through polyarteritis nodosa wake up tired, stiff, and achy. Once systemic disease is suspected, the use of second-order modules allows a directed questioning in which few errors of omission are possible. These modules include questions to identify inflammation, infectious disease, fibromyalgia, rheumatoid arthritis, conditions presenting palindromic arthritis, SLE/Sjögren's/Primary antiphospholipid syndrome (PAPS)/Scleroderma/Myositis module, vasculitis, spondyloarthropathy, and gout, as follows:

Inflammatory module: Fatigue, need to take naps, night sweats, anorexia, weight loss, joint or muscle pain that improves with activity (mechanical conditions get worse with activity).

Infection module: Fever, chills, meningismus, sore throat, skin rash, urogenital discharge. Consider time of year; travel history; a possible portal of entry such as insect bite, skin infection, urogenital infection, recent accidental or surgical wound, and sexual exposure.

Fibromyalgia module: Fatigue, generalized achiness, inefficient sleep, chronic headaches, temporomandibular joint (TMJ) dysfunction, spastic colitis, irritable bladder, multiple drug intolerances, history of depression.

Rheumatoid arthritis module: Small joint involvement such as metacarpophalangeals, proximal interphalangeals, and metatarsophalangeals; symmetry; persistence of symptoms for 6 or more weeks.

Palindromic rheumatism module: Self-limited arthritis or periarthritis that lasts hours to a few days in each individual joint, jumps from joint to joint, and recurs for at least 3 months.

SLE/Sjögren's/Primary antiphospholipid syndrome(PAPS)/ Scleroderma/Myositis module: Alopecia; rash (face, upper chest, fingers, legs); livedo reticularis (blotchy skin); tight skin; fingertip ulcers; Raynaud's (a clearly demarcated white discoloration of digits upon cold exposure); leg ulcers; sicca syndrome (dry eyes, mouth, vagina); oral or nasal ulcers; parotid gland enlargement; dysphagia; dyspnea; pleuritic pain; paresthesias; proximal muscle weakness; history of migraine, stroke, anemia, thrombocytopenia, urine abnormalities, (false) positive serology for syphilis, epilepsy, miscarriages, or thrombophlebitis.

Vasculitis module: Fever; recent headaches; visual decline; jaw claudication (masseter cramp upon chewing); tongue or gum pain or paresthesias; recent deafness; otitis media; nasal discharge, especially if bloody; sinusitis; petechiae (palpable purpura on examination); livedo reticularis; hematuria; skin ulcers; muscle pain; abdominal pain; peripheral neuropathy (especially a wrist drop or a foot drop); stroke.

Spondyloarthropathy module: Early morning and nocturnal low back pain; lumbosacral stiffness that lasts hours upon arising; shifting sciatica (alternating sides); enthesitis (pain or swelling at Achilles tendon or plantar fascia insertion); conjunctivitis; iritis; oral or genital ulcers; antecedent diarrhea or urethritis; history of psoriasis or inflammatory bowel disease (IBD); family history of ankylosing spondylitis, iritis, IBD, or psoriasis.

Gout module: History of kidney stones, arterial hypertension, use of diuretics, or exposure to lead; presence of myeloproliferative disease; family history of gout.

CHAPTER 2

Physical Examination

Musculoskeletal examination may be routine and unrewarding or satisfying and helpful. All depends on the examiner's attitude, knowledge of anatomy, understanding of pathology, and especially the use of a directed rather than random examination routine. Joint examination cannot be learned from goniometric charts. Ask any rheumatologist how often, in actual practice, that goniometer on the shelf gets used. Excessive emphasis on degrees of motion chills the beginner and is frowned on by the experienced because even the most detailed goniometric charts ignore variation among normal individuals. Sex, race, and age have an impact on joint motion. Women are more limber than men, Asians and blacks more than whites, and children more than adults.

Joint range can only be learned by examining diverse people with and without rheumatic complaints and always using the same method. In asymptomatic patients a brief musculoskeletal examination may take 1½ to 2 minutes. Individual observations are internalized and subconsciously averaged. Based on that knowledge and experience, deviations from the norm can be readily identified. This seemingly radical advice is nothing new: Clinicians routinely auscultate hearts and lungs and palpate abdomens regardless of symptoms. In so doing they subconsciously create ranges of normal findings. Based on this background, murmurs are identified and enlarged livers are felt without even giving it a thought.

Prior to describing the brief joint examination three important principles of musculoskeletal pathophysiology are reviewed:

Acute Arthritis: Acutely inflamed joints, similar to experimentally distended joints, spontaneously adopt a characteristic position in which intraarticular pressures are lowest for a given volume of effusion. Awareness of these postures, which are shown in Table 2–1, is essential to focus attention on joints and to distinguish periarticular from articular inflammation.

PATIENT 1: A young woman presented to the emergency room with fever, rigors, and an acutely inflamed right knee (Figure 2–1). Septic arthritis was initially considered, but six attempted knee aspirations yielded no fluid. A more experienced observer noticed that, inconsistent with septic arthritis, the involved limb could be brought painlessly to full extension (Figure 2–2) and suggested the possibility of septic prepatellar bursitis. Aspiration of the prepatellar bursa yielded 0.5 cc of turbid fluid. Smears showed gram positive cocci arranged in chains, and group A streptococci grew on culture. A CT scan obtained 1 hour later (Figure 2–3) revealed a large subcutaneous fluid collection at the outer aspect of the joint. The air bubbles, from 1 cc of air injected in the prepatellar bursa, are proof of the rupture of the bursal sac. The fluid collection was drained with a pigtail catheter, the knee was immobilized with a plaster splint (Figure 2–4), and intravenous penicillin was begun. Drainage ceased in 4 days. A slow improvement led to full recovery within 2 months.

In addition, in acute arthritis range of motion is limited, active and passive ranges of motion are equal, pain occurs in all directions of motion, there is capsular tenderness, and accessible joints are tender, warm, and swollen.

Distal Pain Radiation: Pain is felt locally in superficial joints but extends distally in the limb (deep pain) in deep joints such as the shoulder (Figure 2–5) and hip (Figure 2–6). Confusion may arise if the distal radiation is considered evidence of local disease.

PATIENT 2: An elderly man who was on the waiting list for bilateral knee replacement was referred for evaluation of back pain. His spine was stiff and he could hardly move the neck. Hips only had a jog of extremely painful motion. Interestingly, rather than in the vicinity of the hip, pain was perceived in the anterior knee. Finally, by having the patient lie supine near the edge of the examining table, both knees could be brought without difficulty from full extension to at least 90 degrees flexion, which further ruled out a knee origin of his pain. As expected, an AP pelvic radiograph revealed bilateral sacroiliac joint fusion and destroyed hips. Ankylosing spondylitis was diagnosed and bilateral total hip (rather than knee) replacement gave the patient over 10 years of acceptable function.

TABLE 2–1

SPONTANEOUS POSITIONS ADOPTED BY JOINTS IN ACUTE ARTHRITIS

Metacarpophalangeal: ulnar deviation, semiflexion
Wrist: neutral
Elbow: semiflexion (30–75°)
Shoulder: abduction (30–60°)
Hip: flexion (30–65°)
   external rotation (15°)
   abduction (15°)
Knee: semiflexion (30–60°)
Ankle: plantar flexion (15°)
Subtalar: neutral

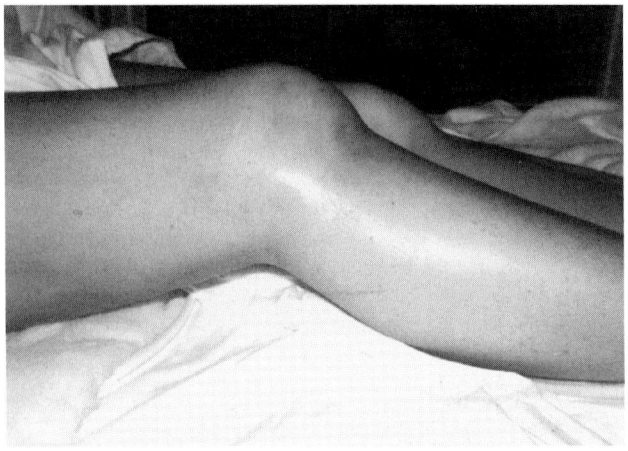

FIGURE 2–1. *Patient 1.* The presumed diagnosis in this young woman was acute arthritis of the right knee. (From Canoso JJ, Barza M. Soft tissue infections. Clin Rheum Dis 19:293–307, 1993. By permission of W. B. Saunders.)

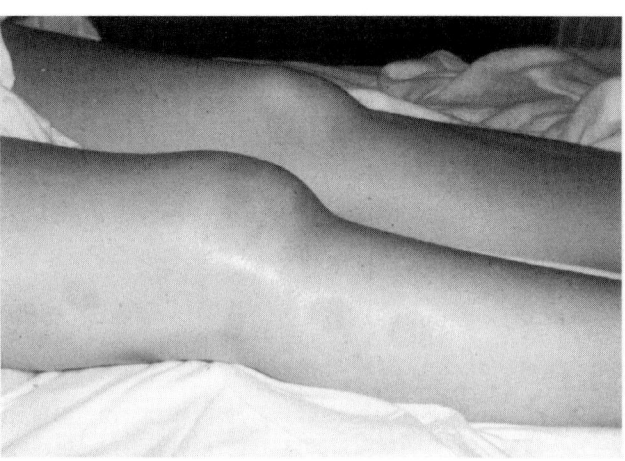

FIGURE 2–2. *Patient 1.* However, the knee could be fully extended, suggesting extraarticular inflammation. There was extensive pitting edema as well as fluctuance and tenderness in the prepatellar area. Thin pus aspirated from the prepatellar bursa eventually grew group A streptococcus.

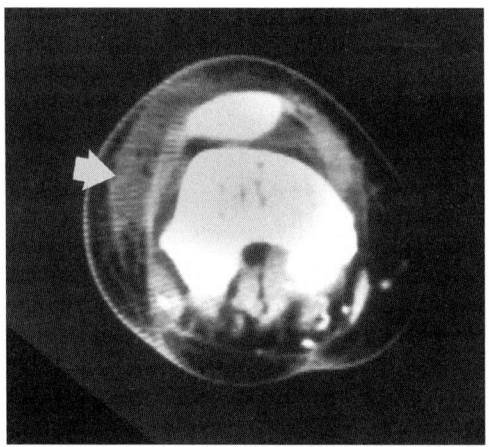

FIGURE 2–3. *Patient 1.* CT scan showed fluid collection in the subcutaneous tissue (arrow) plus air bubbles from 1 mL of air injected in the prepatellar bursa at the time of aspiration, proving bursal rupture.

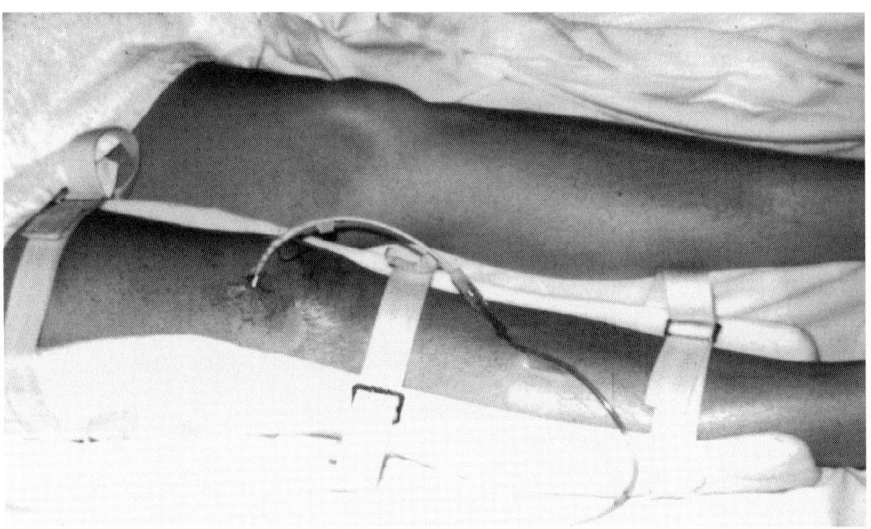

FIGURE 2–4. *Patient 1.* Cavity was drained using a pigtail catheter, and a posterior resting splint was applied. Recovery was uneventful with parenteral and then oral antibiotics.

Tenosynovitis or Arthritis? In tenosynovitis, such as digital flexor tenosynovitis, passive flexion is greater than active flexion (similar findings may be caused by tendon rupture, muscle weakness, and denervation).

PATIENT 3. A woman with long-standing rheumatoid arthritis slowly developed an incomplete fist. On examination, on attempted flexion, several fingers in each hand did not reach the palm. To distinguish flexor tenosynovitis from interphalangeal joint arthritis, the examiner gently helped finger flexion. Some of these fingers had complete passive flexion plus subtle diffuse swelling of the flexor tendon sheath. In the others no further flexion occurred and the PIPs were tender. Well-targeted steroid injections greatly helped this patient's hand function.

The *brief examination* of the musculoskeletal system (which should be used in all routine complete physical examinations) includes gait inspection as the patient walks into the room, maneuvers based on active and passive joint motion, a search for fibromyalgic tender points, and a summary assessment of muscle strength.

Patients should be fully undressed including shoes and socks and have the examining gown open to the back. The sequence and content of the brief musculoskeletal examination is shown in Table 2–2. Figure 2–7 shows the location of tender points in fibromyalgia. Tender point examination has become an essential component of the physical examination.

In patients with regional complaints (hand, wrist, elbow, shoulder, neck, back, hip, knee, ankle/subtalars, feet), the *detailed examination* is based on an analysis of active, passive, and resisted motion. Details of this examination are discussed in the regional rheumatic diseases section. An effort should always be made, in assessing painful or swollen joints, to identify extraarticular components such as tenosynovial, bursal, or enthesial involvement. Optimal therapeutic response can only be achieved if these lesions are addressed. Indeed, their treatment may entirely eliminate pain. Examples of concurrent soft tissue lesions include trochanteric bursitis in patients with hip osteoarthritis, anserine bursitis in cases of knee osteoarthritis, posterior tibialis tenosynovitis (which produces pain and swelling in the medial retromalleolar area) in patients with "ankle" arthritis, and Achilles tendinitis and plantar fasciitis in the spondyloarthropathies.

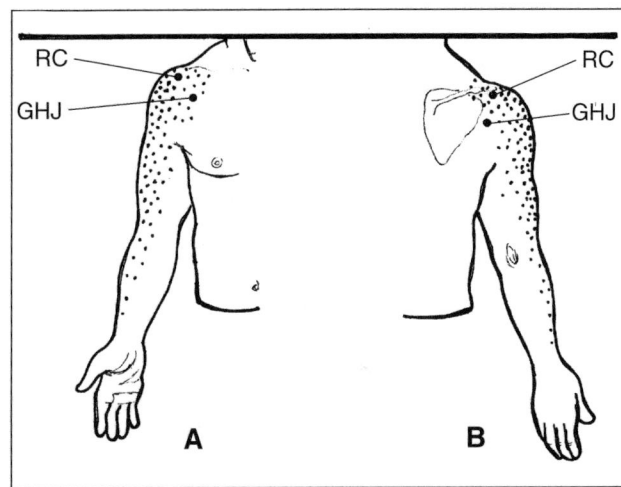

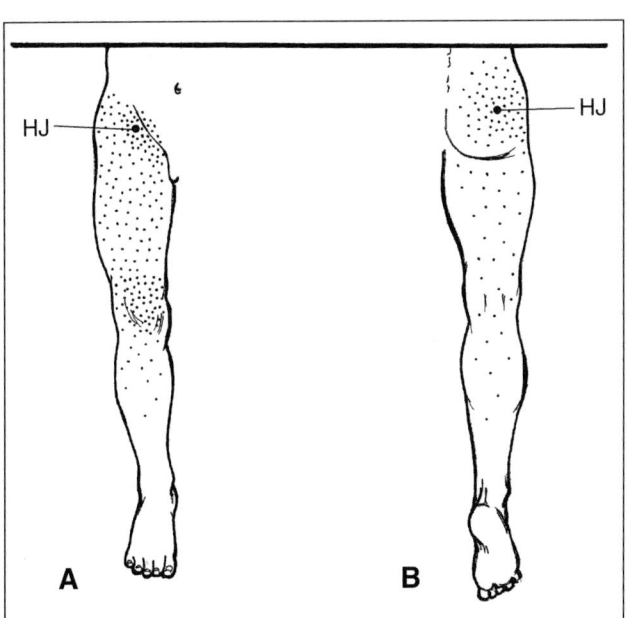

FIGURE 2–5. Pain from deep shoulder structures radiates along C5. When severe, pain may reach the radial forearm and even the hand. GHJ = Glenohumeral joint. RC = Rotator cuff. (After Kellgren JH. In: Scott JT (ed) Copeman's Textbook of the Rheumatic Diseases, 5th ed. Churchill Livingstone, Edinburgh, 62–77, 1978.)

FIGURE 2–6. *L2–4 pain radiation from the hip joint.* Pain may be experienced in the groin, the anteromedial thigh, the anteromedial knee, the trochanteric area, and the buttock. If the extended leg is rotated at the hip and pain is experienced at the knee, the pain source is the hip, not the knee. (After Kellgren JH. In: Scott JT (ed) Copeman's Textbook of the Rheumatic Diseases, 5th ed. Churchill Livingstone, Edinburgh, 62–77, 1978.) A = anterior view. B = posterior view.

TABLE 2–2
BRIEF MUSCULOSKELETAL EXAMINATION*

GAIT

Inspect the patient as he or she walks into the room, sits, stands, and gestures.

JOINTS

Hands

Actively

1. Stretch all fingers, palms down.
2. Turn hands palms up, and (a) bend fingers 2–4 into palmar contact, (b) bring thumbs to base of little finger.

Is there any finger lag? Any deficit in opposition?
If finger lag is present, distinguish tendinous vs. articular.
If deficit in opposition is present, distinguish thenar atrophy (carpal tunnel syndrome) from carpometacarpal joint dysfunction.

Wrists

While holding the patient's forearm with your nondominant hand, *passively*

1. Flex palmarly.
2. Extend dorsally.
3. Deviate radially.
4. Deviate ulnarly.

Any deficit or assymmetry in motion? Any deficit in flexion/extension?
If restriction is present, is there bogginess, effusion, or tenderness at joint line indicative of synovitis?

Elbows

While holding the patient's elbow with your nondominant hand, with your dominant hand *passively*

1. Extend.
2. Flex.
3. Pronate forearm.
4. Supinate forearm.

Is there any deficit of excursion?
If range is limited, assess for swelling and tenderness at the articular lines, indicative of synovitis

Shoulder

While preventing shoulder girdle elevation, *passively*

1. Abduct in the scapular plane, which is 45 degrees forward to the frontal plane.
2. Externally rotate.
3. Internally rotate.

This maneuver, which is designed to disclose articular limitation, will miss tendon problems. If the patient complains of lateral shoulder pain and passive motion is normal, each of the rotator muscles plus the arc of elevation should be tested. If there is superior shoulder pain, acromioclavicular joint, sternoclavicular joint, cervical motion, and diaphragmatic motion (with cough) should be assessed.

Neck

Active motions

1. Flexion
2. Extension
3. Right rotation
4. Left rotation
5. Right lateral bending (bring right ear to shoulder)
6. Left lateral bending (bring left ear to shoulder)

Any deficit or elicited pain should be noted.

Back

With patient standing, *actively*

1. Flex forward.
2. Extend backward.
3. Bend to right.
4. Bend to left.

Note pain and limitation. Include chest expansion and the Schober test if spondylitis is suspected.

(Table 2–2 continued)

TABLE 2–2 (Continued)

Hips

With the patient lying supine, *passively*

1. Flex hip and knee while with your nondominant hand you hold the other knee flat on the table.
2. Now with hip flexed 90 degrees (knee pointing straight up), with your nondominant hand as pivot: (a) deviate foot out (internal hip rotation) (b) deviate foot in (external hip rotation).

Is there any asymmetry or pain?

Knees

1. Passive flexion has already been tested.
2. Passive extension. While your nondominant hand still rests on the anterior knee, your dominant hand brings leg into extension. If patellofemoral crepitus is noted, check for patellar pain with sustained knee flexion test (Figure 28–1) or the "shrug" sign.
3. Check for swelling/effusion with two hands: Your nondominant hand presses down just proximal to patella while thumb and index of your dominant hand, placed at the parapatellar gutters, feel for expansion (fluid displacement).

If effusion is noted, check for a Baker's cyst.
If crepitus or effusion is present, check for lateral and AP (drawer sign) instability (see knee pain section).

Ankles

Passive examination

1. Craddle patient's ankle with your nondominant hand and passively flex and extend the foot (ankle proper) with your dominant hand.
2. Move your nondominant hand a bit more distally and use it to deviate heel in (varus) and out (valgus) (subtalar joint).
3. While still holding the heel, spread your fingers to splint the entire hindfoot. Embrace forefoot with your dominant hand and create a torque motion of inversion and eversion (midtarsal joint).

Is there any pain or limitation at ankle, subtalar, or midtarsal joints? If answer is yes, go to Chapter 29 on foot pain.

Metatarsophalangeal

Active and *passive* motion.

Look for hallux valgus, overlapping fingers, and calluses.

1. Ask patient to plantar flex toes.
2. Ask patient to dorsiflex toes.
3. Press each MTP joint between your index and thumb.

Tenderness *at MTPs* indicates synovitis, *in between MTPs* a probable Morton's neuroma, and *at metatarsals* a probable stress fracture.

BRIEF MUSCLE EXAMINATION[†]

Finger flexors: ask patient to squeeze as strongly as possible your three middle fingers.
Elbow flexors and extensors: with patient's elbow flexed 90 degrees ask patient to flex elbow as strongly as possible, and then extend as strongly as possible, against your resistance.
Shoulders: ask patient to hold arms out and resist you, pressing down just proximal to patient's elbows.
Neck flexors: ask patient to lift forehead against your fingers (if patient is lying supine) or press down chin against your fist (if patient is sitting).
Proximal strength (iliopsoas): with the patient lying supine on the examining table, ask him or her to lift the straight leg as strongly as possible while you resist just proximal to the knee.
Foot plantar flexors: ask patient to press down with the ball of the foot against your hand as if pressing a car pedal.
Proximal strength, global: with patient lying supine ask him or her to sit. Watch if patient has to roll to one side and then push up, which indicates severe proximal weakness.

*If there are no detours, the entire examination takes less than 2 minutes. Any abnormal findings should be pursued as needed. Specific maneuvers for the various joints are found in the appropriate cshapters in Part IV.
[†]I believe that some muscle examination is better than no examination at all provided it is consistently done. If you are going to test strength haphazardly, then I am not sure. For each muscle group tested, rate normal or decreased strength.

It is useful to contrast mechanical versus inflammatory findings in peripheral joint disease. Bony growths at the edges of articular cartilage (osteophytes), effusion, some synovial proliferation, and on occasion remarkable proliferation of intracapsular fat pads characterize osteoarthritic swelling. These joints may be warm but not hot: Acute inflammation in a seemingly osteoarthritic joint suggests superimposed crystal-induced inflammation or infection. Other findings in osteoarthritis include joint crepitation from bone-on-bone contact, nonuniform compartmental narrowing, pain made worst when worn areas are stressed, and uneven limitation of motion. In inflammatory disease such as rheumatoid arthritis, gout, and bacterial infection, swelling results from synovial effusion and proliferation and there is varying warmth,

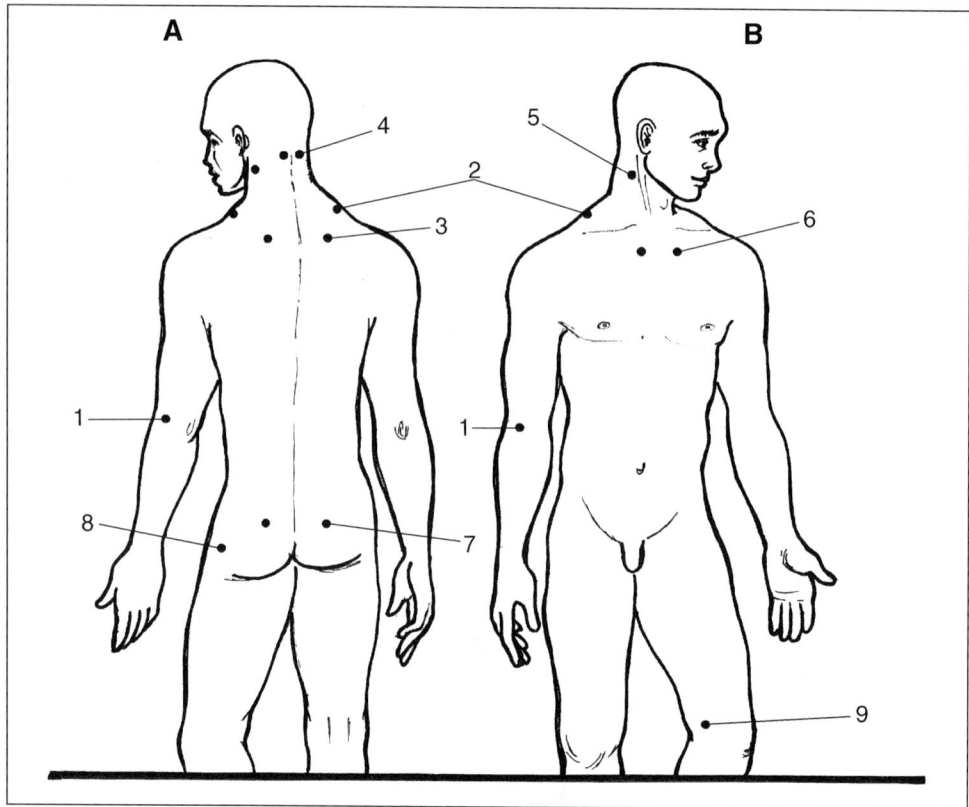

FIGURE 2–7. *Fibromyalgic tender points.* Press firmly (pressure must cause distal nail blanching).
1 = Lateral epicondyle (R&L): the tennis elbow sites, actually 1–2 cm distal to the epicondyle.
2 = Trapezius (R&L): the midpoint of the upper trapezius in a somewhat firm portion of the muscle.
3 = Supraspinatus origin (R&L): above the scapular line, near the medial border of the scapula.
4 = Occiput (R&L).
5 = Low cervical (R&L): at the anterior aspect of intertransverse ligaments C4–5 or C5–6.
6 = Second chondrocostal junction (R&L): close to the origin of the pectoralis major.
7 = Buttock (R&L): In the midpart of the outer quadrant of buttock, in the anterior portion of the gluteus medius.
8 = Greater trochanter (R&L).
9 = Knee (R&L): in the fat pad medial to the knee.
Fibromyalgia criteria: widespread pain (axial plus upper and lower segments plus left- and right-sided pain) in combination with tenderness at 11 or more of the 18 specified sites yielded a sensitivity of 88.4% and a specificity of 81.1% in a study of 293 patients with fibromyalgia and 265 controls. (Wolfe F, Smythe HA, Yunis MB, et al. The American College of Rheumatology 1990 criteria for the classification of fibromyalgia. Arthritis Rheum 33:160–172, 1990.)

capsular tenderness, universal limitation of motion, and universal endpoint pain.

In axial joint disease, differentiation between mechanical and inflammatory disease is based on the history. Pain in mechanical conditions has an abrupt onset, is limited in duration (less than 30 days in over 90% of cases), is aggravated by motion, and has a tendency to reoccur. Morning stiffness is minimal. In contrast, in inflammatory disease such as ankylosing spondylitis, pain and stiffness have an insidious onset, symptoms have often been present for 2 to 3 months at initial evaluation, morning stiffness lasts hours, and there is improvement with activities.

Physical findings in spinal disease, except for possible deformities such as kyphosis due to osteoporotic vertebral collapse or developmental scoliosis, are usually meager. In ankylosing spondylitis (AS) and other spondyloarthropathies, which are characterized by sacroiliitis and inflammation in the outer layers of the intervertebral discs and other spinal structures, lumbar motion is often restricted in all planes.

By convention, lumbar motion in the sagittal plane is assessed by the *Schober test,* which is performed as follows: With the patient standing erect the lumbosacral junction is identified at the intersect of a line connecting both posterosuperior iliac spines (found at the "dimples of Venus") and the spine. Two marks are placed in the midline, one 10 cm proximal and the other 5 cm distal to the lumbosacral junction (15 cm span). The patient is then asked to bend forward and the span between marks is measured. An increment exceeding 4 cm indicates normal motion, between 2 and 4 cm is suspicious, and less than 2 cm indicates definite restriction. Very importantly, grossly abnormal Schobers are not confined to AS. Muscle splinting in acute low back pain, extensive lumbar spondylosis, and diffuse idiopathic skeletal hyperostosis may all drastically restrict lumbar motion.

Chest expansion, which is used as a proxy measurement for dorsal spine motion, measures costovertebral joint motion. To test chest expansion the patient is asked to place both hands behind the neck and exhale fully, measuring the

TABLE 2–3

CONDITIONS THAT CAUSE SACROILIAC JOINT ABNORMALITIES

Ankylosing spondylitis
Reactive arthritis
Psoriatic arthritis
Enteropathic arthritis (Crohn's, ulcerative colitis, intestinal bypass)
Whipple's disease
SAPHO syndrome
Familial Mediterranean fever
Relapsing polychondritis
Septic arthritis
Brucellosis
Tuberculosis
Renal osteodystrophy
Osteomalacia
Osteoarthritis
Diffuse idiopathic skeletal hyperostosis (DISH, or Forestier's disease)
Gout
Hyperparathyroidism
Paget's disease
Paraplegia
Tuberous sclerosis
Metastatic cancer

chest perimeter at the tip of the scapulae. The patient is then asked to inhale maximally and the measurement is made again. A 5 cm or greater increment indicates normal chest expansion. In AS with thoracic involvement, measurements of 2.5 cm or less are frequent. Because limited chest expansion is a late finding in AS and a routine finding in emphysema and thoracic cage conditions, the measurements have limited practical value.

Physical examination of the SI joints is disappointing. Except in acute cases of sacroiliitis, false negative findings are commonplace. Thus, diagnosis of sacroiliitis relies on x-rays and other imaging techniques (see Chapter 4). There are a number of conditions, most of them unrelated to the spondyloarthropathies, that result in sacroiliac joint changes (Table 2–3). In addition, radiographic sacroiliitis may take years to develop. Bone scans show sacroiliitis early, particularly in unilateral cases, but it is often difficult to distinguish bilateral sacroiliitis from the dense uptake around normal SI joints. CT and MRI are quite useful in detecting early sacroiliitis, but the expense involved limits their routine use.

It should be clear by now that in the author's opinion the popular dictum "most important in rheumatologic diagnosis are the history and physical examination" is indeed true.

CHAPTER 3

Pattern Recognition in Rheumatology

Consultants often think less than regular members of the profession give them credit for. Many of the most "esoteric" or "fascinating" diagnoses are made at a glance. How do they do it, by using algorhithms? I don't think so. Consultants use painstakingly learned, experience-derived patterns that narrow diagnostic possibilities down to a minimum. Once they are there they may or not use algorhithms; who knows? A number of commonly observed patterns and their matching conditions are listed in this chapter. Common conditions are described as well as rare ones (discussed in some detail because they do not appear later in the text).

There are, of course, many exceptions to these patterns, and to diagnose them a broad knowledge of internal medicine plus clear thinking is essential. Learn, dear colleague, the rheumatologic patterns that follow, and surprise your friends.

PAINFUL, SWOLLEN HAND(S)

- Gout
- Pseudogout
- Rheumatoid arthritis (RA)
- Remitting seronegative symmetrical synovitis with pitting edema (RS3PE)
- Polymyalgia rheumatica (PMR)
- Mixed connective tissue disease (MCTD)
- Scleroderma
- Rupture of the olecranon bursa
- Medsger's syndrome (neoplasia)
- The puffy hand of drug addiction
- Reflex sympathetic dystrophy (RSD)
- Eosinophilic fasciitis
- Sickle cell (hand-foot syndrome)
- Leprosy
- Factitial (the rubber band syndrome)

Comments: Conditions 1 through 5 produce hand edema in older people. Conditions 4 and 5 occur in older people. The condition is bilateral in RA, RS3PE, and PMR unless neurologic disease paralyzes one hand, in which case the edema affects the good hand. Diffuse swelling with a leathery feeling in both hands suggests MCTD and early scleroderma. In the latter, edema eventually goes away as the skin becomes taut. Raynaud's is prominent in both conditions. Gout and pseudogout cause diffusely swollen hands in older patients with acute arthritis of the wrist, with or without digital synovitis. Rupture of the olecranon bursa, which occurs predominantly in septic bursitis and RA, causes localized inflammatory edema that migrates distally along the ulnar border of the forearm reaching in some cases the dorsum of the hand. In Medsger's syndrome, edema affects predominantly the palmar side of both hands and is later replaced by a variant of Dupuytren contracture. Drug addicts who use the dorsal hand for injection characteristically develop puffy hands. Burning pain and edema characterize the early stages of RSD. This process is generally unilateral. In eosinophilic fasciitis there is an indurated dorsal edema that typically spares the fingers. A puffy, painful hand (and foot) caused by soft tissue and bone ischemia is a well-known feature of sickle cell crises in small children. Lepromatous leprosy often causes bilaterally swollen hands. The diagnosis should be considered in immigrants from endemic areas. Additional skin lesions and neuropathy are usually present. Finally, disturbed individuals may self-induce hand or foot edema by applying a tight rubber band. A faint rubber band pressure mark is sometimes present on examination.

ACUTE ARTHRITIS (painful, swollen, warm joint; a spontaneous position may be adopted, as in Table 2–1)

- Septic arthritis
- Gout*
- Pseudogout[†]
- Pseudoseptic arthritis in rheumatoid or reactive arthritis
- Intraarticular fracture
- Hemarthrosis

*Monosodium urate (MSU) crystals present in synovial fluid (SF).
[†]Ca pyrophosphate dihydrate (CPPD) crystals present in SF.

Comments: The main move here is to aspirate the joint, handling the fluid as in synovial fluid analysis. A bloody SF means hemarthrosis, but gout and pseudogout may also produce hemarthrosis. These should be identified on routine polarizing microscopy. If no crystals are present, place the hemorrhagic fluid in the refrigerator. Fat layering on the top (just like chicken soup) raises the possibility of intraarticular fracture. A high leukocyte count renders the SF turbid in bacterial infection, gout, pseudogout, and pseudoseptic arthritis. Presence of MSU and CPPD crystals indicate gout and pseudogout, respectively, but do not rule out concurrent bacterial infection. If no crystals are found, likely diagnoses are septic arthritis and pseudoseptic arthritis. Make sure a gram stain is done (and exhaustively inspected), and request anaerobic and aerobic cultures. In acute arthritis you must move fast but it helps to first go through the steps mentally. For example, determine if you know how to enter that joint, if all of the required materials are there including two pairs of gloves, a lot of sterile gauze, extra syringes, thin and large-bore needles, and a sterile rubber stopper (to submit the syringe to bacteriology) that may not be in the tray. As important as submitting the fluid is to personally follow it through or have someone in the laboratory you entirely trust to follow it through.

HEMARTHROSIS (bloody synovial fluid obtained in an atraumatic joint aspiration)*

- Excessive anticoagulation
- Hemophilia
- Intraarticular fracture
- Osteonecrosis
- Gout, pseudogout
- Pigmented villonodular synovitis (PVNS)
- Synovial hemangioma
- Synovial metastases

*Hemarthrosis exhibits constant findings: fluid does not clot (but don't find out; always anticoagulate); there are crenated red cells; supernatant is pink or red from hemolysis.

Comments: Patients may bleed into joints from excessive coumadin or heparin anticoagulation. If anticoagulants are not being used, a clotting abnormality may be present.

Hemophiliacs tend to bleed recurrently, with minimal or no trauma, and usually in the same joint(s). In an adult or older person, new-onset coagulopathy may be due to factor VIII inhibitors such as those seen in cases of SLE or multiple myeloma, or fibrinolysis in prostatic and other cancers.

As mentioned, if there is a history of trauma (but also in unconscious or unreliable persons without such a history), the bloody SF should be placed in the refrigerator. If a fat layer forms and initial x-rays are negative, rule out an undisplaced intraarticular fracture by bone scan, CT, or MRI (MRI is best) or by repeating the x-rays 2 weeks later. The problem with this approach is that during this period the affected part must be kept immobilized.

If osteonecrosis was responsible for the bleed (such as in patients on long-term corticosteroids and older patients who are prone to idiopathic osteonecrosis), a similar approach might be taken. As in suspected intraarticular fractures, the author favors a quick diagnosis of osteonecrosis because with appropriate rest or other measures some of these lesions heal.

It should be reemphasized that both gout and pseudogout may cause hemarthrosis. Crystal search may be laborious in a slide flooded with erythrocytes.

Recurrent hemarthrosis occurring in the same joint without trauma or coagulopathy may be caused by a benign intraarticular lesion such as pigmented villonodular synovitis (PVNS) and synovial hemangioma. In PVNS the synovium feels very thickened. In synovial hemangiomas a superficial lesion may be present and phleboliths (calcific bodies within dilated veins) may appear on x-rays. MRI is quite helpful in the diagnosis of PVNS, although it may not discriminate well the lesion from synovial hemosiderosis caused by repeated hemangiomatous bleeds. Diagnosis of both lesions is arthroscopic. Synovial metastases are quite rare. Bone lysis is often present on x-rays. In 50% of cases malignant cells are present on synovial fluid smears.

ARTHRITIS, FEVER, AND A RASH

- Rubella
- Parvovirus B-19
- Gonococcemia
- Meningococcemia
- Lyme borreliosis
- Secondary syphilis
- Adult acute rheumatic fever (ARF)
- Adult Kawasaki disease?
- Vasculitic urticaria
- Acute sarcoidosis
- Adult Still's disease
- Familial Mediterranean fever (FMF)
- Hyperimmunoglobulinemia D and periodic fever syndrome

Comments: Small-joint arthritis, an erythematous macular and papular rash that starts in the face and generalizes within 24 hours, plus retroauricular and posterior neck nodes characterize rubella arthritis, which is particularly common in young women following immunization.

In parvovirus B-19 infection, which is a cause of polyarthritis in adults, the typical "slapped cheeks" rash seen in children is replaced by inconspicuous macules affecting the face or elsewhere. There may be several "lupoid" features to parvovirus infection including thrombocytopenia, positive ANA, and hypocomplementemia. Fortunately, these are only transient and few people are so tested. Great concern may be raised by an imprudently requested ANA.

Gonococcal arthritis, particularly polyarticular febrile cases, feature erythematous macules that evolve into hemorrhagic or hemorrhagic/necrotic pustules. Few lesions are usually present and they tend to involve the upper extremities.

A rather similar clinical pattern occurs in meningococcemia, but here the rash consists of erythematous/petechial papules, sometimes confluent, that may present anywhere. Remember that acute meningococcemia and certainly chronic meningococcemia may not feature meningitis.

The typical erythema migrans of Lyme borreliosis is a single erythematous macule or papule that expands gradually, as it clears in the center, to a diameter of 15 cm or more. There are minimal constitutional symptoms at this stage. The true arthritis of Lyme borreliosis comes later with early generalized or late disease.

The possibility of secondary syphilis should be raised when subacute arthritis associates with brownish red papules in the trunk or scaling papular lesions on palms and soles.

The rare erythema marginatum (EM) of ARF is striking in its appearance: an evanescent rash in which individual lesions expand centrifugally while the center clears. A hot shower makes EM lesions striking. EM has been aptly compared by Taranta to smoke rings, such is its dynamism.

Kawasaki disease is a condition of young children,

although a few adult cases have been reported. There is a high fever, a polymorphous rash in the trunk that may disseminate, palmar and plantar erythema, brawny edema in the dorsum of hands and feet, a strawberry tongue, conjunctival irritation, and cervical adenopathy. Myocarditis in early disease and coronary artery aneurysms and myocardial infarction account for most of the mortality in Kawasaki disease. Arthritis presents in the recovery period and affects large weight-bearing joints.

Vasculitic urticaria is another condition that features arthralgias or arthritis, fever, and a rash in which individual urticarial lesions persist for 24 hours to 3 days. An associated angioedema is frequent.

The typical skin lesion in acute sarcoidosis is erythema nodosum. Skin inflammation may be intense, resembling cellulitis.

The last three conditions listed are intermittent conditions with several overlapping clinical features. Adult Still's disease is seen predominantly in young adults. The condition features high spiking fevers with a rapid return to baseline or below baseline once or twice daily, a discrete salmon-pink macular rash accompanying the fever with elements from 2 to 5 mm in diameter, predominantly in trunk and proximal extremities, and lymphadenopathy. There is high leukocytosis and the ESR is markedly elevated. Whereas in children systemic findings precede the arthritis by weeks or months, adult cases of Still's disease feature concurrent arthritis. Different from childhood cases, adult Still's disease has no association with amyloidosis.

Familial Mediterranean fever (FMF) is an intermittent condition that affects individuals from Mediterranean ancestry and has its onset in late childhood or adolescence. The rare but clinically striking skin lesion of FMF is a very painful, angry-looking pseudoerysipela involving the distal legs. These lesions must be distinguished from the recurrent erysipelas that complicate congenital lymphatic channel hypoplasia. Characteristic manifestations in FMF include fever, large-joint arthritis, serositis, and peritonitis. Leukocytosis and ESR are markedly elevated. Untreated (colchicine), many FMF patients develop amyloidosis.

Hyperimmunoglobulin D syndrome is a rare recently described condition so far identified in Europe that begins in early childhood and features fever, lymphadenopathy, a macular or papular rash in the extremities, abdominal pain, and arthralgias or arthritis of large joints. As in the previous two entities, leukocytosis and ESR are high. An elevated serum IgD (polyclonal) is characteristic of the condition. There is no association with amyloidosis.

PALINDROMIC RHEUMATISM

- Palindromic rheumatoid arthritis (RA)
- Essential palindromic rheumatism
- Crystal synovitis (gout, CPPD pseudogout, calcific periarthritis)
- Lyme borreliosis, stages 2 and 3
- Sarcoidosis
- Whipple's disease
- Acute rheumatic fever
- Reactive arthritis (rare)
- Adult Still's disease
- Familial Mediterranean fever (FMF)
- Hyperimmunoglobulin D syndrome

Comments: Palindromic rheumatism is a fascinating condition in which different joints are affected in sequence, each becoming acutely inflamed for a few hours to a few days after which they once again become normal. It is indeed curious to see a joint that was normal 10 minutes ago and now is warm, tender, and progressively swollen, only to become normal a few hours later. Sometimes inflammation is extraarticular rather than articular.

Of a cohort of patients with palindromic rheumatism, about half will have a positive RF test. Of these, half will go on to develop typical RA within a few years; the others will continue experiencing palindromic attacks.

Of the seronegative cases, some will turn out to have a definable process such as gout, pseudogout, and rarely basic calcium phosphate deposition disease. Sarcoidosis may feature palindromic arthritis over a background of intrathoracic findings. Reactive arthritis occasionally features palindromic arthritis. The condition is suggested by preceding enteric or urogenital infection, coexistent enthesopathy, as well as mucosal and skin changes.

Microbial conditions causing palindromic arthritis include Lyme borreliosis and Whipple's disease. In the latter, relapsing arthritis may go on for years if not decades before lymphadenopathy, diarrhea, and weight loss develop.

Acute rheumatic fever differs from palindromic rheumatism in that individual joints become involved every few days in an additive fashion plus the fever and cardiac findings.

Finally, the previously described adult-onset Still's disease, familial Mediterranean fever, and hyperimmunoglobulin D syndrome are additional conditions that belong to the palindromic rheumatism pattern. Thus, confronted with a patient with palindromic rheumatism the task is, rather than applying a label, to identify the underlying condition. Joint aspiration is essential in these patients.

CHRONIC MONOARTHRITIS

- Mechanical derangement
- Neuropathic (Charcot's) joint
- Rheumatoid arthritis (RA)
- Psoriatic arthritis
- Tuberculous infection
- Foreign body synovitis
- Pigmented villonodular synovitis (PVNS)
- Synovial chondromatosis

Comments: Mechanically damaged joints, for example, an osteochondritic knee or a knee that has suffered a complex meniscal/ligamentous injury, are typically unstable, exhibit coarse crepitation, are chronically swollen from synovial proliferation and effusion, and swelling varies with the use of the joint. Radiographic changes are those of osteoarthritis with bony sclerosis, degenerative cysts, and asymmetric narrowing from cartilage loss. The erythrocyte sedimentation rate (ESR) is normal and joint effusions are typically noninflammatory with leukocyte counts of less than 3000/mm³ and a predominance of mononuclear cells.

In Charcot's joint, instability is greater, crepitation coarser, and effusions often huge contrasting with a virtual absence of pain. Neurologic examination reveals neuropathy. Radiographically there is subluxation, lytic areas, and large ossified intracapsular bodies. It may resemble osteomyelitis or septic arthritis, but the ESR is normal and synovial fluid is noninflammatory with a variable amount of blood. Calcium pyrophosphate dihydrate crystals may be present.

In the remaining conditions arthroscopy and biopsy is the most efficient diagnostic procedure. Both RA and psoriatic arthritis may feature monoarthritis at disease onset. Look for psoriasis at hidden sites (behind ears, scalp, umbilicus, intergluteal fold) and inquire about a family history of psoriasis. Synovial fluid is inflammatory in both conditions with WBCs ranging from 10,000 to 100,000 WBC/mm³ and a predominance of polymorphonuclear cells.

The findings are similar in tuberculosis except that lytic areas are often present on x-rays at initial evaluation.

Foreign body synovitis should be suspected from previous trauma such as a thorn puncture wound or kneeling on a cactus. Patients with PVNS have recurrent bloody or chocolate-colored effusions with WBC counts of less than 20,000/mm³.

Clinical and synovial fluid characteristics in PVNS and synovial hemangioma are often similar. Arthroscopy shows redundant, inflamed synovium in rheumatoid, psoriatic, sarcoid, tuberculous, and foreign body synovitis. Histology allows identification of tuberculosis and sarcoidosis. In foreign body synovitis the offending foreign material is usually identified in the synovectomy specimen. PVNS features marked synovial proliferation and tan-, yellow-, or chocolate-colored nodules and villous proliferation. A histologic diagnosis of PVNS can only be accepted after mycobacterial and fungal infections have been ruled out.

Finally, in synovial chondromatosis the joint is filled with cartilaginous bodies that are often ossified. The fluid is clear, highly viscous, and noninflammatory. Diagnosis and treatment are arthroscopic.

PROTRACTED DISTAL SYMMETRIC POLYARTHRITIS

- Rheumatoid arthritis (RA)
- Systemic lupus erythematosus (SLE)
- Polymyositis (antisynthetase syndrome)
- Certain drug reactions
- Psoriatic arthritis
- Gout
- Pseudogout
- Parvovirus B-19 infection (rare)
- Secondary syphilis (rare)
- Brucellosis (in endemic areas)

Comments: Protracted distal symmetric polyarthritis in over 80% of cases represents RA. Because SLE may also present in this fashion, the appropriate serologic testing for both conditions should be requested. Polymyositis will not be missed if proximal strength is checked. If the patient is taking procainamide, a beta blocker, or quinidine, a drug reaction should be at least considered. These cases feature elevated antinuclear antibodies titers, rheumatoid factor (RF) test may be positive or negative, and antinative DNA and Sm antibodies are negative. Preceding, concurrent, and familial psoriasis should be noted and examination should include areas in which psoriasis may be hidden.

Remember that both gout and pseudogout may present with a pseudo-RA pattern! Arthralgias are common in parvovirus infection, but cases with subacute or chronic arthritis are rare. Diagnosis may be suggested by an initial rash. The condition resolves in a few days in most cases. Autoantibodies and parvovirus testing is not warranted in routine cases.

Secondary syphilis should be investigated if lymphadenopathy and a rash are present. Involvement of the palmar and plantar surfaces is frequent. Look also for oral or perigenital mucous plaques.

Brucellosis caused by *B. melitensis* occurs frequently in Latin America, the Middle East, and Mediterranean countries. Musculoskeletal manifestations occur in over 50% of patients including a rheumatoidlike peripheral arthritis or a spondylitic condition with unilateral SI involvement. Peripheral and axial involvement rarely coexist.

ARTHRITIS AND SUBCUTANEOUS NODULES

- Rheumatoid arthritis (RA)
- Gout
- Pseudogout (rare)
- Sarcoidosis
- Light chain (LA) amyloidosis (primary, multiple myeloma)
- Acute rheumatic fever (ARF)
- Hemochromatosis
- Whipple's disease
- Multicentric reticulohistiocytosis

Comments: In patients with arthritis there is a tendency to consider subcutaneous nodules as proof of RA. While this is true in over 90% of cases, subcutaneous nodules may represent, among others, crystal deposits in chronic gout and pseudogout. If the patient remembers initial episodes of acute arthritis separated by periods of complete health, the likelihood of crystal disease should be strongly considered, but there are RA cases which begin that way (palindromic RA). If the patient has a negative RF, aspirate the nodule as discussed under gout!

In sarcoidosis the RF test is usually negative and chest x-rays show adenopathy and/or reticulonodular disease.

Light chain (LA) amyloidosis should be suspected in an older person with arthritis, bilateral carpal tunnel syndrome, and subcutaneous nodules. A serum protein electrophoresis will reveal a monoclonal spike.

How about ARF? The condition is nowadays rare in the United States, and nodules, uncommon in pediatric cases, are even rarer in adults. But knowing the implications of a missed diagnosis, the condition must be mentioned.

Hemochromatosis and Whipple's disease are rare birds. Both feature a negative RF test, a red flag that should not be overlooked. Hemochromatosis is suspected from concurrent diabetes or cardiomyopathy or a family history that includes one or more of these findings. Whipple's cases often present fever, lymphadenopathy, serositis, weight loss, CNS lesions, and diarrhea. Don't miss these diagnoses; the complications of hemochromatosis are preventable and Whipple's disease is potentially curable (sometimes it can only be arrested). There is now a molecular test for it. Use it in the right setting!

The final condition listed, multicentric reticulohistiocytosis, features small pearled periungeal nodules as well as larger nodules elsewhere. This is a really rare condition that is usually diagnosed by rheumatologists and dermatologists.

DISTAL INTERPHALANGEAL (DIP) JOINT ARTHRITIS

- Osteoarthritis (OA), Heberden's nodes type
- Nodal gout
- Psoriatic arthritis
- Multicentric reticulohistiocytosis

Comments: Almost everyone is aware that in a common form of OA there is a predilection for DIP involvement. The base of the distal phalanx becomes swollen and tender, which gives way, months later, to bony knobs known as Heberden's nodes.

Urate deposits may accumulate about Heberden's nodes. Acute crystal inflammation in this location is known as "nodal gout." A rather similar involvement occurs in DIP psoriatic arthritis. These patients almost regularly feature grossly pitted nails. Rather than sclerosis, subchondral cysts, and cartilage thinning, which are typical of OA x-ray findings, psoriatic DIP arthritis includes centripetal erosions leading to "pseudowidening" of the joint. Once again, look for psoriasis in acral sites and hidden areas.

Multicentric reticulohistiocytosis, mentioned in the previous pattern, also produces erosive changes at the DIPs.

OLIGOARTHRITIS (involvement of 2–3 joints)

- Psoriatic arthritis
- Reactive arthritis
- Lyme borreliosis, stage 3
- Gout
- Pseudogout
- Rheumatoid arthritis (RA)

Comments. Oligoarthritis should make one think automatically of psoriatic arthritis (actively look for the skin lesions) and postdysenteric or postvenereal reactive arthritis. The patient may have, for instance, swelling in one knee, one ankle, and one elbow. Palmar and plantar lesions of reactive arthritis resemble pustular psoriasis. Shallow mucosal ulcerations are virtually painless.

Lyme borreliosis, in the late stage, often features recurrent knee oligoarthritis. Effusions may be huge. Inquire about exposure such as a history of a slowly enlarging rash during a summer beach vacation.

Gout and pseudogout are mentioned because both can resemble all joint conditions. Don't miss a crystal search. The same applies to RA. Interestingly, if in patients with oligoarticular RA the examiner intently presses the MTPs one by one, he or she almost regularly finds symmetric tenderness of which the patient was fully unaware.

SPONDYLITIS

- Ankylosing spondylitis (AS)
- Enteric, urogenital, and other reactive arthritides
- Psoriatic arthritis
- Whipple's disease
- Brucella infection
- Diffuse idiopathic skeletal hyperostosis (DISH), or Forestier's disease*
- Osteomalacia*

*Spondylitis mimickers.

Comments: Characteristic of spondylitis is an inflammatory-type low back pain associated with radiographic changes in the sacroiliac joints and often at higher levels in the spine. The prototypic disease is AS in which there is long-standing low back pain that is relieved by motion, limited lumbar spine motion, plus radiographic sacroiliitis. Similar symptoms are experienced in the reactive arthritides with axial involvement. The telltale sign is a preceding enteric or urogenital infection. Cases that clinically resemble reactive arthritis but lack an antecedent infection are known as undifferentiated spondyloarthropathies.

Psoriatic spondyloartropathy is suggested by the unmistakable psoriatic plaques. As mentioned, psoriasis may be hidden or absent in these patients. The presence of psoriasis in one or both parents should make one think of psoriatic spondylitis.

Whipple's disease and brucellosis are believed to cause spondyloarthropathy by direct infection and perhaps as a reactive phenomenon as well. Brucellosis is suspected when in the proper epidemiologic setting patients develop a febrile illness with peripheral or axial arthritis.

Forestier's disease is an ossifying rather than inflammatory condition. Bridging bone develops along the anterior longitudinal ligament of the spine, causing spinal stiffness. Severe cases feature ossification at tendon attachments causing enthesial pain. The end result in DISH may be quite similar to AS, except that protracted morning stiffness is lacking.

Patients with osteomalacia may feature back and pelvic pain as well as radiographic changes that resemble sacroiliitis. Diagnosis may be suspected from concurrent hypophosphatemic proximal muscle weakness. Low phosphorus levels, low or normal calcium levels, increased alkaline phosphatase, the finding of pseudofractures on x-rays, and low 25(OH)D are diagnostic of vitamin D–deficient osteomalacia.

ENTHESOPATHY

- Reactive arthritis
- Ankylosing spondylitis (AS)
- Psoriatic arthritis
- Bacteremia
- Viremia
- Fluorosis
- X-linked vitamin D–resistant rickets
- Etetrinate treatment
- Forestier's disease (DISH)
- Fluoroquinolone treatment

Comments: Enthesis designates the insertional area of tendon into bone, enthesopathy is a disorder of the enthesis, and enthesitis represents enthesial inflammation. Inflammation of the distal Achilles tendon, the plantar fascia at its attachment in the medial calcaneal tuberosity, and the tibial insertion of the patellar tendon represent typical enthesitides and are seen in reactive arthritis, AS, and psoriatic arthritis. Associated findings in the former include oligoarthritis and perhaps some of the mucocutaneous manifestations of the disease. In AS the patient will have spinal rigidity plus radiographic evidence of sacroiliitis. Patients with psoriatic arthritis and enthesitis usually, but not always, have skin psoriasis. Interestingly, in viremias, such as in AIDS or hepatitis B, and bacteremias, such as in *S. aureus* infection, enthesial pain is frequent.

Certain metabolic disorders including vitamin D–resistant rickets, fluoride intoxication, and etetrinate treatment of psoriasis or severe acne often feature enthesial pain as well as ossification at insertional sites of tendons, ligaments, and joint capsule. Similar findings occur in DISH.

Finally, there is a little understood toxic effect of fluoroquinolones on tendons that includes pain, swelling, and sometimes rupture. The condition most often affects the Achilles tendons, but the epicondylar insertion of wrist extensors (similar to tennis elbow) and the shoulder's rotator cuff may also be involved.

ARTHRITIS AND WEIGHT LOSS

- Severe rheumatoid arthritis (RA)
- RA with vasculitis
- Reactive arthritis
- RA or psoriatic arthritis or ankylosing spondylitis (AS) with amyloidosis
- Cancer
- Enteropathic arthritis (Crohn's, ulcerative colitis)
- HIV infection
- Whipple's disease
- Blind loop syndrome
- Scleroderma with intestinal bacterial overgrowth

Comments: When a patient with arthritis has severe weight loss, several possibilities are raised, none of them insignificant. First, patients with severe RA may have a decrease in lean body mass of more than 10%. These patients, as any chronically starved patient, are at a risk of sudden death. RA patients with this degree of wasting may have systemic complications, in particular systemic vasculitis manifested by palpable purpura, neuropathy or mononeuritis multiplex, or leg ulcers. Patients with uncontrolled reactive arthritis may enter a catabolic state that may take many months to recover from. Some of these patients, with the joint findings overshadowed by wasting, adenopathy, and splenomegaly, may seem to have an evolving lymphoma until someone examines the joints, inspects the glans penis and the oral cavity, and requests SI joint films, establishing the diagnosis.

Another association of weight loss (unless the patient becomes nephrotic) is secondary (AA) amyloidosis complicating RA, psoriatic arthritis, and AS. I am not implying that amyloidosis causes weight loss per se but rather that severe inflammation causes both the amyloidosis (by sustained high serum levels of AA protein) and the weight loss.

Neoplasia, a well-known cause of weight loss, may under some circumstances cause arthritis, for example, in lymphomas. Thus, unexplained weight loss in an arthritic patient, particularly if adenopathy is present, should make the physician consider neoplasia.

Another prominent cause of weight loss is inflammatory bowel disease, which in about 20% of patients leads to arthritis. There is a well-known association between reactive and psoriatic arthritis with HIV infection. In some of the patients arthritis is recognized first. It is therefore important in the evaluation of reactive and psoriatic arthritis patients with progressive weight loss to consider a concurrent HIV infection.

Whipple's disease is rare, as attested by the author's experience of only six cases in a 30 year experience. Four of the six had a massive weight loss. All had articular symptoms but only two had diarrhea. The blind loop syndrome used to feature arthritis in addition to weight loss.

Finally, patients with scleroderma, a condition that may often cause arthritis in early disease, may have profound small-bowel motility disturbances that promote bacterial overgrowth and malabsorption. A scleroderma patient who loses a lot of weight is likely to have this complication.

ARTHRITIS AND A HEART MURMUR

- Subacute bacterial endocarditis (SBE)
- Cardiac myxoma
- Ankylosing spondylitis (AS)
- Reactive arthritis
- Acute rheumatic fever
- Rheumatoid arthritis (RA)
- Systemic lupus erythematosus (SLE) with Libman-Sack endocarditis
- Relapsing polychondritis

Comments: There are patients with valvular heart disease who on evaluation are found to have arthritis (the connection between the two may or not be realized), and there are arthritic patients who in the course of their condition develop a heart murmur. A heart murmur may of course be unrelated to the arthritis, such as murmurs due to valvular calcification, but real associations between valvular disease and arthritis are relatively common. For instance, bacterial endocarditis causes peripheral arthritis and back pain in as many as 50% of cases. These patients may feature, late in the disease, a positive rheumatoid factor test as well as hypocomplementemia. Thus, febrile patients with arthritis and a heart murmur, particularly if back pain is also present, are suspected of having SBE. The same association holds true for cardiac myxoma, a notorious mimicker of systemic disease. Blood cultures and a transesophageal echocardiogram are basic to diagnosing both conditions.

Both AS and reactive arthritis cause, in about 5% of patients, dilatation of the aortic root leading to aortic regurgitation, sometimes retraction of the anterior mitral leaflet causing mitral regurgitation, as well as inflammatory changes in the fibrous portion of the interventricular septum leading to A-V conduction disturbances. Thus, in patients being evaluated for aortic regurgitation, check any available pelvic film for possible sacroiliitis.

Acute rheumatic fever, as noted earlier, is uncommon nowadays, although pockets of disease pop up here and there even in the United States. Mitral regurgitation is often present at initial evaluation and may be reversible. Mitral stenosis develops late, often decades after the initial attack. The association of an additive arthritis and mitral regurgitation should therefore prompt determination of streptococcal antibodies. Rheumatoid arthritis rarely causes heart murmurs, but when it does it is likely that the patient is strongly seropositive and that rheumatoid nodules have formed in the valve leaflets.

In SLE heart murmurs may result from valve necrosis and rupture, Libman-Sack endocarditis (initially an inflammatory lesion), a secondary antiphospholipid syndrome resulting in thrombotic vegetations, or bacterial endocarditis. Lupus patients who are febrile and have a heart murmur should of course have the appropriate blood cultures.

Relapsing polychondritis is a rare condition that is made even rarer by lack of ascertainment. Diagnosis may be missed because appropriate questions may not be asked about nose or ear inflammation, and because the floppy ears that characterize late disease may be missing in the average case. Relapsing polychondritis may dilate the aortic root and cause aortic regurgitation.

ARTHRITIS AND A RASH

- Chronic urticaria
- Vasculitic urticaria
- Systemic lupus erythematosus (SLE)
- Dermatomyositis
- Polymyositis
- Psoriatic arthritis
- Reactive arthritis
- Chronic sarcoidosis
- Sweet's syndrome
- Leprosy

Comments: In chronic urticaria, which associates with angioedema, there are minimal constitutional symptoms and individual urticarial wheals last less than 24 hours. In vasculitic urticaria the itchy lesions last longer and are followed by local hyperpigmentation. Obstructive bronchopulmonary disease, ocular inflammation, and nephritis can be present.

Systemic lupus erythematosus features a variety of rashes; the best known are malar erythema and discoid lupus. The tip-off for the condition is its multisystemic involvement including arthritis, serositis, CNS disease, and renal disease in various combinations. Given consistent clinical findings, diagnosis of SLE is reached by (1) positive SLE-specific serologies such as double-stranded DNA or Sm antibodies, or (2) positive ANA plus the exclusion of mimicking conditions. The primary antiphospholipid syndrome does not cause arthritis, but patients with SLE may present a secondary antiphospholipid syndrome. At least half of these patients feature livedo reticularis, which is a macular netlike reddish blue rash most prominent around the knees and on the thighs. Livedo reticularis may also occur in disseminated intravascular coagulation, cholesterol atheroembolic disease, cryoglobulinemia, polyarteritis nodosa, and other conditions that cause vasospasm or occlusion in perforating arteries as they travel from the subcutaneous tissue to the dermis.

Dermatomyositis rash is erythematous and affects sun-exposed areas including face, neck, and upper chest depending on garments used. It may be quite itchy and photosensitive with prominent superficial edema. Heliotrope rash is a reddish purple periorbital discoloration of upper lids that also look edematous. Gottron's sign is a violaceous papular rash that erases the creases at the knuckles. One or more of these rashes in association with proximal muscle weakness is highly indicative of dermatomyositis, which may or not include arthritis.

In polymyositis, a rash that has been aptly described as "mechanic's hand" is characterized by coarse, fissured skin in opposing surfaces of thumb, index, and middle finger. The area tends to accumulate dirt despite the patient's best efforts. Rheumatoidlike arthritis may be prominent in these patients.

Psoriasis, a lesion that is well known to all primary care physicians, is the hallmark of psoriatic arthritis. Hidden psoriatic lesions should be intently looked for in suspected cases of psoriatic arthritis.

The rash in reactive arthritis includes palmar and plantar pseudopustules (keratoderma blennorrhagica), papular or hyperkeratotic glans lesions (balanitis circinata), and shallow painless erosions in the hard palate.

Chronic sarcoidosis, in which arthritis and tenosynovitis may be prominent, features brownish violet infiltrated skin lesions in the form of papules or plaques. Another well-known but rare sarcoidosis lesion is "lupus pernio," in which there is a diffuse red infiltration of nose, cheeks, and earlobes.

Sweet's syndrome, or acute febrile dermatosis, is characterized by skin lesions that appear abruptly and evolve in several days to several weeks. Lesions are bright red to purple, well demarcated, very painful, tender, and often multiple. The center may be depressed. Fever and leukocytosis are often present. Myalgias, arthralgias, and arthritis are quite frequent. The arthritis is migratory and tends to affect knees, elbows, ankles, and fingers in descending frequency. Diagnosis of

Sweet's syndrome is based on the skin biopsy that shows dense neutrophilic infiltrates in the upper and mid dermis.

Leprosy, a relatively rare condition in the United States where it is virtually confined to Asian or Latin American immigrants, may present with a variety of lesions ranging from a leonine face in lepromatous leprosy to a well-defined anesthetic hypopigmented macule in tuberculoid leprosy. In the Lucio reaction, hyperacute vasculitis features high fever, neuritis, and skin ulcers. Myositis, rheumatoidlike arthritis, and enthesopathy are additional manifestations of lepromatous leprosy. Interestingly, autoantibodies including rheumatoid factor and ANA may be present. The association of facial erythema, polyarthritis, and a positive ANA may suggest a diagnosis of SLE. Tip-offs include the infiltrative appearance of the skin, peripheral neuropathy, and leukocytosis in patients with leprosy.

ARTHRITIS AND MUSCLE WEAKNESS

- Rheumatoid arthritis (RA)
- Ankylosing spondylitis (AS)
- Polymyositis
- Dermatomyositis (DM)
- Systemic lupus erythematosus (SLE), scleroderma, mixed connective tissue disease (MCTD)
- Sarcoidosis
- HIV-associated arthritis
- Whipple's disease

Comments: Rheumatoid arthritis patients become weak from several contributing factors. First, there is the so-called arthrogenic muscle inhibition in which joint inflammation weakens specific muscles, for example, the quadriceps in knee arthritis. Arthrogenic inhibition explains weak hands in finger and wrist arthritis, upper extremity weakness in elbow and shoulder arthritis, and lower extremity weakness, particularly hip and knee extension in hip and knee arthritis, respectively. Thus, weakness caused by arthrogenic inhibition is focal. In addition, corticosteroid use often results in steroid myopathy. Weakness in steroid myopathy is proximal and affects with predilection the iliopsoas muscles. Finally, a general decrease in activities results in generalized weakness. All of these mechanisms must be addressed in treatment planning. True myopathic weakness in an RA-like patient may represent polymyositis of the variety associated with "mechanic's hands," interstitial pulmonary disease, and anti Jo-1 antibodies. It may also represent DM, a diagnosis that is hard to miss if the rash is properly identified.

SLE, scleroderma, and MCTD may feature proximal muscle weakness from associated myositis. These conditions are suggested by the presence of cutaneous sclerosis and Raynaud's in scleroderma/MCTD, and multisystem disease in SLE.

Various forms of arthritis occur in HIV infection, a condition that may cause myopathic weakness directly from HIV myositis or indirectly as a reaction to zidovudine.

Finally, the rare Whipple's disease may features arthritis and myositis. Wasting and lymphadenopathy in a patient with arthritis and myopathic weakness should bring into consideration both HIV infection and Whipple's disease.

ARTHRITIS, SUBACUTE, OR CHRONIC AND PERIPHERAL NEUROPATHY

- Rheumatoid arthritis (RA) with vasculitis
- Polyarteritis nodosa (PAN)
- Wegener's granulomatosis
- Leprosy

Comments: An unequivocal polyarthritis with synovial thickening and effusion suggests that a patient with arthritis and neuropathy indeed has RA as opposed to PAN, in which articular findings are comparatively minor. Although both conditions may cause similar neurologic findings, in large series PAN features predominantly mononeuritis multiplex whereas RA more often causes peripheral neuropathy.

Peripheral neuropathy and arthritis often occur in Wegener's granulomatosis, but ulcerated lesions in the nasal passages, sinuses, or mouth, pulmonary infiltrates, and often renal involvement suggest the diagnosis. A closely related condition, Churg-Strauss's syndrome, causes peripheral neuropathy and arthritis in a context of marked peripheral blood eosinophilia, pulmonary infiltrates, plus a recent or long-standing history of asthma.

Finally, lepromatous leprosy may feature RA-like arthritis and peripheral neuropathy. Diagnosis is suggested by epidemiologic considerations and associated skin lesions.

PROXIMAL JOINT PAIN AND STIFFNESS

- Polymyalgia rheumatica (PMR)
- Osteomalacia
- Multiple myeloma (MM)
- Metastatic cancer
- Light chain (LA) amyloidosis
- Ankylosing spondylitis (AS)
- Frozen shoulder

Comments: PMR is not to be missed because (1) some cases associate with giant cell arteritis, and (2) it is a readily treatable condition. Patients with PMR are older individuals who complain of severe proximal pain and stiffness involving shoulders, neck, hips, and often the lower back. Night rest is interrupted by pain, and morning stiffness and pain are severe and protracted, lasting several hours. The ESR is typically very high and there may be thrombocytosis.

Osteomalacia is another great mimicker. Bone pain from pseudofracture and fractures is typically proximal. Chest wall, shoulder regions, and hip regions are painful. Proximal muscle weakness may also be present from hypophosphatemia. Consider osteomalacia in any older patient with these symptoms.

Multiple myeloma (MM) and disseminated metastatic cancer also have a predilection for older people. Diffuse marrow expansion and widespread bone metastases often result in proximal pain. The ESR is very high, and confusion with PMR is possible. However, malignancy causes osseous tenderness, which is not a feature of PMR.

Amyloidosis of the LA type complicates both MM and

benign monoclonal gammopathies. Amyloid infiltration of joints and muscles causes proximal pain and stiffness. Distinguishing features in amyloidosis include macroglossia, firm synovial masses, and a profound bilateral carpal tunnel syndrome.

Ankylosing spondylitis, because it involves the lumbar and cervical spinal segments, plus the shoulders and hips, may also lead to confusion with PMR. However, in AS patients are younger, there is male predominance, and there is not only pain but also limitation of motion. Frozen shoulder, an initially painful and then restrictive shoulder condition, occurs predominantly in middle-aged or older individuals. Bilateral cases of frozen shoulder may be clinically confused with PMR. Lack of lower body involvement, marked restriction of shoulder motion, and a normal ESR lead away from a diagnosis of PMR.

FIBROMYALGIA

- Fibromyalgia (FM)
- Osteomalacia
- Hypothyroidism
- Viremia (HIV, other)
- Bacteremia
- Narcotic withdrawal

Comments: Fibromyalgia is characterized by chronic generalized pain and symmetric tenderness in a predetermined number of possible tender points. Because osteomalacia may closely resemble FM, it is important in the evaluation of older patients with presumed fibromyalgia to inquire about dietary habits and request appropriate biochemical determinations.

Hypothyroidism is a great mimicker in rheumatology and its clinical spectrum includes fatigue, diffuse soft tissue tenderness, and constipation. The author has picked up several cases of hypothyroidism masquerading as FM. Thyroid-stimulating hormone (TSH) determination is one of the few legitimate tests in the evaluation of fibromyalgia. Fibromyalgia should not be diagnosed in acutely ill patients because fibromyalgic (and enthesial) tenderness is common in both viremia and bacteremia.

If you have the chance, examine FM points in patients undergoing alcohol or opiate withdrawal. Reversible fibromyalgic tenderness is a major component in their musculoskeletal pain.

Suggested Reading

Drenth JPH, Haagsma CJ, van de Meer JWM, International Hyper-IgD Study Group. Hyperimmunoglobulinemia D and periodic fever syndrome. Medicine (Baltimore) 73:133–144, 1994.

Pouchot J, Sampalis JS, Beaudet F, et al. Adult Still's disease: Manifestations, disease course, and outcome in 62 patients. Medicine (Baltimore) 70:118–136, 1991.

Reginato AJ, Schumacher HR Jr, Baker DG, et al. Adult onset Still's disease: Experience with 23 patients and literature review with emphasis on organ failure. Sem Arthritis Rheum 17:39–57, 1987.

Sohar E, Gafni J, Pras M, et al. Familial Mediterranean fever. A survey of 470 cases and a review of the literature. Am J Med 43:227–253, 1967.

CHAPTER 4

Imaging Studies

This is an area in which plenty of money is wasted. The usual error is one of commission. Pain does not show on x-rays, and radiographic findings in early rheumatic disease are either normal or nonspecific. A heel spur seen in a patient with plantar heel pain may give the clinician the wrong impression that the cause of symptoms has been found. Radionuclide bone scans may be irrelevant to the case because increased focal uptake here and there due to asymptomatic osteoarthritis is a common finding in normals from adult age on. Similarly, minor abnormalities without clinical significance such as disc bulgings and rotator cuff defects are commonplace in magnetic resonance imaging (MRI) studies. In this chapter some of the indications and limitations of commonly used imaging procedures are reviewed.

Radiography

Radiographic studies are important in rheumatology, but a clear distinction should be made between interesting information and useful information. The studied area may be in the soft tissues, in joints, or in bones. Views should be obtained according to the disease process.

Soft Tissue X-Rays: Abnormal findings include localized soft tissue swelling (which is well detected clinically), calcification, phleboliths, and gas. Soft tissue x-rays are useful in acute tendinitis, certain types of bursitis, patients with enthesial inflammation, in cases in which a soft tissue angioma is suspected, and to demonstrate the presence of interstitial gas in necrotizing fasciitis and gangrene. In patients with acute tendinitis such as in a scleroderma patient with acute flexor digital tenosynovitis or in acute rotator cuff tendinitis, the presence of amorphous calcium deposits establishes a diagnosis of basic calcium phosphate (BCP) tendinitis. Similar findings may occur in some instances of traumatic subcutaneous bursitis. A lateral view of the hindfoot in plantar ankle flexion is particularly useful in patients with pain and swelling at one or both of the Achilles tendons as it may reveal tendon thickening, effusion in the retrocalcaneal bursa, and erosions in the back of the calcaneous, all indicative of spondyloarthropathy. The presence of rounded calcified bodies in patients with a slowly enlarging soft tissue mass is highly suggestive of an angioma. On the other hand, irregular calcifications in a rapidly enlarging mass may be indicative of synovial sarcoma. Finally, soft tissue x-rays may be used to identify soft tissue gas in suspected cases of necrotizing fasciitis and gangrene. In general, however, with the exceptions noted, soft tissue x-rays are unrewarding.

Joints: Abnormal findings include diffuse or compartmental joint "space" (cartilage) narrowing; chondrocalcinosis; intraarticular calcified bodies; erosions (inflammatory, osteochondritic, compressive); osteonecrosis; fragmentation; lysis; joint "space" widening; displacement of fat pads; capsular expansion; and effusion shadows. Joint x-rays are important in the staging of rheumatoid arthritis (RA), other inflammatory joint conditions, and osteoarthritis (OA).

Bones: Abnormal findings include periostitis and paraarticular bone conditions including osteoid osteoma, Paget's disease, cysts, and tumors.

Rheumatoid Arthritis

A. Findings include periarticular osteopenia, marginal erosions, diffuse joint "space" narrowing, effusions, subluxations (MCPs, MTPs, atlantoaxial).
B. Special views according to joints.
   Hand and wrist: AP and oblique (catcher's view) of both hands including wrists.
   Elbow: AP and lateral at 90 degrees flexion.
   Shoulder: AP in internal and external rotation.
   Cervical spine: A lateral view in flexion. If atlanto-odontoid subluxation is present, add open mouth view.
   Hip: AP and external rotation.
   Knee: AP and lateral.
   Foot: AP and lateral.
C. *Considerations:* Request hand and foot films in all patients, initially and at 1 to 2 year intervals to determine disease progression during the initial 5 years of disease. Other joints should be studied if symptomatic. Bilateral views are useful as internal controls.

Osteoarthritis

A. Findings include asymmetric cartilage loss (medial, lateral, or patellofemoral compartmental narrowing in the knee; central or superior narrowing in the hip; etc.).
B. Special views according to joints same as in RA with the following exceptions: special views for first carpometacarpal (CMC) joint in first CMC OA; a standing view of both knees in knee OA.
C. *Considerations:* Studies should be confined to symptomatic joints.

Gout

A. Early cases show only nonspecific soft tissue swelling. Late cases exhibit radiographically dense paraarticular

soft tissue masses (tophi) and punched out erosions with an "overhanging ledge." Earliest late findings occur in the first MTP joint.
B. Special views in patients with late gout and structural damage of individual joints should be as in OA.
C. *Considerations:* Clearly, x-rays in early gout are unhelpful and should not be requested. Patients may arrive late in the disease, sometimes with the wrong diagnosis of RA or OA. Under these circumstances x-rays are extremely useful for diagnosis.

Chondrocalcinosis

A. Findings may be focal, usually traumatic or basic calcium phosphate (BCP) deposition, or systemic, as in calcium pyrophosphate dihydrate (CPPD) deposition disease, BCP, and calcium oxalate deposition disease. Systemic disease is shown by widespread involvement of joints, particularly those that possess fibrocartilage.
B. Individual symptomatic joints should be studied as in OA. To determine systemic chondrocalcinosis, obtain hand (AP of both hands including wrists), knee (AP and lateral of both knees), and pelvis (AP) films. Look for calcific deposits at the triangular ligament of the wrist, hyaline cartilage and menisci in the knee films, and symphisis pubis.
C. *Considerations:* Chondrocalcinosis is a radiologic term that implies cartilage calcification. Various types of calcium crystals may deposit, each with a different clinical implication (see Chapter 18 on gout, CPPD, and BCP disease).

Spondyloarthropathy (ankylosing spondylitis, reactive arthritis, psoriatic spondyloarthropathy, inflammatory bowel disease [IBD]–associated spondyloarthropathy)

A. Findings include sacroiliitis, osteitis pubis, syndesmophytes, erosions, and enthesopathy. In sacroiliitis there is irregularity, erosion, bone bridging, and eventually bony fusion in one or both sacroiliac joints. Syndesmophytes are bony bridges between vertebrae at the outer layers of the intervertebral disc. Enthesopathy implies inflammatory changes at ligament and tendon insertions. There may be focal erosion and postinflammatory ossification appearing as an irregular, fluffy bony spur.
B. Radiographic changes at the sacroiliac joints take several months to years to develop. Thus, x-rays taken early in the disease course will be negative. Bone scintigrams are helpful in early stages if the sacroiliitis is asymmetric. Symmetric increased uptake may be difficult to distinguish from the normally dense uptake near the sacroiliac joints. CT scans and MRI are excellent to detect early changes that usually occur in the iliac side of the joint; however, the procedures are expensive and definite documentation of sacroiliitis may not be needed if additional findings are present. To detect sacroiliitis with minimal expense and gonadal radiation, obtain a single AP view of the pelvis with 20 to 30 degrees of cephalad inclination (Figure 4–1).
C. *Considerations:* In reactive and psoriatic spondyloarthropathy, sacroiliitis tends to be unilateral. In AS and IBD-associated spondyloarthropathy, in contrast, changes are usually bilateral and symmetric. Gross paraspinal beaked syndesmophytes, usually unilateral, typically associate with reactive and psoriatic spondylitis. Thin anterior syndesmophytes are the rule in AS and IBD-related spondyloarthropathy.

Special Situations

Suspected Baker's cyst: Ultrasound works best. MRI and CT are expensive; arthrography is painful and may lead to complications.
Suspected internal derangement off the knee: MRI.
Articular or paraarticular mass: Obtain plain x-rays to rule out a primary bone lesion. MRI shows characteris-

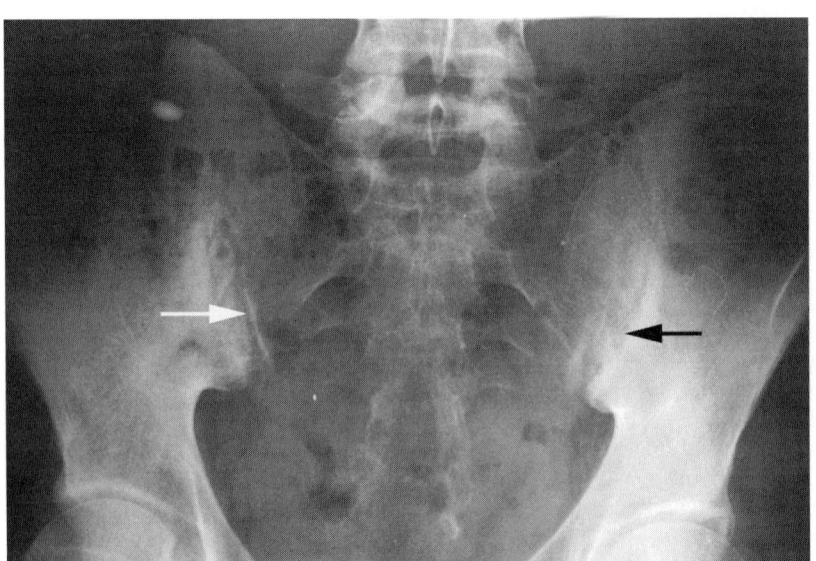

FIGURE 4–1. An anteroposterior (AP) view of the pelvis with 30 degrees cephalad inclination of the beam is excellent to evaluate sacroiliac joints in a single film, sparing the patient from the radiation involved with oblique views. The AP view also provides some idea about the hips. The patient, who is 30 years of age, has reactive arthritis. There is narrowing and irregularity in both sacroiliac joints, particularly the left (arrows).

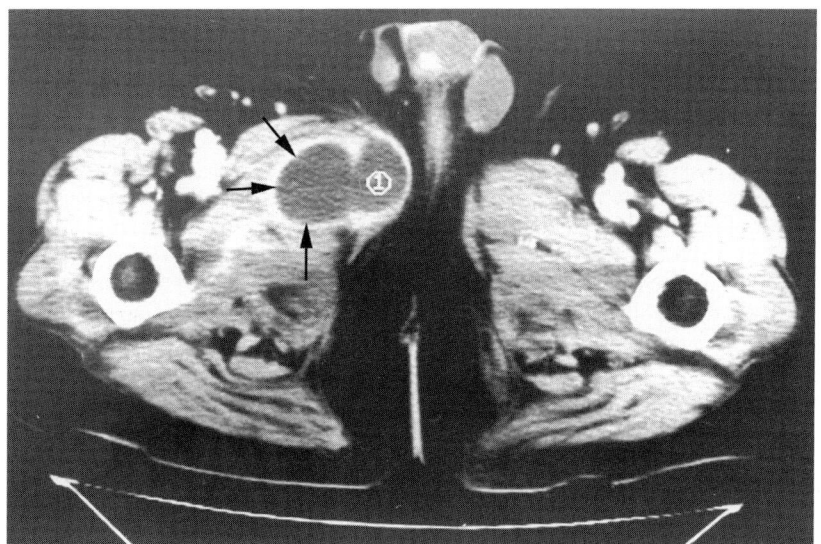

FIGURE 4–2. *Patient 4.* Helical CT scan with contrast shows a large, bilocular intramuscular cavity in right medial upper thigh. There is frank enhancement in the surrounding tissue. The lesion proved to be an abscess caused by *S. epidermidis*.

tic findings in pigmented villonodular synovitis (PVNS).

Frozen shoulder: Plain x-rays to rule out bone lesion, subluxation, and an obstructive large calcified mass. Chest x-rays in a smoker.

Suspected calcific tendinitis: Plain x-rays.

Shoulder impingement syndrome: Plain x-rays to diagnose calcific mass, acromial anomalies. If recurrent, and if decompressive surgery is under consideration, MRI to determine tendon rupture (that may modify surgical approach).

Acute low back pain: No x-rays except in patients with a "red flag" (clinical suspicion of malignancy, osteomyelitis, spondylitis, fracture).

Spinal metastasis: MRI to determine extent of disease and impending neural impingement.

Spinal stenosis (as suggested by neurogenic claudication): Plain AP and lateral lumbar spine x-rays. MRI or CT in preoperative cases.

Acute neck pain: No x-rays except in patients with a red flag (clinical suspicion of malignancy, osteomyelitis, fracture, clinically suggested odontoid or lateral masses lesion).

Cervical myelopathy (as suggested clinically): Plain AP and lateral of cervical spine. MRI to determine cord status.

Frequently Encountered Problems

Dark films. Visualization of soft tissues, essential in enthesopathy and late gout, is not possible.

Light films. Unsuited for the detection of periarticular osteopenia and early erosions.

Unnecessary films. They add expense and radiation. Common examples include lumbosacral spine films in acute low back pain, cervical spine films in acute neck pain, AP, oblique, and extension cervical spine films, oblique views of the hand and foot, shoulder axillary views (useful in subluxation), wrist films (wrists are adequately seen for rheumatologic purposes in hand films), ankle or foot films in ankle sprains not fulfilling Ottawa rules.

Computed Tomography (CT)

This technique, which involves a fair amount of radiation as well as expense, is important to define cortical bone. CT is useful in diagnosing osteomyelitis, particularly in chronic cases in which a bone sequestrum may be present. Also, CT allows better visualization of spinal facet joints than MRI does. Soft tissue masses are also well defined, particularly when the study is done with contrast. An improvement over standard CT is the helical CT, which has improved efficiency and has greatly reduced the radiation dose to obtain multiplanar or three-dimensional reconstructions.

PATIENT 4. A 64-year-old man who 1 month before had undergone reconstructive surgery for urethral stenosis presented with pain in the anteromedial proximal right thigh. He was afebrile. Some local puffiness was present, but no induration or fluctuance was noted. Hip motion was free and painless and no hernial sac was palpable in the inguinal area. An echo showed normal venous and arterial flow and no abscess. He was treated with naproxen 500 mg tid. Ten days later he presented febrile, having had rigors, and marked swelling and induration were now present at the previously painful area. A helical CT with contrast showed a multilocular cavity with enhancement at its margin (Figure 4–2). A large multilocular intramuscular abscess was drained surgically. The root of the abscess was adjacent to the urethra. *S. epidermidis* grew from the pus.

Metallic implants (such as joint prostheses) greatly distort CT images but have little effect on MRI. However, because of a shorter exposure time plus lower operating costs, CTs are far more available than MRIs. This represents an advantage only if CT findings are to be diagnostically useful. To give two examples, although CT can be used, spinal stenosis and spinal metastases are better defined with MRI. To be cost effective and minimize risks, the choice of imaging procedure in a given clinical situation should be discussed with an experienced radiologist.

Magnetic Resonance Imaging (MRI)

Magnetic resonance imaging is an expensive but unsurpassed tool to define internal derangement in knee and other joints, osteonecrosis of the hip, intra- and para-articular masses, rotator cuff tears, spinal stenosis, cervical myelopathy, bony metastases, osteomyelitis, recurrent carpal tunnel syndrome, and soft tissue lumps that could represent a malignant tumor (Table 4–1).

PATIENT 5. An 87-year-old woman with severe coronary artery disease and neurogenic claudication due to spinal stenosis was admitted to the hospital with a protracted episode of angina pectoris. CPK levels remained normal and no EKG changes developed. On the second hospital night severe medial right knee pain developed spontaneously. No effusion was noted. There was true bony tenderness around the medial tibial plateau proximal to the anserine bursa and anterior to the medial collateral ligament. The patient, who before was fully ambulatory, was now unable to place the foot on the ground. Prior to her discharge the next day, knee x-rays were obtained and were read normal (Figure 4–3). The following day an MRI was obtained. A large subchondral fracture was present (spontaneous osteonecrosis) (Figure 4–4). She was treated with bed rest and knee protection with a walker. One month later a band of sclerosis had appeared at the fracture site (Figure 4–5). Now, after 6 months she is fully ambulatory and only minimal residual sclerosis is present on follow-up knee films.

TABLE 4–1
JOINT AND SOFT-TISSUE IMAGING BY MRI

	Appearance	
	On T1	On T2
Fat	Bright	Bright or gray
Bone marrow	Bright	Bright or gray
Cortical bone	Black	Black
Intervertebral disk	Gray	Bright (n. pulposus)
Degenerated disk	Black	Black
Vessels	Black	Black
Muscle	Gray	Gray
Meniscus	Black	Black
Torn meniscus	Bright (tear)	Bright (tear)
Synovial fluid	Gray	Bright
Extravasated blood	Black	Bright
Ganglia	Black	Bright
Ligament	Black	Black
Tendon	Black	Black
Torn tendon	Black	Bright (tear)
Nerve	Gray	Black

In T1, fat can be suppressed (rendered black), allowing adjacent synovial effusion and water deposition at torn sites in menisci or tendons to stand out.
Bright = hyperintense = high signal.
Gray = isointense*.
Black = hypointense = low signal.
*The reference tissue in the limbs is muscle.

If a soft tissue lump appears cystic on palpation, ultrasound should be used first. Smooth cystic lesions do not suggest malignancy and further evaluation may not be required. There are minimal health hazards from MRI, the most significant being isolation anxiety, which presents in 5% to 10% of patients and can be prevented with a sedative. Contraindications to MRI include a cardiac pacemaker, implanted neural stimulators, cochlear implants, intraocular metal, a stainless steel Harrington rod (used for the correction of scoliosis), and old intracranial aneurysm surgical clips. As mentioned, current joint implants are not ferromagnetic and are not a contraindication for MRI studies. Image distortion is less with MRI than with CT. Magnetic resonance imaging may be used in many other conditions of the musculoskeletal system, but preference should be given to less expensive and less time-consuming techniques such as ultrasound and CT if equivalent information can be obtained.

Ultrasound

No ionizing radiation is involved and studies are relatively inexpensive. Ultrasound studies are important in the diagnosis of cystic lesions such as iliopsoas bursa distensions (iliopsoas bursitis may result in prominent lower extremity edema or femoral nerve palsy) and in the diagnosis of Baker's cysts (which among other complications may compress veins and nerves or rupture leading to the syndrome of "pseudothrombophlebitis"). Truly cystic lesions give a regular echo; beware of inhomogeneous masses that may represent a soft tissue sarcoma. Deep soft tissue masses, such as pyomyositis, can also be well shown by echo. Another use of ultrasound is to determine the integrity of rotator cuff tendons. MRI is superior in this setting, however, because it offers a more detailed and complete view of the tendon plus an outline of the impinging structures such as the acromion and the acromioclavicular joint. Ultrasound studies are widely used in pediatric rheumatic disease. Not only are they helpful to identify joint and tenosynovial effusions within a general area of inflammation, but children truly enjoy seeing on the screen their inner parts in action.

Radionuclide Bone Scan

Early (vascular phase) bone scans are useful to detect hypervascular areas such as in early sympathetic dystrophy or synovitis. Late (bone) uptake shows synovitis, bone accretion around osteoarthritic joints, stress fractures, and spinal osteophytes. Bone scans are extremely useful in the diagnosis of osteomyelitis, Paget's disease, primary bone tumors with the possible exception of multiple myeloma, and metastases. There are occasional patients whose symptoms suggest synovitis but have normal findings on physical examination, laboratory studies, and x-rays. In this setting, increased radionuclide uptake in symptomatic joints suggests that synovitis is indeed present. This should be a *rare* indication to request a radionuclide bone scan.

Bone Densitometry

Bone densitometry is usually done by DXA or DEXA, which stands for dual-energy x-rays absorptiometry, or by com-

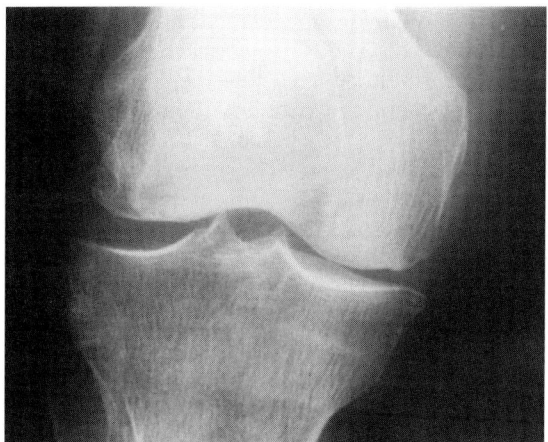

FIGURE 4–3. *Patient 5.* This elderly patient had, for 2 days, acute bony pain in right upper anteromedial tibia. An AP film of the knee is normal.

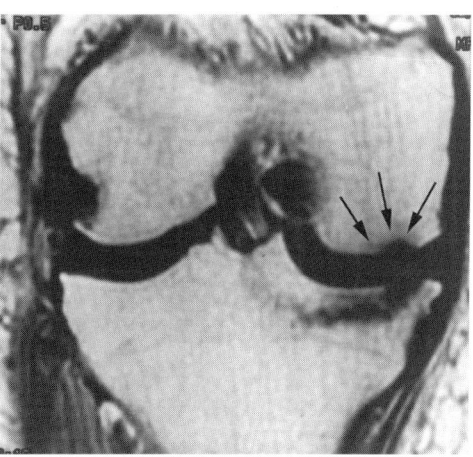

FIGURE 4–4. *Patient 5.* An MRI of the right knee was obtained the next day, and a large subchondral fracture is seen under the medial tibial plateau. There is also a small osteochondritic lesion in the medial femoral condyle facing the tibial lesion (arrows).

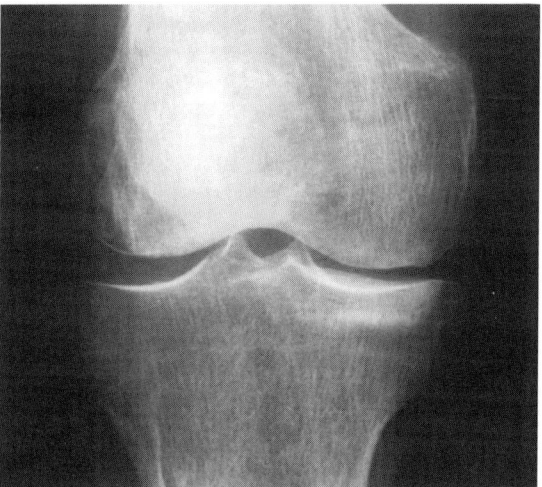

FIGURE 4–5. *Patient 5.* One month later a thick band of sclerotic bone is seen at the site of the fracture. X-rays obtained 6 months after the initial study were normal. The patient had full recovery.

puted tomography. DXA implies a very small radiation dose and it takes only 5 to 15 minutes for the entire procedure. CT densitometry exposes the patient to more radiation, takes longer to be performed, and is more expensive. Medicare reimburses part of the cost and other insurances also cover it. The use of these techniques is discussed in Chapter 22. Guidelines for requesting bone densitometry may be found in the appendix.

Electrodiagnosis and Muscle Biopsy

Electrodiagnosis is a term that encompasses the recording of electrical activity of muscle or electromyography (EMG) and nerve conduction studies (NCS). *Electromyography* is essential in the evaluation of suspected inflammatory or metabolic muscle disease. The procedure studies electrical activity at rest, motor unit action potentials recruited on minimal contraction of the muscle, the recruitment pattern as a maximal contraction is approached, and the anatomic distribution of the observed abnormalities, that is, whether they are confined to a nerve, a portion of a plexus, a specific spinal segment, proximal muscles, or proximal plus peripheral muscles.

In a very ill patient with classic dermatomyositis rash, a consistent EMG is all that is needed to initiate therapy. In most situations, however, because of greater specificity, a *muscle biopsy* is obtained contralaterally in a symmetric muscle to the one showing EMG changes. If the clinical suspicion is myositis or vasculitis (such as polyarteritis nodosa), H&E and other routine tissue stains will suffice. If a metabolic myopathy is suspected, however, the rheumatologist or primary care physician must make sure the neuropathologist and the surgeon talk to each other ahead of the procedure so the specimen will not be ruined for histochemistry and electron microscopy.

Nerve conduction studies (NCS) are usually requested (1) to establish the pattern (mononeuritis multiplex vs. polyneuropathy) and type (demyelinating vs. axonal) of neuropathy, and (2) to prove compression neuropathies such as carpal tunnel syndrome (CTS) and tarsal tunnel syndrome prior to decompressive surgery. The author considers it questionable to operate on a patient with symptoms of CTS and normal NCS findings because the condition may be mild, intermittent, and therefore amenable to further conservative treatment. Even more questionable is to perform surgery without having had the test performed, since compression may be at some other level, a different type of neuropathy may be present, and so on. On he other hand, if a conservative treatment is planned the expense and pain of going through a NCS cannot be justified.

Mononeuritis multiplex may be demyelinating (approximately one-third of cases) or axonal (two-thirds of cases). Polyarteritis nodosa, rheumatoid vasculitis, and SLE cause axonal mononeuritis multiplex. Only half of cases of axonal mononeuritis multiplex, however, occur in association with an autoimmune disease. Nerve conduction studies include motor latency (the time latency to the target muscle), sensory conduction, and more sophisticated studies such as the H reflex, the F wave, and evoked cortical potential recordings including visual, brain stem, auditory, and somatosensory evoked potentials. Both the H reflex and the F wave are used to detect proximal pathology, such as radiculopathy. Finally, repetitive nerve stimulation before and after exercise is essential in the diagnosis of neuromuscular junction disease such as myasthenia gravis (repetitive stimulation blocks transmission, followed by increased transmission) and the Lambert-Eaton syndrome (repetitive stimulation facilitates transmission).

CHAPTER 5

Laboratory Studies

CBC is most important; anemia in rheumatic disease patients may be a marker of chronic inflammation, blood loss, hemolysis, or marrow suppression; leukopenia and lymphopenia add to a diagnosis of SLE and also HIV infection; thrombocytosis is a marker of inflammation in rheumatoid arthritis, reactive arthritis, giant cell arteritis, polymyalgia rheumatica, polyarteritis nodosa, and Wegener's granulomatosis. It is also a marker of myeloproliferative disorders, conditions that cause gout as well as erythromelalgia.

Alkaline phosphatase, alanine aminotransferase (ALT), and aspartate aminotransferase (AST) may increase from concurrent hepatitis in mixed cryoglobulinemia or from toxic hepatitis in patients receiving nonsteroidal anti-inflammatories (NSAIDs) or methotrexate. However, in certain clinical situations with abnormal "liver" enzymes, a *CPK/aldolase* determination reveals that myositis rather than hepatitis is responsible for the increased ALT and AST levels (there are plenty of these enzymes in muscle).

PATIENT 6. A 65-year-old man was referred for evaluation of arthralgias, general debilitation, and marked elevation of serum ALT and AST. Autoimmune hepatitis and mixed cryoglobulinemia had been leading diagnostic considerations. On examination skin was normal and liver and spleen were not palpable. Neck and hip flexors were weak with relative sparing of distal strength. Pronounced muscle weakness prevented the patient from rising unaided from the examining table. Myositis was suspected and CPK and aldolase determination was requested. Both were elevated about 50 fold and alkaline phosphatase was normal. Muscle biopsy confirmed the diagnosis of polymyositis, and a dramatic response to high-dose corticosteroids followed.

Urinalysis and serum creatinine level are critical indicators of kidney involvement in rheumatic disease (nephritis in SLE and the vasculitides; amyloidosis in RA and the spondyloarthropathies) or NSAIDs or cyclosporine nephropathy. Periodic routine laboratory testing is important to detect silent blood loss and to determine liver and kidney status in patients treated long term with potentially toxic medications.

A *serum uric acid (UA) level* should be obtained when gout is suspected, although normal values are frequently encountered during acute gout. Indeed, it has been shown that a brisk decrease, rather than an increase, in serum UA in a chronically hyperuricemic patient acts as a trigger of acute gout. A 24 hour urine UA and creatinine determination (to assure completeness of collection) is important to detect the 10% of gout patients who are hyperexcretors. These patients are at a greater risk of urolithiasis, tophaceous deposits, frequent gout attacks, and destructive gouty arthropathy. Although some authorities recommend 24 hour urine UA determination only when a UA-lowering drug is being considered (to avoid the error of giving, for instance, probenecid to a hyperexcretor), the author requests the test following the first attack of crystal-documented gout.

To collect the urine properly the patient empties his or her bladder at a defined time, for example, at 8 a.m., and from this time on each voided volume is collected, the last collection being at 8 a.m. the following day. When the patient feels an urge to defecate, the urine should be collected first. This advice appears to be, and most likely is, unnecessary. It is included to remind you that patients often don't know how to proceed and they need to be instructed in advance.

The *erythrocyte sedimentation rate (ESR)* is a very useful test in the diagnosis and follow-up of giant cell arteritis (GCA) and as a marker of severe disease in RA. However, the ESR is not very sensitive to disease activity changes in RA and being so nonspecific, ESR elevations may be due to a comorbid infectious, inflammatory, or neoplasic disease (Table 5–1).

The *C-reactive protein (CRP)*, a test relatively little used in the United States, helps discriminate SLE flares in which results are normal or near normal from intercurrent infection

TABLE 5–1

FACTORS THAT INFLUENCE THE ERYTHROCYTE SEDIMENTATION RATE (ESR)

Increase	Decrease	No Effect
Anemia	Polycythemia	Body temperature
Inflammatory disease	Sickle cell disease	Recent meal
Female sex	Spherocytosis	Aspirin
Pregnancy	Acanthocytosis	NSAIDs
Hypercholesterolemia	Anisocytosis	Extreme leukocytosis
High room temperature	Microcytosis	High-dose corticosteroids
		Hypofibrinogenemia
		> 2 hour delay in running test
		Bile salts
		Congestive heart failure
		Cachexia

From Sox HC, Liang MH. The erythrocyte sedimentation rate: Guidelines for rational use. Ann Intern Med 104:515–523, 1986.

that markedly increases CRP (with the caveat that SLE flare and infection often go hand in hand). Because CRP levels change faster than the ESR, CRP is a better indicator of adequate steroid dose in conditions in which you definitely want to know, such as GCA.

Synovial Fluid (SF) Analysis

This test deserves special recognition; it is essential for diagnosis in septic arthritis and the crystal-induced synovitides and provides direct evidence of inflammatory rather than degenerative joint disease. Also, if an unconscious patient has a tightly swollen joint that proves to be a hemarthrosis, place an aliquot in the refrigerator and inspect 1 hour later: If the fluid is crowned by a fat layer, just like chicken soup, an intraarticular fracture is quite likely. Table 5–2 provides the range of SF findings in various rheumatic conditions; Table 5–3 summarizes bursal fluid findings in common bursitides. Details of aspiration for specific joints and bursae are spelled out in the appendix. However, some general principles are discussed here.

Knee aspirations are usually done by primary care physicians. Joints with a more difficult access, except in unusual circumstances, should be aspirated by a rheumatologist or orthopedist. Hips are notoriously difficult to tap except under fluoroscopic guidance. Since hip aspirations are usually done to rule out septic arthritis and septic arthritis of the hip is by definition surgical (granted that some have been successfully drained with an indwelling catheter placed under fluoroscopic control), the procedure should always involve an orthopedic surgeon.

Bursal aspiration is a straightforward procedure well within the scope of primary care physicians. The olecranon bursa is easier to aspirate than the prepatellar.

If no fluid is obtained it is wiser to enlist the help of a rheumatologist or an orthopedic surgeon rather than declaring "no fluid present." Some comments on "dry taps" and "QNS" are pertinent here. To put it bluntly, a dry tap often means needle misplacement: Reposition the needle and give a few more tries. If fluid still cannot be obtained, ask for help. There are several types of error possible. One is that there is no fluid simply because a normal solid structure was entered. A classic one is the infrapatellar fat pad, an adipose lump placed between the patellar tendon and the knee joint. This lump is quite large in some patients to the point of being confused with prepatellar bursitis. An experienced colleague will recognize the structure and say "that's fat."

TABLE 5–2
SYNOVIAL FLUID FINDINGS IN VARIOUS CONDITIONS

	Color	Viscosity	WBC/mm^3*	% PMNs†	Crystals	Culture
Normal fluid	Clear	+++++	63 (13–150)	7 (0–25)	None	Negative
Osteoarthritis	Clear or hematic	++++	1291 (1–34,000)	31 (1–99)	None‖	Negative
Systemic lupus erythematosus turbid	Clear to turid	++++	3,416 (0–14,200)	39 (0–93)	None	Negative
Rheumatoid arthritis	Turbid	+, ++	15,721 (100–181,000)	67 (1–95)	None	Negative
Reactive arthritis	Turbid	+, ++	14,447 (3,300–43,200)	72 (26–96)	None	Negative‡
Acute rheumatic fever	Turbid	++, +++	12,218 (600–60,000)	50 (2–98)	None	Negative
Gout	Turbid	+ to +++	20,064 (20–102,000)	79 (2–100)	MSU	Negative
Pseudogout	Turbid	++, +++	26,334 (50–290,400)	82 (7–100)	CPPD	Negative
Septic arthritis (non-GC)	Turbid to pus	+, ++	100,000 (15,000–432,000)	90 (80–97)	None	Positive
GC arthritis	Clear to pus	++ to ++++	68,391 (150–250,000)	89 (60–100)	None	Positive or negative§

*Mean (range).
†Median (range).
‡Chlamydia often present in synovial membrane.
§Gonococcal DNA present by PCR in synovial membrane.
‖Occasionally CPPD or BCF crystals.
CPPD crystals = calcium pyrophosphate dihydrate crystals.
MSU crystals = monosodium urate crystals.
BCF crystals = basic calcium phosphate crystals.
From Cohen AS, Goldenberg D. Synovial fluid. In: Alan S. Cohen (ed) Laboratory Diagnostic Procedures in the Rheumatic Diseases, 3rd ed. Grune & Stratton, Orlando, 1–54, 1985.

TABLE 5–3
SUBCUTANEOUS BURSITIS BURSAL FLUID FINDINGS

	WBC count/mm³*	% PMNs†	Crystals	Culture
Traumatic bursitis	350 (0–24,500)	5 (0–98)	None	Negative
Gout	2,375 (650–12,000)	40 (2–98)	MSU	Negative
Septic bursitis	13,500 (1000–425,000)	94 (30–100)	None	Positive
Rheumatoid bursitis	2,500 (200–25,200)	30 (2–86)	Cholesterol in 50%	Negative

*Mean (range).
†Median (range).
From Canoso JJ. Bursal membrane and fluid. In: Alan S. Cohen (ed) Laboratory Diagnostic Procedures in the Rheumatic Diseases, 3rd ed. Grune & Stratton, Orlando, 55–76, 1985.

A second error is altogether missing the fluid-containing cavity. Prime examples are prepatellar bursa effusions mistaken for joint effusions and olecranon bursa effusions thought to represent elbow effusions. In both instances, placing the needle intraarticularly will of course result in a dry tap. An experienced colleague will say "you missed the target."

A third error is correctly inserting the needle in the effused joint without being able to withdraw fluid. This may happen because the needle is too thin, for example, a #22 needle to drain a purulent or a riciform effusion, or because the needle tip landed in a fat pad or adjacent muscle. As an example, a knee may be entered too proximally. While this would not be a problem if you know the exact location of the suprapatellar bursa (the proximal synovial extension beneath the distal quadriceps), failure may result from inserting the needle too deep into the fat pad or too superficially within muscle. Also, the knee may be entered too distally with the needle tip landing in the infrapatellar fat pad. In either case an experienced colleague might say "let me give a try."

Joint and bursal aspirations require proper sterilization of the skin, the use of gloves that need not be sterile, and adherence to the rules of universal precautions. Although anesthetic infiltration is done with a thin needle, the aspiration itself should be with a #18 or larger needle if infection is suspected or a #20 needle if the purpose is diagnosis of suspected inflammatory or crystal-induced disease. If gonococcal infection is likely, the specimen should be plated at the bedside on agar chocolate and carried warm to microbiology. All samples should be promptly submitted for routine culture and analysis. Suspicion of anaerobes, such as in acute arthritis following a joint prosthesis, requires immediate transfer to anaerobic medium. Most synovial aspirations are done to determine whether crystals are present or not. Few primary physicians' laboratories have a polarizing microscope (although one can be readily improvised) and in small hospitals laboratory personnel may not be proficient in crystal identification. When in doubt, the primary care physician should find out if a rheumatologist is available to review the specimen.

Remember that corticosteroid crystals, present in all preparations for intraarticular use, may look just like gout or pseudogout crystals under the polarizing microscope. Cell counts and differential are of course very useful diagnostically, but if a SF sample is left sitting on a counter for several hours, even if well anticoagulated, WBC counts will be spuriously low (such as 500/mm³ instead of an initial 60,000/mm³). Aspirations performed late at night are particularly likely to have this fate.

Technique of Synovial Fluid Analysis

Immediately upon obtaining the fluid, 1 to 3 mL should be anticoagulated in EDTA (purple-top tube) for WBC count and differential. The tube must be shaken energetically to achieve effective anticoagulation (any fibrin clot will precipitously reduce the WBC count). Next, a drop of fluid should be placed on a clean microscope slide and covered with an equally clean coverslide for crystal search. Finally, the syringe should be capped with a sterile rubber cap and submitted for bacteriologic studies as clinically indicated.

A critical step is to do a thorough and informed crystal search. A polarizing microscope should ideally be used, but not all hospitals or laboratories have one. However, with some practice, patience, and by turning the room lights off to gain discrimination, crystals can be easily detected with a regular microscope by dimming the light and lowering the condenser to achieve a phase effect. Although extracellular crystals may represent dirt on the slide, intracellular crystals are always significant. On regular light monosodium urate (MSU) crystals appear as thin rods that often stick out from the cell contour on both ends (Figure 5–1A). Calcium pyrophosphate dihydrate (CPPD) crystals are usually much smaller and chubbier than MSU crystals and only rarely stick out from the cell (Figure 5–1B). It is sometimes difficult, because they may be so small, to distinguish CPPD crystals from refringent vacuoles. Basic calcium phosphate crystals are amorphous and appear as debris (Figure 5–1C). The rare oxalate crystals are envelope shaped and unmistakable (Figure 5–1D). In a young man with acute arthritis and absence of chondrocalcinosis on x-rays, MSU-looking intracellular cystals confirm gout whereas in an older person with radiographic chondrocalcinosis, CPPD-looking crystals confirm pseudogout (with the caveat that 8% of pseudogout patients have coexistent gout).

There are, however, many situations in which precise crystal identification is essential for patient management. Determining the type of crystal can only be done with a polarizing microscope by using compensated polarized light. As most people know, a polarizing lens on the ocular end of the microscope cuts light by half. If another polarizing lens is placed over the light source at right angles from the upper polarizing lens, the 50% of light that passed through the first polarizing lens is cut off, turning the field black. If crystals (MSU, CPPD, corticosteroid) are present in the slide, however, light passing the distal lens will be bent by the sample so the crystals will stand up bright and sharp on a black background.

So far, little will has been done to distinguish MSU from CPPD crystals except that the former are much brighter than the latter. The critical difference between these crystal species can only be appreciated by inserting a first-order compensator plate between the distal polarizing lens and the specimen. Due

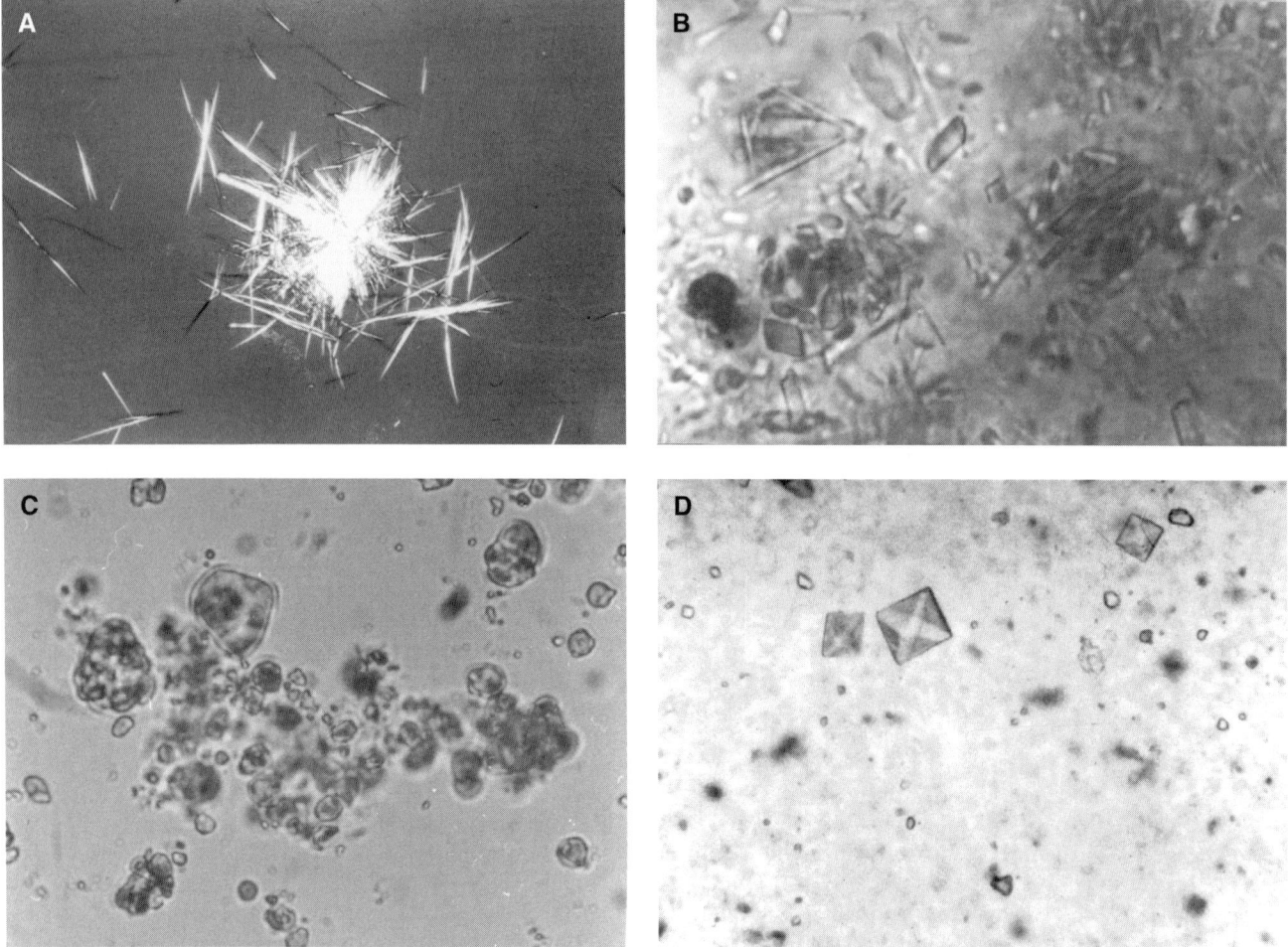

FIGURE 5–1. *Four species of crystals. A,* Needle-like monosodium urate crystals showing a characteristic of intense birefringency and negative elongation. Compensated polarized light × 300. *B,* A clump of calcium pyrophosphate dihydrate crystals. These crystals are shorter and chubbier than MSU crystals. *C,* Hydroxyapatite crystals in synovial fluid aspirated from an osteoarthritic knee. These crystals are nonbirefringent (they cannot be seen using polarized light) but stain well with Alizarin red, a nonspecific stain for calcium. *D,* Oxalate crystals in synovial fluid from a patient on chronic hemodialysis. *A* with polarized light; *A–D* on 400×. (Courtesy of Dr. Antonio Reginato, Cooper Medical Center, Camden, NJ.)

to inherent optical characteristics, the first-order compensator, placed at 45 degrees to both polarizing lenses, turns the black background red. The compensator has an optical axis called the alpha axis. Crystals in the sample are randomly arranged. Crystals that parallel to the compensator's axis appear yellow and perpendicular to it appear blue are by convention negatively birefringent. This, for practical purposes (unless the patient received intraarticular steroids), means gout. Conversely, crystals that parallel to the compensator axis are blue and perpendicular to it are yellow are said to be positively birefringent, which usually means CPPD pseudogout.

Summarizing, MSU crystals are long, strongly birefringent, and negatively birefringent; CPPD crystals are short, weakly birefringent, and positively birefringent. What to do in the middle of the night if a polarizing microscope is not available or no one is around to set it up? Take a good look with a regular microscope according to the directions just given and establish whether intracellular crystals are present as well as their general appearance. It is also important to prepare a wet smear by sealing the coverslide with nail polish and placing it in a refrigerator. Taking these precautions the smear will remain viable for a few days, which is enough time to have it reviewed by a rheumatologist or an expert laboratory technician. Some SF determinations such as viscosity, mucin clot, and glucose and protein content add unnecessary cost to the procedure.

PATIENT 7. A 62-year-old man, a horse trainer, was referred for evaluation of an obscure symmetric distal polyarthritis of 2 years duration. Studies had shown moderate normochromic anemia, a marked increase in ESR, some degree of renal insufficiency, low-grade proteinuria, normal serum protein electrophoresis, negative RF and ANA, and trace positive cryoglobulins in his serum. A renal biopsy obtained elsewhere was nondiagnostic, showing mesangial proliferation and vascular fibrosis. On examination the patient was a debilitated, unkempt man with synovial thickening and tenderness at the MCPs, PIPs, wrists, and ankles. There was diffuse MTP synovitis with the peculiarity that tenderness was most prominent in the big toes. Admission laboratory results included Hct 35%, Westergren ESR 100 mm/1 hour, serum creatinine 1.6 mg/dl, serum UA 8.5 mg/dl (N 6–8 mg/dl), and urinalysis 1+ protein without formed elements in the sediment. Low-grade polyarticular gout was suspected and several joints were aspirated. Traces of fluid were obtained from a wrist, an MCP, and a great toe MTP. Cell count in wrist fluid was 4000/mm^3 with 100% mononuclear cells. Synovial fluid smears from all three joints revealed intra- and extracellular MSU crystals, proving the suspected diagnosis of gout. Because gout could be overlapping with other rheumatic disease the patient was treated with oral colchicine 0.6 mg per hour for 8 doses followed by colchicine 0.6 mg once daily. Within 3 days of treatment all joints became asymptomatic. One month later allopurinol was added and 1 year later joint examination was normal, Hct was 40%, ESR was 12 mm/1 hour, creatinine was 1.4 mg/dl, urinalysis was normal, and the patient was carrying on with his life at the race track.

Improvised Compensated Polarizing Microscopy Set: A very useful and inexpensive compensated polarizing microscopy set can be improvised by using polarizing sunglasses, an ordinary microscope slide, and clear cellophane tape, as follows:

1. A first-order compensator plate is built by covering both sides of the microscope slide with clear cellophane tape.
2. After disassembling the polarizing sunglasses, one lens (PA) is placed over the light source.
3. The other polarizing lens (PB) is to be held by hand on top of the microscope's ocular.

To operate the system, rotate the ocular polarizing lens until a black background is obtained. Then, rotate the improvised compensator plate placed above PA (at 45 degrees to both polarizing lenses) so as to obtain a pink background. The axis of this compensator is parallel to the streak lines on the cellophane. To make sure the system works, inspect a known MSU sample, such as material obtained from a tophus, and ascertain that crystals oriented alongside the microscope slide look yellow and crystals that are perpendicular to it look blue.

Suggested Reading

Canoso JJ. Bursal membrane and fluid. In: Alan S, Cohen (ed). Laboratory Diagnostic Procedures in the Rheumatic Diseases, 3rd ed. Grune & Stratton, Orlando, 55–76, 1985.

Cohen AS, Goldenberg D. Synovial fluid. In: Alan S. Cohen, Editor, Laboratory Diagnostic Procedures in the Rheumatic Diseases, 3rd ed. Grune & Stratton, Orlando, 1–54, 1985.

Fagan TJ, Lidsky MD. Compensated polarized light microscopy using cellophane adhesive tape. Arthritis Rheum 17:256–261, 1974.

Schmerling RH, Delbanco TL, Tosteson AN, et al. Synovial fluid test. What should be ordered? JAMA 264:1009–1014, 1990.

Schumacher HR Jr, Reginato AJ. Atlas of Synovial Fluid Analysis and Crystal Identification. Lea & Febiger, Philadelphia, 1991.

CHAPTER 6

Immunologic Studies

Rheumatoid Factor (RF)

Rheumatoid factors are autoantibodies directed against aggregated IgG. Routine RF determination quantifies IgM RF. Useless if taken in isolation, in the proper clinical context a positive RF test is an important diagnostic aid in RA. In addition, RA patients with very high RF titers tend to have more severe articular and systemic disease. RF determinations help in the investigation of Sjögren's syndrome and provide a clue in the diagnosis of mixed cryoglobulinemia. A positive RF is common in untreated subacute bacterial endocarditis, leprosy, and other chronic infections. Also, about 5% of normal young individuals and a much higher rate of normal older individuals have a positive RF test. Obviously, if one were to study RF in a population sample, more false positives than true positives for rheumatic disease would be found simply because the added rate of RF-associated rheumatic disease in the population at large is less than 3%.

Antinuclear Antibodies (ANA)

Done on Hep-2 cells, a positive ANA test is found in the overwhelming majority of SLE patients. Clinical correlates of lupus autoantibodies are shown in Table 6–1. Specific patterns of fluorescence associate with particular antibodies: a peripheral pattern with double-stranded DNA antibodies (Figure 6–1A), a fine-speckled pattern with anti-Ro and anti-La antibodies among others (Figure 6–1B), a homogeneous pattern with antihistone antibodies (Figure 6-1C), and a centromeric pattern with anticentromeric antibodies.

Less than 5% of SLE patients have a negative ANA. These patients tend to have anti-Ro antibodies or anti-single-stranded DNA antibodies. Also, positive ANAs may turn negative when lupus patients are treated aggressively and in lupus nephritis with chronic renal failure. In addition to SLE, positive ANAs are seen in mixed connective tissue disease (100% if included in disease definition), scleroderma (80%–95%), Sjögren's syndrome (50%–90%), and RA (20%–30%); many patients receiving procainamide, isoniazid, or hydralazine; occasionally in infectious diseases such as HIV, tuberculosis, and leprosy; in a significant number of patients with autoimmune hepatitis or malignant disease; and, as expected from the way the test is calibrated, in about 5% of normal people. An ANA test should be performed when there is *clinical* suspicion of SLE or other connective tissue disease rather than as a screening test.

PATIENT 8. A young woman was self-referred to the clinic for a further opinion on the treatment of recently diagnosed SLE. She complained of fatigue, migraines, alopecia, morning stiffness, arthralgias, and Raynaud's phenomenon. An ANA determination done elsewhere was positive and hydroxychloroquine treatment was under consideration. The patient was asked to describe rather than enunciate her symptoms, which she did with some disgust. The "migraine" was described as a band around her head, the "Raynaud's" consisted of a mottled bluish discoloration of fingers upon

TABLE 6–1

CLINICAL CORRELATES OF LUPUS AUTOANTIBODIES

Lupus Autoantibody	Clinical Association
Anti-nRNP (or U1RNP)	Myositis
	Raynaud's phenomenon
	Milder lupus
Anti-Sm	Isolated central nervous system disease
	Nephritis
Anti-P	Depression
	Psychosis
Antihistone	Drug-induced lupus
Anti-DNA	Nephritis
Anti-Ro (SSA)	Lymphopenia
	Pneumonitis
	Photosensitivity
	Nephritis (in the absence of anti-La)
	Purpura
	Rheumatoid factor
	Congenital heart block
	Neonatal lupus dermatitis
	Neonatal cholestasis
	Complement component C^2 deficiency
Anti-La (SSB)	Absence of nephritis
	Sjögren's syndrome
	Congenital heart block
	Neonatal lupus dermatitis
	Neonatal cholestasis
	Subacute cutaneous lupus erythematosus
Anticardiolipin, circulating anticoagulant, or false positive VDRL	Thrombosis
	Miscarriage
	Thrombocytopenia
	Hemolytic anemia
Anti-beta^{-2} glycoprotein 1	(same)
Anti-RA33	Erosive arthritis

Modified from Harley JB. Autoantibodies are central to the diagnosis and clinical manifestations of lupus. J Rheumatol 21:1183–1185, 1994. (Twelve of 33 SLE patients had anti-RA33 and of these, 5 had erosive disease, as opposed to none without anti-RA33.)

cold exposure, the "arthralgias" denoted pressure pain in the lateral elbows and inner knees, and by "alopecia" she meant a fair amount of hair left on her comb each morning. Findings on physical examination were normal except widespread, symmetrically placed tender points. Tenderness was most prominent in the lateral elbows and inner knees. Laboratory results brought by the patient included a 1:40 (borderline) homogeneous-pattern ANA done on Hep-2 cells and normal CBC, urinalysis, and ESR. The patient was told that her condition was fibromyalgia rather than SLE, but reassurance did not work; she soon saw another rheumatologist. *Corollary*: in a patient without clinical evidences of SLE or other connective tissue disease, ANA determination is contraindicated.

To reemphasize, every normal individual stands a 5% chance of having a low titer (1:40 to 1:80), usually homogeneous positive ANA. Once an uncalled for positive ANA has been obtained, patient's and physician's concern is unavoidable. The consultant may dismiss the ANA outright or may request additional studies prior to dismissing the ANA. The costs and anxiety generated by an imprudently obtained ANA are considerable. A note should be added regarding legitimately requested ANAs (clinical features that suggest connective tissue disease) which, on Hep-2 cells, are reported as showing a cytoplasmic pattern of fluorescence. The presence of antisynthetase (polymyositis) or antimitochondrial (primary biliary cirrhosis) antibodies should be suspected.

Anti-Ro (SSA) and anti-La (SSB) antibodies measured by different methods are common in Sjögren's syndrome and also in SLE. A condition known as *subacute cutaneous lupus erythematosus* features high anti-Ro titers in most patients. In addition, anti-Ro antibodies are often present in SLE patients with negative ANA. Photosensitivity in SLE correlates highly with the presence of anti-Ro antibodies. Anti-Ro and anti-La antibodies cross the placenta and, by binding to antigens expressed in certain fetal tissues (conduction system of the heart, skin, biliary tract), cause the rare *neonatal lupus syndrome*.

Anti-double-stranded DNA (dsDNA) antibodies can be measured by a variety of techniques of which the gold standard is a radioimmunoassay, the Farr technique. ELISA techniques have a high rate of false positive results from single-stranded DNA segments bound to the plastic plates. A positive dsDNA test is highly specific for SLE and therefore very useful for diagnosis when few clinical manifestations are present, for example, isolated glomerulonephritis. Active lupus nephritis usually occurs in a context of high-titer dsDNA antibodies and falling complement levels.

Anti-Sm antibodies (named after a patient, Smith, in whom the antibody was first isolated) are also highly specific for SLE, although they are present in only 25% of patients.

Antiribonucleoprotein (RNP) Antibodies

High titers of RNP antibodies, currently known as anti-U1 RNP antibodies, are seen in mixed connective disease (MCTD), a condition that many observers consider a transi-

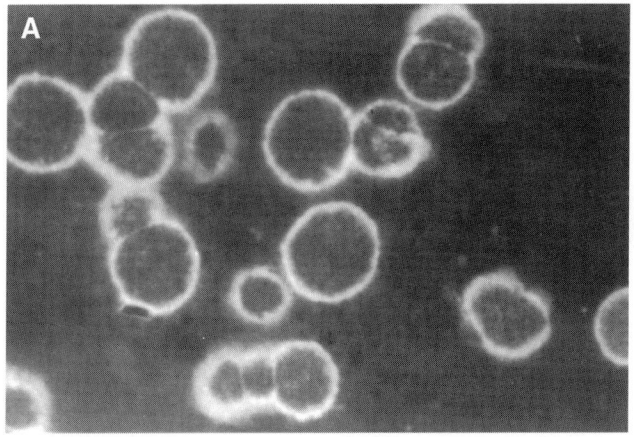
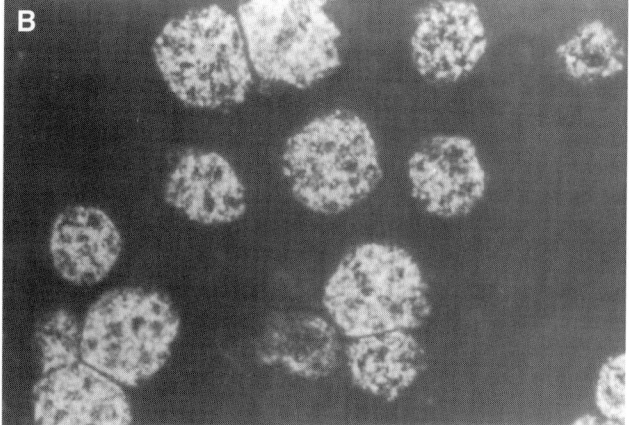
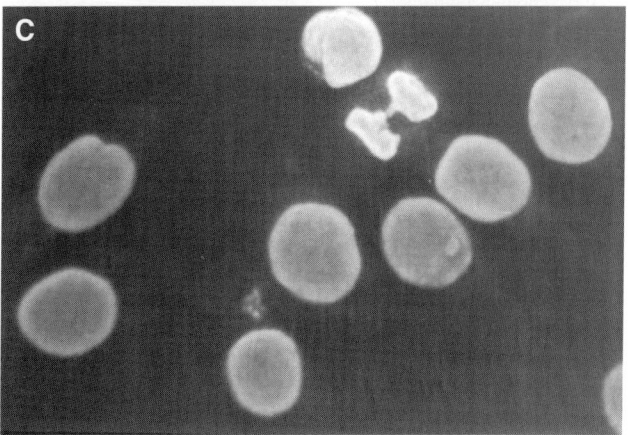

FIGURE 6–1. *Antinuclear antibodies detected by immunofluorescence using as substrate Hep-2 cells. A, Peripheral pattern; B, speckled pattern; C, homogeneous pattern. 1000×.*

tional state rather than a discrete disease entity. When patients with MCTD are followed for years they often develop scleroderma, SLE, or RA.

Antiphospholipid antibodies (APA), or antibodies against alpha2-glycoprotein 1, of which APA may be a surrogate marker, are believed to cause the antiphospholipid antibody syndrome (APS). APS may occur in patients with SLE (secondary APS) or as a primary condition known as PAPS.

Antiphospholipid antibodies may be detected in serum samples by an enzyme-linked immunosorbent assay (ELISA) for IgG or IgM anticardiolipin antibodies (positive in 80% of APS), as a false positive VDRL (present in 20% of APS), or as a positive lupus anticoagulant (LA) assay (positive in 40% of APS). Accepted tests for the LA include the dilute activated partial thromboplastin time (APTT), the kaolin clotting time test, and the Russell viper venom time test. Because LA associates with thrombophilia rather than bleeding, the clinical meaning of the designation is opposite to what it says. When APS is suspected, a serum and a plasma sample should be obtained for APA and LA studies. Because of its low sensitivity a VDRL test should not be requested. Anti-alpha2-glycoprotein 1 antibodies should be studied in patients with clinical manifestations of PAPS who are negative for APA and LA tests. As shown in Table 6–2 many conditions cause thrombophilia.

Antiphospholipid antibodies that appear in infection (such as HIV) or are drug induced (such as in patients receiving chlorpromazine) do not use alpha2-glycoprotein 1 as a cofactor and do not cause an hypercoagulable state.

Anti-neutrophil-cytopasmic antibodies (ANCA) may be one of two types as determined by indirect immunofluorescence: They may produce diffuse cytoplasmic fluorescence (c-ANCA) or perinuclear fluorescence (p-ANCA). Proteinase 3 is the antigen in the former and myeloperoxidase in the latter. Both types of ANCA may be determined by an ELISA technique as well. Although perinuclear fluorescence is nonspecific, cytoplasmic fluorescence has important disease associations including Wegener's granulomatosis in which 95% of patients (less than 50% in the limited forms) exhibit high titers, systemic necrotizing small-vessel vasculitis (microscopic polyarteritis nodosa), and a crescentic necrotizing glomerulonephritis. The latter may represent a forme fruste of Wegener's granulomatosis. While the diagnostic value of c-ANCA is beyond doubt, there is still controversy as to its value to predict or reflect disease activity.

Complement Studies

Falling serum complement levels (C_3, CH50) along with high titers of dsDNA antibodies characterize active SLE and often herald the onset of lupus nephritis. Hereditary C_2 deficiency, plus the already described anti-Ro/SSA antibody, associate with ANA-negative SLE and subacute cutaneous lupus erythematosus. Diagnosis of hereditary C_2 deficiency is suggested by a persistently low CH50 and a normal C_3 in a clinically stable patient. Given this setting it is legitimate to request C_2 determination. A low C_2 level in both parents is confirmatory of the condition. Low complement levels usually reflect complement system activation such as seen in some types of vasculitis, mixed cryoglobulinemia, sepsis, and subacute bacterial endocarditis. Palpable purpura in these conditions reflects PMN accumulation influenced by immunecomplex deposition or venular expression of adhesion molecules under the influence of locally released IL1.

Immune Complexes

Immune complexes determinations have little, if any, diagnostic value. What is important is the cause of, rather than the presence of, immune complexes. The clinician faces a clinical syndrome, not a test result.

Cryoglobulins and Cryofibrinogen

The same considerations as with immune complexes apply. As an example, if a palpable purpura is present, regardless of the presence of cryoglobulins, one should consider sepsis; SBE; hepatitis A, B, and C; vaccine- or drug-induced vasculitis; a primary vasculitis such as Wegener's granulomatosis, connective tissue disease such as SLE or Sjögren's; and malignancy such as lymphoma, multiple myeloma, and Waldenstrom's macroglobulinemia. In some situations a premature identification of cryoglobulins may obfuscate the clinician's mind, as in the case that follows.

PATIENT 9. A 60-year-old man was referred for evaluation of a 1 month history of malaise, anorexia, weight loss, low back pain, a petechial rash, plus a positive cryoglobulin test obtained elsewhere. An abdominal aneurysm had been resected 3 months before. An autoimmune condition, probably an essential cryoglob-

TABLE 6–2
CONDITIONS ASSOCIATED WITH AN INCREASED RISK OF THROMBOEMBOLISM

Atrial fibrillation
Estrogen use (replacement or contraception)
Pregnancy
Immobilization: congestive heart failure, myocardial infarction, stroke, postsurgical convalescence
Cancer: pancreas, lung, ovaries, testes, urinary tract, breast, stomach
Surgical trauma: orthopedic, thoracic, abdominal, and genitourinary procedures
Antiphospholipid syndrome with one or more of the following:
    Lupus anticoagulant
    Anticardiolipin antibodies
    Anti-beta-2 glycoprotein 1 antibodies
    Protein C deficiency
    Protein S deficiency
Antithrombin III deficiency
Resistance to activated protein C
Dysfibrinogenemia
Protein C deficiency
Protein S deficiency
Abnormal plasminogen or plasminogen activator mechanisms
Heparin cofactor II deficiency
Increased plasminogen activator inhibitor
Behçet's disease
Thromboangiitis obliterans
Homocysteinuria

ulinemia or vasculitis, were the leading diagnostic considerations. The patient appeared chronically ill. He was afebrile. A florid palpable purpura involved the dorsum of hands (some of these lesions were bullous), lower extremities, and buttocks. A faint aortic regurgitation murmur was present. The back was held rigid. No bony tenderness was noted. A small-vessel vasculitis, a tumoral cryoglobulinemia such as seen in multiple myeloma or lymphoma, and, given the murmur and the back pain, subacute bacterial endocarditis were considered on admission. By the second hospital day the patient continued to be afebrile and six admission blood cultures remained negative. Given his poor general condition, corticosteroid treatment was considered. However, by the next day all of the blood cultures grew *Enterococcus*. Cardiac echoes including a transesophageal study were negative. The patient was treated for bacterial endocarditis, and all abnormalities resolved with the exception of the heart murmur. A positive cryoglobulins test had delayed diagnosis for almost 2 weeks. Fortunately, corticosteroids never got started.

As this case exemplifies, the presence of cryoglobulins should not change the diagnostic steps a clinician must take. There are several situations, however, in which cryoglobulin determination is important:

1. Mixed cryoglobulinemia clinically characterized by recurrent palpable purpura and petechiae, Raynaud's phenomenon, subtle evidences of hepatitis, hyperglobulinemia, high levels of RF, and low serum complement components as seen in hepatitis B and C.
2. Cryoglobulins per se may lead to serious manifestations including leukocytoclastic vasculitis and renal insufficiency.
3. Monoclonal components present in some cryoprecipitates may be benign or may be indicative of multiple myeloma. A widely used classification of cryoglobulinemias is shown in Table 6–3.

Finally, cryofibrinogenemia should be suspected when patients present cold sensitivity, livedo reticularis, skin ulcers, acral purpura, and gangrene. Technical difficulties, mainly a faulty blood collection, may interfere with cryoglobulins and cryofibrinogen determination. An important point: Let the laboratory know you are requesting these tests; a technician should be dispatched to receive the specimens (a red-top tube for cryoglobulins and a lavender EDTA tube for cryofibrinogen) and carry them to the laboratory in a warm container. To determine cryoglobulins the blood is allowed to clot at 37° C and the serum is separated by centrifugation. The supernatant is removed, in a Wintrobe tube, and kept in the refrigerator at 1° C. The tube is inspected for precipitation after 1 and 7 days. At the final reading the specimen is centrifuged, which provides a cryocrit. An immunoelectrophoresis on the precipitate completes the study. A similar procedure after centrifugation of the EDTA tube is used to determine presence and amount of cryofibrinogen.

Lyme Borreliosis Antibody Test

Unfortunately, false positive results by indirect immunofluorescence (IF) and also by enzyme-linked immunosorbent assay (ELISA) greatly outnumber true positives in nonendemic areas. A positive ELISA test is most helpful when the clinical suspicion of Lyme borreliosis is medium high, strengthening the diagnosis. On the other hand, a borderline or negative serology in the face of suggestive evidence of late disease, for example, relapsing knee arthritis or encephalopathy, calls for a Western blot, a proliferative assay, or an actual search of *B. burgdorferi* DNA by the polymerase chain reaction (PCR) in synovial fluid. To overcome the nonspecificity of ELISA and IF tests it is recommended by the Centers for Disease Control (see appendix) that every equivocal or positive ELISA test be confirmed by Western blot. If the blot is positive the test is reported as positive. If the blot is negative the test is reported as negative. Lyme borreliosis tests should be done in reliable reference laboratories to avoid as far as possible encountering false positive results.

HLA Determinations

HLA determinations of the DR locus and specifically the DR4 alleles that are markers of severe RA in whites remain to this day a research tool. Interestingly, determination of these markers in blacks would be of no use, since the "bad" DR4 alleles are not overrepresented in severe RA in blacks. The diagnostic value of HLA-B27 determination in spondyloarthropathy has been a matter of controversy. An agreed on important use of the test is in the assessment of patients with symptoms suggestive of spondyloarthropathy who cannot have pelvic films (pregnant women, for instance) and when sacroiliac joint films are negative or equivocal, a situation that often arises within the first 2 years of disease. HLA-B27 positivity in these settings strongly supports a diagnosis of spondyloarthropathy. Another indication for HLA-B27 determination is in the diagnosis of spondyloarthropathy in children and women, since these groups have less axial and more peripheral joint involvement than adult males. Finally, HLA-B27 positivity helps diagnosing reactive arthritis when

TABLE 6–3

CLASSIFICATION OF CRYOGLOBULINEMIAS

Types	Components	Disease Associations
I	Monoclonal IgM *or* IgG	Waldenström's macroglobulinemia Lymphoma Myeloma MGUS*
II (mixed)	Monoclonal cold-reactive IgM, IgG, *or* IgA *plus* polyclonal IgG	Hepatitis C virus Hepatitis B virus? Sjögren's syndrome Lymphoma
III (mixed)	Polyclonal cold-reactive IgM *or* IgM in combination with IgG or IgA or both *plus* Polyclonal IgG	Connective tissue disease Hepatitis C virus

*MGUS = monoclonal gammapathy of undetermined origin. May develop into overt lymphoma.
Adapted from Brouet JC, et al. Biologic and clinical significance of cryoglobulins: A report of 86 cases. Am J Med 57:775–788. 1974.

enthesitis is present (such as uni- or bilateral Achilles tendinitis) in absence of spinal or peripheral joint disease. On the other hand, a positive HLA-B27 result in the wrong setting such as in patients with mechanical low back pain (there is a 5%–7% chance of being HLA-B27 positive in the general population) only creates confusion.

PATIENT 10. A 40-year-old man was evaluated for almost painless progressive limitation of his neck and lower back evolving over a number of years. There had been no GI or genitourinary symptoms. On examination the patient's neck was held in slight flexion with only nodding movements possible. There was minimal motion at the costovertebral joints (chest expansion 1 cm), and the lumbar segment had no measurable lengthening on attempted flexion (Schober 0, nl 6–8 cm). An AP film of his pelvis with 30 degrees cephalad inclination showed fused SI joints and bamboo-type fusion between L4–5 and L5–S1. Routine laboratory studies were requested but not an HLA-B27, which would not have added if positive, or subtracted if negative, to a diagnosis of classical ankylosing spondylitis.

In summary, similar to other tests, HLA-B27 determination should only be requested when the test is likely to afford useful information above and beyond that gathered from the history, physical examination, and x-rays.

Suggested Reading

American College of Rheumatology Ad Hoc Committee on Clinical Guidelines. American College of Rheumatology guidelines for the initial evaluation of the adult patient with acute musculoskeletal symptoms. Arthritis Rheum 39:1–8, 1996.

Centers for Disease Control. Proceedings of the Second National Conference on Serologic Diagnosis of Lyme Disease. Association of State and Territorial Public Health Laboratory Directors, Washington, DC, 1994, 1–111.

Rao JK, Weinberger M, Oddone EZ, et al. The role of antineutrophil cytoplasmic antibody (c-ANCA) testing in the diagnosis of Wegener granulomatosis. Ann Intern Med 123:925–932, 1995.

Shmerling RH, Delbanco TL. The rheumatoid factor: An analysis of clinical utility. Am J Med 91:528–534, 1991.

Sox H, Liang M. The erythrocyte sedimentation rate. Guidelines for rational use. Ann Intern Med 104:515–523, 1986.

Von Mühlen CA, Tan EM. Autoantibodies in the diagnosis of systemic rheumatic diseases. Sem Arthritis Rheum 24:323–358, 1995.

Ward MM. Review: Evaluative laboratory testing: Assessing tests that evaluate disease activity. Arthritis Rheum 38:1555–1563, 1995.

CHAPTER 7

Questionnaires and Other Assessment Instruments; Criteria

It may appear surprising that functional questionnaires, global assessments, disease activity indices, disease severity indices, and disease damage indices are included among methods of assessing rheumatic disease. However, it has been shown both in SLE and RA that such instruments are extremely useful not only in assessing disease but in predicting outcomes. This is so because questionnaires gather actual life events (symptoms, signs, organ damage) whereas most laboratory tests only measure isolated biochemical or immunologic variables. Rheumatologists are increasingly incorporating these research tools into routine clinical practice. Primary care physicians would do well to know what these instruments are, the reason they are used, and how to interpret results. For example, the SLE Disease Activity Index (SLEDAI) (Table 7–1) better detects small degrees of clinical activity than a battery of laboratory tests including ESR, anti-dsDNA antibodies, C_3, C_4, and circulating immune complexes. Additional SLE-related indices that will be increasingly encountered in the medical literature include the Index of Disease Severity for SLE (Table 7–2) and the SLE Damage Index (Table 7–3).

Among function questionnaire instruments the Health Assessment Questionnaire (HAQ) (Table 7–4) has had a major impact in clinical research and has been translated and validated in several languages. The American College of Rheumatology has proposed a core set of disease activity measures to be used uniformly in clinical trials. Interestingly, of the eight measurements three are global assessments (pain as assessed by the patient using a visual analogue scale and disease activity as assessed by both the patient and the physician by using a 5 point categorical scale). Two measurements are derived from physical examination: tender joint count and swollen joint count assessed in 68 joints or in 20 joints (by using groups of joints rather than individual joints), which appears to work just as well. One measurement is the patient's assessment of physical function as determined by HAQ (determining the HAQ takes 10 minutes) or the Arthritis Impact Measurement Scales (AIMS) (determining the AIMS takes 15–20 minutes). One measurement is a laboratory test, either ESR by the Westergren technique or C-reactive protein level. The final measurement, which is to be used in disease-modifying drug trials of longer than 1 year duration, is radiography or other imaging technique to assess structural damage.

This is the language in which clinical trials in rheumatology are and will be reported, which is a substantial departure from individual measurements that may be objective but have little relevance to the patient.

Another frequently used scale is the functional classification of RA (Table 7–5). Since this classification is frequently used by insurance companies, primary physicians would do well to learn how to use it with an individual patient.

When confronted with criteria such as the ACR Classification Criteria for Systemic Lupus Erythematosus, primary care physicians may be puzzled by the meaning of *classification*. They may ask themselves whether classification is tantamount to diagnosis, and if not, what classification criteria are used for. In answer to the first question the stated purpose of classification criteria (such as the lupus criteria, the vasculitis criteria, etc.) is to allow categorization of (already diagnosed) patients to achieve relatively homogeneous groups for epidemiologic, therapeutic, or other studies rather than diagnosing disease. Thus, patients who fulfill criteria may be included in these studies whereas patients who lack them may not.

If classification criteria are to be applied to already diagnosed patients, then additional criteria must be available to diagnose disease. This is not usually the case, although it varies among conditions. In some conditions diagnosis is made by fulfilling a single criterion. This criterion must have a high specificity and a high predictive value such as crystal identification in crystal-induced arthritis or microbial isolation, whether a bacterium, a fungus, a spirochete, or a virus, in microbial arthritis.

But how is diagnosis made in basic conditions such as osteoarthritis, SLE, and spondyloarthropathy? Clinical, radiologic, and arthroscopic findings are characteristic in osteoarthritis and spondyloarthropathy. In SLE there are no established diagnostic criteria; diagnosis is usually made by (1) consistent clinical findings, (2) positive ANA (high sensitivity and low specificity), and (3) exclusion of mimicking conditions *or* consistent clinical findings *plus* positivity in highly specific tests such as anti-dsDNA and/or anti-Sm.

Suggested Reading

Bloch DA, Moses L, Michel BA. Statistical approaches to classification. Methods for developing classification and other criteria rules. Arthritis Rheum 33:1137–1144, 1990.

Bombardier C, Gladman DD, Urowitz M, et al. and the Committee on Prognosis Study in SLE. Derivation of the SLEDAI: A disease activity index for lupus patients. The Committee on Prognosis Studies in SLE. Arthritis Rheum 35:630–640, 1992.

TABLE 7–1
DISEASE ACTIVITY INDEX FOR LUPUS PATIENTS (SLEDAI)*

Weight	SLEDAI Score	Descriptor	Definition
8	_____	Seizure	Recent onset. Exclude metabolic, infectious, or drug causes.
8	_____	Psychosis	Altered ability to function in normal activity due to severe disturbance in the perception of reality. Include halucinations, incoherence, marked loose associations, impoverished thought content, marked illogical thinking, bizarre, disorganized, or catatonic behavior. Exclude uremia and drug causes.
8	_____	Organic brain syndrome	Altered mental function with impaired orientation, memory, or other intellectual function, with rapid onset and fluctuating clinical features. Include clouding of consciousness with reduced capacity to focus, and inability to sustain attention to environment, plus at least two of the following: perceptual disturbance, incoherent speech, insomnia or daytime drowsiness, or increased or decreased psychomotor activity. Exclude metabolic, infectious, or drug causes.
8	_____	Visual disturbance	Retinal changes of SLE. Include cytoid bodies, retinal hemorrhages, serous exudate or hemorrhages in the choroid, or optic neuritis. Exclude hypertension, infection, or drug causes.
8	_____	Cranial nerve disorder	New onset of motor or sensory neuropathy involving cranial nerves.
8	_____	Lupus headache	Severe, persistent headache; may be migranous, but must be nonresponding to narcotic analgesia.
8	_____	CVA	New-onset cerebrovascular accident(s). Exclude arteriosclerosis.
8	_____	Vasculitis	Ulceration, gangrene, tender finger nodules, periungual infarction, splinter hemorrhages, or biopsy or angiogram proof of vasculitis.
4	_____	Arthritis	More than 2 joints with pain and signs of inflammation (i.e., tenderness, swelling, or effusion).
4	_____	Myositis	Proximal muscle aching/weakness, associated with elevated creatine phosphokinase/aldolase or electromyogram changes or a biopsy showing myositis.
4	_____	Urinary casts	Heme-granular or red blood cell casts.
4	_____	Hematuria	>5 red blood cells/high power field. Exclude stone, infection, or other cause.
4	_____	Proteinuria	>0.5 g 24 hours. New onset or recent increase of more than 0.5 g/24 hours.
4	_____	Pyuria	>5 white blood cells/high power field. Exclude infection.
2	_____	New rash	New onset or recurrence of inflammatory-type rash.
2	_____	Alopecia	New onset or recurrence of abnormal, patchy, or diffuse loss of hair.
2	_____	Mucosal ulcers	New onset or recurrence of oral or nasal ulcerations.
2	_____	Pleurisy	Pleuritic chest pain with at least 1 of the following: rub, effusion, or pleural thickening.
2	_____	Pericarditis	Pericardial pain with at least 1 of the following: rub, effusion, or electrocardiogram or echocardiogram confirmation.
2	_____	Low complement	Decrease in CH50, C3, or C4 below the lower limit of normal for testing laboratory.
2	_____	Increased DNA binding	>25% binding by Farr assay or above normal range for testing laboratory.
1	_____	Fever	>38° C. Exclude infectious causes.
1	_____	Thrombocytopenia	<100,000 platelets/mm^3.
1	_____	Leukopenia	<3000 white blood cells/mm^3. Exclude drug causes.

*SLEDAI: Data collection sheet. Maximal possible score 105; maximal score observed 45.
From Bombardier C, Gladman DD, Urowitz MB, et al. Derivation of the SLEDAI. A disease activity index for lupus patients. Arthritis Rheum 35:630–640, 1992.

Buchbinder R, Bombardier C, Yeung M, et al. Which outcome measures should be used in rheumatoid arthritis clinical trials? Arthritis Rheum 38:1568–1580, 1995.

Fortin PR, Abrahamowicz M, Danoff D. Small changes in outpatient lupus activity are better detected by clinical instruments than by laboratory tests. J Rheumatol 22:2078–2083, 1995.

Fries JJ, Spitz P, Kraines RG, et al. Measurement of patient outcome in arthritis. Arthritis Rheum 23:137–145, 1980.

Gladman D, Ginzler E, Goldsmith C, et al. The development and initial validation of the SLICC/ACR damage index for SLE. Arthritis Rheum 39:363–369, 1996.

Katz JD, Senécal J-L, Rivest C, et al. A simple severity of disease index for systemic lupus erythematosus. Lupus 2:119–123, 1993.

Pincus T, Brooks RH, Callahan LF. Prediction of long-term mortality in patients with rheumatoid arthritis according to simple questionnaire and joint count measures. Ann Intern Med 120:26–34, 1994.

TABLE 7-2
A DISEASE SEVERITY INDEX FOR SYSTEMIC LUPUS ERYTHEMATOSUS

The following four items each receive one point:

1. Lowest recorded hematocrit to date = 30%–37%
2. History of proteinuria (2+ or more)
3. Highest recorded creatinine to date = 1.3–3
4. Four to six ARA criteria for SLE satisfied to date

The following six items each receive two points:

1. History of cerebritis (seizure or organic brain syndrome)
2. History of pulmonary disease (lupus pneumonitis, pulmonary hemorrhage or pulmonary hypertension)
3. Lowest recorded hematocrit to date < 30%;
4. Highest recorded creatinine to date > 3
5. Biopsy-proven diffuse proliferative glomerulonephritis
6. Seven or more ARA criteria for SLE satisfied to date

Maximum score possible is 13.

After Katz JD, Senécal J-L, Rivest C, et al. A simple severity of disease index for systemic lupus erythematosus. Lupus 2:119–123, 1993.

TABLE 7-3
SYSTEMIC LUPUS INTERNATIONAL COOPERATING CLINICS (SLICC) SLE DAMAGE INDEX

Item	Score	
OCULAR (either eye, by clinical assessment)		
Any cataract ever	1	
Retinal change *or* optic atrophy	1	
NEUROPSYCHIATRIC		
Cognitive impairment or major psychosis (e.g., memory deficit, difficulty with calculation, poor concentration, difficulty in spoken or written language, impaired performance level)	1	
Seizures requiring therapy for 6 months	1	
Cerebral vascular accident ever (score 2 if > 1)	1	2
Cranial or peripheral neuropathy (excluding optic)	1	
Transverse myelitis	1	
RENAL		
Estimated or measured GFR < 50%	1	
Proteinuria 24 hours equal or more than 3.5 g	1	
or		
End-stage renal disease (regardless of dialysis or transplantation)	3	
PULMONARY		
Pulmonary hypertension (right ventricular prominence, or loud P2)	1	
Pulmonary fibrosis (physical and x-ray)	1	
Shrinking lung (x-ray)	1	
Pleural fibrosis (x-ray)	1	
Pulmonary infarction (x-ray)	1	
CARDIOVASCULAR		
Angina *or* coronary artery bypass	1	
Myocardial infarction ever (score 2 if more than once)	1	2
Cardiomyopathy (ventricular dysfunction)	1	
Valvular disease (diastolic murmur, or a systolic murmur > 3/6)	1	
Pericarditis for 6 months, or pericardiectomy	1	
PERIPHERAL VASCULAR		
Claudication for 6 months	1	
Minor tissue loss (pulp space)	1	
Significant tissue loss ever (e.g., loss of digit or limb) (score 2 if > 1 site)	1	2
Venous thrombosis with swelling, ulceration, or venostasis	1	
GASTROINTESTINAL		
Infarction or resection of bowel below duodenum, spleen, liver, or gall bladder ever (score 2 if > 1 site)	1	2
Mesenteric insufficiency	1	
Chronic peritonitis	1	
Stricture *or* upper gastrointestinal tract surgery ever	1	
MUSCULOSKELETAL		
Atrophy or weakness	1	
Deforming or erosive arthritis (including reducible deformities, excluding avascular necrosis)	1	
Avascular necrosis (score 2 if > once)	1	2
Osteoporosis with fracture or vertebral collapse (excluding avascular necrosis)	1	
Osteomyelitis	1	
SKIN		
Scarring chronic alopecia	1	
Extensive scarring or panniculum other than scalp and pulp space	1	
PREMATURE GONADAL FAILURE	1	
DIABETES (regardless of treatment)	1	
MALIGNANCY (exclude dysplasia) (score 2 if > one site)	1	2

Damage occurring since onset of lupus, ascertained by clinical assessment and present for at least 6 months unless otherwise stated. Repeat episodes mean at least 6 months apart to score 2. The same lesion cannot be scored twice.

From Gladman D, Ginzler E, Goldsmith C, et al. The development and initial validation of the SLICC/ACR damage index for SLE. Arthritis Rheum 39:363–369, 1996.

TABLE 7-4
HEALTH ASSESSMENT QUESTIONNAIRE (HAQ)

	Without Difficulty?	With Difficulty?	With Some Help from Another Person?	Unable to Do

1. Dressing and Grooming
   Are you able to:
   a. get your clothes out of the closet and drawers
   b. dress yourself, including handling of closures (buttons, zippers, snaps)
   c. shampoo your hair
2. Arising
   Are you able to:
   a. stand up from a straight chair without using your arms for support
3. Eating
   Are you able to:
   a. cut your meat
   b. lift a full cup or glass to your mouth
4. Walking
   Are you able to:
   a. walk outdoors on flat ground
5. Hygiene
   Are you able to:
   a. wash and dry your entire body
   b. use the bathtub
   c. turn faucets on and off
   d. get on and off the toilet
6. Reach
   Are you able to:
   a. comb your hair
   b. reach and get down a 5 lb. bag of sugar that is above your head
7. Grip
   Are you able to:
   a. open push-button car doors
   b. open jars that have been previously opened
   c. use a pen or pencil
8. Outside Activity
   Are you able to:
   a. drive a car (for reasons other than arthritis I do not drive___)
   b. run errands and shop
9. Sexual Activity
   Are you able to
   a. have sex (I am not involved in a sexual relationship____)

Note: Functional ability is measured by nine general component categories (dressing and grooming, arising, eating, walking, hygiene, reach, grip, outside activity, and sexual activity), each of which consists of one or more specific questions. For example, "Are you able to shampoo your hair?" is one question asked in the dressing and grooming component. Each question is scored from 0 to 3 based on the following scale: "without difficulty" = 0, "with difficulty" = 1, "with some help from another person or with a device" = 2, and "unable to" = 3. The highest score in any question within a component is the score for that component. The index is calculated by adding the scores and dividing by the total number of components answered.

From Fries JF, Spitz P, Kraines RG, et al. Measurement of patient outcome in arthritis. Arthritis Rheum 23:137–145,1980.

TABLE 7-5
AMERICAN COLLEGE OF RHEUMATOLOGY REVISED CRITERIA FOR CLASSIFICATION OF FUNCTIONAL STATUS IN RHEUMATOID ARTHRITIS

Class I: Completely able to perform usual activities of daily living (self care, vocational, and avocational).
Class II: Able to perform usual self-care and vocational activities, but limited in avocational activities.
Class III: Able to perform usual self-care activities, but limited in vocational and avocational activities.
Class IV: Limited in ability to perform usual self-care, vocational, and avocational activities.

From Hochberg MC, Chang RW, Dwosh I, et al. The American College of Rheumatology 1991 revised criteria for the classification of global functional status in rheumatoid arthritis. Arthritis Rheum 35:498–502, 1992. Usual self-care activities include dressing, feeding, bathing, grooming, and toileting. Avocational activities (recreational and/or leisure) and vocational (work, school, homemaking) activities are patient desired and age and sex specific.

CHAPTER 8

Methods of Treatment

This chapter reviews drugs used in the treatment of rheumatic and musculoskeletal conditions; physical medicine measures; and orthopedic procedures including soft tissue surgery (such as carpal tunnel release), arthroscopy, conservative surgery, and total joint replacement. Techniques of joint aspiration and injection are described in the appendix.

Pharmacologic

Nonsteroidal Anti-Inflammatory Drugs (NSAIDs)

These agents are most useful in acute, subacute, and chronic inflammatory noninfectious conditions. A partial listing of conditions includes gout, rheumatoid arthritis (RA), reactive arthritis, as well as some regional painful syndromes particularly when amorphous calcification is present. In RA, NSAIDs are analgesic and anti-inflammatory but do not alter disease progression. A combination of NSAIDs is no more effective but has a greater risk of toxicity than maximal doses of a single agent. Commonly used NSAIDs are shown in Table 8–1.

Aspirin is the least expensive NSAID but is cumbersome to take as well as highly ulcerogenic. Nonacetylated salicylates such as choline magnesium trisalicylate, salsalate, and sodium salicylate lack the acetyl moiety that ruins the enzyme cyclooxygenase. As a result, platelets are unaffected, gastric toxicity is low, and adverse renal effects are probably less severe than with other NSAIDs. Nonacetylated salicylates deserve greater use particularly in SLE with borderline thrombocytopenia, osteoarthritis that is unresponsive to acetaminophen, and generally when an anti-inflammatory is needed in a patient who appears to be at a greater risk of NSAIDs side effects.

An advantage of all salicylates over other NSAIDs is that blood levels can be measured. The newer NSAIDs are less toxic than the pioneer phenylbutazone (its use for any indication should be discouraged because of its potential to induce aplastic anemia) and indomethacin, which is also highly ulcerogenic, often causes distressing CNS toxicity, and may also induce bone marrow aplasia. Indomethacin is particularly useful in patients with spondyloarthropathy and in acute gout.

Each new NSAID tends to be more expensive and margin-

TABLE 8–1
ANALGESICS AND NONSTEROIDAL ANTI-INFLAMMATORY AGENTS

Drug	Protein Binding	Half-life	Effect on Platelets	GI Toxicity	Kidney Toxicity in At-Risk Patients
Acetaminophen	20–50%	2 hours	None	Minimal	Increases risk of ESRD
Aspirin	80–92%	15 minutes 15–20 hours as salicylate	Irreversible*	High	Probably none
Nonacetylated salicylates	80–90%	4–15 hours	None	Minimal	Probably none
Nabumetone	99%†	3–4 hours		Low	Possible
Ibuprofen	98%	2 hours	Transient	Low	Possible
Sulindac	93–98%	16–18 hours	Transient	Median	Possible
Naproxen	97.6–99.5%	12–15 hours	Transient	High	Yes
Piroxicam	99%	30–86 hours	Transient	High	Yes
Diclofenac	99%	1–2 hours	Transient	High	Yes
Indomethacin	99%	3–11 hours	Transient	High	Minimal

*New platelets must be formed to correct aggregation defect.
†The biotransformation product 6-methoxy-2-naphthylacetic acid.
Patients at risk of renal insufficiency: elderly, dehydrated, preexistent renal disease

ally less toxic than the previous ones. The most frequent and serious toxicity of NSAIDs is GI toxicity. Aspirin, indomethacin, piroxicam, sulindac, and tolmetin are well known for their aggressive gastrotoxic properties. Gastrointestinal symptoms may be reduced by taking these agents with meals. Due to various effects, most significantly a depletion of tissue prostaglandin in the gastroduodenal mucosal lining, NSAIDs cause superficial erosion with occult bleeding and peptic ulcer. Minor dyspetic symptoms and diarrhea occur in 10% to 50% of patients. It has been estimated that serious GI complications such as a perforated ulcer, severe bleeding, and gastric outlet obstruction occur in 2% to 4% of patients who take NSAIDs for 1 year.

In Silverstein's study (Table 8–2), risk factors for severe GI complications included old age (greater than 75 years), cardiovascular disease, and a history of peptic ulcer or bleeding. The risk of serious complications within 6 months of NSAIDs treatment was 0.4% for patients with none of the risk factors, 1% for those having one risk factor, and 9% for patients who had all four risk factors. Magnesium-aluminum hydroxide 10 to 20 mL as needed to a total dose of 60 mL a day, sulfacrate, and histamine-2-receptor antagonists such as cimetidine and ranitidine are effective in relieving dyspeptic symptoms but have not been shown to prevent NSAIDs-induced ulcers. A protective role of proton pump inhibitors such as omeprazole remains to be shown. The concurrent administration of the synthetic prostaglandin misoprostol reduces the risk of serious (stomach and duodenum) complications by about 40%.

Drawbacks of this medication include its high cost and diarrhea as a side effect. Diarrhea may be prevented by starting the misoprostol at a low dose, that is, 100 µg bid or qid and slowly raising the dose. Given its unequivocal gastrointestinal protective effect, misoprostol should be used in individuals at high risk of complications. In patients with an average risk the less toxic NSAIDs—nabumetone, ibuprofen, or nimesulide—should be used first. If these agents prove ineffective one of the other agents should be used beginning with naproxen or diclofenac and leaving indomethacin to last. Treatment of dyspepsia should be with any of the agents mentioned.

Caution should be exerted when NSAIDs are used in patients with known or suspected renal disease. Risk factors for nephrotoxicity include old age, concurrent diuretic use, renal insufficiency with serum creatinine of 2 mg/dl or higher, nephrotic syndrome, arteriosclerotic cardiovascular disease, sodium depletion, and liver cirrhosis. In these settings, decreased synthesis of vasodilatory prostaglandins may lead to acute, reversible renal failure. It has been said that nonacetylated salicylates and sulindac are safer than other NSAIDs in patients with reduced renal perfusion. There are, however, reported cases of renal insufficiency with the use of these agents. Other renal syndromes resulting from NSAID use include fluid retention, potassium retention and hyperkalemia, the nephrotic syndrome (in association with interstitial nephritis), and very rarely papillary necrosis.

Elderly patients who take NSAIDs may exhibit subtle mental changes particularly in recall memory and occasionally overt psychosis or gross cognitive impairment, which is reversible upon discontinuation of the drug. Propionic acid derivatives such as ibuprofen, naproxen, ketoprofen, and fenoprofen appear to be more detrimental to recall memory than other NSAIDs.

TABLE 8–2

RISK FACTORS OF GASTROINTESTINAL ULCER IN PATIENTS RECEIVING NSAIDs

Definite risk factors
   Age over 70
   History of peptic ulcer or upper GI bleed
   Cardiovascular disease
   High-dose NSAIDs
   Combined use of NSAIDs
   Concomitant corticosteroid therapy
   Duration of therapy less than 3 months
Possible risk factors
   Smoking
   Alcohol use
   Helicobacter pilori infection
   Female sex

From Silverstein FE, Graham DY, Senior JR, et al. Misoprostol reduces serious gastrointestinal complications in patients with rheumatoid arthritis receiving nonsteroidal anti-inflammatory drugs. Ann Intern Med 123:241–249, 1995; and Lichtenstein DR, Syngal S, Wolfe MM. Nonsteroidal anti-inflammatory drugs and the gastrointestinal tract. The double-edged sword. Arthritis Rheum 38:5–18, 1995.

Another important, albeit rare, toxicity of NSAIDs is meningismus. This complication has been reported predominantly in SLE with the use of ibuprofen. Other NSAIDs may cause meningismus as well.

Allergic manifestations of NSAIDs include urticarial skin rashes, asthma, and nasal polyposis. These effects are shared by aspirin and the newer NSAIDs but not by nonacetylated salicylates, which may be safely administered. Stevens-Johnson's syndrome or toxic epidermal necrolysis may occur in oxicam- (piroxicam, tenoxicam) treated patients.

Finally, hepatotoxicity characterized by asymptomatic elevation of liver enzymes is a known complication of NSAIDs, particularly in older patients. The most important precaution in patients taking NSAIDs is to make them aware of possible complications and associated symptoms. Guidelines for monitoring the use of NSAIDs are shown in the appendix. Pharmacologic characteristics of commonly used NSAIDs are displayed in Table 8–1.

Suggested Reading

American College of Rheumatology Ad Hoc Committee on Clinical Guidelines. American College of Rheumatology 1995 Guidelines for the management of rheumatoid arthritis. Arthritis Rheum 39:713–722, 1996.

Greene JM, Winickoff RN. Cost-conscious prescribing of nonsteroidal anti-inflammatory drugs for adults with arthritis. Arch Intern Med 152:1995–2001, 1992.

Lichtenstein DR, Syngal S, Wolfe MM. Nonsteroidal antiinflammatory drugs and the gastrointestinal tract. Arthritis Rheum 38:5–18, 1995.

Roujeau J-C, Kelly JP, Naldi L, et al. Medication use and the risk of Stevens-Johnson syndrome or toxic epidermal necrolysis. N Engl J Med 333:1600–1607, 1995.

Saag KG, Rubenstein LM, Chrischilles EA, et al. Nonsteroidal antiinflammatory drugs and cognitive decline in the elderly. J Rheumatol 22:2142–2147, 1995.

Silverstein FE, Graham DY, Senior JR, et al. Misoprostol reduces serious gastrointestinal complications in patients with rheumatoid arthritis receiving nonsteroidal anti-inflammatory drugs. Ann Intern Med 123:241–249, 1995.

Analgesics versus NSAIDs

For certain conditions, in particular osteoarthritis, there appears to be no advantage in using a NSAID over the inexpensive acetaminophen. Severe nocturnal pain and flares that may be crystal related justify the use of NSAIDs in osteoarthritis. Acetaminophen may also be combined with NSAIDs for added analgesia in situations such as acute low back pain. Unfortunately, there appears to be an association between chronic use of acetaminophen and the development of end-stage renal failure. It would appear that in the short term or in the episodic treatment of pain, acetaminophen is safer than NSAIDs, but it seems fair to say that its long-term safety has not been established.

Muscle Relaxants

This category includes diazepam, a benzodiazepine; cyclobenzaprine, a tricyclic agent; and agents such as carisoprodol and methocarbamol. The use of diazepam should be discouraged because of its addicting potential and because it may worsen depression.

Cyclobenzaprine is a weak muscle relaxant and its major use is in the treatment of chronic pain including fibromyalgia (see later). Because of its sedating and muscle-relaxing properties, it is often used as an adjunct to analgesics or NSAIDs in patients with protracted low back or neck pain. An important side effect of cyclobenzaprine, particularly in older individuals, is sinus tachycardia. Carisoprodol and methocarbamol, considered primary muscle relaxant drugs, are also mild sedatives. They may be helpful in acute low back pain associated with severe muscle spasm.

Tricyclic Antidepressant Drugs

These appear to be out of place in this section, but ask any rheumatologist the top ten medications he or she uses and a tricyclic agent will be there. Tricyclic antidepressants, in particular amitriptyline, cyclobenzaprine, and doxepin, are often helpful in the treatment of fibromyalgia and the myofascial syndromes. They are also a good adjunct in RA and other chronic conditions in which joint pain, by interfering with sleep, triggers fibromyalgia. Amitriptyline and cyclobenzaprine have both serotonergic and noradrenergic effects.

Tricyclic antidepressants do not create physical dependency or lose efficacy over time. Because of their anticholinergic effects, they may create problems in patients who already have dry mouth and dry eyes (a frequent concomitant in fibromyalgia).

A sedative effect is particularly prominent in the first few weeks of treatment, and for this reason tricyclic agents should be taken just before bedtime. If the patient complains of prolonged morning grogginess the agent should be taken earlier in the evening.

As mentioned, cyclobenzaprine may induce worrisome sinus tachycardia when high doses are used. Tricyclic antidepressants are risky in patients with cardiac arrhythmias.

Unfortunately, because of a high sensitivity to anticholinergic effects, only half of fibromyalgia patients remain on these drugs long enough to fairly assess effectiveness (at least several weeks). Indeed, only 30% of "intent to treat" fibromyalgia patients are improved. Desipramine, a tricyclic agent with noradrenergic action only, has proven as effective as amitriptyline in the control of pain in diabetic neuropathy. The author has used it with some success in fibromyalgia patients who suffered intolerable anticholinergic effects on other tricyclic agents. Fluoxetine, an antidepressant with serotonergic action only, is ineffective in fibromyalgia. Better medications are sorely needed to treat fibromyalgia.

Suggested Reading

Carette S. FM 20 years later: What have we really accomplished? J Rheumatol 22:590–594, 1995.

Carette S, Bell MJ, Reynolds WJ, et al. Comparison of amitriptyline, cyclobenzaprine, and placebo in the treatment of fibromyalgia. Arthritis Rheum 37:32–40, 1994.

Max MB, Lynch SA, Muir J, et al. Effects of desipramine on pain in diabetic neuropathy. N Engl J Med 326:1250–1256, 1992.

Capsaicin

Capsaicin is a natural alkaloid extracted from capsicum, the hot pepper plant. The effect of topically applied capsaicin on sensory terminals is double. Initially, it causes a local burning sensation due to release of substance P and other neuropeptides. With the chronic application of the substance, that is, applying the capsaicin-containing cream qid, a state of neuropeptide depletion is achieved that results in analgesia in a variety of conditions, particularly soft tissue problems and osteoarthritis.

It is of course difficult to explain an effect of a nonabsorbable, surface-applied substance on a joint. Also, the stingy nature of the compound makes it difficult to conduct valid double-blind studies. However, the compound is in general use, seems to work in many instances, and lacks significant side effects.

Capsaicin is sold in several strengths, 0.025%, 0.075%, and 0.25%. The first two are used qid and the last, bid. Accidental application of the compound on the eye, genitalia, and anal area must be avoided.

Suggested Reading

Matucci-Cerinic M, McCarthy G, et al. Neurogenic influences in arthritis: Potential modification by capsaicin. J Rheumatol 22:1447–1449, 1995.

Placebo Effect as a Therapy

As physicians, we are often pleased to use a particular medication that has a 30%, 40%, even 70% record of effectiveness for a given process. And we are often astonished to find out, when proper studies are completed, that the effectiveness of the drug in question was similar to a placebo. When assessing results of a controlled trial we should pay more attention to and assess with the same fairness the response to the placebo and the response to the so-called active drug. The effectiveness of placebos is indeed substantial, not to be dismissed, and occasionally useful. A good thing about placebos, as compared with active drugs that don't work for a particular condition beyond a placebo effect, is that true placebos are chemically inactive and have milder side effects than active drugs.

PATIENT 11. A 60-year-old right-handed switchboard operator was referred because of long-standing right parascapular pain with radiation to shoulder and upper arm. The patient had been seen by several physicians for the preceding 3 years, and a variety of diagnoses had been made including muscle spasm, a myofascial syndrome, and bursitis. Routine chemistries, ESR, chest x-ray, tangential views of the scapula, a bone scan, and an MRI had been normal or negative. Twice she had been on medical leave with some improvement but pain promptly recurred upon returning to work. Analgesics, NSAIDs, massage, ultrasound, and laser therapy had afforded minimal relief. The only treatment that had resulted in asymptomatic periods of up to 2 months had been local infiltrations with a mixture of xylocaine and methylprednisolone acetate of which she had four within the last year.

Physical examination was normal with the exception of point tenderness in the soft tissues between the tip of the scapula and the spine. Firm pressure on this point failed to reproduce the shoulder or arm pain. There was right-sided pain upon bending the neck to the left as well as bringing the scapulae closer together, suggesting that pain originated within the trapezius. It was also apparent that short of a job modification, little could be expected in her case.

After explaining to her my assessment, I agreed to her request of another infiltration, only this time I would use a new, powerful albeit nonsteroidal drug, bupivacaine. Pain relief was complete. Within a few weeks a receptionist position was made available for her at her company and there has been no recurrence of pain. The same effect was achieved by giving her bupivacaine, a local anesthesic with a longer action (about 3 hours) than xylocaine (about 30 minutes), as with xylocaine mixed with a long-acting corticosteroid.

Suggested Reading

Turner JA, Deyo RA, Loeser JD, et al. The importance of placebo effects in pain treatment and research. JAMA 271:1609–1614, 1994.

Gout Medications

Two types of medications are used in gout. The first, which includes oral NSAIDs, oral colchicine, I.V. colchicine, and I.M. ACTH or triamcinolone acetonide, are potent anti-inflammatories that are highly effective in acute gout.

Because it causes diarrhea in over 70% of patients, oral colchicine is a poor choice as compared with the other agents. Intravenous colchicine has negligible GI toxicity, but deaths have occurred following its use in dehydrated elderly individuals as well as in patients with liver or renal failure. I suggest staying away from it.

Intramuscular agents have the advantage of full compliance. Also, they are quite useful in the patient with dyspepsia or a history of ulcer or GI bleed. The mystique that surrounds I.M. ACTH is probably unwarranted; triamcinolone acetonide is more readily available and also cheaper.

The second type of medication is used to decrease serum and synovial uric acid (UA) levels. As a result, monosodium urate (MSU) crystals clustered within synovial tissue and elsewhere are leached out. Because acute gout is caused by MSU crystals from broken down synovial clusters that enter the joint, once synovial microtophi are removed, acute gout can no longer develop. The natural history of tophi is continuous growth. Left unchecked, tophi-studded joints often become destroyed by chronic inflammation. Another serious complication of tophaceous gout is the now exceptional "gouty nephropathy," a condition featuring arterial hypertension and chronic renal insufficiency. Many other complications of tophi may arise such as neural compression at the spine.

Thus, there are two good reasons to use UA-lowering agents: (1) to terminate recurrences of acute gout, and (2) to prevent tissue damage and disfiguration from tophaceous deposits. Two categories of UA-lowering agents exist on the market: allopurinol, which blocks UA formation and therefore its tissue, fluids, and urine load, and probenecid and sulfinpyrazone, which force the kidney to excrete increased amounts of UA.

Because the latter exert their effect on the renal tubule, a properly working kidney (serum creatinine < 2 mg/dl) is a prerequisite for their action. Also, because uricosurics increase the urine UA concentration, they cannot be used in individuals with a history of urolithiasis and in patients with a high basal UA excretion (about 10% of gout patients). It is generally believed that recurrent gout may be triggered when patients initiate a UA-lowering agent. To prevent this complication prophylactic oral colchicine is customarily added for 6 months in patients without tophi or until resorption of superficial tophi has occurred. The UA-lowering agent should be continued for life.

Glucocorticoids

Glucocorticoids may be life saving in SLE and the necrotizing vasculitides and are vision saving in giant cell arteritis. They are also very useful taken in low doses in the treatment of polymyalgia rheumatica, rheumatoid arthritis (RA), and systemic lupus erythematosus. The frequent and severe toxicities associated with high-dose glucocorticoids are seldom questioned. After all, they are used for major conditions that have a catastrophic outcome if left untreated.

There are often problems, however, with the long-term use of low oral doses, which are difficult to reduce and hard to discontinue. Although metabolic toxicity is less than with higher doses, patients may still develop osteoporosis, cataracts, diabetes mellitus, and possibly osteonecrosis.

Regarding osteoporosis, prednisone doses of 10 mg per day or less administered for 20 weeks in patients with RA caused an 8.2% decrease in lumbar trabecular bone mineral density (2.1% in cortical bone) as compared with patients receiving placebo. This bone loss was incompletely reversed by steroid discontinuation. Interestingly, in a recent study in RA patients the bone mineral loss induced by prednisone at a mean daily dose of 5.5 mg per day could be prevented by the daily addition of calcium 1 g plus vitamin D 500 IU. This is an important observation because in a recent study of early RA the addition of prednisolone 7.5 mg per day reduced, compared to patients receiving placebo, the rate of bone erosion at 2 years.

Some prediction of steroid complications may be obtained from the history, for example, a family history of diabetes; presence of diabetes, arterial hypertension, or glaucoma; and presence of osteoporosis or osteoporosis risk factors. Pros and cons of glucocorticoid therapy should be

TABLE 8–3
COMPLICATIONS OF GLUCOCORTICOID THERAPY

Present in most patients; early effects
    Insomnia
    Emotional lability
    Increased appetite or weight gain or both
Common in patients with risk factors or other drug toxicities
    Arterial hypertension
    Diabetes mellitus
    Peptic ulcer disease
    Acne vulgaris
Predictable long-term effects minimized by conservative dose regimens
    Iatrogenic Cushing
    Adrenal insufficiency
    Increased risk of infection
    Osteoporosis
    Osteonecrosis
    Myopathy
    Impaired wound healing
Insidious and delayed effects
    Skin atrophy
    Cataracts
    Atherosclerosis
    Growth retardation
    Fatty liver
Rare and unpredictable
    Psychosis
    Pseudotumor cerebri
    Glaucoma
    Epidural lipomatosis with spinal stenosis syndrome
    Pancreatitis

Modified from Boumpas DT, Chrousos GP, Wilder RL, et al. Glucocorticoid therapy for immune-mediated diseases: Basic and clinical correlates. Ann Intern Med 119:1198–1208, 1993.

openly discussed with patients and a notation entered in the record. Baseline bone densitometry is recommended for patients with osteoporosis risk factors, and baseline eye examination, particularly ocular pressures, should be obtained in patients who are 65 years of age or older. A medical alert bracelet should be worn by patients on chronic corticosteroid therapy. Table 8–3 lists the various glucocorticoid side effects arranged by frequency and timing.

Suggested Reading

American College of Rheumatology Ad Hoc Committee on Clinical Guidelines. Guidelines for monitoring drug therapy in rheumatoid arthritis. Arthritis Rheum 39:723–731, 1996.
Boumpas DT, Chrousos GP, Wilder RL, et al. Glucocorticoid therapy for immune-mediated diseases: Basic and clinical correlates. Ann Intern Med 119:1198–1208, 1993.
Buckley L, Leib E, Cartularo K, et al. Calcium and vitamin D supplementation prevents bone loss secondary to low-dose corticosteroid treatment of patients with rheumatoid arthritis. Arthritis Rheum (suppl) 38:S358, 1995.
Kirwan JR, and the Arthritis and Rheumatism Council Low-Dose Glucocorticoid Study Group. The effect of glucocorticoids on joint destruction in rheumatoid arthritis. N Engl J Med 333:142–146, 1995.
Laan RFJM, van Riel PLCM, van de Putte LBA, et al. Low-dose prednisone induces rapid reversible axial bone loss in patients with rheumatoid arthritis. Ann Intern Med 119:963–968, 1993.
Nesher G, Sonnenblick M, Friedlander Y. Analysis of steroid-related complications and mortality in temporal arteritis: A 15-year survey of 43 patients. J Rheumatol 21:1283–1286, 1994.

Slow-Acting (Remittive) Agents for Rheumatoid Arthritis (RA), Sjögren's, and Spondyloarthropathy

Fortunately, the introduction of methotrexate (MTX) in small weekly oral doses has substantially changed the outlook in RA. Methotrexate may also be used in psoriatic arthritis and is an alternative to sulfasalazine in the treatment of serious ankylosing spondylitis and reactive arthritis. Methotrexate use requires stringent clinical and laboratory surveillance, the main adverse effects being a tendency to opportunistic infections, acute (hypersensitivity?) interstitial pneumonitis, and the very rare development of cirrhosis (Table 8–4).

Primary care physicians should learn how to distinguish the first two and how to prevent, as far as possible, the occurrence of the third. I routinely obtain baseline chest x-rays and pulmonary function tests including DLCO. Many times an RA patient on MTX develops cough and a fever due to intercurrent URI; under those circumstances it is reassuring to know that the DLCO, which is the first parameter to change in MTX and PCP pneumonitis, remains normal. Cough, fever, dyspnea, and a decreased DLCO should make the primary physician discontinue MTX and take measures, with the help of a pulmonary consultant, to distinguish PCP from MTX pneumonitis, which usually requires bronchoscopy and BAL. Once the former has been ruled out, the latter can be presumptively diagnosed. Diagnostic proof is afforded by the spontaneous or prednisone-aided resolution of findings.

A fourth possible confounding factor is pneumonitis caused by the underlying disease itself. RA pneumonitis tends to be a chronic, afebrile process that differs from the acute or subacute pneumonitides previously discussed. Risk factors for complications of MTX therapy include alcohol intake, length of therapy, diabetes, obesity, a mean corpuscular volume greater than 100 implying subclinical folate deficiency, preexistent pulmonary disease, and possibly the presence of psoriasis. The American College of Rheumatology has given guidelines for the prevention of MTX liver toxicity (see appendix).

TABLE 8–4
SIDE EFFECTS OF LOW-DOSE ORAL METHOTREXATE

1. Gastrointestinal: anorexia, nausea, stomatitis, diarrhea
2. Neurologic: headache, dizziness, fatigue, mood alterations
3. Hepatic: cirrhosis
4. Hematologic: leukopenia, thrombocytopenia, pancytopenia
5. Pulmonary: interstitial pneumonitis
6. Opportunistic infections: herpes zoster, fungal, pneumocystitis
7. Lymphoma: reversible EB virus–associated lymphoma
8. *Methotrexate is teratogenic*

Risk factors: 1, 2: folate deficiency; 3: alcohol use, old age, long-term therapy; 4: unrecognized renal insufficiency, folate deficiency, coexistent infection, concurrent use of probenecid or trimethoprim-sulfamethoxazole; 5: unknown.

Patients with psoriatic arthritis may be more liable to MTX liver toxicity than patients with RA. Indeed, in a serial biopsy study of RA patients treated long term with oral MTX, only minor alterations were found with a mean follow-up of 8.2 years. In this cohort, patients were routinely asked about their compliance with the recommendation of completely abstaining from alcohol, and AST and serum albumin levels were monitored every 4 to 6 weeks. If they had any elevation of AST they were asked to reduce the MTX dose by 2.5 mg. A less serious but more frequent side effect of MTX is GI toxicity including stomatitis, nausea, and indigestion suggesting folate deficiency. Concurrent folate supplementation 1 mg per day with initial determination of blood folate and serum B_{12} (because folate supplementation may unmask or aggravate B_{12} deficiency) substantially reduces GI toxicity without negating its antiarthritic efficacy. Hematologic toxicity may be caused by myelosuppression or folate deficiency.

Other highly effective medications that can be used in RA as alternatives to MTX include injectable gold and azathioprine. Gold treatment is attended by a high rate of skin and mucosal reactions, the development of autoimmune thrombocytopenia in 1% to 3%, renal toxicity with proteinuria or hematuria, and bone marrow suppression in less than 1% of cases. Patients receiving parenteral gold should be monitored with CBC and differential to detect eosinophilia that is predictive of skin toxicity, and urinalysis for the early detection of membranous nephropathy. Oral gold has a lower rate of toxicity but is also less effective. The main concern with the long-term use of azathioprine is its potential to induce lymphomas in renal transplant recipients.

In RA, the risk of lymphoma in patients taking azathioprine has not proved greater than the risk other RA patients have. The main toxicity of azathioprine is myelosuppression, which is expressed clinically as sepsis, bleeding, and severe anemia. Concurrent use of allopurinol or the presence of renal insufficiency requires a dose reduction to one-half or one-third of the usual azathioprine dose. ACE inhibitors should be avoided. Azathioprine is considered a good alternative agent to use in RA and also in polymyositis.

Hydroxychloroquine and sulfasalazine are safer but weaker agents that are used in mild RA and in patients who refuse or cannot take MTX, injectable gold, or azathioprine. With hydroxychloroquine patients become legitimately concerned when they hear about its potential ocular toxicity. In reality, this is a rare event that tends to be overemphasized by physicians unfamiliar with the drug. Risk factors for ocular toxicity include a cumulative dose of 800 g and age greater than 70. With a simple ophthalmologic evaluation performed at baseline and then every 6 months, the chronic use of the drug is quite safe. More common side effects of hydroxychloroquine, which are usually mild, involve the CNS, skin, GI tract, and musculoskeletal system. These effects, as well as their management, are shown in Table 8–5. Hydroxychloroquine should not be used in patients with renal insufficiency, since neurotoxicity and vacuolar cardiomyopathy leading to heart failure may occur. With the preceding precautions kept in mind, there is no safer and less costly medication than hydroxychloroquine for the treatment of mild RA, mild SLE, and Sjögren's syndrome.

Sulfasalazine is as effective as hydroxychloroquine in RA and is also a useful agent in the treatment of ankylosing spondylitis, enteropathic arthritis (the arthritis associated with Crohn's disease and ulcerative colitis), psoriatic arthritis, and reactive arthritis. The sulfapiridine moiety of sulfasalazine appears to account for its antiarthritic properties. Allergic rashes and gastrointestinal intolerance are the leading causes of sulfasalazine discontinuation. Myelosuppression is rare but represents the most serious toxic effect of sulfasalazine. Fortunately, most patients tolerate the compound well.

Second-line agents for RA should be recommended by a rheumatologist. Early consultation is essential to provide optimal treatment to patients with RA. Also, rheumatologists should review these patients periodically, perhaps every 3 to 6 months to determine treatment response and offer advice on occupational therapy, physical therapy, and orthopedic surgery issues that may emerge.

In the meanwhile, it is the general physician who will be called for a "chest cold" that may represent pulmonary MTX toxicity or a sore throat that may be the initial symptom of gold-induced or sulfasalazine-induced agranulocytosis. Primary physicians following RA patients should familiarize themselves with the peculiarities of second-line agents and early identification of serious toxicity. Most importantly, patients must be made aware of warning signs so they seek prompt advice. Guidelines recommended by the American College of Rheumatology for the monitoring of patients receiving second-line medications for RA are shown in the appendix.

TABLE 8–5

COMMON SIDE EFFECTS OF HYDROXYCHLOROQUINE OR CHLOROQUINE THERAPY

1. CNS: headache, nervousness, insomnia
2. Skin: urticaria, rash, increased skin pigmentation
3. GI: abdominal cramps or distention, nausea, diarrhea, heartburn
4. Musculoskeletal: feeling flulike or achy

Management: Hold the medicine for 72 hours; restart one-half of the original dose, administering half in the morning and half in the evening. If the skin rash is urticarial or lichen planus like, discontinue the drug.

Modified from Wallace DJ. Antimalarial agents and lupus. Rheum Dis Clin 20:243–263, 1994.

Suggested Reading

American College of Rheumatology Ad Hoc Committee on Clinical Guidelines. Guidelines for the management of rheumatoid arthritis. Arthritis Rheum 39:717–722, 1996.

American College of Rheumatology Ad Hoc Committee on Clinical Guidelines. Guidelines for monitoring drug therapy in rheumatoid arthritis. Arthritis Rheum 39:723–731, 1996.

Cash JM, Klippel JL. Drug therapy: Second-line drug therapy for rheumatoid arthritis. N Engl J Med 330:1368–1375, 1994.

Dougados M, van der Linden S, Leirisalo-Repo M. Sulfasalazine in the treatment of spondyloarthropathy: A randomized, multicenter, double-blind, placebo-controlled study. Arthritis Rheum 38:618–627, 1995.

Godeau B, Coutant-Perronne V, Huong DLT, et al. Pneumocystis carinii pneumonia in the course of connective tissue disease: Report of 34 cases. J Rheumatol 21:246–251, 1994.

Kremer JM, Kaye GI, Kaye NW, et al. Light and electron microscopic analysis of sequential liver biopsy samples from rheumatoid arthritis patients receiving long-term methotrexate therapy: Follow-up over long treatment intervals and correlation with clinical and laboratory variables. Arthritis Rheum 38:1194–1203, 1995.

Morgan SL, Baggott JE, Vaughn WH, et al. Supplementation with folic acid during methotrexate therapy for rheumatoid arthritis. Ann Intern Med 121:833–841, 1994.

Weinblatt ME. Methotrexate for chronic diseases in adults. N Engl J Med 332:330–331, 1995.

Cytotoxic Agents

Cyclophosphamide and other alkylating agents are useful in the treatment of polyarteritis nodosa, Wegener's granulomatosis, diffuse proliferative lupus nephritis, and rheumatoid arthritis complicated by necrotizing vasculitis or impending ocular perforation. These conditions are usually handled by rheumatologists, but primary care physicians concurrently following the patients may be the first to encounter minor or serious drug toxicity, sometimes years after the agent was discontinued.

Main concerns associated with the use of cyclophosphamide include bone marrow suppression, infection, permanent sterility due to ovarian failure, hemorrhagic cystitis, and the late emergence of neoplasms involving predominantly, but not confined to, the urinary tract.

Bladder toxicity is most frequently seen in patients treated with oral cyclophosphamide. The increased risk of bladder cancer in these patients continues for at least 20 years after discontinuation of the drug. On the other hand, bladder cancer has not been reported as a complication of intravenous cyclophosphamide. This may be due to lower total doses, sporadic administration, plus the use of mesna, which reacts chemically with the urotoxic cyclophosphamide metabolite, acrolein. Guidelines for the monitoring of patients on these agents are shown in the appendix.

Suggested Reading

American College of Rheumatology Ad Hoc Committee on Clinical Guidelines. Guidelines for monitoring drug therapy in rheumatoid arthritis. Arthritis Rheum 39:723–731, 1996.

Talar-Williams C, Hijazi YM, McClellan MW, et al. Cyclophosphamide-induced cystitis and bladder cancer in patients with Wegener's granulomatosis. Ann Intern Med 124:477–484, 1996.

Experimental Treatments of RA

Experimental treatments include minocycline, cyclosporine, combination therapy, monoclonal antibodies, oral immunization with type II collagen, and intravenous immunoglobulins. The use of these treatments clearly belongs in the domain of rheumatologists.

Minocycline administered at a dose of 50 mg p.o. twice a day has a mild but unequivocal beneficial effect in patients with rheumatoid arthritis. The drug is safe, its major adverse effect being dizziness in about 5% of patients. Minocycline compares favorably with other agents, such as hydroxychloroquine, that are useful in mild RA.

Another drug useful in RA is cyclosporine; doses must not exceed 5 mg/kg/day if significant renal toxicity (a raise in serum creatinine > 30% above baseline) is to be avoided.

The combined use of second-line (remittive) agents in RA is usually considered when a NSAID plus low-dose prednisone plus maximal doses of a second-line agent fail to control disease activity. Combinations used include MTX plus hydroxychloroquine; MTX plus sulfasalazine; MTX plus cyclosporine; MTX plus sulfasalazine plus hydroxychloroquine; MTX plus azathioprine; and MTX plus hydroxychloroquine plus azathioprine in reported series rather than a controlled trial. In the MTX plus cyclosporine trial, the combination of the two agents was superior to MTX alone. In the MTX plus sulfasalazine plus hydroxychloroquine trial, the combination of the three agents was more effective than the use of one or two of the individual agents. In the MTX plus azathioprine trial, the combination of the two agents did not increase efficacy.

Monoclonal antibodies are in the experimental phase and results of a few controlled trials in RA have been unimpressive. A possible exception is the use of antitumor necrosis alpha antibodies. Results of oral immunization with type II collagen have also been less than optimal.

The very expensive intravenous immunoglobulins have a proven value in Kawasaki's disease in which they decrease the rate of coronary artery aneurysms. They have also been used acutely in dermatomyositis leading to temporary improvement and appear to be useful in the primary antiphospholipid syndrome (PAPS), positive antineutrophil cytoplasmic antibody nephritis, IgA nephropathy, and myasthenia gravis. There are anecdotal reports of their use in SLE and RA. The expense of intravenous immunoglobulins in these conditions is hardly justifiable.

Suggested Reading

Landewé RBM, Dijkmans BAC, van der Woude FJ, et al. Long-term low-dose cyclosporine in patients with RA: Renal function loss without structural nephropathy. J Rheumatol 23:61–64, 1996.

Tilley BC, Alarcón GS, Heyse SP, et al. Minocycline in rheumatoid arthritis. A 48-week, double-blind, placebo-controlled trial. Ann Intern Med 122:81–89, 1995.

Tugwell P, Pincus T, Yocum D, et al. Combination therapy with cyclosporine and methotrexate in severe rheumatoid arthritis. N Engl J Med 333:137–141, 1995.

Wilske K, Yocum D (ed). Rheumatoid arthritis: The status and future of combination therapy. J Rheumatol 23 (suppl 44):1–110, 1996.

Physical Medicine

It is good practice to identify occupational therapists (OTs) and physical therapists (PTs) in the community who have experience and an expressed interest in the treatment of rheumatic disease patients because most OT and PT offices deal predominantly with sports-related injuries, an altogether different field. Emphasis of PT should be on developing a home exercise program. Once the regime has been mastered by the patient, periodic visits to the therapist are important for supervision and to step up the program. OTs stress joint protection and energy conservation, pain relief by nonpharmacologic means such as a home paraffin tank, and the prescription of adaptive devices that make life easier for many rheumatic disease patients. Aerobic training should be attempted in patients whose lower extremities are relatively unimpaired. Patients should be encouraged to use the pool programs offered through the local Arthritis Foundation. Some communities are fortunate enough to have a physiatrist. These highly trained physicians have the skills to assess the patients' function in relation to their home and community environments and expectations, to supervise comprehensively the progress of PT and OT interventions, and to make referrals to various community and government agencies.

Primary care physicians should have a working knowledge of PT and OT in order to provide sound instruction (1) to patients afflicted by self-limited conditions (such as crystal-induced arthritis involving the wrist or knee), (2) in situations in which PT and OT referrals cannot be implemented, and (3) for the long-term conditioning of older patients without rheumatic disease. Primary care physicians should be able to teach patients the correct use of a cane and crutch walking, as well as giving sound advice on adequate footware, pillow, and mattress.

Finally, primary care physicians should involve themselves in the prevention of sports-related and workplace-related overuse injuries. Injury prevention requires education, proper warm-up and stretching, as well as an exercise program to increase overall flexibility, strength, and endurance. Bed rest has deleterious effects on the musculoskeletal system including negative nitrogen balance, increased calcium loss, muscle wasting and weakness, and loss of endurance. These effects are compounded by regional muscle inhibition caused by joint inflammation plus the osteoporosis and tendinous deterioration that occur with aging. Immobility dramatically enhances all negative influences on the musculoskeletal system.

Emphasis should be placed on motion rather than rest. Thus, initial physical treatment of synovitis includes active and passive range of motion, isometric muscle contractions, and temporary splintage. As the patient improves, emphasis is placed on muscle strengthening and endurance exercises. Swimming is the ideal exercise to increase endurance. Walking across water in chest-high water is just as effective as swimming for patients with painful involvement of their shoulders. Cycling is also possible in many patients with predominantly upper extremity arthritis. The exercise program should progress slowly but surely while joints are monitored for any increase in inflammation.

As a general rule, postexercise pain that persists more than 2 hours indicates overexercise. Also, an increase in joint effusions should indicate a temporary decrease in active exercises while maintaining in full strength the isometric exercises program. The appendix contains exercise instructions for the hand, shoulder, neck, back, hips, and knees. Emphasis is placed on stretching, range of motion, and isometric exercises. These and other instructions may be photocopied and provided to patients with specific instructions indicated (number of repetitions, how many times to perform the exercises each day, etc.).

Chiropractic Manipulation

Chiropractic medicine has a demonstrated role in speeding up recovery in self-limited conditions such as acute neck and low back pain. No long-term beneficial effects have so far been shown. Treatment is based on manipulation aimed at bringing the joint through its full anatomic, rather than merely physiologic, range of motion.

Chiropractors have a positive attitude, confidence in their interpretation of symptoms, and talk to patients sympathetically and authoritatively. These characteristics, more than any merits of their treatments, may explain the high acceptance chiropractors receive from their patients. Perhaps a lack of those very characteristics, rather than ineffectiveness, explains some of the beating we practitioners of orthodox medicine receive.

Since chiropractic maneuvers may be dangerous in patients with a brittle spine, it is of paramount importance that patients be referred to experienced professionals. In particular, manipulation should be avoided in patients with ankylosing spondylitis and a fused spine or extensive idiopathic skeletal hyperostosis as well as in patients with an unstable neck such as in a RA patient with atlantoaxial subluxation.

Suggested Reading

Bigos SJ, et al. Acute Low Back Problems in Adults. Clinical Practice Guideline Number 14. AHCPR Publication No. 95-0642. Agency for Health Care Policy and Research, Rockville, MD, December 1994.

Orthopedic Surgery

Some of the most significant advances in the treatment of rheumatic diseases have come from orthopedics. These include, among others, metatarsal head resection, metatarsophalangeal joint prostheses, cervical spine stabilization, and repair of ruptured tendons in RA; joint replacement in RA and osteoarthritis; and the surgical treatment of carpal tunnel syndrome, lateral epicondylitis, rotator cuff disease, and spinal stenosis. The primary care physician, assisted by the rheumatologist, will sense when orthopedic procedures are needed, make the referral, and work with the surgeon to achieve compliance with postoperative exercises and the required prophylactic measures.

Among orthopedic procedures few have rivaled the impact of arthroscopy. The technique is invaluable to repair a torn meniscus; section and smooth out a hypertrophic plica; release a tight lateral retinaculum (fibers from the quadriceps that attach to the lateral patella); decompress a shoulder impingement; obtain adequate specimens for histologic diagnosis of pigmented villonodular synovitis, tuberculous arthritis and fungal arthritis; and treat loculated joint infections, among others.

Arthroscopy has greatly reduced morbidities associated with arthrotomy including disfiguration and pain from surgical scars, secondary infection, and protracted postoperative muscle atrophy. Unfortunately, arthroscopy has morbidities of its own including nerve paralysis, iatrogenic infection, and compartmental syndromes from tissue leakage of the distending fluid. These, plus the costs involved, which are at least as high as with open surgery, should make one judicious about the ever growing indications of arthroscopy.

Joint arthroplasties have had a tremendous impact on rheumatic disease care. Hip and knee arthroplasties have been successful in returning to self-sufficiency those patients who would otherwise be bedridden or wheelchair bound. Because of the inherent longevity of hip prostheses, young age of the patient is a relatively minor obstacle for their insertion. Knee prostheses, however, have a limited life (about 10 years) so their use before the age of 60 is judged unwise. Obesity is a major determinant of knee osteoarthritis and also a cause of premature prosthetic wear. Weight reduction is therefore essential prior to inserting a knee prosthesis. Shoulder prostheses have also been highly successful. Also, patients with the condition known as rotator cuff arthropathy (Milwaukee shoulder) who cannot be offered total shoulder replacement because the rotator cuff is destroyed may still be treated with a large-head humeral hemiarthroplasty that articulates with both the acromion and the glenoid fossa. Wrist arthroplasties, although not optimal, are better than a fused wrist particularly in younger patients and when disease is bilateral. Metacarpophalangeal joint prostheses help mechanical pain and cosmesis more than function. They are definitely indicated, as an example, in patients with hemochromatosis and severe osteoarthritis in the second and third MCP joints. Elbow and ankle prostheses have had lesser success. In referring patients for orthopedic consultation an opinion should always be requested about conservative options such as soft tissue procedures and osteotomies that by changing biomechanics often relieve pain and improve joint function.

1. *Indications for surgery.* The usual indication for surgery is unrelieved mechanical pain. Secondary osteoarthritic changes in a chronically inflamed joint eventually result in bone-on-bone contact and irregular articulating surfaces. Initially, mechanical pain may be controlled by analgesic medications and walking aids such as a cane or crutches. As time goes on, however, rest pain sets in, disturbing night rest. A disrupted sleep as well as too much pain on necessary daily activities such as getting in or out of a car are clear indications to consider joint prostheses. Another important indication is pain and instability threatening independent living in an older person.

2. *Operative clearance.* Preoperative clearance for total joint replacement includes prior treatment of skin and urinary tract infections, carious teeth, and if possible prostatic hypertrophy. Potentially contaminated skin lesions such as psoriasis or eczema at the operative site must be cleared prior to the procedure.

3. *Antibiotic coverage.* It has been standard practice for the past 15 years to cover total arthroplasties with a first-generation cephalosporin, usually cefazolin or cephalothin 1 g I.V. 2 hours before surgical incision followed by 1 g I.V. q 8 hours for 1 to 2 days. The use of antibiotic prophylaxis is just one of the factors that have decreased the rate of postoperative sepsis following arthroplasties. Additional factors include improvements in operating room discipline (fewer people, less traffic, improved barrier draping, and use of sterile suction units); technical dexterity (decreased operating time); and a better preoperative evaluation, as discussed in number 2. Patients receiving methotrexate should have the drug discontinued 2 weeks before the procedure. This is a controversial recommendation not only in terms of whether MTX adds or not to the risk of infection, but also because RA usually flares 2 to 3 weeks after MTX discontinuation.

4. *Anticoagulation.* Hip and knee procedures are often complicated by venous thrombosis. Total hip and knee replacement patients are given subcutaneous low molecular weight heparin or warfarin beginning the night of admission, and the anticoagulation is usually continued 6 weeks following surgery.

5. *Antibiotic prophylaxis.* Patients who received a joint prosthesis have a foreign body that favors hematogenous infection following procedures with a high risk of bacteremia. These include long procedures and surgery in infected areas, including peridontal disease. No antibiotic prophylaxis is recommended for other dental, genitourinary, or gastrointestinal procedures.

6. *Postoperative gout.* Gout patients, regardless of reason for admission, often develop acute gout while on the ward. In some the attack supervenes because suppressive medications such as colchicine or a NSAID are discontinued. In others the culprit appears to be a sudden drop of serum urate levels as dehydration and/or acidosis are corrected. Be that as it may, acute arthritis in a hospitalized patient usually represents gout or pseudogout. Joint aspiration is essential not only to confirm crystal-induced arthritis but to exclude sepsis by gram stain and aerobic and anaerobic cultures (remember that crystal synovitis and bacterial infection may coincide).

7. *Postoperative rehabilitation.* Postoperative rehabilitation actually begins 1 week prior to surgery when the patient is instructed on crutch-assisted gait. Generally speaking, exercises are an essential component of postoperative care. Following hip surgery the patient is placed on pillow suspension traction for 24 hours and isometric gluteal and quadriceps exercises are started. On the second postoperative day the patient performs range of motion (ROM) exercises and is encouraged to sit at the edge of the bed. A quick progression of exercises follows and independent crutches ambulation is implemented by the sixth or eighth day. An OT consult should be obtained prior to discharge to determine the need of assistive devices such as a raised toilet seat, long-handled shoehorns, and elastic shoelaces. In total knee replacement, continued passive motion begun in the recovery room has had encouraging early results. Otherwise, patients are started early on active assisted flexion exercises with the help of a physical therapist. Patients are allowed to walk with a walker or crutches by the second or third postoperative day. Following knee arthroscopy, straight leg raises and isometric quadriceps exercises should begin in the immediate postoperative phase.

Suggested Reading

Anderson RJ. The orthopedic management of rheumatoid arthritis. Arthritis Care Res 9:223–229, 1996.

Fitzgerald RH. Infected total hip arthroplasty: Diagnosis and treatment. J Am Acad Orthop Surg 3:249–262, 1995.

Zimlich RH, Fulbright BM. Current status of anticoagulation therapy after total hip and total knee arthroplasty. J Am Acad Orthop Surg 4:54–62, 1996.

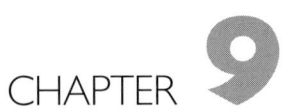

Special Situations in Rheumatic Disease Therapy

Rheumatic Diseases and Pregnancy

Rheumatic diseases and pregnancy have a conflicting relationship. Certain rheumatic diseases are detrimental to pregnancy, and pregnancy definitely alters rheumatic disease expression and places constraints on therapy (see appendix).

Regional Pain Syndromes

Pregnancy results in carpal tunnel syndrome in approximately 20% to 30% of women during the third trimester. Symptoms tend to be mild and are fully reversible following delivery. Treatment should be conservative with a wrist splint in the neutral position.

Pregnant women often develop lumbalgia. This is unavoidable from the increased functional lordosis needed to balance the extra anterior weight. Another cause of low back pain is osteitis condensans ilii, a condition that may be suspected clinically but is diagnosed retrospectively when an area of sclerosis in the iliac bone adjacent to the sacroiliac (SI) joint is found on x-rays. The joint margins are normal, as is the sacrum adjacent to the SI joint. Following delivery, women may have sciatica as a result of a pyriformis muscle syndrome (see Part IV). Also, there may be vague, toothache-like hip pain from transient osteoporosis of the hip. This condition, considered a variant of sympathetic dystrophy, runs a self-limited course in several months.

Because x-rays and other imaging techniques are best avoided during pregnancy, diagnosis may remain tentative as long as septic arthritis is excluded by a lack of fever and hip splinting or by ultrasound-guided hip aspiration. Following delivery, a de Quervain's tenosynovitis often develops from lifting the baby. The condition resolves with the husband's help, the use of a splint, or a local steroid infiltration.

Systemic Rheumatic Diseases

There is still controversy on the effects of pregnancy on SLE. It is now clear that in the absence of active nephritis and with a normal blood pressure, pregnant SLE patients have only a mild increase in lupus flares. The risk of toxemia is increased. Fertility is not affected by SLE. However, lupus patients have an increased rate of early (less than 14 weeks) pregnancy losses as well as a high risk of growth retardation and prematurity. To this should be added middle trimester losses in patients with a secondary antiphospholipid syndrome.

Only about 50% of pregnant lupus patients deliver a full-term baby. Lupus pregnancies are by definition high-risk pregnancies that call for the highest of obstetrical and rheumatologic skills. Lupus activity during pregnancy is best controlled with low to medium prednisone doses (10–20 mg per day). Patients with antiphospholipid antibodies and a history of fetal loss should receive low-dose aspirin throughout pregnancy.

Patients with a history of thrombosis should receive aspirin plus low molecular weight heparin. Lupus and Sjögren's patients with pathogenic SSA (anti-Ro) and SSB (anti-La) antibodies are at an increased risk of having babies with the neonatal lupus syndrome. The frequency of neonatal lupus syndrome in the offspring of these patients is small, however, and pregnancies should not be discouraged.

Interestingly, RA usually improves during pregnancy only to resume activity in the postpartum period. This feature of RA allows discontinuation of potentially dangerous medications in most patients. As in SLE, RA activity during pregnancy is best controlled with small doses of corticosteroids (10–15 mg per day). Antirheumatic drugs may be immediately resumed postpartum if the baby is fed with formula. Otherwise, a short-acting NSAID such as ibuprofen may be used immediately before each breast feeding plus low-dose prednisone. Sulfasalazine may be the least problematic of the second-line medications in this setting.

Scleroderma patients have increased esophageal problems, particularly regurgitation, during pregnancy. There may be difficulties in conception, intrauterine growth retardation, and low birth weights. D-penicillamine, a common form of treatment in scleroderma, is formally contraindicated during pregnancy.

Pregnancies in ankylosing spondylitis are uneventful. The course of pregnancy in other rheumatic diseases has been less studied. The appendix contains guidelines of the American College of Rheumatology on the potential effects of antirheumatic medications on pregnancy and lactation.

Rheumatic Disease in Old Age

Regional Pain Syndromes

Shoulder problems, lumbar and cervical spinal conditions, hip osteoarthritis (OA), and knee OA are leading causes of pain and disability in the elderly population. Common shoulder problems include the frozen shoulder or shoulder periarthritis, and chronic degenerative tendinitis involving the rotator cuff. The Milwaukee shoulder is a feared complication of advanced rotator cuff disease. Degenerative spinal stenosis with neurogenic claudication is frequent in old age, the task of the clinician being to distinguish this condition from vascular claudication.

Primary care physicians should be conversant with the diagnosis and management of hip and knee osteoarthritis, including the various nonpharmacologic therapeutic choices, because NSAIDs pose a significant risk in the older population. A working knowledge of walking aids and indications for total joint replacement is essential for physicians who care for elderly patients.

Systemic Conditions

Osteoporosis, osteomalacia, elderly-onset RA, polymyalgia rheumatica (PMR), late-onset SLE, tumor-associated arthritis, myositis, and drug-induced syndromes constitute the bulk of systemic rheumatic diseases in the elderly. All of these conditions are discussed in the appropriate sections. A few points are stressed here.

Many older patients who seldom go outdoors and do not consume dairy products have osteomalacia rather than osteoporosis. Treatment in these patients must include vitamin D as well as calcium supplementation. Elderly-onset RA, a closely related condition known as RS3PE, and PMR have overlapping features and may indeed represent subsets of the same condition. Giant cell arteritis (GCA) complicates approximately 10% of cases of PMR. GCA may be subdued in PMR patients treated with low-dose corticosteroids, but it may still cause blindness if unrecognized and insufficiently treated. Elderly-onset RA and late-onset SLE are no longer considered benign conditions. Seropositive RA frequently follows a destructive course, and the mortality of late-onset SLE is high.

CHAPTER 10

Rheumatic Manifestations of Endocrine, Hematologic, and Malignant Disease

Endocrine Disorders

Endocrine conditions often feature rheumatologic syndromes (Table 10–1). In some patients, musculoskeletal manifestations appear first. A high index of suspicion for endocrine disease has allowed the author to detect a number of endocrine conditions under the disguise of rheumatologic disease. *Seronegative polyarthritis* may be mimicked by hypothyroidism, acromegaly, and hyperparathyroidism. Myxedematous arthropathy includes arthralgias, myalgias, cylindrical leg edema, and bilateral carpal tunnel syndrome. CPK may be elevated. Thyroid replacement results in slow (weeks to months) correction of symptoms. Acromegaly features joint stiffness and pain in the extremities and back. Carpal tunnel syndrome is a prominent association in active disease. Radiographically the height of the intervertebral discs is increased initially and there may be degenerative changes in the glenohumeral joint (shoulder involvement is rare in idiopathic OA). Periosteal resorption in hyperparathyroidism may result in a pseudo RA. Hand x-rays characteristically show ragged periosteal resorption in the radial side of the middle phalanges in the second and third fingers. *Fibromyalgia* may occur in hypothyroidism, hyperthyroidism, and chronic adrenal insufficiency. Fibromyalgic pain may also appear when chronic glucocorticoid therapy is being reduced too fast, and in patients newly placed on pharmacologic glucocorticoid doses.

As an example, a patient with UC treated with glucocorticoids develops musculoskeletal pain as the steroid dosage is reduced. Inflammatory bowel disease–related arthritis is considered. However, physical examination reveals fibromyalgic tender points rather than arthritis. The steroid dosage is increased and symptoms promptly go away. A very slow steroid reduction is then undertaken and fibromyalgic pain does not recur.

Finally, exogenous glucocorticoids may cause or increase existing fibromyalgic pain. Smythe et al. have shown that glucocorticoids cause a general decrease in pain threshold particularly in the tibial regions (Smythe's tender shins syndrome). Finally, a slight increase in fibromyalgic tenderness was noted in patients taking the active drug in a placebo-controlled trial of low-dose corticosteroids in fibromyalgia. In the author's view, rather than creating de novo fibromyalgia, thyroid hormone and glucocorticoid fluctuations bring up subclinical or unrecognized fibromyalgia.

PATIENT 12. A young woman, a physician's wife, finally decided to consult after 2 months of living a bed-to-chair existence because of diffuse achiness and lack of stamina. Symptoms had gradually developed over the past 2 years. She had initially attended some psychotherapy sessions. Recently, physician friends had suggested the possibility of fibromyalgia. Past medical history was significant for a bout of depression while the patient was in college. On examination she appeared both depressed and exhausted; general examination including muscle strength was normal; and musculoskeletal examination revealed disseminated fibromyalgic tender points. Laboratory studies obtained elsewhere included normal CBC, ESR, CPK, and aldolase. Antinuclear antibodies and rheumatoid factor tests were negative. Thyroid tests were requested and revealed a marked elevation of TSH and depression of free T4. On thyroid hormone replacement the patient improved her mood, stamina, and achiness, and became once again functional. The fibromyalgic tenderness improved but did not go away.

TABLE 10–1

MUSCULOSKELETAL MANIFESTATIONS OF ENDOCRINE DISEASE

1. Acromegaly
   - Polyarthralgias
   - Carpal tunnel syndrome
   - Back pain (degenerative disease)
   - Myopathy
2. Hyperthyroidism
   - Fibromyalgia
   - Frozen shoulder
   - Back pain (osteopenia)
   - Myopathy
3. Hypothyroidism
   - Fibromyalgia
   - Polyarthralgias/arthritis
   - Carpal tunnel syndrome
   - Frozen shoulder
   - Myopathy
4. Chronic adrenal insufficiency
   - Fibromyalgia
   - Arthralgias
   - Joint effusions
5. Cushing
   - Painful tibias syndrome
   - Exacerbation of fibromyalgia
   - Joint effusions
   - Back pain (osteopenia)
   - Osteonecrosis
   - Myopathy
6. Hyperparathyroidism
   - Pseudogout (CPPD crystals)
   - Polyarhalgias/arthritis
   - Brown tumors
   - Back pain (osteopenia)
7. Diabetes
   - Cheiroarthropathy
   - Dupuytren's contracture
   - Trigger finger
   - Frozen shoulder
   - DISH
   - Diabetic osteoarthropathy (Charcot's joint; diabetic osteolysis)

CPPD = calcium pyrophosphate dihydrate.
DISH = diffuse idiopathic skeletal hyperostosis.

Back pain and osteopenia occur in endogenous and exogenous Cushing's, hyperthyroidism, hyperparathyroidism, and hypogonadism. The initial change in acromegaly, as stated earlier, is an increased height in intervertebral discs. As the disease progresses, however, the intervertebral discs collapse leading to severe anterior and posterior arch spinal degeneration.

Avascular necrosis of bone is a well-known complication of corticosteroid therapy, while it is relatively infrequent in spontaneous Cushing's syndrome. A high index of suspicion is required to diagnose osteonecrosis in patients with an underlying joint condition. As an example, hip pain developing in a lupus or RA patient on chronic corticosteroid therapy while other joints are stable, improving, or in remission should prompt investigation. A useful clue in early avascular necrosis of the hip is severe pain with a virtually normal range of motion. Later in the course of the disease, as the femoral head collapses, hip motion will be both restricted and painful.

Crystal-induced arthritis, particularly CPPD deposition disease, may complicate hypothyroidism and hyperparathyroidism. Thyroid replacement in the former and parathyroidectomy in the latter have no effect on the chondrocalcinosis. Indeed, parathyroidectomy is often followed by a transient increase in the frequency of pseudogout.

Diffuse idiopathic skeletal hyperostosis (DISH) associates with diabetes mellitus in 50% of patients. A similar association is seen in vitamin D–resistant rickets, fluorosis, and prolonged etretinate therapy for acne.

Myopathy is featured by both hypothyroidism (increased CPK) and hyperthyroidism (normal CPK). Myopathy, usually affecting first the iliopsoas muscles (weakness of hip flexion), is a well-known complication of endogenous and exogenous Cushing's syndrome.

Finally, proximal muscle weakness is a well-known feature of acromegaly. *Carpal tunnel syndrome* may be caused by diabetes, hypothyroidism, and acromegaly among many other nonendocrine etiologies.

Systemic fibrosis is a common feature in poorly controlled insulin-dependent and adult-onset diabetes. The condition features one or more of the following: Dupuytren's contracture, trigger finger that typically involves multiple digits, carpal tunnel syndrome, frozen shoulder, which is often bilateral, and the well-known diabetic cheiroarthropathy in which patients have incomplete contact of the hands in the praying position.

Finally, *neuropathic arthropathy* is seen in diabetes complicated by peripheral neuropathy as well as in several other conditions in which the sensory input is deficient including syringomyelia, tabes dorsalis, amyloidosis, leprosy, chronic renal failure, and congenital indifference to pain.

Hematologic Disease

There are well-known associations between hematologic disease and rheumatic complaints. For the sake of brevity only the rheumatologic manifestations of sickle cell disease and hemophilia are discussed.

In *sickle cell disease,* for unknown reasons, erythrocytes become bound to endothelium and then sickle, obstructing the microcirculation. Tissue hypoxia follows, leading to necrosis and inflammation. Well-known rheumatologic manifestations of sickle cell disease resulting from ischemia include the foot-hand syndrome that occurs in children, painful crises, and avascular necrosis of bone. In addition, the poorly vascularized bone in sickle cell disease is unusually prone to infection.

Painful crises are due to ischemia, which eventually results in avascular necrosis of bone in 10% to 40% of patients. The femoral head is the most frequent site and involvement is usually bilateral. Onset of symptoms occurs at an average age of 25. By the age of 30, bilateral hip replacement is usually required. Results of arthroplasty are generally poor with a chance of revision of 30% by 4.5 years follow-up. Joint effusions are a frequent finding in bone crises. Muscle infarction, clinically manifested by indurated, tender muscle may also follow. Methylprednisolone in intravenous boluses has been effective in shortening duration of painful crises. There is also evidence that hydroxyurea treatment decreases the frequency of painful crises in sickle cell disease.

As mentioned, osteomyelitis is frequent in sickle cell disease. Usual pathogens include *S. aureus* and salmonella. Treatment includes bone debridement and prolonged antibiotics. As it could be expected, differentiation between painful crises and osteomyelitis may be difficult. Recommendations to identify bone infection in in patients with sickle cell disease are shown in Table 10–2.

A frequent and disabling complication of *hemophilia* is hemarthrosis. The condition may be congenital or acquired because of the presence of anti–factor VIII antibodies. A clue to diagnosis may be an unexplained hemarthrosis or soft tissue hematoma associated with a prolonged partial thromboplastin time and a normal prothrombin time indicative of a disorder of the intrinsic limb of the coagulation cascade. Spontaneous bleeding occurs in patients with less than 1% of factor VIII activity, requires some trauma between 1% to 5%, and complicates major trauma or surgery in patients with 5% to 50%. Interestingly, hemarthrosis tends to recur in the

---

TABLE 10–2

MANAGEMENT OF SUSPECTED BONE INFECTION IN SICKLE-CELL DISEASE

1. Admit patient to hospital
2. Obtain complete blood cell count and erythrocyte sedimentation rate (ESR); if leukocyte count and ESR* are elevated, osteomyelitis must be considered.
3. Obtain blood cultures.
4. Determine febrile agglutinins and culture stools for salmonella species.
5. Consult hematologist and infectious disease specialist.
6. Obtain plain bone radiographs. Repeat in 10–14 days if initial findings are negative.†
7. Obtain technetium or gallium scintigram. These tests do not distinguish osteomyelitis from bone infarction but they serve to detect multiple sites of infection and osteomyelitis involving the pelvis and spine.
8. Any bone thought to be infected should be aspirated for culture.

*Author's comments: A normal ESR does not necessarily exclude osteomyelitis or other serious infection in patients with sickle cell disease.
†It may be cost effective to obtain MRI if the clinical picture is suggestive and initial x-rays are negative.
After Epps CH Jr, Bryant DD III, Coles MJ, et al. Osteomyelitis in patients who have sickle-cell disease: Diagnosis and management. J Bone Joint Surg 73A;1281–1284, 1991.

same joint(s). Severe degenerative changes with prominent cyst formation and deformity follows, calling for the highest of orthopedic skills.

Malignant Disease

There are many possible relationships between *cancer and rheumatic disease*. Patients with leukemia, particularly the acute leukemias and the blastemic phase of chronic leukemias, may have arthritis. Leukemic arthritis may be acute or subacute and oligo- or polyarticular. Leukemic cells are infrequent in synovial fluid. There is characteristic tenderness at the metaphyses of long bones, ribs, and sternum. Antileukemic therapy brings rapid symptomatic relief.

Lymphomas may cause articular symptoms from paraarticular bone involvement in B-cell lymphomas and from lymphomatous synovitis, which closely resembles RA in T-cell lymphomas. Bone metastases from solid tumors cause skeletal pain, pathologic fractures, and sometimes neural compression. Carcinomatous synovitis is definitely uncommon. The knee is usually involved, paraarticular osteolysis is often present on x-rays, and effusions are hemorrhagic. Malignant cells have been found in only 50% of reported cases. In addition, lymphomas and solid tumors cause rare nonmetastatic rheumatologic syndromes including "cancer arthritis," fascial fibrosis (Medsger's syndrome), lupus-like illness, dermatomyositis, probably some cases of scleroderma, hypertrophic osteoarthropathy (HO), and gout.

Cancer arthritis is described as an asymmetric seronegative arthritis that develops explosively in an older patient with an overt or occult malignancy. Gout and pseudogout must be excluded. Response to successful tumor resection has been variable.

Lupus-like illnesses have been described in association with lymphoid leukemia, lymphomas, thymoma, and some solid tumors. Medsger's syndrome features bilateral palmar swelling followed by Dupuytren's contacture and joint restriction in an individual with ovarian, cervix, lung, or other cancer. Marked thrombocytosis is often present. The syndrome may precede the clinical appearance of the malignancy for months to 2 years. Dermatomyositis but not polymyositis associates with malignancy in 15% to 20% of adult cases. Most patients with an associated malignancy are over 50. An association between scleroderma and breast and lung cancer has been described. Hypertrophic osteoarthropathy may be explosive in onset in patients with lung carcinoma. An association between HO and other malignant tumors such as nasopharyngeal carcinoma, esophageal cancer, and hepatocarcinoma has also been described.

Finally, gout is a known association of the myeloproliferative disorders in which purine metabolism is grossly enhanced. Twenty-four-hour urine excretion of UA is increased in these patients. Certain clinical and laboratory features should raise the suspicion of underlying malignancy: excessive anemia (Hct < 20) and thrombocytopenia in a child with presumed juvenile RA (acute leukemia); a monoarthritis with bone lysis on x-rays (metastatic cancer); a Baker's cyst that remains hard in knee semiflexion (sarcoma); a patient with PMR whose bones are tender (metastases, multiple myeloma); thrombocytosis in a patient with dermatomyositis (underlying cancer); thrombocytosis in a patient with lupus (ovarian cancer); hand swelling, acute Dupuytren's, and joint contractures (ovarian and other carcinomas).

From an opposite viewpoint, patients with RA, particularly those with Felty's syndrome, are at an increased risk of developing malignant lymphoma. The same may be true for SLE. Primary Sjögren's syndrome often gives way to a B-cell lymphoma. Patients with hepatitic C infection and cryoglobulinemia have an increased risk of hepatocarcinoma and non-Hodgkin's lymphoma.

CHAPTER 11

Disability Issues

Vocational Rehabilitation

Even though rheumatic diseases are the second most important cause of work disability payments in the United States, and work disability occurs in 50% of patients with RA, vocational rehabilitation resources are grossly underutilized by rheumatic disease patients. Bringing up disability issues is quite difficult, and therefore the opportunity should not be missed when patients express concern or ask a relevant question.

Primary care physicians should become familiar with community resources available to rheumatic disease patients including programs sponsored by the federal and state governments, the Arthritis Foundation, and private parties. Rheumatologists, social workers, the local chapter of the Arthritis Foundation, and the state rehabilitation commission may be contacted to obtain useful information about these programs.

In general terms, as a patient perceives a possible job loss the first resource to explore is the patient's employer. A change in job description with the same employer may or may not be possible.

The next step is referral to the local state-federal vocational rehabilitation agency. This agency provides career counseling and vocational testing services at no cost to

---

TABLE 11-1

REHABILITATION SERVICES ADMINISTRATION CRITERIA FOR SEVERE DISABILITY STATUS FOR CLIENTS CLASSIFIED UNDER THE CODE "ARTHRITIS AND RHEUMATISM"

Individuals classified in 1 of these 4 categories are considered to be severely disabled:
1. Arthritic condition has produced 1 of the following:
    a. Impairment involving 3 or more limbs
    b. Impairment involving 1 upper and 1 lower limb on the same side
    c. Impairment of both upper extremity limbs and need for assistance from another person or devices for activities of daily living
    d. Impairment of lower limbs to a degree that bilateral assistance devices are required, or the individual is unable to use public transportation
2. Recipient of Social Security Disability Insurance (SSDI)
3. Recipient of Supplemental Security Income
4. Functional loss and limitation from 1 or more conditions:
    a. Substantial loss or limitation, including inability to use public transportation, perform sustained work activity for 6 hours or more, climb 1 flight of stairs, or walk 100 yards on level ground without pausing, has disfigurement or deformity such as to cause social rejection, or unintelligible speech.
    b. Need for multiple services over an extended period of time.

From Allaire SA, et al. Management of work disability. Arthritis Rheum 36:1663–1670, 1993.

TABLE 11-2

SOCIAL SECURITY ADMINISTRATION GUIDELINES FOR DISABILITY

I. Arthritis of a major weight-bearing joint
   With history of persistent joint pain and stiffness and signs of severe limitation of motion of the affected joint on current clinical examination. With:
   A. Gross anatomic deformity of hip or knee (e.g., subluxation, contracture, bony or fibrous ankylosis, instability) with radiographic evidence of either severe joint space narrowing or significant bony destruction and severely limiting ability to walk and stand; or
   B. Reconstructive surgery or surgical arthrodesis of a major weight-bearing joint and return to full weight-bearing status did not occur, or is not expected to occur, within 12 months of onset.
II. Arthritis of one major joint in each arm
   With history of persistent joint pain and stiffness, signs of severe limitation of motion of the affected joints on current physical examination, and radiographic evidence of either severe joint space narrowing or significant bony destruction. With:
   A. Abduction and forward flexion (elevation) of both arms at the shoulder, including scapular motion, restricted to less than 90 degrees; or
   B. Gross anatomic deformity and enlargement or effusion of the affected joints.
III. Disorders of the spine
   A. Arthritis manifested by ankylosis or fixation of the cervical or dorsolumbar spine at 30 degrees or more of flexion measured from the neutral position with radiographic evidence of:
      1. Calcification of the spinal ligaments; or
      2. Bilateral ankylosis of the sacroiliac joint with abnormal apophyseal articulation.
   B. Osteoporosis, generalized (established by radiograph), manifested by pain and limitation of back motion and paravertebral muscle spasm with radiographic evidence of nontraumatic vertebral compression fracture(s).
   C. Other vertebral disorders (e.g., herniated nucleus pulposus, spinal stenosis) with the following persisting for at least 3 months despite prescribed therapy and expected to last 12 months. With both:
      1. Pain, muscle spasm, and significant limitation of motion in the spine; and
      2. Appropriate radicular distribution of significant muscle weakness and sensory and reflex loss.

Modified from Disability Evaluation under Social Security: A Handbook for Physicians. U.S. Department of Health and Human Services, Social Security Administration. Publication No. (SSA) 79–10089, August 1979.

clients, regardless of financial status, as well as additional services such as medical treatment, surgery, physical therapy, vocational training, and transportation at no cost if financial need can be demonstrated. To qualify for these services severe disability must be documented from information provided by the patient's physician or a medical examiner paid by the agency. Severe disability criteria, as they relate to rheumatic diseases, are listed in Table 11–1.

Another resource available in several states is the job program of the Arthritis Foundation. This program, funded by Projects with Industry of the Rehabilitation Services Administration, provides training in essential skills including résumé writing, interviewing, handling of disease symptoms on the job, and participation in a job search club. Primary care physicians should become familiar with these important community resources.

Social Security Disability

Individuals with physical impairments may be eligible for Social Security Disability Insurance (SSDI) or Supplemental Security Income (SSI). To qualify for SSDI the applicant must have contributed to the Social Security Trust for a predetermined number of quarter years that depends on the applicant's age at onset of disability. SSI, on the other hand, is funded through general tax revenues and therefore independent of an applicant's contributions. The list of arthritis and disorders of the spine criteria that an applicant must meet to qualify for SSDI is shown in Table 11–2.

Individuals not meeting criteria may still be eligible for SSDI or SSI by using the concept of "residual functional capacity," which is the ability to perform work-related tasks despite physical or mental limitations. The Social Security Administration supplies a book that describes in detail the listing of impairments. Needless to say, a detailed description of the patient's clinical findings is essential to reduce the likelihood of denials in meritorious cases.

Suggested Reading

Allaire SH, Partridge AJ, Andrews HF, et al. Management of work disability: Resources for vocational rehabilitation. Arthritis Rheum 36:1663–1670, 1993.

U.S. Department of Health and Human Services, Social Security Administration. Disability Evaluation under Social Security: A Handbook for Physicians. Publication No. (SSA)79-10089, August 1979.

PART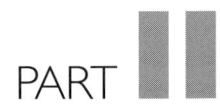

CONNECTIVE TISSUE DISORDERS

CHAPTER 12

Rheumatoid Arthritis

Rheumatoid arthritis (RA) is the prototype chronic inflammatory disease of joints. The implications of RA to the patient and to society are staggering. Women and men are affected by RA in the prime of their lives. Rheumatoid patients live their lives with painful, stiff, and often distorted joints. Systemically, RA has the potential to produce wasting and irreversibly damage organs. Medications used for disease control are far from innocuous and being on the watch for toxicities becomes an integral part of life for the RA sufferer. Approximately half of patients are unable to work within 10 years of onset of illness. Finally, survival is decreased by RA with a mortality similar to lymphomas. This chapter describes the articular aspects of RA and the systemic effects of rheumatoid disease. General aspects of therapy should be reviewed in the appropriate chapters before implementing drug, PT, or orthopedic treatment of RA.

Differential diagnosis as well as minimal criteria for diagnosis is emphasized as opposed to classification criteria that require a specified disease duration. To what extent should radiographic studies be carried out? Which articular, systemic, psychologic, and iatrogenic complications may be expected to occur? What are the trade-offs of the various forms of therapy? When should orthopedic surgeons be called in? Two additional conditions are clustered with the RA-related sections: remitting seronegative symmetrical synovitis with pitting edema (RS3PE) and polymyalgia rheumatica (PMR). Grouping old-age-onset RA, RS3PE, and PMR together makes the differences among them more apparent.

Rheumatoid Arthritis: Articular Aspects

Presentation and Progression

Cause

Rheumatoid arthritis is more common in women than in men with a female to male ratio of 3 to 1. Although most cases develop between the ages of 30 and 60, incidence increases with age. There is uncertainty, however, about the homogeneity of RA in the older age group. "Splitters" have already dissected out several conditions previously thought to be part of RA. Thus, old-age-onset RA (seropositive and seronegative) has been distinguished from polymyalgia rheumatica, the RS3PE syndrome, and old-age spondyloarthropathy. The etiology of RA remains unknown. In addition to a hypothetical triggering (infectious?) agent, important host factors have emerged that are relevant to prognosis. Markers of a more severe prognosis include possessing disease-severity HLA-DR4 genes (which apply to caucasian U.S. patients), rheumatoid factor positivity, higher joint counts, and a low functional capacity. The 1987 revised criteria for the classification of RA are shown in Table 12–1.

Presentation

The distal symmetric pattern of joint involvement in established RA is known to all. However, early disease is notoriously difficult to diagnose. Early RA patients have stiffness, achiness, and some swelling about one or more of the peripheral joints. Parvovirus B-19 and other viruses, however, may cause a similar distal symmetric synovitis. Viral synovitis should be suspected when RA-like symptoms develop, for instance, in a young elementary school healthcare worker. Diffuse hand swelling and subtle manifestations of carpal tunnel syndrome may prevail in old-age-onset RA. Older individuals are prone to developing diffuse hand swelling nonspecifically, however, whether due to RA, PMR, the RS3PE syndrome, spondyloarthropathy, gout, or pseudogout; hence the importance of obtaining hand films to rule out chondrocalcinosis and joint aspiration to more definitively rule out microcrystalline disease. If rheumatoid tenosynovitis appears first, a wrong diagnosis of traumatic

---

TABLE 12–1

THE AMERICAN RHEUMATISM ASSOCIATION 1987 REVISED CRITERIA FOR THE CLASSIFICATION OF RHEUMATOID ARTHRITIS

1. Morning stiffness in and around the joints lasting at least 1 hour before maximal improvement
2. Soft tissue swelling or fluid (not bone overgrowth only) in 3 or more joints observed by physician
3. At least one joint area as above in the PIP, MCP, or wrist joints
4. Symmetric arthritis (involvement of PIP, MCP, or MTP joints is acceptable without absolute symmetry)
5. Subcutaneous nodules observed by a physician
6. Positive test for rheumatoid factor by any test that has been positive in less than 5% of normal controls
7. Radiographic erosions or periarticular osteopenia in hand and wrist x-rays

To classify a patient as having RA, criteria 1 through 4 must have been present for at least 6 weeks.

From Arnett FC, et al. The 1987 revised ARA criteria for classification of rheumatoid arthritis. Arthritis Rheum 315:988, 1988.

posterior tibialis tenosynovitis in a tennis player or a wrist tenosynovitis in an office worker is likely to be made. A chronic monoarthritis is another form of presentation of RA that may be a challenge for clinicians.

Differential diagnosis includes internal derangement of the knee, low-grade infection (consider TB), foreign body synovitis (history helps), and spondyloarthropathy, in particular reactive arthritis and psoriatic arthritis (look at those areas in which psoriasis hides). Palindromic rheumatism designates a jumping type of arthritis. Patients have acute pain and swelling in a joint lasting a few hours to a few days, only to develop similar findings in another joint, and so on. Patients with palindromic rheumatism and a positive RF test often go on, after months or years, to develop RA. In a subset of patients with palindromic rheumatism and positive RF, rheumatoid nodules are prominent, the so-called rheumatoid nodulosis.

PATIENT 13. A 56-year-old man was seen because of a disrupting migratory arthritis occurring anywhere between 7 and 20 days apart. Arthritis affected one joint at a time, symptoms were violent, and within 1 to 3 days the episode was over. Multiple subcutaneous nodules were present on his hands (Figure 12–1). The left knee showed acute inflammation. Synovial fluid aspirated from this knee had 20,000 WBC/mm^3, 90% of PMNs, and no crystals on polarizing microscopy. The rheumatoid factor test was markedly positive. The patient was started on intramuscular gold. Unfortunately, shortly after initiation of treatment the extensor tendons for the fifth and fourth right digits ruptured. Tendon transfer was successfully performed. Four months later joint symptoms had gone away and by the sixth month of therapy the nodules were much reduced in size.

Undue fatigability is common in early RA and patients soon realize that difficulties are worse on waking up, improving slowly during the morning hours. Diagnosis of early RA depends on the index of suspicion, the ability to uncover relevant information by appropriate RA-directed questions, and the exclusion of other inflammatory conditions by negative answers to connective tissue disease– and spondyloarthropathy-directed questions.

Physical examination, if done purposefuly and with attention to detail, usually provides helpful diagnostic clues. An essential finding is the unequivocal detection of joint inflammation, that is, tenderness, painful limitation in all directions of motion, swelling, and the presence of an effusion. Tenderness may be uncovered at PIPs, MCP, or MTPs, or thickening in characteristically involved synovial sheaths (flexor carpi radialis or extensor carpi ulnaris), bringing the patient closer to the pattern of distal symmetric joint involvement characteristic, but by no means specific of RA. As the disease progresses additional joints become overtly involved and the typical articular pattern of RA eventually develops.

Laboratory studies are often helpful: Thrombocytosis and an increased ESR or CRP speak of inflammatory disease. Rheumatoid factor is present in approximately 50% of cases at disease onset. The ANA, which should be obtained because in most cases of systemic lupus erythematosus (SLE) joints are affected first, is positive in 30% of cases, albeit in low titer and with a homogeneous pattern of fluorescence. Patients who have a positive ANA should be further studied with complement (C_3, CH50) and specific lupus antibodies (dsDNA, Sm) determination. Different from SLE, complement levels in RA are normal or elevated and dsDNA and Sm antibody tests are negative. Rheumatoid factor negative patients should be closely scrutinized for alternative conditions that mimic early RA. Prominent among these are the spondyloarthropathies, hypothyroidism and the rare conditions hemochromatosis and light chain (LA) amyloidosis.

Radiographic studies in early RA show only paraarticular soft tissue swelling. Paraarticular osteopenia (washed-out bone) is the next finding to develop. The characteristic small

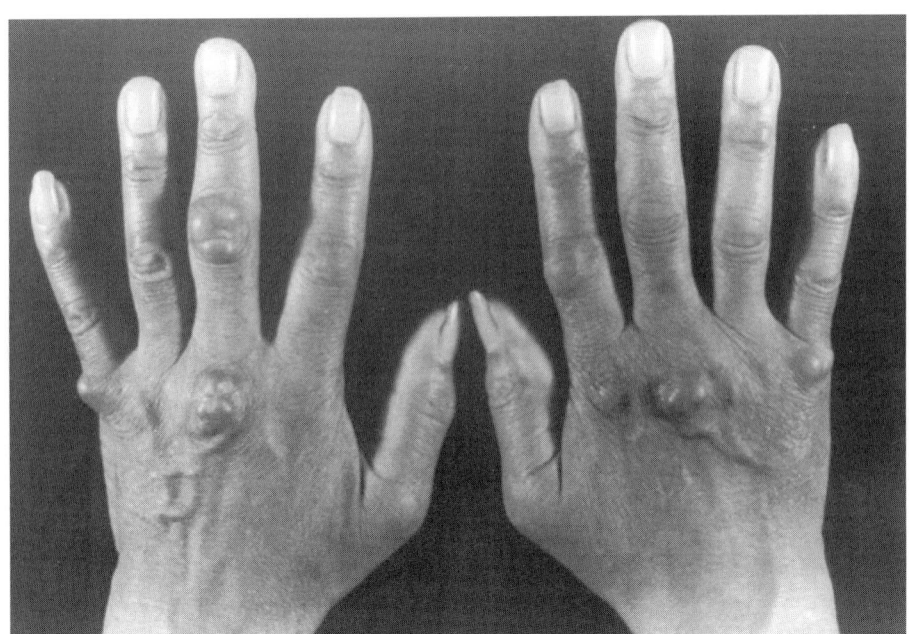

FIGURE 12–1. Patient 13. This man with seropositive palindromic arthritis developed subcutaneous nodules in his hands, followed by tendon ruptures.

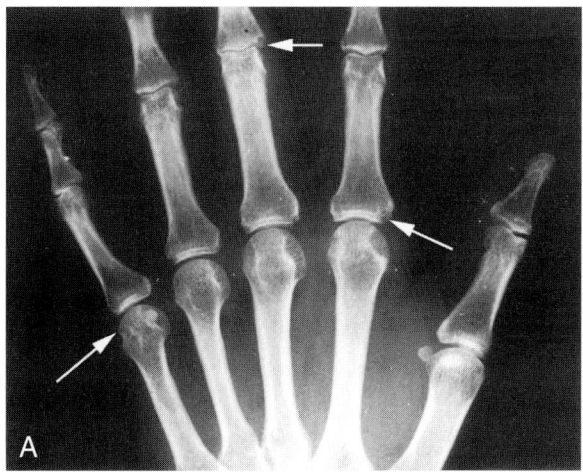 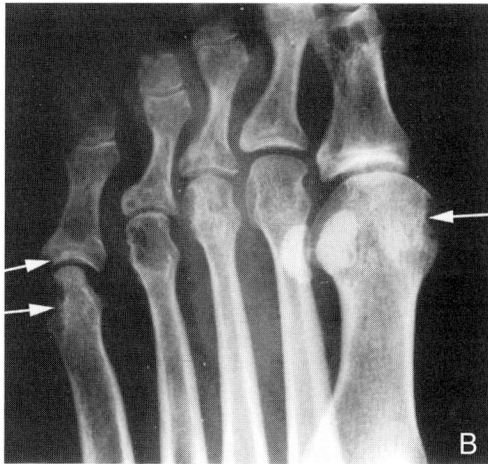

FIGURE 12–2. *Rheumatoid arthritis.* A, Periarticular osteopenia and marginal erosions in MCPs and a PIP (arrows). B, In the same patient, marginal erosions at metatarsal heads.

marginal bone erosions and cartilage thinning appear later but usually within 2 years of disease onset.

Radiographic findings in RA should be contrasted with those in osteoarthritis (OA): (1) Rheumatoid erosions are initially small, located at the corners of a joint where synovial tissue directly layers bone, and involve osteopenic bone that accounts for their fuzzy margins (Figure 12–2). In osteoarthritis, there are no marginal erosions but well-demarcated cysts within sclerotic (dense) subchondral bone (Figure 12–3). (2) Cartilage thinning in RA and other inflammatory conditions is characteristically diffuse within a joint. Osteoarthritic cartilage loss is uneven within a joint.

Synovial fluid analysis is desirable before a diagnosis of RA is positively made. Any accessible synovial effusion should be aspirated for diagnosis, for example, to document chronic sterile synovitis and to rule out other diagnoses such as RA-like gout or pseudogout. Synovial fluid in RA is inflammatory to highly inflammatory with WBC counts ranging from 10,000 to 100,000 cells/mm^3 (closer to the lower end in early disease), predominance of PMS, absence of crystals, and a negative culture result. Since polyarticular MSU gout and CPPD pseudogout may mimic RA to perfection, a detailed search for crystals is essential in postpuberal males as well as in postmenopausal females.

Diagnosis

Summary of Diagnosis

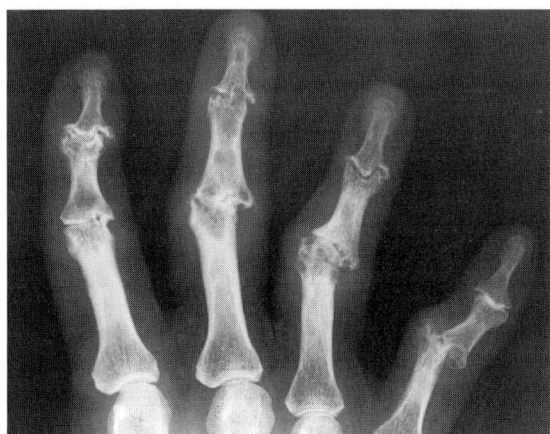

FIGURE 12–3 *Erosive osteoarthritis.* Detail of hand films of a 46-year-old woman with destructive osteoarthritis of proximal and distal interphalangeal joints. There was a family history of hand osteoarthritis. There was no psoriasis, the ESR was normal, and rheumatoid factor test was negative. The involved joints show cartilage loss, sclerosis, cyst formation, and ulnar subluxation of proximal interphalangeal joints 2, 3, and 4.

> **RHEUMATOID ARTHRITIS**
>
> - History and physical examination to seek symmetry and distal involvement and to rule out other rheumatic diseases such as microcrystalline disease, CTDs, spondyloarthropathy, and certain infections.
> - CBC: Thrombocytosis is frequent; anemia is rare in early disease; leukocytosis in very acute cases; leukopenia occasionally present in association with splenomegaly.
> - ESR, CRP: Usually elevated depending on extent and degree of joint inflammation.
> - RF positive in 50% at onset and 90% within 2 years.
> - ANA positive in 30%, low titer, homogeneous pattern.
> - In ANA-positive cases, determine complement and specific lupus antibodies dsDNA and Sm (in RA, complement is elevated or normal; dsDNA and Sm antibodies are negative).
> - If a joint effusion is present, aspirate to rule out crystal disease and to confirm aseptic polymorphonuclear inflammation. Infections rarely mimic RA. Depending on circumstances, secondary syphilis, parvovirus B-19 infection, rubella infection, or tuberculosis may have to be ruled out.

Natural History

Expected Outcome

Rheumatoid arthritis remits permanently in some patients. Criteria for complete clinical remission of RA are shown in Table 12–2. This favorable outcome is extremely rare in an office setting but may be common in the community at large. Whether these cases represent true RA or a self-limited condition such as reactive arthritis or viral arthritis, which may fulfill clinical RA criteria, can only be conjectured.

In the bulk of patients, however, rheumatoid arthritis is either a relapsing disease with minimal or no residual damage (palindromic-type RA), a relapsing disease with progressive residual damage, a slowly progressive disease, or a rapidly destructive disease known as "malignant RA." Palindromic-type RA and malignant RA are the least common types. It has been observed that the initially involved joints lay out a pattern that remains true during disease course. Said in other words, new joint involvement is unusual after the first 2 years of disease. The same can be said about erosion sites. Persistently inflamed joints sooner or later develop the signature of late RA: irreversible bone, cartilage, and fibrous tissue changes. Late RA develops from hydrostatic forces; synovial tissue bulk; bone erosion; capsule, ligament, and tendon failure; muscle and soft tissue contractures; and reducible and then fixed compensatory changes in distal joints. All of these changes are abhorrent to the rheumatologist and should be abhorrent to primary physicians as well. Ulnar deviation, swan-neck deformities, boutonniere deformities, and the like are overstressed during medical training as characteristic of RA. In fact, they only reflect late or failed therapy for RA.

Physicians should also realize that outcome in RA is far worse than thought previously in terms of function and life expectancy. Erosive disease develops in the initial 1 to 2 years. A full 50% of RA patients are unable to work within 10 years of onset of disease; hence current emphasis in identifying "bad" RA cases from the outset based on clinical findings, nutrition, ESR, RF, function questionnaires, and, with the reservations noted, HLA-DR typing. Prompt aggressive therapy is more than justified in these cases.

Treatment

Methods

Treatment of RA includes pharmacologic agents, PT, and a keen watch for orthopedic problems. Needless to say, effective therapy in RA implies aggressive early treatment before erosions and cartilage loss have a chance to develop. As rightfully emphasized by the ACR Committee of Guidelines for the Management of RA, the majority of care of an RA patient should be provided by a single physician. Also, who will be in charge of monitoring drug therapy must be clearly established. Patients should be instructed on monitoring themselves for toxic effects. A close collaboration between the primary care physician and the rheumatologist is of paramount importance in the care of RA patients.

Drug Therapy in Early RA: It may be initially difficult to determine whether a patient has RA or other type of inflammatory joint disease. Nonsteroidal anti-inflammatory drugs because of their nonspecific action and relative safety represent a good treatment choice during this period of uncertainty. Among NSAIDs the nonacetylated salicylates, nabumetone, and ibuprofen are safer in frail patients as well as in patients who are at a higher risk of GI toxicity. Coumadinized patients present a problem. In this group, ibuprofen and naproxen have a good record of tolerance, although PTs should be repeated weekly for several weeks, since dose adjustments may need to be done.

Elderly patients are very sensitive to central nervous system effects of NSAIDs; mental confusion and incontinence may develop in this age group. Gastric toxicity has been discussed in the NSAIDs section. With the exceptions noted, patients with suspected RA should be placed on full doses of a strong NSAID such as diclofenac 75 mg bid or naproxen 500 mg bid or tid.

Most patients improve on these agents as determined by less pain, a shorter duration of morning stiffness, and reduction in swelling. Although patients feel and function better, this by no means indicates that disease is or will be under control. Treatment with NSAIDs alone is inadequate except during the period of diagnostic uncertainty, which should not be allowed to extend for more than a few weeks.

Once RA has been diagnosed, oral methotrexate (MTX) should be initiated without delay. Contraindications to MTX use include alcohol consumption (patients are required to abstain completely from alcohol) and serologic evidence of hepatitis B or C. Depending on age and patient size (older people and smaller people require a smaller initial dose), patients are started on MTX 5 to 10 mg (2 to 4 tablets) per week. MTX may be taken in a single dose or cycled over 24 hours before, with, or after meals, always on the same day of the week and at the same time to set a routine. Dose increments should be by 2.5 mg every 6 weeks until clear-cut response has been obtained or a 20 mg weekly dose has been reached. Unimproved patients should be switched to intramuscular MTX starting with the previous ineffective dose,

---

TABLE 12–2

THE AMERICAN RHEUMATISM ASSOCIATION CRITERIA FOR COMPLETE CLINICAL REMISSION IN RHEUMATOID ARTHRITIS

A minimum of five of the following requirements must be fulfilled for at least 2 consecutive months in a patient with definite or classic RA:*

1. Morning stiffness not to exceed 15 minutes
2. No fatigue
3. No joint pain
4. No joint tenderness or pain on motion
5. No soft tissue swelling in joints or tendon sheaths
6. Erythrocyte sedimentation rate (Westergren's) less than 30 mm/hour (females) or 20 mm/hour (males)

*Exclusions: Clinical manifestations of active vasculitis, pericarditis, myositis, or unexplained recent weight loss or fever secondary to RA prohibit a designation of complete clinical remission.

From Pinals RS, Masi AF, et al. Preliminary criteria for clinical remission in rheumatoid arthritis. Arthritis Rheum 24:1308, 1981.

that is, 17.5 mg weekly, since I.M. administration increases absorption from 60% to 80%, to 100%.

Alternatives to the use of MTX include intramuscular gold and azathioprine. Intramuscular gold is administered weekly initially and subsequently every 2 to 4 weeks. Test doses of 10 and 25 mg are administered in the initial 2 weeks. Subsequently, 50 mg weekly doses are administered until toxicity, improvement, or a cumulative 1000 mg to 1500 mg dose has been reached. Azathioprine is used at a dose of 2 mg per kilogram of body weight.

Patients with mild RA may be treated with sulfasalazine or hydroxychloroquine. Sulfasalazine is administered at a dose of 1.5 to 3 g per day preferably using enteric-coated tablets. Hydroxychloroquine is started at a dose of 200 mg bid. Monitoring for both drugs was discussed in the introduction. A failure to improve within a 6 month period is an indication to step up therapy, usually recommending MTX.

Although rheumatologists dislike using corticosteroids in early RA, if symptoms are disabling on full NSAIDs doses (it only takes a week to find out), prednisone 5 to 10 mg per day may be added as a "bridging medication." Patients should be informed of the reasons for this treatment, the risks involved, and that a dose reduction will be undertaken within a few weeks until discontinuation. Clearly stated goals and a structured reduction schedule are essential in preventing corticosteroid dependency. A negative calcium balance can be expected during this period. In addition, any systemic absorption of corticosteroid infiltrations will add to the bone mineral loss. Patients on bridging corticosteroids should receive calcium 1000 mg and vitamin D 500 IU as a daily supplementation. Once a satisfactory MTX dose has been reached, usually 12.5 to 17.5 mg per week, the steroid reduction should be started by removing 1 mg every 2 weeks. A smooth reduction is facilitated by using 1 mg prednisone tablets. Patients often worry about the sudden increase in pills and need to be reassured that the total amount of medication has actually decreased. Corticosteroid infiltrations should not be used during this initial period but rather be left for joints or tendon sheaths that lag behind in their improvement. Corticosteroid doses and techniques of injection and infiltration are given in the appendix.

Unfortunately, the rare postinjection septic arthritis occurs more frequently in RA than in other conditions. Beware of "postinjection flares" in rheumatoid joints and of joint deterioration after a successful response. Suspect joints should be aspirated for WBC and differential, gram stain, and culture. Postinjection septic arthritis is usually caused by *S. aureus,* an agent readily detectable on gram stain. If the gram stain is positive, appropriate antibiotics should be immediately started and a decision made on the method of draining: serial needle aspirations, tidal lavage, or arthroscopy. If no bacterias were seen, antibiotics should be started and discontinued if culture results are negative.

Physical Therapy (PT) in Early RA: Maintaining or improving limb function, rather than just fixing the diseased joints, should be the goal in any patient with articular disease. Physical therapy, which in the context of this chapter encompasses both occupational therapy (OT) and (PT), is essential in the treatment of early RA and should be implemented from the outset by requesting OT and PT evaluation. Emphasis should be placed on patient education, techniques of joint protection, and in providing a home PT progam to be implemented 7 days a week with periodic evaluations and reinforcements. This differs from PT as performed in sports injuries–geared practices in which patients receive treatment packages that include ultrasound, massage, muscle stimulation, laser applications, and exercises that require special machinery while little emphasis is placed on teaching exercises to be performed at home by the patient.

Unequivocally, without PT the most sophisticated pharmacologic treatment of RA is sadly incomplete. The PT program need not be complicated. Basically, patients are encouraged to use freely noninflamed joints while inflamed joints are both rested and exercised. This is an apparent rather than real contradiction. Rest has strong analgesic and anti-inflammatory effects, but motion is required to prevent joint stiffness, cartilage atrophy, and muscle wasting. With an appropriate balance of rest and motion both forms of PT can be used to the patient's advantage.

Rest in acutely inflamed joints is best achieved with the use of removable splints that may be ready made or custom made. Ready-made splints seldom fit the part smoothly and are ill suited for serious splintage. Of the custom-made splints the stronger plaster splints are heavy and messy to make except when OCL (Eudora, Kansas) or a similar cloth-confined plaster is used. Plaster splints are the choice for knee immobilization. Lightweight molded plastic splints are comfortable to use but also expensive. They are ideal for wrist splinting. The beneficial effects of splints are best shown in the wrist where immobilization affords instant analgesia (house officers are invariably astonished when uncontrollable wrist pain, refractory even to opiates, ceases as a splint is applied).

To prevent the detrimental effects of prolonged immobilization, the splint should be removed two or three times daily and the joint actively or passively moved through the painless range three or four times to help cartilage nutrition, stretch ligaments and muscles, and encourage venous and lymphatic return. Isometric exercises for quadriceps muscles, hamstring muscles, buttock muscles, and abdominal wall muscles should be taught. These exercises are performed two to three times daily and consist of five to six strong isometric contractions held for 6 seconds (see the appendix). Needless to say, isometric quadriceps exercises are essential in preventing quadriceps atrophy when the knee joint is inflamed. Acutely inflamed joints should be splinted steadily for 1 to 2 days followed by night splinting for 3 to 4 weeks.

All RA patients should be instructed on additional rest, including a nap if possible, before tackling the evening activities. A prolonged warm shower or immersion bath upon arising in the morning (after taking the morning medications) goes a long way in providing analgesia and improving joint stiffness. Hand exercises are then performed in the sink under tepid water followed by general flexibility and stretching exercises and isometric exercises as described in the appendix.

Patients with RA benefit greatly from pool exercises and they should inquire at the local Arthritis Foundation about the availability of such a program. If pool programs are unavailable locally, encourage patients to use a heated pool at least four times a week. Plain walking across water, floating, and swimming if possible are all excellent exercises. Patients who are able to cycle should be encouraged to enter a physical conditioning program.

Expected Response

Following the program just outlined, most patients experience some degree of improvement. Initial improvement reflects the additive effects of rest, NSAIDs, and low-dose corticosteroids. As treatment progresses the beneficial effect of disease-modifying drugs is added. Of these drugs MTX, sulfasalazine, and azathioprine have a relatively prompt action (4–6 weeks). With intramuscular gold, improvement is delayed 3 to 6 months. Disease remission (no symptoms, no inflammatory findings on examination, a normal ESR) is uncommon; some degree of residual inflammation will remain in most patients and occasional flares will break through the improvement brought about by the basic treatment.

Disease flares may be handled by increasing NSAID dosage, steroid infiltration in localized areas of inflammation, the addition of low-dose corticosteroids if these have not been started, an increase in MTX dose, the addition of another disease-modifying medication, or a complete change in disease-modifying medications. Second-line agents should be continued in patients who attained remission. The condition is not cured; it only became dormant. Discontinuation of the second-line agent will be followed in most cases by renewed disease activity.

Treatment of RA requires knowledge, empathy, resourcefulness, flexibility, optimism, an understanding of the patient's home, work, and recreational environment, readiness to seek advice from others, and, above all, patience. Treatment programs should not be abandoned before they have a chance to work. Is the NSAID dose sufficient? Is the second-line agent dose sufficient? Is the patient doing the right amounts of rest and exercise? Are there aggravating factors in the home or at work? Since only a few RA patients escape from untoward effects of medications, a high index of suspicion must be kept at all times. Particularly frequent are the erosive gastropathy in patients on NSAIDs and minor liver enzyme elevations in patients receiving methotrexate. Unfortunately there is a small group of RA patients with relentless disease in whom a rapid deterioration of joints as well as systemic organ damage may be expected.

When to Refer

There is no question that RA patients fare best when followed by an expert. Thus, all patients with suspected RA should have the benefit of an early rheumatologic evaluation. PT and OT consultations should also be obtained to outline the best possible treatment program. Patients with mild disease may be followed by primary care physicians as long as there is periodic rheumatologic assessment and the rheumatologist is involved in major treatment decisions. Cases with severe disease (joints stubbornly inflamed, destructive disease, major systemic involvement) should be followed primarily by a rheumatologist. Patients should be clearly informed of who in the medical team is going to provide the primary care.

Guidelines for the Disorder

The American College of Rheumatology has published several guidelines on RA (see the appendix):

1. Guidelines to monitor liver toxicity in patients treated with MTX.
2. Guidelines for the management of RA.
3. Guidelines to monitor treatment of RA.
4. Guidelines to establish remission of RA.

Resources Available

The local office of the Arthritis Foundation should be contacted for information on the aquatic program and available educational materials (see appendix for information regarding the national office of the Arthritis Foundation).

Key Points

RHEUMATOID ARTHRITIS

- Rheumatoid arthritis is a potentially disabling condition that markedly reduces life expectancy.
- Treatment of RA should be implemented early and be aggressive.
- Physical therapy is an integral component of the treatment program.
- Nonsteroidal anti-inflammatories relieve symptoms but have little effect on disease progression.
- Low-dose corticosteroids appear to decrease the rate of erosion at a significant metabolic and structural cost.
- Second-line agents have a delayed effect on RA. They consolidate improvement and unusually cause remission.
- Corticosteroid infiltrations are useful in joints that lag behind in improvement and to prevent rupture of Baker's cysts.
- Primary care physicians should work closely with rheumatologists for best treatment results.

Suggested Reading

American College of Rheumatology Ad Hoc Committee on Clinical Guidelines. Guidelines for the management of rheumatoid arthritis. Arthritis Rheum 39:713–722, 1996.

Harris ED. Clinical features of rheumatoid arthritis. In: Kelley MN, Harris ED Jr, Ruddy S, et al. (eds). Textbook of Rheumatology. W.B. Saunders, Philadelphia, 874–911, 1993.

Pincus T, Brooks RH, Callahan LF. Prediction of long-term mortality in patients with rheumatoid arthritis according to simple questionnaire and joint count measures. Ann Intern Med 120:26–34, 1994.

Van der Heide A, Jacobs JWG, Bijlsma JWJ, et al. The effectiveness of early treatment with "second line" antirheumatic drugs. A randomized, controlled trial. Ann Intern Med 124:699–707, 1996.

Rheumatoid Arthritis: Systemic Manifestations

RA patients suffer nonspecific complications of chronic inflammation (fever, anemia, thrombocytosis, muscle atrophy, weight loss, amyloidosis); complications from arthritis

TABLE 12–3
SYSTEMIC MANIFESTATIONS OF RHEUMATOID ARTHRITIS

Fever
Leukocytosis
Leukopenia (usually with splenomegaly)
Thrombocytosis
Increased ESR, CRP, and SAA
Weight loss
Cachexia
Systemic amyloidosis (rare)
Lymphadenopathy
Atlantoaxial subluxation with or without medullary compression
Compressive neuropathies from arthritis/tenosynovitis
Rheumatoid nodules (subcutaneous, visceral)
Sicca syndrome
Episcleritis
Nodular scleritis
Cricoarythenoid arthritis
Pleuritis (dry, effusive, cholesterol)
Pleural or intrapulmonary rheumatoid nodules
Pulmonary interstitial disease (fibrotic, inflammatory)
Bronchiolitis, with or without organizing pneumonia
Bronchiectasias
Pericarditis: acute dry or effusive, with or without tamponade; chronic effusive; or effusive/fibrotic with pericardial constriction
Cardiac valve nodules
Vasculitis: small vessel with periungual infarction, palpable purpura type, PAN-like necrotizing vasculitis with mononeuritis multiplex and leg ulcers

in critical locations (carpal tunnel, cricoarytenoid joint, atlantoaxial joint); and systemic complications from immune complex disease (rheumatoid nodules, serositis, rheumatoid lung, vasculitis). A list of systemic complications of RA is shown in Table 12–3.

Presentation and Progression

Cause

Rheumatoid tissue releases lymphokines, in particular interleukin-1 (IL-1) and tumor necrosis factor, that cause fever, anemia, thrombocytosis, muscle atrophy, and weight loss. In addition, interleukin-6 and tumor necrosis factor tell hepatocytes to increase serum amyloid A (SAA) levels with the potential to induce amyloidosis; fibrinogen, which increases the ESR; and CRP, which can be directly measured. Immune complexes containing IgG rheumatoid factors are complement fixing and have the potential, along with activated T-cells, to initiate systemic interstitial and vascular inflammation and necrosis.

Finally, increased tenosynovial bulk causes the carpal tunnel syndrome and synovial growth elsewhere, which results in findings such as hoarseness or upper airway obstruction when the cricoarytenoid joints are involved, brain stem compression syndromes from atlanto-odontoid joint instability, and a variety of compression neuropathies from articular or tenosynovial synovitis.

Presentation

Fever is unusual in RA except in acute early disease, the so-called *pseudoseptic arthritis* in which abrupt flares of hip or knee rheumatoid synovitis clinically resemble septic arthritis, cases complicated by necrotizing vasculitis, or as a drug fever.

Anemia is quite common; contributing factors include marrow suppression from chronic inflammation or myelosuppressive drugs, erosive gastropathy from the use of NSAIDs, and folate deficiency in MTX-treated patients who are not receiving folate supplementation.

Felty's syndrome represents a subset of RF-positive RA in which severe neutropenia associates with an enlarged spleen. Surprisingly, many patients with Felty's do not suffer recurrent pyogenic infections. Other patients do, and in those cases splenectomy decreases the rate of infections. It has been noted that some second-line medications, in particular parenteral gold and MTX, may raise leukocyte and neutrophil counts in Felty's patients.

Muscle atrophy and *weight loss* reflect the combined impact of arthrogenic muscle inhibition, disuse atrophy, plus the systemic catabolic effects of IL-1 and tumor necrosis factor. The resulting general debilitation may be quite severe.

Amyloidosis of the SA type as a complication of RA is uncommon in the United States but is relatively common in Europe and Japan. The reasons for this difference are unknown. Amyloidosis should be suspected when RA patients develop proteinuria with or without splenomegaly.

Other causes of proteinuria must be ruled out such as interstitial nephritis caused by NSAIDs; gold or D-penicillamine immune complex glomerulonephritis in patients so treated; SLE erroneously diagnosed as RA; diabetic nephropathy if the patient has diabetes; light chain (Bence Jones) proteinuria if the patient has developed B-cell lymphoma or multiple myeloma (the incidence of lymphoma is raised in RA); or an independent cause of proteinuria.

Carpal tunnel syndrome results from tenosynovial bulk pressing on the median nerve (see Part IV, Musculoskeletal Conditions [Regional Rheumatic Diseases]).

Cricoarytenoid arthritis presents with hoarseness, which is worse in the early morning, paralleling peripheral joint stiffness.

Atlantoaxial subluxation, which often associates with lower cervical segments' instability is a potentially life-threatening condition that should be suspected when RA patients complain of suboccipital pain. Pain radiation to the occiput and sides of the neck is common. Neck motion may cause flashes of pain along the upper extremities, spine, and lower extremities (Lehrmitte's sign) in cases with cord compression. Finally, sudden death is a rare complication of severe atlantoaxial subluxation. Diagnosis of atlantoaxial subluxation is made on a lateral radiograph of the neck obtained in flexion. As compared with films obtained in neutral or extension, there is a widened gap (> 3mm; usually > 7mm in symptomatic individuals) between the anterior part of the odontoid and the posterior surface of the anterior arch of the atlas. Cases of RA with symptomatic atlantoaxial subluxation should be evaluated neurosurgically.

Palpable *rheumatoid nodules* are present in approximately 30% of cases and represent a classic finding in RA (Figure

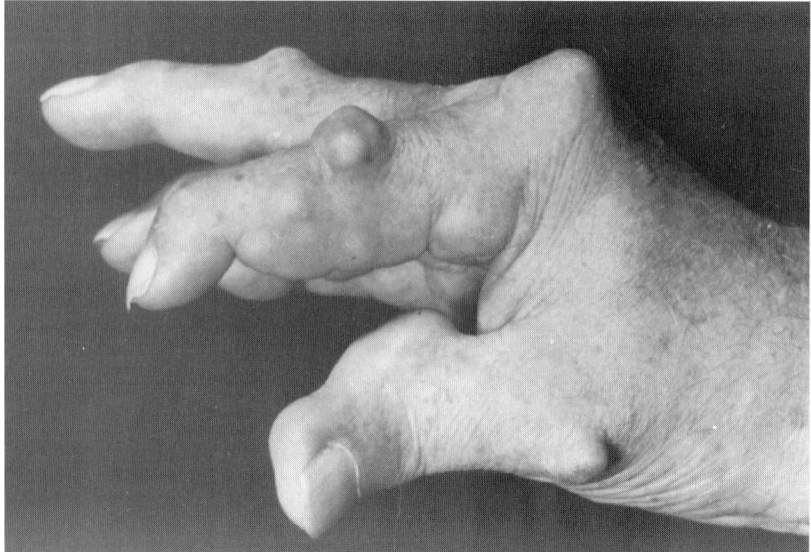

FIGURE 12–4. Rheumatoid arthritis. Hand of a 60-year-old man with seropositive rheumatoid arthritis. There are fixed deformities and gross rheumatoid nodules. This man is very active and does heavy labor. He has minimal pain. Hand films show erosions, some of them cystic, and sclerosis rather than osteopenia. Patients like him are said to have "typus robustus" rheumatoid arthritis.

12–4). Nodules tend to occur in pressure areas such as the extensor surface of elbows and forearms and the Achilles tendons. They may also involve pleural or pericardial surfaces, lung parenchyma, heart including cardiac valves, and the meninges. Rheumatoid nodules are firm or hard in consistency, usually painless, and deeply seated in the subcutaneous tissue. Periosteal attachment is common. Rheumatoid nodules must be distinguished from nodular formations in other diseases that feature arthritis such as sarcoidosis, monosodium urate gout, calcium pyrophosphate dihydrate pseudogout, light-chain amyloidosis, hemochromatosis, multicentric reticulohistiocytosis, and Whipple's disease. With the exception of sarcoidosis, which features RF in 30%, RF is negative in these conditions. Interestingly, rheumatoid nodules may develop de novo during the course of MTX treatment. These nodules, which appear in approximately 9% of MTX-treated patients, differ clinically from those caused by the disease itself: They tend to be very superficial (dermal rather than subcutaneous) and the predominant location is in contact areas of opposing fingers such as the index and thumb. They may develop elsewhere, however, including the lung parenchyma.

Ocular involvement in RA includes a secondary Sjögren's syndrome in 20% to 30% of patients; episcleritis appearing as a red, congested, slightly raised, tender scleral area in patients with high-titer rheumatoid factor and active extraarticular disease; and the dreaded nodular scleritis in which necrotic rheumatoid granuloma may lead to eye perforation (Table 12–4).

Pleuritis and *pericarditis* may be subclinical or clinically apparent. Serosal involvement is present in most cases of RA at autopsy but only a minority have recognized clinical disease, that is, pleuritic pain, rub, effusion, or pleural scarring. Rheumatoid pleural effusions tend to be unilateral, torpid, and are frequently asymptomatic. Pleural fluid is a predominantly mononuclear exudate with a very low glucose from decreased blood-to-pleura transfer and markedly decreased complement suggesting immune complexes disease. Pericarditis, which is also common pathologically but rare as a cause of symptoms, may present acutely with fever, pain, and a pericardial rub. Pericardial tamponade may rarely occur in these patients. Chronic rheumatoid pericarditis may also be effusive resulting in a large, often clinically silent pericardial sac, or effusive and fibrotic causing constriction of the heart. Chronic rheumatoid effusions, both pleural and pericardial, may be turbid or milky from myriad large, plate-shaped, negatively birefringent cholesterol crystals.

Parenchymal pulmonary involvement in RA includes pleural-based or intrapulmonary rheumatoid nodules, interstitial pulmonary disease, bronchiolitis obliterans with or without organizing pneumonia, and bronchiectasias. All forms of rheumatoid lung are more frequent in cigarette smoking patients. Single rheumatoid nodules need to be distinguished from primary lung neoplasms and multiple nodules from metastatic disease. Interstitial disease is uncommon clinically but is found in approximately 30% of patients by chest x-rays and simple pulmonary function tests. In addition, RA patients may have MTX- or gold-induced inflammatory interstitial disease. Bronchoscopy and BAL should be performed before establishing a diagnosis of MTX pneumonitis because opportunistic infections, in particular *P. carinii* pneumonitis, may complicate the course of immunosuppressive therapy in RA.

Rheumatoid vasculitis is relatively uncommon. Vessels of different caliber may be involved. A benign occlusive vasculopathy of the periungual vessels appearing as dark spots that subsequently peel off and a small-vessel vasculitis of the lower extremities presenting as a palpable purpura are the most common types of RA vasculitis. An infrequent type is a polyarteritis nodosa-like necrotizing vasculitis that features perimalleolar ulcers, splinter hemorrhages, bullous eruption, digital gangrene, various types of neuropathy including mononeuritis multiplex, and rarely gut or myocardial infarction. All forms of rheumatoid vasculitis are more frequent in patients with high-titer rheumatoid factor and additional features of extraarticular disease such as episcleritis, serositis, distal polyneuropathy, and Felty's syndrome. Initiation of

TABLE 12–4
DIFFERENTIAL DIAGNOSIS OF CONDITIONS THAT CAUSE ARTHRITIS AND EYE LESIONS

	Conjunctivitis	Keratitis	Scleritis	Iritis	Posterior Uveitis	Retinal Lesions
Rheumatoid arthritis		+	+			
JRA*				+		
Sjögren		+				
Lupus						+
Scleroderma						+
Necrotizing vasculitides						+
Wegener's granulomatosis		+		+	+	+
Giant cell arteritis						+
Takayasu						+
Reactive arthritis	+			+		
Ankylosing spondylitis				+		
Psoriatic arthritis				+		
Ulcerative colitis				+		
Crohn's†				+	+	
Behçet†				+	+	+
Sarcoidosis†		+		+	+	+
Microbial endocarditis†						+
Syphilis		+		+		
Lyme disease				+		
Whipple's				+	+	

*JRA = juvenile rheumatoid arthritis: oligoarthritis of lower extremities, chronic anterior uveitis, positive ANA.
†With or without arthritis.

steroids or a sudden change in steroid dose is said to cause necrotizing rheumatoid arteritis, but a steroid step up is more likely to occur in progressing disease, and disease often flares as steroids are reduced. Different from true polyarteritis nodosa, rheumatoid necrotizing arteritis features chronic synovitis, lacks renal involvement, and only rarely involves the gut.

Diagnosis

Summary of Diagnosis

> **RHEUMATOID ARTHRITIS: SYSTEMIC MANIFESTATIONS**
>
> - Systemic RA features one or more of the following: weight loss, high-titer RF, rheumatoid nodules, episcleritis, pulmonary interstitial disease, pleuritis, pericarditis, leg ulcers, palpable purpura, periungual skin infarctions, bullous eruption, digital gangrene, and neuropathy.
> - Identification of systemic RA is observer dependent. A careful history and physical examination repeated over time should focus on weight, lacrimary secretion (Schirmer's test; see Chapter 13), lymph nodes, skin status, chest status, spleen size, muscle strength, tendon reflexes, and skin sensation.
> - Compressive complications of RA include cricoarytenoid arthritis, various neuropathies, and medullary compression from atlantoaxial subluxation. Inquire about voice changes, sore throat, paresthesias, and cervical pain with radiation to extremities.
> - Voice changes and unexplained sore throat call for ENT evaluation.
> - Obtain a lateral film of the cervical spine in flexion as a baseline and repeat the study to detect atlantoaxial subluxation if the patient develops neck or occipital pain or neurologic findings. If abnormalities are found, request neurosurgical consultation.

Natural History

Expected Outcome

Systemic disease in RA usually indicates severe disease and associates with high titers of rheumatoid factor. The course of systemic RA varies with the individual manifestations. Fever readily corrects with anti-inflammatory treatment but improvement in anemia and thrombocytosis is slow, since it takes several months to a year to control disease activity. The rare systemic amyloidosis has a chronic course; amyloid deposition should be halted with disease remission. Rheumatoid nodules may acquire disfiguring proportions and, by creating pressure points, result in ulceration and secondary olecranon bursa infection. Episcleritis has no consequences to the eye but has a tendency to recur paralleling disease activity. Secondary Sjögren's is often minimally symptomatic in RA. Glandular enlargement, pulmonary interstitial lymphocytic pneumonitis, and pseudolymphoma or lymphoma are rare in RA-related Sjögren's. Episcleritis occurs in patients with additional manifestations of systemic RA such as vasculitis and serositis. Nodular scleritis is a more serious ophthalmologic complication of RA as it may cause eyeball perforation and visual loss.

Most cases of rheumatoid pleuritis and pericarditis are subclinical or have a mild course. Large effusions pose a diagnostic problem (infection and neoplasm must be ruled out) and may be difficult to control. Interstitial pulmonary disease has a chronic, stable, or slowly progressive course and may result in bronchiectasis and respiratory insufficiency. Pulmonary rheumatoid nodules are often a cause for concern but rarely create problems such as bullae or a bronchopleural fistula.

Periungual and palpable purpura-type vasculitis has a benign course, but necrotizing arteritis may result in severe neuropathic weakness, extensive skin infections, and rarely bowel perforation or myocardial infarction. A particularly poor prognosis triad includes extensive neuropathy of any type, vasculitic skin lesions, and a depressed complement. This form of vasculitis is rare, however. Overall, the excess mortality due to rheumatoid vasculitis is small.

Regarding compressive complications, cricoarytenoid arthritis is more of a nuisance and only exceptionally does it cause stridor; untreated carpal tunnel syndrome runs a progressive course and may lead to hand disability; atlantoaxial subluxation, especially if noted serendipitously, may be nonprogressive. Symptomatic cases must be evaluated neurosurgically to make sure that serious brain stem compression does not follow.

Treatment

Methods

Systemic RA is treated according to the individual manifestations. Optimization of basic treatment may be sufficient to control weight loss, chronic inflammation-induced anemia, thrombocytosis, some Felty's cases (leukopenia may improve on MTX or gold), some of the pleuropulmonary manifestations, and minor forms of vasculitis. Pericardial tamponade requires a pericardial window and a tapering course of high-dose steroids. Constrictive pericarditis calls for pericardiectomy; neither steroids nor immunosuppressive agents will loosen the fibrosis.

Necrotizing vasculitis is an indication to increase steroids and to reconsider stronger or combined second-line therapy, that is, cyclophosphamide or the addition of azathioprine. Cricoarytenoid arthritis may benefit from corticosteroid inhalations and, if unrelieved, by a brief course of oral steroids. Carpal tunnel syndrome often responds to corticosteroid infiltrations and a wrist splint in neutral. Surgical release in persisting cases usually includes synovectomy. Atlantoaxial subluxation is treated with C1–2 stabilization.

Expected Response

Response to treatment in systemic and compressive RA is generally satisfactory.

When to Refer

It is strongly advised that patients with systemic RA be promptly referred to, and primarily followed by, a rheumatologist. Persisting carpal tunnel syndrome should trigger rheumatology consultation. Atlantoaxial subluxation calls for joint assessment by a rheumatologist and a neurosurgeon.

Key Points

> **RHEUMATOID ARTHRITIS: SYSTEMIC MANIFESTATIONS**
>
> - Weight loss, chronic disease anemia, thrombocytosis, and a high ESR and/or CRP in RA indicate a severe, ongoing inflammatory response. The addition of low-dose corticosteroids should be considered in these instances.
> - Small-vessel vasculitis improves with a step up of basic treatment plus low-dose corticosteroids.
> - Necrotizing vasculitis, extensive neuropathy, and depressed complement levels call for high-dose corticosteroids and the possible addition of an immunosuppressive.
> - Symptomatic atlantoaxial subluxation requires prompt neurosurgical evaluation.
> - In associated Sjögren's, replace tears and insist on dental prophylaxis.
> - Felty's syndrome often improves with MTX or intramuscular gold. Leukocyte colony stimulating factor may help in intercurrent infection. Recurrent infections are an indication for splenectomy.
> - Amyloidosis is a rare complication of RA in the United States but is relatively frequent in Europe and Japan.
> - Pericardial tamponade usually requires a pericardial window.
> - Constrictive/effusive pericarditis is treated by pericardiectomy.

Suggested Reading

Anaya JM, Diethelm L, Ortiz LA, et al. Pulmonary involvement in rheumatoid arthritis. Sem Arthritis Rheum 24:242–254, 1995.

Bacon PA, Kitas GD. The significance of vascular inflammation in rheumatoid arthritis. Ann Rheum Dis 53:621–623, 1994.

Puechal X, Said G, Hilliquin P, et al. Peripheral neuropathy with necrotizing vasculitis in rheumatoid arthritis. A clinicopathologic and prognostic study of thirty-two patients. Arthritis Rheum 38:1618–1629, 1995.

Shadick NA, Fanta CH, Weinblatt ME, et al. Bronchiectasis. A late feature of severe rheumatoid arthritis. Medicine (Baltimore) 73:161–170, 1994.

Voskuyl AE, Zwinderman AH, Westedt ML, et al. The mortality of rheumatoid vasculitis compared with rheumatoid arthritis. Arthritis Rheum 39:266–271, 1996.

Watts RA, Carruthers DM, Scott DGI. Isolated nail fold vasculitis in rheumatoid arthritis. Ann Rheum Dis 54:927–929, 1995.

Rheumatoid Arthritis in the Elderly

Elderly-onset RA features an acute or subacute onset of symptoms, shoulder involvement is frequent, and prominent hand edema is often present. Conditions that share these findings include remitting seronegative symmetric synovitis with pitting edema (RS3PE), polymyalgia rheumatica (PMR), and late-onset spondyloarthropathy. Because the four conditions have different clinical implications (e.g., 15% of patients with polymyalgia rheumatica develop giant cell arteritis), an attempt should be made to establish a definite diagnosis.

Presentation and Progression

Cause

The higher prevalence of shoulder involvement in the elderly may relate to a high background of degenerative shoulder changes in this age group. The pathogenesis of the hand edema is unknown. Factors may include decreased mobility and lesser tissue coherence as if the loosened and wrinkled senile skin were particularly prone to fill with edema fluid. Table 12–5 contrasts features of late-onset RA, PMR, and RS3PE.

Presentation

Onset of RA is usually abrupt in elderly patients. Although peripheral joint synovitis, including MCPs, PIPs, and wrists, is the rule, shoulder complaints may be dominant. Hand edema is common. Lower extremity joints are less frequently involved than in the younger age group. As an example, MTP arthritis occurs in 90% of younger RA patients and in only 50% of late-onset RA. Approximately half of patients are RF positive. Late-onset spondyloarthropathy should be suspected in patients with enthesopathy (Achilles tendinitis, plantar fasciitis) and when inflammatory-type low back pain is present. Clinical findings in PMR, RS3PE, seronegative late-onset RA, and late-onset spondyloarthropathy may be quite similar.

Seropositive RA cases have a progressive and destructive course. As discussed under crystal-induced synovitides, both gout and CPPD pseudogout may have a rheumatoid-like appearance in the elderly. Also, certain solid tumors, particularly colon and lung cancer, may feature a rather similar paraneoplastic polyarthritis. Chest x-rays and a search for occult blood in the stools are important to rule out malignancy in presumed late-onset RA.

Diagnosis

Summary of Diagnosis

> **ELDERLY-ONSET RHEUMATOID ARTHRITIS**
> - Abrupt-onset polyarthritis involving predominantly upper extremity joints.
> - Shoulder involvement is common.
> - Lower extremity findings may be spared; only 50% of cases have MTP arthritis.
> - Fifty percent of cases are RF positive.
> - The condition must be distinguished from PMR, RS3PE syndrome, late-onset spondyloarthropathy, crystal synovitis, and malignancy-related arthritis.
> - Obtain chest x-rays and check stools for occult blood.
> - Joint aspiration is essential to rule out mimicking crystal synovitis.

TABLE 12–5

DIFFERENCES AND SIMILARITIES BETWEEN LATE-ONSET RHEUMATOID ARTHRITIS, POLYMYALGIA RHEUMATICA, AND REMITTING SERONEGATIVE SYMMETRICAL SYNOVITIS WITH PITTING EDEMA (RS3PE)

	Late-Onset Rheumatoid Arthritis	Polymyalgia Rheumatica	RS3PE
Age of onset	Over 60 years	Over 50 years	Over 60 years
Sex distribution (F/M)	1/1	2.5/1	1/4
Mode of onset	Acute or subtle	Acute	Acute
Predominant joint pattern	Peripheral joints in upper extremities, shoulders	Shoulders, lower back, hips, knees	Hands, wrists, shoulders, knees
Distal edema	May be present	May be present	Present
Rheumatoid factor positivity	Positive in 50%	Negative	Negative
HLA association	DR4	?	B7 in United States; no association with HLA-B antigen in France
Course	Severe in RF (+) Mild in RF (–)	Self-limited 1–3 years. Giant cell arteritis in 15%–20%	Self-limited 1–2 years. May be followed by RA, spondyloarthropathy, or connective tissue disease
Response to low-dose corticosteroids	Poor in RF (+) Good in RF (–)	Good	Good

Natural History

Expected Outcome

Elderly seronegative RA has a rather benign course. In contrast, seropositive cases tend to be locally and systemically aggressive. Invalidation and premature death often occur.

Treatment

Methods

Treatment of elderly-onset RA should take into account age-related factors. Because older patients often tolerate NSAIDS poorly, preference should be given to milder agents such as nabumetone and ibuprofen. By allowing greater mobility, low-dose prednisone, 5 to 10 mg per day, may be critical to maintain independent living. Because older patients tend to be vitamin D and calcium deficient, 1 g of calcium plus calcitriol 0.25 µg should be routinely added to slow down progression of steroid-induced osteoporosis and to avert the risk of osteomalacia. The author has been eager to use MTX in elderly patients with RA. Because effective doses tend to be small in this age group (7.5–10 mg/week), treatment should be started at 5 mg once a week with 2.5 mg dose increments every 3 weeks until improvement has occurred or a 15 mg weekly dose has been used without improvement for 3 weeks, at which point both diagnosis and therapy should be reconsidered. Needless to say, folate supplementation is essential in this age group. A recommendation that applies to all patients with RA but is particularly relevant to older patients is to obtain vitamin B_{12} and folate levels prior to initiating MTX. Subclinical B_{12} deficiency should be detected, since with the use of folate the hematologic aspects of B_{12} deficiency will be prevented but neurologic disease may progress unchecked.

Rehabilitation measures should be applied early to attain the goal of maintaining independence. Formal occupational and physical therapy evaluation should be requested. Patients should be provided assistive devices, and safety modifications may have to be implemented in their homes. To name just a few, Velcro buttons, elastic shoelaces, long-handled shoehorns, bulky handles for utensils, bedside commode, shower bench, and rails go a long way toward making life easier and safer for these patients. Energy conservation measures and stretching, strengthening, and endurance exercises should also be emphasized.

Expected Response

Treatment response is dramatic in many cases of elderly-onset RA, particularly in the seronegative group. Unfortunately, disease course tends to be rapidly progressive and malignant in patients with seropositive RA.

When to Refer

After rheumatologic evaluation most cases of seronegative elderly-onset RA can be handled by primary care physicians. Severe seropositive cases should be followed in close cooperation with a rheumatologist.

Key Points

> **ELDERLY-ONSET RHEUMATOID ARTHRITIS**
> - Seronegative elderly-onset RA tends to have a benign course.
> - Seropositive cases, however, tend to be progressive and invalidating.
> - Seropositive elderly-onset RA should be treated early and aggressively.
> - Seronegative cases should be clearly distinguished from crystal-induced synovitis and malignancy-related arthritis. Ruling out PMR and RS3PE may be difficult if not impossible.
> - Symptoms and findings of giant cell arteritis should be frequently investigated in patients with presumed late-onset seronegative RA.
> - Spontaneous disease remission after one to a few years indicates the condition was either PMR or RS3PE, rather than RA.

Suggested Reading

Michet CJ Jr, Evans JM, Fleming KC, et al. Common rheumatologic diseases in elderly patients. Mayo Clin Proc 70:1205–1214, 1995.

van Schaardenburg D, Breedveld FC. Elderly-onset rheumatoid arthritis. Sem Arthritis Rheum 23:367–378, 1994.

Polymyalgia Rheumatica (PMR)

Polymyalgia rheumatica is a common systemic inflammatory disorder in the older age group. The condition must be distinguished from other systemic rheumatic disorders, malignant disease, and metabolic disease.

Presentation and Progression

Cause

The cause of PMR is unknown; epidemiologic studies have failed to demonstrate seasonal or secular patterns in this condition. Prevalence of PMR in the population over 50 years is 0.6%, which is roughly half the prevalence of RA. Women are affected twice as frequently as males (Table 12–5). Interestingly, 15% of patients with PMR have giant cell arteritis (GCA) and 30% of GCA patients have PMR (see Chapter 16). GCA may precede, be concurrent, or follow the clinical onset (and treatment) of PMR.

Presentation

In an older person the sudden onset of malaise plus shoulder, neck, hip, and thigh stiffness and pain should raise the suspicion of PMR. Symptoms are typically worse during the night and in the early morning hours. Headache, jaw claudication, or other cephalic symptoms may indicate an associated GCA. Physical examination reveals pain on passive motions of the shoulder and hip suggestive of synovitis. Small knee effusions may be present. Carpal tunnel syndrome is a frequent association. Uni- or bilateral hand edema occurs in 10% of patients.

Muscle weakness is not a feature of PMR, but proximal muscle strength may be inhibited by pain. Fever and severe weight loss should raise the suspicion of infective endocarditis or a solid tumor. Ribs and sternum should be examined for tenderness indicative of multiple myeloma. Hypothyroidism and osteomalacia should also be considered in the differential. Thus, laboratory evaluation should include CBC, platelet count, ESR/CRP, alkaline phosphatase, ALT, CPK, TSH, Ca, P, rheumatoid factor, ANA, and serum protein electrophoresis. The presence of thrombocytosis, a very high ESR (in up to 20% the ESR is normal), and elevation of liver enzymes (in particular the serum alkaline phosphatase) in one-third of cases, plus absence of evidence of an underlying disease support the diagnosis of PMR. Synovial fluid analysis reveals mild inflammation with WBC 1000 to 20,000/mm^3 and a predominance of mononuclear cells. Studies of synovial membrane have shown mild nonspecific lymphocytic synovitis. Except in the minority of GCA-associated cases, diagnosis of PMR is clinical. Most authorities agree that temporal artery biopsy in patients without GCA symptoms is not required.

Diagnosis

Summary of Diagnosis

POLYMYALGIA REUMATICA

- Age older than 50.
- Female/male ratio 2.5 to 1.
- Proximal pain and stiffness.
- Severe nocturnal symptoms.
- Protracted a.m. stiffness.
- Evidence of GCA in 15% of cases; request temporal artery biopsy if there are suggestive findings.
- Very high ESR in 80%, thrombocytosis, elevated LFTs in 30%.
- Normal CPK, serum protein electrophoresis, TSH, Ca, and P.
- Negative blood cultures and normal cardiac echo if fever is present.

Natural History

Expected Outcome

Polymyalgia rheumatica is a self-limited condition that burns out after 1 to 3 years of activity. There are no complications of the disease other than the ocular and other ischemic manifestations in cases associated with GCA. GCA may become apparent after initiation of therapy for PMR at a time when the ESR is normal or minimally elevated. This notion underscores the need to keep a close tab on PMR patients with visits no longer than 2 weeks apart in the first months of therapy and on a monthly basis thereafter.

Treatment

Methods

Cases without clinical evidence of GCA may be treated with NSAIDs or low-dose prednisone. One approach is to administer full doses of a potent NSAID such as naproxen or diclofenac for 1 to 2 weeks. If no improvement ensues, the NSAID is discontinued and low-dose corticosteroids are begun. Initial prednisone dose should be 10 or 15 mg per day administered as a single morning dose. Once the patient becomes asymptomatic and the ESR normal, a slow dose reduction should be undertaken by removing 1 mg every 2 to 4 weeks. Residual symptoms with only a minimal elevation of ESR may be controlled by adding a mild NSAID such as nabumetone or ibuprofen. There is seldom a need to use alternative medications such as hydroxychloroquine or methotrexate. The addition of one of these agents should be considered in protracted cases that require 10 mg or more of prednisone daily for several months and when the metabolic complications of the corticosteroid are feared.

Expected Response

On low-dose prednisone symptoms subside over 1 to 2 weeks. The ESR usually normalizes in 2 to 4 weeks.

Complications

Complications of protracted corticosteroid treatment are common during PMR treatment, in particular an accelerated bone mineral loss with aggravation of osteoporosis. However, if prophylactic precautions are taken, that is, calcium plus vitamin D supplementation (see corticosteroid-induced osteoporosis), and the steroid is kept at the lowest effective dose, clinical complications are rare.

When to Refer

Suspected cases of PMR should be referred to a rheumatologist for diagnostic confirmation and treatment advice. Once evaluated, provided there is no clinical evidence of GCA, patients with PMR may be followed by primary care physicians. Needless to say, any physician following a case of PMR should become conversant with the natural course and possible complications of the condition.

Key Points

POLYMYALGIA RHEUMATICA

- A self-limited condition featuring proximal synovitis predominantly in the hip and shoulder joints.
- A normal ESR may be a cause of delayed diagnosis and treatment.
- Fifteen percent of cases have an associated GCA.
- Clinical GCA may precede, be concurrent with, or follow onset of PMR.
- Temporal artery biopsy is not required in absence of GCA symptoms.
- The vast majority of PMR cases are uncomplicated and therefore benign.
- Initial treatment of PMR should be with NSAIDs. In most instances low-dose corticosteroids will be required.

- Prophylaxis of steroid-induced osteoporosis should be implemented early.
- A frequent and thorough follow-up allows an early detection of complicating GCA.

Suggested Reading

Chung T-Y, Hunder GG, Ilstrup DM, et al. Polymyalgia rheumatica: A 10-year epidemiologic and clinical study. Ann Intern Med 97:672–680, 1982.

Ferraccioli GF, Salaffi F, De Vita S, Casatta L, Bartoli E. MTX in PMR: Preliminary results of an open, randomized study. J Rheumatol 23:624–628, 1996.

Helfgott SM, Kieval RI. Polymyalgia rheumatica in patients with a normal erythrocyte sedimentation rate. Arthritis Rheum 39:304–307, 1996.

Salvarani C, Gabriel S, Hunder GG. Distal extremity swelling with pitting edema in polymyalgia rheumatica. Arthritis Rheum 39:73–80, 1996.

Salvarani C, Gabriel SE, O'Fallon WM, et al. Epidemiology of polymyalgia rheumatica in Olmsted County, Minnesota, 1970–1991. Arthritis Rheum 38:369–373, 1995.

Remitting Seronegative Symmetrical Synovitis with Pitting Edema (RS3PE)

This recently described condition is controversial. Marked distal edema is a constant feature of RS3PE but is also a frequent finding in old-age synovitis regardless of etiology (RA, gout, CPPD pseudogout). A diagnosis of RS3PE should only be accepted after thorough consideration of alternative diagnoses.

Presentation and Progression

Cause

The cause of RS3PE as a separate entity is unknown. There is good evidence that on follow-up some cases evolve into known conditions such as RA or spondyloarthropathy.

Presentation

Salient features of RS3PE include age older than 60, male predominance, an abrupt onset of symptoms, florid symmetric distal polyarthritis, and the presence of diffuse pitting edema in the involved areas. The latter is the most peculiar feature of RS3PE although, as noted later, is not specific for the condition. Laboratory findings include a very high ESR, a negative RF test, and an increased prevalence of the HLA-B7 antigen found in the United States but not in France. A unilateral condition involving exclusively the moving side has been seen in patients with hemiparesis. Although pseudogout and gout can be ruled out based on x-ray findings (absence of chondrocalcinosis) and joint aspiration (absence of CPPD and MSU crystals), it is difficult to distinguish RS3PE from RA and polymyalgia rheumatica. A definite diagnosis may have to be deferred to the patient's course. The distal pattern of joint involvement in RS3PE and RA is opposite to the proximal pattern in polymyalgia rheumatica; furthermore, polymyalgia rheumatica runs a self-limited course allowing interruption of treatment after 1 to 3 years. Distinguishing late-onset RA and RS3PE is more difficult because in a retrospective study done in France the latter may merge into RA, spondyloarthropathy, or other disease.

Summary of Diagnosis

REMITTING SERONEGATIVE SYMMETRICAL SYNOVITIS WITH PITTING EDEMA (RS3PE)

- Age over 60.
- Male predominance.
- Abrupt onset.
- Distal synovitis.
- Distal pitting edema.
- Consider gout, CPPD, RA, spondyloarthropathy.
- Obtain hand x-rays, a pelvic film to rule out sacroiliitis, UA level, RF, and joint aspiration.
- Obtain serum protein electrophoresis to rule out multiple myeloma.

Natural History

Expected Outcome

Spontaneous resolution usually occurs within 18 months. In the French experience many of the patients eventually developed RA or spondyloarthropathy. Some went on to connective tissue disease.

Complications of RS3PE are few; the author has seen acute carpal tunnel syndome requiring emergency decompression and a rare case of tendon rupture.

Treatment

Methods

Patients with SR3PE are treated in the same fashion as late-onset RA and polymyalia rheumatica. A nonsteroidal anti-inflammatory agent such as nabumetone, ibuprofen, or naproxen should be used first. If symptoms are not fully controlled within 1 to 2 weeks, hydroxychloroquine may be added. Because hydroxychloroquine has such a delayed action, prednisone 7.5 or 10 mg daily may be used as a bridging medication. Alternatively, reduced doses of MTX (7.5–10 mg per week) may be added. Calcium and vitamin D supplementation is an essential adjunct if steroids are used.

Expected Response

The condition is usually brought under control within a few weeks. Given its self-limiting course, discontinuation of therapy after 1½ to 2 years is a realistic goal.

When to Refer

Patients with suspected RS3PE would benefit from rheumatologic consultation. Wrist aspiration to rule out crystalline disease is not done easily and should be performed by someone with experience. Also, as mentioned earlier, it may be difficult to extricate RS3PE from RA and polymyalgia rheumatica. Once a firm diagnosis is made and treatment is under way, patients may be followed by the primary care physician.

Key Points

REMITTING SERONEGATIVE SYMMETRICAL SYNOVITIS WITH PITTING EDEMA (RS3PE)

- Accuracy in diagnosis is essential (rule out crystal disease and make an effort to separate RS3PE from late-onset RA and PMR).
- Although it was originally described as a self-limited disease transition to RA, spondyloarthropathy or connective tissue disease may occur, at least in the French experience.
- The evidence in support of the previous statement is retrospective. Differences in genetic background may also be involved.
- Treatment of RS3PE and late-onset RA is similar.
- Response to treatment is excellent, at least in the short term.

Suggested Reading

McCarty DJ, O'Duffy JD, Pearson L, et al. Remitting seronegative symmetrical synovitis with pitting edema. JAMA 254:2763–2767, 1985.

Schaeverbeke T, Fatout E, Marcé S, et al. Remitting seronegative symmetrical synovitis with pitting oedema: Disease or syndrome? Ann Rheum Dis 54:682–684, 1995.

CHAPTER 13

Systemic Lupus Erythematosus (SLE), Primary Antiphospholipid Syndrome, and Sjögren's Syndrome

Systemic lupus erythematosus (SLE) is a multisystem, relapsing disease with the potential to involve skin, mucosae, serosae, lungs, heart, kidneys, joints, the central and peripheral nervous system, and blood elements. There is an array of laboratory abnormalities, especially blood cytopenias, plus the presence of multiple autoantibodies.

The most prevalent immunologic finding in SLE is a positive ANA. ANA-negative SLE is rare (less than 5% with current techniques) and tends to be seen in patients with anti-Ro (SSA), anti-single-stranded DNA antibodies, or congenital C_2 deficiency. A randomly obtained positive ANA is rarely indicative of, or predictive of, SLE. Positive ANAs occur in a host of additional conditions, particularly RA, scleroderma, and Sjögren's. Also, ANAs are positive in 5% or more of normal individuals depending on the age. An imprudently obtained positive ANA (such as in a patient with fibromyalgia) becomes a source of concern and expense. In a patient with consistent clinical findings, however, a positive ANA strongly favors SLE. Further diagnostic certainty is provided by (1) a positive test for SLE-specific antibodies dsDNA or Sm (40% of cases), (2) fulfilling additional SLE classification criteria at the time of evaluation or on follow-up, and (3) exclusion of mimicking conditions.

There is a large set of conditions, led by subacute bacterial endocarditis, that should at least be considered before establishing a diagnosis of SLE. A diagnostically important but often forgotten finding in SLE is the presence of ready-made LE cells in Wright stains of pleural, pericardial, synovial, and peritoneal effusions. Younger readers may wonder what LE cells are. They are PMNs that have phagocytosed an entire altered nucleus that now appears as a homogeneous purple inclusion body displacing the PNN nucleus to the periphery of the cell. In the LE test, which is rarely requested today because ANAs on Hep-2 cells are far more sensitive (95% as opposed to 60%), the LE cell phenomenon occurs "in vitro": Bare nuclei from mechanically fragmented cells bind antinuclear antibodies, fix and activate complement, and attract viable PMNs that phagocytose the altered free nuclei resulting in the "LE cell." Cavitary effusions in SLE have all the ingredients to produce "in vivo" LE cells: free nuclei from broken-down cells, viable PMNs, ANAs, and complement. Finding spontaneous LE cells may be particularly important when patients are admitted, as an example, on Friday night.

The test costs nothing if you yourself inspect the smear. A confirmatory ANA is, of course, requested.

SLE is overwhelmingly more frequent in women with a female/male ratio of 10 to 1. Two-thirds of cases appear during the childbearing years and only one-third in the pediatric and old-age groups. An unexplained increased incidence of SLE has been noted among blacks and Hispanics.

There are no agreed upon diagnostic criteria for SLE. The widely used American College of Rheumatology (ACR) SLE classification criteria (Table 13–1) have been designed for patient classification for clinical trials and epidemiologic studies rather than diagnosis. They are a useful guide, however, to use during the process of diagnosis. There are conditions such as the primary antiphospholipid syndrome, subacute bacterial endocarditis, and leprosy in which patients may fulfill more than the required four SLE classification criteria. Conversely, SLE may be confidently diagnosed in patients fulfilling only two criteria if these criteria are anti-dsDNA antibodies and red cell casts on urine sediment. Indeed, cases of bona fide SLE fulfilling less than the required four classification criteria appear to have the same degree of significant organ involvement as cases that fulfill four or more criteria.

Conspicuously absent from the SLE classification criteria are some of the very manifestations that make clinicians consider SLE including prolonged fever, malaise, alopecia, Raynaud's phenomenon, and a relapsing disease course. Important as they are clinically, these manifestations lacked the required specificity to make it to the classification criteria.

It is now well established that tissue damage in SLE is mostly immune complex mediated. Antibodies entering intact cells are also involved, particularly in the pathogenesis of the renal lesion. The multiplicity of autoantibodies in SLE is explained by two overlapping mechanisms: (1) a somewhat restricted polyclonal antibody response, and (2) an antigen-driven antibody response probably triggered by nucleosomal antigens. Genetic, hormonal, and environmental factors are heavily involved in disease pathogenesis. Genetic predisposition to SLE is conferred by the HLA-B8, DR2, and DR3 alleles as well as C_2 and C_{4A} deficiency. Prominent among environmental factors is ultraviolet light exposure, particularly ultraviolet B (290 to 320 nm). In addition to sunlight, ultraviolet B radiation is emitted by unshielded white fluorescent lamps. Ultraviolet exposure may not only cause exacerbation of cutaneous lesions but also systemic disease activity.

TABLE 13–1

THE AMERICAN RHEUMATISM ASSOCIATION 1982 REVISED CRITERIA FOR THE CLASSIFICATION OF SYSTEMIC LUPUS ERYTHEMATOSUS

CRITERION (Definition)

1. *Malar rash* (fixed erythema, flat or raised, over the malar eminences, tending to spare the nasolabial folds)
2. *Discoid rash* (erythematous raised patches with adherent keratotic scaling and follicular plugging; atrophic scarring may occur in older lesions)
3. *Photosensitivity* (skin rash as a result of unusual reaction to sunlight, by patient history or physical observation)
4. *Oral ulcers* (oral or nasopharyngeal ulceration, usually painless, observed by a physician)
5. *Arthritis* (nonerosive arthritis involving 2 or more peripheral joints, characterized by tenderness, swelling, or effusion)
6. *Serositis* ([a] pleuritis—convincing history of pleuritic pain or rub heard by a physician or evidence of pleural effusion OR [b] pericarditis—documented by ECG or rub or evidence of pericardial effusion)
7. *Renal disorder* ([a] persistent proteinuria greater than 0.5 gram per day or greater than 3+ if quantitation not performed OR [b] cellular casts—may be red cell, hemoglobin, granular, tubular, or mixed)
8. *Neurologic disorder* ([a] seizures—in the absence of offending drugs or known metabolic derangements, e.g., uremia, ketoacidosis, or electrolyte imbalance OR [b] psychosis—in the absence of offending drugs or known metabolic derangements, e.g., uremia, ketoacidosis, or electrolyte imbalance)
9. *Hematologic disorder* ([a] hemolytic anemia—with reticulocytosis OR [b] leukopenia—less than 4000/mm^3 on 2 or more occasions OR [c] lymphopenia—less than 1500/mm^3 on 2 or more occasions OR [d] thrombocytopenia—less than 100,000/mm^3 in the absence of offending drugs)
10. *Immunologic disorder* ([a] positive LE cell preparation OR [b] anti-DNA: antibody to native DNA in abnormal titer OR [c] anti-Sm: presence of antibody to Sm nuclear antigen OR [d] false positive serologic test for syphilis known to be positive for at least 6 months and confirmed by *Treponema pallidum* immobilization or fluorescent treponemal absorption test)
11. *Antinuclear antibody* (an abnormal titer of antinuclear antibody by immunofluorescence or an equivalent assay at any point in time and in the absence of drugs known to be associated with "drug-induced lupus" syndrome)

Note: The proposed classification is based on 11 criteria. For the purpose of identifying patients in clinical studies, a person shall be said to have systemic lupus erythematosus if any 4 or more of the 11 criteria are present, serially or simultaneously, during any period of observation.

Outcome in SLE depends on demographic, socioeconomic, and vital organ involvement. The condition has a worse prognosis in patients with a low socioeconomic level, older patients (> 50 at diagnosis), and in patients with kidney damage, lung damage, thrombocytopenia, and very active disease. The toxicity of the drugs required for disease control must also be added. Prognosis in SLE has vastly improved over the past three decades presumably as the combined result of earlier detection, effective corticosteroid and immunosuppressive treatment, availability of antibiotics, newer antihypertensive agents, improvements in intensive care, and organ transplantation. Overall, a 90% survival may be expected at 10 years. Frequent causes of death include infection, active SLE, and acute vascular events, in particular atheromatous myocardial infarction. Mortality in SLE conforms to a bimodal pattern with early deaths (less than 5 years from diagnosis) being due predominantly to active SLE and infections and late deaths being caused by infection, premature vascular disease, and end organ failure. SLE is a treacherous condition in which treatment strategies must be frequently adjusted to unexpected events. Except in mild cases, which may be followed by primary care physicians, SLE clearly belongs in the field of rheumatology.

For the purpose of this discussion, which emphasizes diagnosis and management, SLE is arbitrarily divided into mild SLE, renal SLE, neuropsychiatric SLE, pleuropulmonary SLE, discoid LE (DLE) and subacute cutaneous lupus erythematosus (SCLE), pregnancy and SLE, SLE and fever, and drug-induced SLE. Two closely related sections include one on the primary and secondary antiphospholipid syndrome (PAPS and SAPS), a condition that may be confused with SLE, and the other on Sjögren's syndrome.

Suggested Reading

Abu-Shakra M, Urowitz MB, Gladman DD, et al. Mortality studies in SLE. Results from a single center. I. Causes of death. J Rheumatol 22:1259–1264, 1995.

Abu-Shakra M, Urowitz MB, Gladman DD, et al. Mortality studies in systemic lupus erythematosus. Results from a single center. II. Predictor variables for mortality. J Rheumatol 22:1265–1270, 1995.

Calvo-Alén J, Bastian HM, Straaton KV, et al. Identification of patients subsets among those presumptively diagnosed with, referred, and/or followed up for systemic lupus erythematosus at a large tertiary center. Arthritis Rheum 38:1475–1484, 1995.

Ward M, Studenski S. Long-term survival in systemic lupus erythematosus. Arthritis Rheum 38:274–283, 1995.

Mild SLE

Presentation and Progression

Cause

Mild SLE comprises most cases of the condition as seen in a primary care setting. The reasons why SLE may be mild in some patients and a devastating condition in others can only be speculated on.

Usual Symptoms and Signs

Clinical manifestations in mild SLE are highly variable. Patients may or not (most do) fulfill the required four or more ARA SLE classification criteria. Symptoms include low-grade fever, malaise, fatigue, alopecia, rash, Raynaud's phenomenon, arthralgias, and pleuritic pain. Visual symptoms, migraines, and decreased memory are frequent in this setting. Findings on examination include malar rash (about 50%); discoid lupus (less than 10%); upper eyelid, periungual, and mottled palmar erythema (very much observer-dependent findings); vasculitic lesions (Figure 13–1), painful or painless oropharyngeal or nasal ulcerations (10% to 30%); lymphadenopathy; arthralgias; generally nonerosive yet sometimes deforming arthritis; pleural or pericardial rub; and splenomegaly.

Leukopenia, lymphopenia, and a normal or slightly decreased platelet count may be present. Serum creatinine

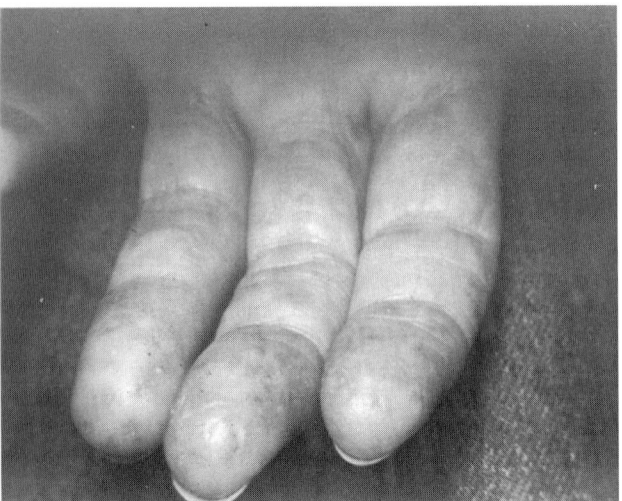

FIGURE 13-1. *Systemic lupus erythematosus.* Many episodes of small-vessel vasculitis resulted in pitted scars and loss of digital pulp.

and urinalysis are normal. Immunologic studies reveal a positive ANA with a predominantly diffuse or speckled pattern of fluorescence, normal or modestly elevated levels of dsDNA or Sm antibodies, and normal or slightly depressed C_3, C_4, or CH50 complement determinations. Thus, by definition patients with mild SLE lack significant renal, CNS, pulmonary, and hematologic disease.

Diagnosis

Summary of Diagnosis

> **SLE**
> - Multisystem involvement by history and physical examination.
> - CBC, platelet count, serum creatinine, ALT, CPK, urinalysis with detailed examination of sediment, TSH.
> - Chest x-rays.
> - Consider alternative diagnoses: connective tissue diseases, infection, neoplasm.
> - ANA determination on Hep-2 cells (sensitivity).
> - Serum C_3, C_4; CH50; dsDNA, Sm (specificity).

Natural History

Expected Outcome

Protracted flares and remissions are the rule in mild SLE. Flares may follow a pattern that repeats over time. Increasing hair loss, malaise, a mounting ESR, a falling complement, and higher levels of dsDNA antibodies are often premonitory of a flare. Disease flares may include arthralgias or arthritis involving small joints of the hand, wrists, elbows, knees, and ankles; a more pronounced rash; small-vessel vasculitis; or pleuritic pain with a pleural or pericardial rub. These may occur as single manifestations or in a cluster. As the flare subsides the previous state of health is resumed without accruing organ damage. Although the usual course of the condition is to remain circumscribed to non-life-threatening events there are occasional patients in whom glomerulonephritis or CNS disease develops. Disease progression is more likely to occur in the first 3 years following diagnosis. Thus, patients with early mild SLE should be followed frequently, perhaps every month until time proves that the condition is stable.

History and physical examination should emphasize detection of possible SLE involvements (see history taking in introduction). Laboratory determinations should include CBC, platelet count, ESR, serum creatinine, urinalysis, serum C_3 and CH50, and dsDNA antibodies. Each of these tests serves a specific purpose (some might argue that the ESR should not be included; I do). On the other hand, studies that are not likely to help should not be requested. These include immune complexes determination and serial ANA, RF, VDRL, and serum protein electrophoresis. In mild SLE blood parameters should be normal or slightly decreased. The ESR fluctuates with disease activity; stable normal values are the goal. Serum creatinine should not increase. Only a minimal proteinuria or a few RBCs without red cell casts should be allowed. Complement levels should not fall and dsDNA antibodies should not rise.

The importance of a carefully done urinalysis every time the patient visits the office cannot be overemphasized. There is no substitute for the focused attention the primary care physician, rheumatologist, or nephrologist applies in performing this basic study. A minimal urine evaluation includes a dipstick determination for protein and hemoglobin and, most importantly, an adequately performed urine sediment. To this end the urine is spun 5 minutes at 2000 to 3000 rpm in a conical tube. After centrifugation the supernatant is removed except the final 1 mL by tilting the tube. The tube, now held vertical, is gently tapped two or three times with the pulp of a finger to resuspend the sediment. A drop of this concentrate is placed on a clean slide and covered with a clean coverslide. Finally the sample is inspected with the condenser set low and a dim light first at $10\times$ and then at $40\times$ in a darkened room.

Treatment

Methods

A physician who treats SLE patients must be informed, sensitive to the well-founded concerns of the patient, compulsive in implementing a detailed follow-up, conservative when no life-threatening involvements are encountered, and daring when decisive action is required. Mild SLE cases with predominantly skin and joint involvement respond well to simple measures. These patients can and should be followed by primary care physicians with only occasional input from a rheumatologist. Patients may change, however, and primary care physicians should be ready to seek consultation or transfer the patient in the event of deterioration. Needless to say, ongoing flexible relationships among primary care physician, rheumatologist, and nephrologist are essential in the long-term care of SLE patients.

General Recommendations: (1) Patients with mild SLE should be reassured about the benign nature of the condition in terms of physical disability and life expectancy. Minimal or no organ damage accrues in most cases even after decades of disease. Cognitive dysfunction detectable by sophisticated neurophysiologic testing with little effect on most patients' lifestyle is one exception. Another exception are occasional nonerosive joint deformities (Jaccoud's arthritis) that seldom acquire the severity seen in RA. Patients should be made aware, however, that changes in the condition may occur in the first few years of disease and a close follow-up is essential for early detection and appropriate therapy. (2) Patients should be informed of pregnancy-related issues (see section on pregnancy in lupus) and the very small likelihood of transmitting the disease to the offspring: Although antinuclear antibodies are present in 20% of first-degree relatives of SLE patients, autoimmune disease occurs in less than 10%, which includes cases of autoimmune thyroid disease. Patients often feel reassured by knowing that disease concordance in homozygous twins is less than 30%. (3) An accompanying depressive component, which is understandably present in many SLE patients, should be identified and treated. (4) All unnecessary medications should be discontinued. (5) Patients should be given advice on how to protect themselves from ultraviolet light. Pharmaceutical industry advances on high-grade sun filters and blockers do not obviate the need to implement common sense measures that add significant protection: Patients should wear, if possible, a hat and long-sleeve shirt. If a trip to the beach is contemplated or if patients want to swim or practice outside sports, sun exposure should be avoided in the hours of greatest brightness (10 a.m. to 4 p.m.). And even so they should use a hat and a filter or blocker on the entire exposed skin (see appendix). There is evidence that unfiltered fluorescent light (bare fluorescent lamps) emit significant ultraviolet B radiation that may be sensed by photosensitive patients. The usual acrylic diffuser of fluorescent lamps eliminates this problem by decreasing both the ultraviolet B output and the ultraviolet B/ultraviolet A ratio. (6) Although estrogen use doubles the risk of developing SLE, estrogen treatment of perimenopausal and postmenopausal patients has not been shown to aggravate SLE. Perimenopausal SLE patients should therefore be encouraged to use estrogens with progesterone for the prevention of both osteoporosis and coronary artery disease, conditions known to be aggravated by corticosteroid use. (7) Follow-up of mild SLE patients by primary care physicians assures that all routine health maintenance examinations will be timely done.

Medications: Drugs used in mild SLE should be effective in suppressing inflammation and also safe. The disease itself has few serious complications, and physicians should avoid falling into the "treatment is worse than the disease" trap. Most of the research done on treatment of SLE has focused on severe manifestations of the disease, in particular lupus nephritis. There have been few studies on the treatment of mild SLE. The recommendations that follow are based on collective experience and common sense, although supporting studies are quoted where applicable.

Inflammation, the basic lesion in SLE, brings up the use of anti-inflammatory agents. Nonacetylated salicylates such as choline magnesium trisalicylate 1500 mg bid or salsalate 1 g bid in this setting make special sense for several reasons: First, gastric irritation is unusual with these agents; second, because SLE patients are potentially thrombocytopenic, one should choose agents that do not interfere with platelet aggregation; third, nonacetylated salicylates have little effect on glomerular filtration, and this may be important if an occasional patient has subclinical kidney disease. Similar benefits apply to nabumetone, a mild pro-drug anti-inflammatory agent taken in a single or divided dose of 1000 to 2000 mg per day.

Other NSAIDs may, of course, be used in SLE. They all possess an inhibitor effect on platelets, are gastrotoxic, and have the potential to reduce glomerular filtration. The purported renal safety of sulindac has been disputed. In addition, NSAIDs may cause meningismus with ibuprofen being the most frequently incriminated agent. All NSAIDs are potentially hepatotoxic, and patients with SLE appear to be at a higher risk for this complication. Fortunately the condition is mild and asymptomatic.

In addition to an anti-inflammatory agent the use of hydroxychloroquine (HQ) should be considered. Indeed, in the author's practice, most mild SLE patients are on chronic HQ therapy. This medication, started at 400 mg per day for 1 month and continued at 200 mg per day, appears to have a stabilizing effect indefinitely on the condition. Larger doses may be required such as 400 mg per day for 2 years subsequently decreased to 200 mg per day. Hydroxychloroquine improves skin lesions, articular manifestations, serositis, and may have a beneficial effect on fatigue and cognitive dysfunction. The beneficial effect on joints has been documented in a double-blind trial of hydroxychloroquine discontinuation in which patients who received a placebo fared worse than those who continued the active drug. An additional beneficial effect of HQ, which inhibits platelet aggregation and adhesion, is to contribute to the prevention of thromboembolic complications for patients with a secondary antiphospholipid syndrome. For the time being and until more is known about the antithrombotic efficacy of HQ at the doses used (which are one-quarter of the doses used for short-term anticoagulation in patients with total hip replacement reported by Charnley), SLE patients with the antiphospholipid syndrome should be placed on anticoagulation irrespective of the use of HQ.

The usual precautions in patients on HQ treatment include an initial ophthalmologic evaluation and periodic reevaluations at 6 to 12 month intervals. As it turns out, ophthalmologic testing varies with the interests of the ophthalmologist. A common routine is to administer visual fields and acuity, color vision tests, an Amsler grid, and a fundus examination.

The therapeutic effect of HQ takes place slowly beginning after a lag time of 6 weeks and reaching full effect after 3 to 6 months. When HQ is discontinued, disease flares predictably occur within 1 to 3 months.

In the event of pregnancy experts' opinions are divided. Some believe it safer for the mother and the fetus to continue the HQ through pregnancy rather than discontinuing it, which risks a lupus flare with the attendant risk of fetal loss. Other authorities recommend stopping the drug when the patient finds out she is pregnant and use steroids if the condition flares. According to the FDA, the drug is rated C in use-in-pregnancy ratings. Breast feeding while taking HQ is contraindicated. This means that risk cannot be ruled out but potential benefits may justify the potential risk.

Disease fluctuations uncontrolled with the use of a nonacetylated salicylate in the therapeutic range (plasma levels of 15 to 30 mg/dl), or nabumetone, or other NSAID if desired plus HQ may be treated by doubling the HQ dose for 1 to 2 months or by adding low-dose corticosteroids.

Prednisone doses used in mild SLE are in the range of 10 to 20 mg per day, preferably below 20 to decrease the risk of osteonecrosis. Unfortunately, bone mineral loss is significant even with 7 to 10 mg per day doses. Prophylaxis of osteoporosis with calcium and vitamin D supplementation (see corticosteroid-induced osteoporosis) is a must in female or male SLE patients receiving corticosteroids. Once the desired therapeutic effect has been achieved, a slow dose reduction should be undertaken, for example, 1 mg every week or two. The use of 1 mg tablets is very practical for steroid reduction. Certain SLE manifestations are exquisitely sensitive to dose changes. The author has seen, for instance, a patient whose platelet counts consistently decreased from 80,000 to 90,000/mm^3 to 30,000 to 40,000/mm^3 when the prednisone dose was reduced from 5 to 4 mg per day, and vice versa, an experiment that was repeated several times until a stable dose of 5 mg was settled on. More often patients require 10 to 15 mg of prednisone per day to remain symptom free.

Low-dose methotrexate as used in RA has been employed with success as a steroid-sparing agent in mild SLE. The use of methotrexate, with a schedule similar to that used in RA, should be considered when steroids have caused significant side effects (psychosis, cataracts, osteonecrosis, difficult to control arterial hypertension) as well as in patients who are unwilling to take them.

Expected Response

Remember that nonacetylated salicylates, similar to all salicylates, have a 5 to 7 day lag before a plateau is reached. Also, as higher serum salicylate levels are achieved, saturation of metabolic pathways magnifies small-dose increments. Thus, dose increments should not be done at less than 1 week intervals and even then very cautiously. A salicylate level of 20 to 25 mg/dl should be aimed for. Nabumetone also has a slow action and reaches steady state only after 3 to 7 days. Hydroxychloroquine has a 3 to 4 month delay until its full effect is reached. Severe symptoms may require a "bridging" use of corticosteroids, usually started at 10 to 15 mg per day and continued for 2 to 4 weeks followed by the slow decrement just described.

Complications

Complications of nonacetylated salicylates include gastric irritation and symptoms of salicylism, for example, deafness and buzzing in the ears. Nabumetone has few side effects, the main being an insufficient anti-inflammatory action. Prednisone, even in low doses, causes bone mineral loss. Women with one or more risk factors for osteoporosis are at an even higher risk. Another major risk of corticosteroid use in SLE is osteonecrosis. Doses greater than 20 mg per day administered for more than 1 month may cause osteonecrosis. Higher doses administered for a longer period of time will be more likely to induce osteonecrosis. Because hip involvement is rare in SLE synovitis, the appearance of hip pain in any corticosteroid-treated SLE patient should be viewed with suspicion. Indeed, active synovitis should not preclude the early identification of hip osteonecrosis in SLE.

When to Refer

In my opinion, formed over many years of interaction with primary care physicians, patients with mild, stable SLE may be followed by their primary care physicians on a 1 to 2 month schedule with a rheumatologist reviewing the cases every 6 months to 1 year. A fluid interaction between the primary care physicians and rheumatologists is essential in the care of these patients, as is their early referral when safety boundaries are crossed, for example, hematologic (thrombocytopenia or hemolytic anemia), pulmonary, neurologic (any suspicious finding), renal (any evidence of renal disease), or other. Rheumatologists, by the nature of their training, are in the best position to evaluate these more seriously ill patients and seek further referrals if needed.

Resources Available

The Lupus Foundation of America is an important self-help and charitable organization that should be joined by all SLE patients for support and information. See the appendix for address.

Key Points

> **MILD SLE**
>
> - Probably the most common form of SLE.
> - Transition to a more serious SLE is more likely to happen in early disease (less than 3 years after diagnosis).
> - Treatment should be conservative using sound general advice and low-toxicity medications.
> - The combination of nonacetylated salicylates plus hydroxychloroquine is often successful in these patients.
> - If low-dose corticosteroids are used, they should be in addition to, rather than instead of, the previous regime, and at each visit dose reduction should at least be considered.
> - Calcium and vitamin D supplementation is essential in corticosteroid-treated patients.
> - Corticosteroid reduction should be made by the milligram; this may lead to discontinuation or to the use of the lowest effective dose.

Suggested Reading

Boumpas DT, Fessler BJ, Austin HA III, et al. Systemic lupus erythematosus: Emerging concepts. II: Dermatologic and joint disease, the antiphospholipid antibody syndrome, pregnancy and hormonal therapy, morbidity and mortality, and pathogenesis. Ann Intern Med 123:42–53, 1995.

Mills JA. Medical progress: Systemic lupus erythematosus. N Engl J Med 330:1871–1879, 1994.

Rihner M, McGrath H Jr. Fluorescent light photosensitivity in patients with systemic lupus erythematosus. Arthritis Rheum 35:949–952, 1992.

Wallace DJ. Antimalarial agents and lupus. Clin Rheum Dis 20:263, 1994.

Renal SLE

Routine kidney biopsy studies have shown that some degree of kidney involvement is universal in SLE. Fortunately, in about half of the patients, findings are limited to minor mesangial changes without pathologic or clinical evidence of glomerulonephritis (GN). In the remaining half GN occurs some time during the course of SLE, and within this group three-quarters have a component of tubulointerstitial disease. Significant renal disease as well as other organ involvement in SLE dictates the need for specialized care. A well-informed primary care physician should be cognizant of the main features of lupus renal disease for early identification and referral.

Presentation and Progression

Findings described under mild SLE may all be present in patients with renal lupus. The spectrum of associated findings depends on when in the natural course of SLE renal disease sets in or is identified. As an example, there are patients in whom kidney involvement appears first, without other manifestation of SLE, as an isolated nephrotic syndrome (membranous GN). On evaluation the patient is noted as having a positive ANA, which is not sufficient to establish diagnosis, plus positive dsDNA or Sm antibodies that allows a diagnosis of SLE to be made. A similar situation occurs in patients presenting with diffuse proliferative GN. More frequently, however, renal involvement is noted on initial evaluation of a patient suspected of having SLE. Finally, renal abnormalities may be absent at diagnosis and only appear on follow-up. These cases are initially thought to have mild SLE, hence the importance of a frequent and careful surveillance of urinalysis in lupus patients.

Cause

Renal disease in SLE compromises variably the glomeruli and the interstitium. Within the glomeruli immune complexes may deposit in the mesangium, the subendothelium, and the subepithelial region. Mesangial deposits have a lesser import and appear even in biopsies obtained from patients without clinical renal disease. Subendothelial deposits are regularly present in focal and diffuse proliferative GN and are markers of severe disease. Subepithelial deposits correlate highly with membranous GN. Finally, tubulointerstitial disease associates with immune deposits in the tubular basement membrane. The World Health Organization pathologic classification of renal SLE is shown in Table 13–2.

Presentation

Patients may have, as mentioned, any combination of clinical and laboratory SLE findings plus urinalysis and kidney function abnormalities. Unfortunately, because of technical problems and compensatory mechanisms, serum creatinine and creatinine clearance may not reflect accurately, at least initially, the extent of renal damage. There are well-defined pathologic entities with a significant prognostic import: mesangial, focal proliferative, diffuse proliferative, and membranous. To this should be added information gained from a detailed assessment of acute and chronic changes (Table 13–3). Correlation of clinical and pathologic changes can only be made with approximation. Thus, mild urinary findings (mild proteinuria and hematuria) correlate with mild renal disease such as mesangial or mild focal proliferative GN but may also occur in early severe focal proliferative GN or diffuse proliferative GN. There are, in addition, cases of mesangial or focal proliferative GN that change to diffuse proliferative or membranous GN at

TABLE 13–2

THE WORLD HEALTH ORGANIZATION CLASSIFICATION OF LUPUS NEPHRITIS

Class I. No abnormalities
  (a) Nil by all techniques
  (b) Deposits demonstrable by electron or immunofluorescence microscopy
Class II. Mesangial glomerulonephritis
  (a) Mesangial widening and/or mild hypercellularity
  (b) Moderate hypercellularity
Class III. Focal proliferative glomerulonephritis
  (a) Active necrotizing lesions
  (b) Active and sclerosing lesions
  (c) Sclerosing lesions
Class IV. Diffuse proliferative glomerulonephritis
  (a) Without segmental lesions
  (b) With active necrotizing lesions
  (c) With active and sclerosing lesions
  (d) With sclerosing lesions
Class V. Membranous glomerulonephritis
  (a) Pure membranous glomerulonephritis
  (b) Associated with lesions class II (a or b)
  (c) Associated with lesions class III (a–c)
  (d) Associated with lesions class IV (a–d)

TABLE 13–3

ACTIVITY AND CHRONICITY INDICES IN LUPUS NEPHRITIS

ACTIVITY INDEX (range 0–24)	CHRONICITY INDEX (range 0–12)
Glomerular Changes	**Glomerular Changes**
Glomerular hypercellularity	Glomerular sclerosis
Leukocyte infiltration	Fibrous crescents
Karyorrhexis/fibrinoid necrosis	
Cellular crescents	**Tubulointerstitial Changes**
Hyaline thrombi, wire loops	Tubular atrophy
	Interstitial fibrosis
Tubulointerstitial Changes	
Tubulointerstitial inflammation	

Each feature is scored 0 to 3+ (absent, mild, moderate, severe). Indices are composite scores for individual lesions in each category of activity or chronicity. Scores for necrosis/karyorrhexis and cellular crescents are multiplied by a factor of 2, assuming they are more ominous.

a later date. On the other hand, proteinuria, an active urinary sediment containing red cell casts, and functional abnormalities, such as an increased serum creatinine or a decreased creatinine clearance, is more consistent with diffuse proliferative GN. These considerations underscore the importance of biopsing the kidney when lesion type is uncertain and to determine potentially reversible changes.

A clinicopathologic correlation of the World Health Organization classification of lupus nephritis allows the following statements to be made:

Class I, normal, or minimal change: Only a few patients fall into this category.
Class II, or mesangial GN: It may be clinically silent (normal urinalysis) but is more frequently characterized by mild proteinuria and hematuria. In a few cases mesangial changes are severe and lead to renal insufficiency.
Class III, or focal proliferative nephritis: It is characterized by proteinuria (rarely nephrotic syndrome), hematuria, and rarely arterial hypertension and renal insufficiency.
Class IV, or diffuse proliferative GN: It features hematuria, heavy proteinuria (over 50% have the nephrotic syndrome), and renal insufficiency in most.
Class V, or membranous GN: It is characterized clinically by nephrotic-range proteinuria that is almost regularly present, hematuria in 50%, and arterial hypertension. Renal insufficiency at onset is rare.

Diagnosis

Summary of Diagnosis

> **RENAL SLE**
> - Diagnosis of renal SLE rests on an accurate and repeated assessment of urinalysis, particularly a well-examined urinary sediment.
> - Red cell casts indicate active lupus nephritis.
> - Renal function tests lag behind, and tend to underestimate, pathologic changes.
> - Beware of decreasing C_3 and CH50 and rising titers of dsDNA antibodies: Renal disease may be on the horizon.
> - Kidney biopsy is useful for: (1) uncovering severe focal proliferative or diffuse proliferative GN with only minor changes on urinalysis and a normal renal function, and (2) determining the activity index (reversibility) of the renal lesion.

Natural History

Expected Outcome

Prognosis and therapy in SLE largely depend on the presence and degree of kidney involvement. Transitions from mild SLE to renal SLE as well as from limited renal involvement to severe lupus nephritis are more likely to occur within the first few years of illness. Thus, at the time of diagnosis, a lupus patient has a 50% chance of already having, or subsequently developing, renal disease. On the other hand, patients who have escaped renal disease for 3 to 5 years have only a small chance of acquiring renal disease later in the course of SLE. A suppressive effect on the disease occurs in the late stages of renal insufficiency: Clinical manifestations of SLE dampen and even the ANA may turn negative.

Untreated, diffuse proliferative lupus nephritis leads to renal insufficiency with a 5 year survival of only 25%. Complications of membranous GN include the nephrotic syndrome (risk of death from thrombosis or infection) and arterial hypertension (risk of stroke or cardiac death). Current treatment methods have dramatically improved prognosis in lupus nephritis, with a 5 year survival of about 70%. Interestingly, the tubulointerstitial index and the condition of renal vessels (lupus vasculopathy) have emerged in recent years as major determinants of prognosis in renal SLE.

Treatment

Methods

Treatment of mild renal lupus (class II, III) is with steroid doses sufficient for the extrarenal manifestations of the lupus such as prednisone 10 to 20 mg per day. In severe nephritis, including class IIIa and IV, there is no question that both corticosteroids and immunosuppressive medications need to be administered. A commonly used regime includes prednisone 60 mg per day for 1 to 2 months. Upon reassessment, unimproved patients are begun on intravenous cyclophosphamide boluses given monthly for 6 months and quarterly for 2 years. The prednisone dose is reduced. The coadministration of mesna with the cyclophosphamide plus ample hydration clearly reduce bladder toxicity. In membranous GN a renal biopsy is essential. Presence of activity is an indication for aggressive treatment such as in diffuse proliferative GN. On the other hand, in a purely membranous lesion every-other-day high-dose corticosteroids may be tried.

Expected Response

Therapeutic response in severe lupus nephritis is slow. Regression of lesions to a milder histologic form, such as transition from class IV to class V GN, has been repeatedly documented.

Complications

The high-dose corticosteroids used in lupus nephritis necessarily result in iatrogenesis. Most severe and best recognized is osteonecrosis. Cataracts, osteoporosis, accelerated atherosclerosis, and diabetes are additional complications of glucocorticoid treatment of renal SLE. Intravenous cyclophosphamide is substantially safer than when administered orally. This is particularly true for the bladder dysplasias and bladder cancer. About 25% of young women treated with I.V. cyclophosphamide develop irreversible ovarian failure. An additional risk created by immunosuppression is fatal opportunistic infection involving the lung or central nervous system.

When to Refer

Patients with renal SLE need close specialized care. Major decisions need to be made regarding renal biopsy, corticosteroid dose, use of immunosuppressive medications, and changes in an ongoing treatment program. In addition, medications used in severe renal, neuropsychiatric, or hematologic lupus unavoidably lead to serious iatrogenesis. Minimizing complications, such as the early identification and treatment of osteonecrosis, is best accomplished in specialized clinics. Patients with mild stable renal disease may be followed by a nephrologist or rheumatologist. A nephrologist, working in close collaboration with a rheumatologist, is in the best position to care for SLE patients with significant renal disease.

Key Points

> **RENAL SLE**
>
> - Prognosis in SLE largely depends on the presence or absence of severe renal disease.
> - Absence of nephritis at diagnosis should not give a sense of security; renal disease may ensue on follow-up.
> - Histologic transitions occur in 10% to 45% of cases: from nonrenal to renal, from class II or III to class IV, and from class V to class IV (ascending severity); and from class IV to class V (descending severity) as a result of corticosteroid and immunosuppressive treatment.
> - Aggressive treatment of lupus nephritis decreases irreversible scarring and delays or halts progression of renal insufficiency.

Suggested Reading

Boumpas DT, Austin HA, Fessler BJ, et al. Systemic lupus erythematosus: Emerging concepts. I: Renal, neuropsychiatric, cardiovascular, pulmonary, and hematologic disease. Ann Intern Med 122:940–950, 1995.

Golbus J, McCune JW. Lupus nephritis. Classification, prognosis, immunopathogenesis, and treatment. Clin Rheum Dis 20:213–242, 1994.

Neuropsychiatric SLE

Neuropsychiatric manifestations are believed to occur in about 75% of SLE patients. Of these, less than one-third are severe. Neuropsychiatric lupus ranges from cognitive dysfunction to stroke, and from aseptic meningitis to Guillain-Barré's syndrome (Tables 13–4 and 13–5). A general classification of SLE-related neuropsychiatric disease must include, as in other organ involvements in this condition, four general types of events: (1) lesions or disturbances directly caused by the lupus, (2) secondary events from lupus involvement in organs or systems (such as stroke from arterial hypertension caused by renal disease or cerebral embolization from valvular vegetations), (3) iatrogenic complications of treatment such as depression, arterial hypertension, and accelerated atherosclerosis caused by corticosteroids as well as CNS infections from immunosuppression, and (4) coincidental neuropsychiatric disease. Thus, in neuropsychiatric lupus many factors are involved, clinical manifestations are varied, and often there is uncertainty regarding diagnostic attribution (i.e., are these findings due to the lupus?).

TABLE 13–4

NEUROPSYCHIATRIC MANIFESTATIONS IN SYSTEMIC LUPUS ERYTHEMATOSUS

DIFFUSE CEREBRAL DYSFUNCTION

Organic amnestic/cognitive dysfunction (20%)
Psychosis (10%)
Major affective disorder (< 1%)
Dementia (rare)
Altered consciousness

FOCAL CEREBRAL DYSFUNCTION

Cranial neuropathies (rare)
Seizures (grand mal, focal, temporal lobe, petit mal) (15%)
Cerebrovascular accidents (5%)
Transverse myelitis (1%)

MOVEMENT DISORDERS

Chorea (3%)
Athetosis (rare)
Parkinson-like (rare)
Cerebellar ataxia (rare)

PERIPHERAL NEUROPATHY

Symmetric sensorimotor (10%)
Mononeuritis multiplex (rare)
Chronic, relapsing neuropathy (rare)
Guillain-Barré syndrome (extremely rare)
Autonomic neuropathy (extremely rare)

MISCELLANEOUS

Headache (common)
Aseptic meningitis (rare)
Normal pressure hydrocephalus (rare)
Pseudotumor cerebri (rare)
Cerebral venous thrombosis (extremely rare)
Myasthenia gravis (rare)
Eaton-Lambert syndrome (rare)

Adapted from West SG, Emlen W, Wener MH. Neuropsychiatric lupus erythematosus: A 10-year prospective study on the value of diagnostic tests. Am J Med 99:153–163, 1995; Boumpas DT, Austin HA, Fessler BJ, et al. Systemic lupus erythematosus: Emerging concepts. I. Renal, neuropsychiatric, cardiovascular, pulmonary, and hematologic disease. Ann Intern Med 122:940, 1995; and Hinchey J, Chaves C, Appigiani B, et al. A reversible posterior leukoencephalopathy syndrome. N Engl J Med 334:494–500, 1996.

Presentation and Progression

Cause

Neuropsychiatric lupus is caused by a variety of mechanisms of which some are only partially understood. (1) Antineuronal antibodies and antiribosomal-P protein antibodies have been shown to associate with diffuse neuropsychiatric SLE. (2) Autopsy specimens often show bland intimal proliferation of small vessels. (3) Associated thrombi and microinfarctions may be caused by these vascular changes or an associated antiphospholipid syndrome. (4) Small and large cerebral hemorrhages are also common. (5) Reversible posterior leukoencephalopathy syndrome (white matter edema) may cause altered mental functioning, seizures, and loss of vision in patients with arterial hypertension, renal failure, and/or on immunosuppressive agents. (6) A true cerebral vasculitis is rare, but both Libman-Sack's endocarditis and

TABLE 13–5

PATHOGENESIS OF NEUROPSYCHIATRIC MANIFESTATIONS IN SYSTEMIC LUPUS ERYTHEMATOSUS

1. Neural SLE itself
   (a) Microvascular disease (immune complex, antiphospholipid antibodies, TTP)
   (b) Cerebral edema
   (c) Macrovascular disease (major vessel arteritis—rare—, arterial thrombosis or embolus in antiphospholipid syndrome)
   (d) Neuronal dysfunction (antineuronal antibodies, antiribosomal P antibodies)
2. SLE lesion in another organ
   (a) Renal insufficiency
   (b) Libman-Sack or antiphospholipid endocarditis emboli
3. Complications of SLE therapy
   (a) Corticosteroid-induced psychosis, arterial hypertension, accelerated atherosclerosis)
   (b) Immunossuppressive agents (cerebral abscesses, meningitis, vertebral osteomyelitis with epidural progression)
4. Independent neuropsychiatric disease: any

valvular vegetations from a secondary antiphospholipid syndrome may cause embolic infarction. (7) A gross focal lesion may represent cerebral abscess from immunosuppression or hypertensive hemorrhage due to renal insufficiency and/or corticosteroid use. (8) Finally, independent causes of CNS disease must be taken into consideration such as the development of a meningioma.

Presentation

The most common neuropsychiatric manifestation of SLE, which may occur in both mild and severe disease, is a cognitive disturbance that includes memory loss, difficulties in problem solving, apathy, and in more serious cases disorientation, agitation, stupor, and even coma. Cognitive disturbance may be identified clinically in about 20% of patients and by formal psychologic testing in close to 70%. Lupus psychosis, which may be difficult to distinguish from steroid psychosis, occurs in about 20% of cases. Rarely lupus dementia results from cumulative lupus lesions or multiple cerebral infarctions in patients with an associated antiphospholipid syndrome. A common manifestation of SLE per se that may also be caused by an associated antiphospholipid syndrome is an atypical migraine. Fortification specters such as wavy or zigzag lines crossing the visual field and seen with the eyes open or closed are common in this setting. Other types of scotomas, such as negative scotomas and scintillating scotomas, are also seen. Seizures in SLE are often multifactorial including electrical disturbances caused by the lupus itself, steroid use, renal insufficiency, arterial hypertension, or CNS infection. Major strokes are rare and tend to be hemorrhagic or embolic. Lupus meningitis is uncommon. More frequently meningismus is caused by NSAIDs, particularly ibuprofen, or infection in immunosuppressed patients. Transverse myelitis is a fortunately rare complication of SLE that is closely linked with the presence of antiphospholipid antibodies. Neuromuscular conditions such as myasthenia gravis and Eaton-Lambert's syndrome rarely occur. A variety of peripheral nerve lesions, particularly a symmetric sensorimotor neuropathy, appear in approximately 20% of lupus patients.

Diagnosis

Summary of Diagnosis

NEUROPSYCHIATRIC LUPUS

- A broad range of central and peripheral nervous system abnormalities may occur in SLE.
- Accuracy in diagnosis, that is, determining that the condition is indeed due to the lupus, is essential for treatment.
- CNS infection must be considered, particularly in immunosuppressed patients.
- Watch for clinical manifestations of an associated antiphospholipid syndrome (livedo reticularis, heart murmur, history of venous or arterial thrombosis, migraines).
- Perform formal neuropsychologic testing in patients with cognitive dysfunction. Depression, hypothyroidism, and other cases of pseudodementia must be sought in these patients.
- Patients with arterial hypertension, renal failure, or immunosuppressives may have a reversible syndrome that comprises headache, altered mental functioning, abnormalities in visual perception including cortical blindness, and seizures.
- CSF findings (present in 50%), for example, increased protein and slight lymphocytic pleocytosis, are nonspecific but speak of active CNS involvement. CSF examination is essential to rule out infection.
- EEG findings (present in 50% to 80%) are diffuse and nonspecific.
- MRI findings (present in 80%) are nonspecific: single or multiple, small or large high-intensity lesions on T2-weighted scans. Some of these lesions are rapidly reversible.
- Cerebral angiography is usually normal.
- Transesophageal echocardiography is essential in patients with possible micro or macro cerebral embolism.

Natural History

Expected Outcome

Outcome in neuropsychiatric lupus is as diverse as the nature and location of the CNS lesions. Cases due to subcortical edema are dramatic both clinically and on CT or MRI, but findings are rapidly reversible with appropriate therapy. Cognitive dysfunction may be stable or may progress slowly; a parallelism with lupus activity and corticosteroid use has been both found and denied. Focal lesions, some of them due to edema, often regress. Embolic infarctions characteristically recur, and multiple added infarctions, such as seen in patients with valvular lesions, may rarely cause dementia.

Treatment

Methods

There are so far no controlled studies on the treatment of neuropsychiatric lupus. Although many psychotropic and anticonvulsant drugs are known to cause ANAs and even clinical lupus, they still can be used in the treatment of SLE-related neuropsychiatric disease. Recurrent embolic lesions, whether caused by Libman-Sack's endocarditis or an associated antiphospholipid syndrome (differentiation between the two is only possible in early lesions), may be prevented by high-grade anticoagulation plus low-dose aspirin (see antiphospholipid syndrome section). High-dose oral corticosteroids are used in suspected evolving CNS lupus disease. Severe focal lesions of a presumed vasculitic nature may be treated by pulse methylprednisolone boluses, 1 g I.V. on 3 subsequent days alone or in association with pulse intravenous cyclophosphamide.

In contrast, patients with the posterior leukoencephalopathy syndrome should have blood pressure controlled and immunosuppressants temporarily removed, which is rapidly followed by clinical improvement. Selecting cases for such an aggressive treatment calls for the highest of clinical skills. An important confounding variable is steroid psychosis. If an SLE patient develops psychosis while on steroids it is legitimate to double the dose and assess response. In active lupus cerebritis the patient will improve; in steroid-induced psychosis there will be little or no change. Patients with residual neurologic dysfunction (for instance, from multiple infarctions) cannot benefit from corticosteroids or immunosuppression.

When to Refer

Lupus patients with suspected neuropsychiatric disease should be referred for rheumatologic and neurologic evaluation. In mild cognitive dysfunction no specific treatment is needed and the patient may be followed by the primary care physician. In most instances, however, specialized care is required by a rheumatologist and a neurologist.

Key Points

> **NEUROPSYCHIATRIC LUPUS**
>
> - Neuropsychiatric lupus has diverse locations, pathogeneses, and significance.
> - Secondary, iatrogenic, and unrelated neurologic processes challenge the clinician's diagnostic skills.
> - Once neuropsychiatric lupus is diagnosed, the next problem is to choose treatment.
> - Pharmacologic treatment of psychiatric disease and seizures should not exclude drugs that are known to cause ANA and even SLE.
> - Recurrent embolic or thrombotic disease in patients with Libman-Sack's endocarditis or an associated antiphospholipid syndrome may be halted by high-grade anticoagulation plus low-dose aspirin.
> - The posterior leukoencephalopathy syndrome improves rapidly with blood pressure control.
> - Psychosis in a corticosteroid-treated patient may be caused by the steroid or the lupus: Double the steroid dose to find out.
> - Scar-related dementia is unresponsive to corticosteroids or immunosuppression.
> - Once infection, embolic disease, and other non-lupus CNS conditions have been ruled out, corticosteroids with or without an immunosuppressive may be started.

Suggested Reading

Boumpas DY, Yamada H, Patronas NJ, et al. Pulse cyclophosphamide for severe neuropsychiatric lupus. QJ Med 81:975–984, 1991.

Devinsky O, Petito CK, Alonso DR. Clinical and neuropathological findings in systemic lupus erythematosus: The role of vasculitis, heart emboli, and thrombotic thrombocytopenic purpura. Ann Neurol 23:380–384, 1988.

Hinchey J, Chaves C, Appigiani B, et al. A reversible posterior leukoencephalopathy syndrome. N Engl J Med 334:494–500, 1996.

Lavalle C, Pizarro S, Drenkard C, et al. Transverse myelitis: A manifestation of systemic lupus erythematosus strongly associated with antiphospholipid antibodies. J Rheumatol 17:34–37, 1990.

Toubi E, Khamashta MA, Panarra A, et al. Association of antiphospholipid antibodies with central nervous system disease in systemic lupus erythematosus. Am J Med 99:397–401, 1995.

West SG, Emlen W, Wener MH. Neuropsychiatric lupus erythematosus: A 10-year prospective study on the value of diagnostic tests. Am J Med 99:153–163, 1995.

Pleuropulmonary SLE

A variety of respiratory system lesions may occur in SLE (Table 13–6). Taken together they appear at one time or another in about 75% of patients. Pleuropulmonary lupus may be a presenting manifestation of the disease, part of the clinical cluster at the time of diagnosis, or an additional site of involvement during patient follow-up. There are also changes that are secondary to lupus involvement elsewhere such as pleural effusions caused by nephrotic syndrome, uremia, thromboembolism, or cardiac failure. Very importantly, opportunistic lung infections may occur in SLE from the immunosuppression caused by the disease itself or the medications used. Finally, pleuropulmonary changes may represent independent comorbidities from tobacco smoking and other environmental toxics. Thus, similar to neuropsychiatric lupus, diagnosis of lupus pleuropulmonary disease requires thoughtful consideration of primary, secondary, iatrogenic, and coincidental conditions.

Presentation and Progression

Cause

The various components of the respiratory system may be involved in SLE. Pleural involvement reflects serosal immune complex deposition and complement activation. Parenchymal disease may be caused by acute injury to the vascular/alveolar unit in acute pneumonitis, alveolar hemorrhage, and reversible hypoxemia caused by neutrophil aggregates; chronic interstitial injury in inflammatory alveolitis and chronic fibrosis; and small airway inflammation in bronchiolitis obliterans with or without organizing pneumonia. Small and large vascular lesions may be caused by lupus

TABLE 13-6
PLEUROPULMONARY MANIFESTATIONS OF SYSTEMIC LUPUS ERYTHEMATOSUS

1. Pleuritis or pleuropericarditis (rule out infection, CHF, uremia, pulmonary embolism)

FREQUENCY: 45%–60%

Pleuritic pain
Cough
Dyspnea
Fever
Pleural effusion, uni- or bilateral
Pericardial effusion may coexist

Diagnosis: thoracentesis for general characteristics of the fluid (exudate vs. transudate), smears, cultures

2. Acute lupus pneumonitis (rule out infection, alveolar hemorrhage, pulmonary embolism)

FREQUENCY: 1%–4%

Dyspnea
Cough
Pleuritic pain
Hypoxemia
Fever

Diagnosis: fiberoptic bronchoscopy and BAL for general appearance of the aspirate, smears, cultures, transbronchial biopsy

3. Interstitial lung disease (rule out other causes of ILD)

FREQUENCY: about 3%

Dyspnea, progressive
Cough, nonproductive
Rales
Bibasilar interstitial or reticulonodular infiltrates on chest x-ray

Diagnosis: High-resolution CT to determine focal alveolar opacities (ground glass) vs. interstitial fibrosis (macroscopic honeycomb cysts)

4. Pulmonary hemorrhage (rule out CHF, pneumonia, uremia, pulmonary embolism)

FREQUENCY: rare

Dyspnea
Cough
Hemoptysis (inconstant)
Pleuritic pain
Hypoxemia
Fever
A falling hematocrit

Diagnosis: bronchoscopy and BAL; gross blood and hemosiderin-laden macrophages in pulmonary hemorrhage

5. Bronchiolitis obliterans (BO) and bronchiolitis obliterans with organizing pneumonia (BOOP) (rule out infection, drug effects)

FREQUENCY: rare

Acute or subacute
Fever
Cough
Dyspnea
Pulmonary hyperinflation (BO) or focal alveolar infiltrates with air bronchograms or diffuse interstitial or reticulonodular infiltrates (BOOP)

Diagnosis: transbronchial biopsy or open lung biopsy

6. Diaphragmatic dysfunction (rule out pleural or parenchymal disease causing restrictive disease)

FREQUENCY: unclear; may be 1% or more

Dyspnea
Reduced lung volumes (shrinking lung syndrome)

Diagnosis: physiologic studies

7. Pulmonary hypertension (rule out pulmonary embolism and thrombosis of major pulmonary veins)

FREQUENCY: rare; associations include Raynaud's, renal disease, RNP antibody, positive RF, positive anticardiolipin antibodies

Dyspnea
Fatigue
Chest pain
Accentuated pulmonary sound
Right ventricular heave
Systolic murmur
Right-sided failure

Diagnosis: ventilation perfusion scans, echocardiography, pulmonary angiography

---

arteritis or in situ thrombosis or embolization in patients with an associated antiphospholipid syndrome. Pulmonary hypertension may be the end result of both types of lesions. Finally, diaphragmatic and intercostal muscle dysfunction due to myositis or pleural adhesions may cause hypoventilation in patients with SLE.

Presentation

Pleuritis, usually with effusion, is the most common pleuropulmonary manifestation of SLE, occurring in 60% of patients. Additional systemic manifestations such as fever, alopecia, oral ulcers, arthritis, and leukopenia usually coexist, providing a clue to diagnosis. The process is often bilateral, and the pericardium may be involved as well. Patients have pleuritic pain and sometimes dyspnea. Uni- or bilateral pleural rubs, sometimes with a pericardial rub, may be present on examination. Neck veins and respiratory variations of blood pressure should be closely watched in patients with pleuropericarditis for early identification of pericardial tamponade. Pleural effusions, small or moderate in size, are usually present on chest x-rays. Pleural fluid in SLE is typically an exudate with WBC counts ranging from several hundreds to 15,000 cells/mm^3. The prevailing cells are PMNs initially and mononuclears later in the disease course. Glucose concentrations are normal or moderately decreased (above 50% of serum values) and complement levels are typically low. Spontaneous LE cells are present in approximately 60% of lupus effusions. Transudative pleural effusions may occur in lupus patients reflecting nephrotic syndrome, renal insufficiency, cardiac failure, and pulmonary thromboembolism. Other etiologies of pleuritis must also be considered. Parapneumonic effusions and empyemas are generally unilateral, the glucose level is drastically decreased, and there is peripheral leukocytosis. Malignant effusions also tend to be unilateral, the fluid is often hemorrhagic, and malignant cells are often present on smear. The main differential diagnosis, however, is with pulmonary thromboembolism, which may mimic lupus pleuritis almost to perfection, the correct diagnosis being suggested by a ventilation-perfusion scan.

Pulmonary hemorrhage and *acute lupus pneumonitis* each occur in less than 5% of SLE patients. Both conditions have an abrupt onset and feature fever, dyspnea, hypoxemia, and dense uni- or bilateral alveolar infiltrates. Additional findings in pulmonary hemorrhage include hemoptysis in 50% of cases and a sudden drop in blood hemoglobin greater than 3 g/dl in virtually all patients. Bronchoscopy with bronchoalveolar lavage helps in distinguishing these conditions and in the exclusion of infection. Gross blood and hemosiderin-laden macrophages in the aspirates characterize pulmonary hemorrhage. Purulent secretions and the appropriate smears, stains, and cultures assist in the diagnosis of *microbial pneumonia*. Of particular importance in this setting, particularly in patients treated with high-dose corticosteroids and other immunosuppressive agents, is not to miss *P. carinii*, tuberculous, or fungal infection. Absence of gross blood or purulence in the aspirated secretions and negative Grocott's methenamine silver and auramine-rhodamine stains support a diagnosis of acute lupus pneumonitis.

Chronic interstitial disease is a rare complication of SLE that causes progressive dyspnea, a dry cough, and Velcro-type bibasilar rales. Differentiation between alveolitis and fibrosis in these cases has been facilitated by high-resolution CT.

Bronchiolitis obliterans with or without organizing pneumonia is also rare in SLE. Patients have progressive dyspnea, cough, and fever. X-rays show hyperinflation in pure bronchiolitis obliterans and focal alveolar, interstitial, or reticulonodular infiltrates when organizing pneumonia is present. Diagnosis is histologic and requires bronchoscopy and transbronchial (or open) biopsy.

Finally, patients with SLE may feature the *"shrinking lung syndrome"* in which there is a decreasing lung volume plus basal atelectasis caused by respiratory muscle weakness and/or pleural adhesions. Diagnosis of diaphragmatic weakness in this setting requires involved physiologic and neurophysiologic testing.

Diagnosis

Summary of Diagnosis

PLEUROPULMONARY SLE

- Lupus pleuritis tends to be bilateral and often associates with pericarditis.
- Spontaneous LE cells may be present in pleural (and pericardial) fluid.
- Chest x-rays may suggest parenchymal, vascular, and neuromuscular lupus involvement.
- Differentiation among early pulmonary hemorrhage, acute lupus pneumonitis, and microbial pneumonia (particularly *P. carinii*, tuberculous, fungal, and mixed infections) is facilitated by bronchoscopy and BAL.
- Fibrotic and alveolar-type interstitial disease can be distinguished by CT.
- Pulmonary hypertension may occur from microvascular disease or major vessel thrombi. Large perfusion defects in ventilation-perfusion scans suggest the latter.
- A precise diagnosis of respiratory muscle weakness requires involved physiologic techniques and often remains unproven.

Natural History

Lupus pleuritis tends to be a recurrent problem that responds well to therapy. Acute lupus pneumonitis may be lethal if not aggressively treated. Even more serious is pulmonary hemorrhage in which mortality is almost uniform if aggressive treatments are not used. Chronic interstitial disease features a slow deterioration in pulmonary function. The alveolitic forms of the condition are amenable to therapy. Bronchiolitis obliterans per se, in contrast with cases with organizing pneumonia, responds poorly to corticosteroids and immunosuppressive medications. Finally, unrecognized and untreated neuromuscular dysfunction may cause respiratory failure and death.

Treatment

Methods

Lupus pleuritis responds well to small to moderate doses of oral corticosteroids. Acute lupus pneumonitis requires high-dose corticosteroids such as prednisone 1 to 2 mg/kg. Inflammatory chronic interstitial disease and bronchiolitis obliterans with organizing pneumonia tend to respond to corticosteroids. Pulmonary hemorrhage is treated with I.V. methylprednisolone 1 g for 3 consecutive days followed by high doses of oral prednisone that are tapered over several weeks. Cyclophosphamide boluses and plasmapheresis are often concurrently used. Although no controlled trials have been conducted, aggressive combination therapy appears to reduce mortality from 90% to about 30%. In successfully treated cases resorption of infiltrates is extremely rapid and is usually complete within 2 to 4 days. The alveolitis-type interstitial disease often responds to oral corticosteroids.

When to Refer

Other than cases of clear-cut lupus pleuritis that rapidly respond to therapy and stable interstitial disease, the management of pulmonary SLE belongs in the combined field of pulmonary medicine and rheumatology.

Key Points

PLEUROPULMONARY SLE

- Varied lesions; sooner or later one or more of them will occur in the majority of patients.
- Lupus pleuritis is highly symptomatic but mild in terms of response to therapy.
- Pulmonary hemorrhage and acute lupus pneumonitis are life-threatening conditions.

- Interstitial disease progresses slowly, is readily detected by auscultation, and alveolar cases (these can be distinguished by CT) are treatable with corticosteroids.
- Bronchiolitis obliterans with organizing pneumonia is also responsive to corticosteroid therapy.
- Pulmonary hypertension is rare; it may occur from microvascular occlusive disease or from major artery embolism or thrombosis. The latter are amenable to treatment with anticoagulant therapy.
- Neuromuscular respiratory failure is often responsive to high-dose corticosteroid agents.

Suggested Reading

Kahl LE. The spectrum of pericardial tamponade in systemic lupus erythematosus. Arthritis Rheum 35:1343–1349, 1992.

Orens JB, Martínez FJ, Lynch JP III. Pleuropulmonary manifestations of systemic lupus erythematosus. Clin Rheum Dis 20:159–193, 1994.

Schwab EP, Schumacher HR Jr, Freundlich B, et al. Pulmonary alveolar hemorrhage in systemic lupus erythematosus. Sem Arthritis Rheum 23:8–15, 1993.

Yale SH, Limper AH. *Pneumocystis carinii* pneumonia in patients without acquired immunodeficiency syndrome: Associated illnesses and prior corticosteroid therapy. Mayo Clin Proc 71:5–13, 1996.

Discoid LE (DLE) and Subacute Cutaneous Lupus Erythematosus (SCLE)

These potentially disfiguring conditions remain largely limited to the skin, which sets them apart from SLE.

Presentation and Progression

Cause

The exquisite photosensitivity of SCLE, and to a lesser extent DLE, suggests that ultraviolet radiation is involved in causation. There is indeed evidence that ultraviolet radiation results in surface exposure of the cytoplasmic antigens SSA (Ro), SSB (La), Sm, and ribonucleoprotein antigens, which potentially makes them immunogenic. SCLE appears to be mediated by humoral immunity; cellular immunity may be responsible for DLE. Both lesions may occur within the context of SLE; discoid lesions are present in less than 10% of patients and SCLE in a smaller proportion of cases.

Presentation

Discoid LE may present as single or multiple plaque (indurated) lesions involving predominantly exposed skin: face, scalp, and ears. Epidermal atrophy, telangiectasia, scaling, and hyper/hypopigmentary changes characterize this lesion. In scalp lesions, different from SLE, alopecia is permanent (scarring alopecia). Patients who have additional DLE lesions below the neck are said to have generalized DLE.

Subacute cutaneous LE involves predominantly the extensor aspect of the upper extremities, upper back, and upper chest (Figure 13–2). Lesions may be papulosquamous or polycyclic, with a ratio of 2 to 1. Epidermal atrophy and pigmentary changes are common, and induration does not occur. Interestingly, about one-third of patients with SCLE also have lesions consistent with DLE.

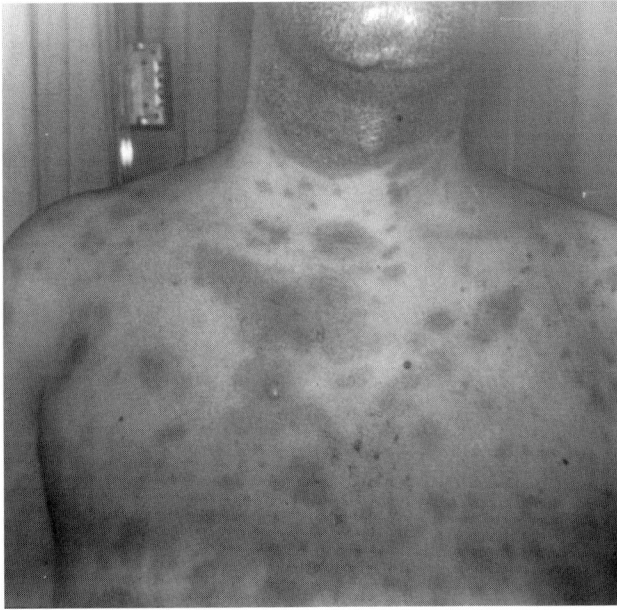

FIGURE 13–2. *Subacute lupus erythematosus.* This man, who first presented with aseptic meningitis, later developed round or oval erythematous lesions, some with central clearing, small-joint arthritis, and high titers of SSA/anti-Ro antibodies. A feature of his case was extreme photosensitivity.

Diagnosis

Summary of Diagnosis

> **DISCOID LE (DLE) AND SUBACUTE CUTANEOUS LE (SCLE)**
>
> **DLE**
> - Well-demarcated plaque with epidermal atrophy, follicular plugging, telangiectasis, and pigmentary changes.
> - Face, scalp, and ears are the most frequent locations.
> - Additional below-the-neck lesions in 40%.
> - ANA positive in 10% of patients.
> - Skin biopsy is characteristic.
>
> **SCLE**
> - Papulosquamous or polycyclic nonindurated, nonscarring lesions; permanent pigmentary changes are frequent.
> - Extensor surface of arms, upper chest, and upper back.
> - Mild systemic features (may fulfill ARA criteria) in 30% to 50%.
> - Anti-SSA (Ro) antibodies present in 70%.
> - Skin biopsy is characteristic.

Natural History

Expected Outcome

Untreated DLE runs a chronic course and can be quite disfiguring, such as the irreversible loss of the scalp hair. Cases with positive ANA may go on to develop systemic disease. Subacute cutaneous LE has a chronic, relapsing course with frequent residual pigmentary changes. Although many of the patients have mild systemic symptoms, transition to serious disease is quite uncommon. Cases featuring extensive papulosquamous disease, particularly in males as well as those associated with Sjögren's and vasculitis, may have a more severe course.

Treatment

Methods

Sun protection (see appendix) is essential in patients with DLE and SCLE. Topical and intralesional steroids may be used. Hydroxychloroquine in the doses recommended for mild SLE is highly effective for both lesions. In resistant cases, chloroquine may be used instead. Dapsone has been used with benefit in antimalarial-resistant SCLE.

When to Refer

Patients with facial and scalp DLE or with extensive SCLE are best handled by dermatologists. Mild SCLE should be evaluated by a dermatologist or rheumatologist for diagnostic confirmation and then followed by the primary care physician.

Key Points

DISCOID LE (DLE) AND SUBACUTE CUTANEOUS LE (SCLE)

- Both conditions may be strictly cutaneous or may associate with SLE.
- Alopecia caused by DLE is permanent (scarring alopecia).
- Cases of DLE with positive ANA may progress to SLE, although not necessarily.
- Cases of SCLE that fulfill ACR criteria for SLE tend to have mild, predominantly cutaneous, highly photosensitive disease.
- Male cases of SCLE with extensive papulosquamous rash are at a higher risk of severe systemic disease.
- Antimalarial agents are effective in the majority of patients with DLE or SCLE.

Suggested Reading

Callen J, Klein J. Subacute cutaneous lupus erythematosus. Clinical, serologic, immunogenetic, and therapeutic considerations in seventy-two patients. Arthritis Rheum 31:1007–1013, 1988.

Cohen MR, Crosby D. Systemic disease in subacute cutaneous lupus erythematosus: A controlled comparison with systemic lupus erythematosus. J Rheumatol 21:1665–1669, 1994.

Laman SD, Provost TT. Cutaneous manifestations of lupus erythematosus. Clin Rheum Dis 20:195–212, 1994.

Mond CB, Peterson MGE, Rothfield NF. Correlation of anti-Ro antibody with photosensitivity rash in systemic lupus erythematosus. Arthritis Rheum 32:202–204, 1989.

Pregnancy and SLE

The complex interactions between lupus and pregnancy may have damaging effects on the mother and the fetus. Both SLE and the antiphospholipid syndrome, present in 5% to 10% of lupus patients, increase the risk of pregnancy loss. Shared clinical findings make it difficult to distinguish active lupus nephritis from pregnancy-induced hypertension or preeclampsia. In addition, pregnancy per se features clinical and laboratory findings that may be interpreted as manifestations of active SLE. Finally, babies born to mothers who possess in their serum the anti-Ro antibody may exhibit the neonatal lupus syndrome. Overall, however, in the absence of active lupus nephritis and with appropriate supervision, a successful outcome may be expected in most lupus patients' pregnancies.

Presentation and Progression

Cause

The problem pregnancies of SLE patients are only partially understood. Placental infarcts and immune damage account for the additional risk of fetal loss in patients with an associated antiphospholipid syndrome. Maternal anti-Ro antibody transfers across the placenta, binds to Ro antigen present in fetal skin and the cardiac conduction system, and causes the neonatal lupus syndrome.

Presentation

Whereas normal pregnant women have a 10% risk of fetal loss, the risk in pregnant lupus patients increases to approximately 40%. Pregnancy losses in both instances occur overwhelmingly during the embryonal period (less than 12 weeks gestation). In contrast, in lupus patients with an associated antiphospholipid syndrome the excess fetal loss predominates in the second trimester. Lupus nephritis and the high-dose corticosteroids used in its therapy add a substantial risk of arterial hypertension and preeclampsia. In addition, pregnant SLE patients feature a high risk of prematurity and intrauterine growth retardation.

Interestingly, pregnancy per se results in clinical and laboratory findings that may be mistaken for lupus activity. These include alopecia, facial and palmar erythema, carpal tunnel syndrome, arterial hypertension, seizures, anemia, thrombocytopenia, increased ESR, and proteinuria. Distinguishing pregnancy-associated hypertension or toxemia from active lupus nephritis is essential to institute appropriate therapy.

Diagnosis

Summary of Diagnosis

PREGNANCY AND SLE

- Lupus pregnancy is a high-risk pregnancy.
- Expert monitoring of both the lupus and the pregnancy is essential to maximize chances of success.
- Determine the presence of antiphospholipid antibodies and anti-Ro(SSA) and anti-La(SSB) antibodies in the mother, and if the latter two are positive, measure

- their activity against the 52-kd and 48-kd antigens, respectively.
- Lupus findings such as alopecia, facial and palmar erythema, carpal tunnel syndrome, arterial hypertension, anemia, thrombocytopenia, increased ESR, and proteinuria may also be caused by pregnancy.
- CBC, platelet count, serum creatinine, urinalysis (with a detailed sediment), anti-dsDNA, and alternative complement components should be serially followed.
- Fever, true rash, oral ulcers, lymphadenopathy, arthritis, serositis, palpable purpura, urine sediment RBC casts, alternative pathway hypocomplementemia, and increased levels of anti-dsDNA antibodies remain valid indicators of lupus activity during pregnancy.

Natural History

Expected Outcome

Poorly controlled SLE, particularly with active nephritis, a history of fetal loss, presence of the antiphospholipid syndrome, and arterial hypertension, used to cast a grim outlook on fetus viability and indicated a high risk of potentially lethal complications in the mother. This ominous scenario has changed with the advent of improved treatment programs for SLE and the antiphospholipid syndrome, the availability of fetal monitoring, and advances in obstetric and neonatal medicine.

Complications of pregnancy in lupus patients may occur in the mother and/or the pregnancy. Maternal complications include arterial hypertension and proteinuria, particularly in patients with preexisting hypertension or lupus nephritis; thrombocytopenia, which may be caused by late pregnancy, toxemia, the lupus, or an associated antiphospholipid syndrome; lupus flare; congestive heart failure in patients with renal insufficiency or arterial hypertension; and pulmonary thromboembolism in patients with the antiphospholipid syndrome.

Pregnancy complications are quite frequent, with only about 50% of pregnancies resulting in a full-term infant of normal weight. Complications include an increased embryonal loss due to the lupus, increased middle trimester fetal loss in patients with an associated antiphospholipid syndrome, intrauterine growth retardation and prematurity due to either the lupus or an associated antiphospholipid syndrome, and the neonatal lupus syndrome in babies born to mothers carrying the anti-Ro (SSA)-52kd and anti-La (SSB)-48kd antibodies. However, only a minority of babies born to mothers with pathogenic anti-Ro and anti-La antibodies have the syndrome: Less than 25% have cutaneous manifestations and less than 3% have fetal cardiomyopathy, congenital permanent heart block, or intrauterine fetal death.

Treatment

Methods

Most important in lupus pregnancy is to make sure the SLE has been inactive for at least 6 months prior to conception. Lupus activity during pregnancy is best treated by adding corticosteroids or by increasing their dose. Large oral corticosteroid doses are used in active lupus nephritis. If hypertension is present (differentiating lupus nephritis from pregnancy-related hypertension and toxemia may be difficult and indeed these conditions may coexist), hydralazine, methyldopa, or calcium channel blockers should be used and delivery induced as soon as possible. Fetal myocarditis and atrioventricular block may be treated empirically with dexamethasone (which crosses the placenta), but results are usually disappointing. Most surviving infants with atrioventricular block require a permanent pacemaker.

When to Refer

Pregnant lupus patients should be seen by a rheumatologist and obstetrician in alternate months until the 6th month of pregnancy and in alternate 2 week interals thereafter. Intensive rheumatologic surveillance should be continued at least 3 months following delivery.

Key Points

PREGNANCY AND SLE

- Mothers with pathogenic anti-Ro/La should be monitored with serial fetal EKG and ultrasound.
- Fetal myocarditis or atrioventricular block is an indication for dexamethasone therapy (dexamethasone crosses the placenta).
- Only drugs with a record of safety for both the mother and the fetus should be used.
- If the patient has inactive lupus at the time of conception, is normotensive, has normal serum creatinine, and has no history of pregnancy loss, the chances of a successful pregnancy are virtually average.

Suggested Reading

Lockshin M, Reinitz E, Druzin ML, et al. Lupus pregnancy. Case-control prospective study demonstrating absence of lupus exacerbation during or after pregnancy. Am J Med 77:893–898, 1984.

Petri M, Howard D, Repke J. Frequency of lupus flare in pregnancy. The Johns Hopkins lupus pregnancy experience. Arthritis Rheum 34:1538–1545, 1991.

Urowitz MB, Gladman DD, Farewell VT, et al. Lupus and pregnancy studies. Arthritis Rheum 36:1392–1397, 1993.

SLE and Fever

The interrelationships between SLE and infection are complex. Fever is a prominent finding in lupus flares but just as frequently represents infection. Because infection often associates with, or triggers, lupus activity, fever in a lupus patient should always raise concern and elicit appropriate investigations.

Presentation and Progression

Cause

Lupus fever may reach any level and even associate with shaking chills in absence of microbial infection. However, the presence of shaking chills should be taken as evidence of infection unless proven otherwise by blood and other appropriate cultures. Infections in corticosteroid- and/or immunosuppressant-treated patients are often due to *Staphylococcus aureus;* other agents include *L. monocytogenes, N. meningitidis, Salmonella, M. tuberculosis, Pneumocystis,* viruses such as disseminated *varicella-zoster,* and fungal agents such as *Candida, Nocardia,* and *Aspergillus.* Mixed infections are common, as is overwhelming sepsis.

Fever due to lupus usually associates with other evidence of active disease including skin rash, oral ulcers, arthritis, pleuritis, or palpable purpura. Leukocyte counts may be normal or decreased, there is usually lymphopenia, and serum CRP levels are either normal or minimally elevated.

Conversely, in infection, there is usually leukocytosis and a marked increase in CRP levels. Lupus flares and infection often coexist. It is usually unclear, in cases featuring both lupus activity and infection, whether infection triggers the lupus activity or whether the lupus flare, with its attendant decrease of body defenses, for example, decreased cell-mediated immunity, hypocomplementemia, and decreased bacterial opsonization, fosters the infection. Summarizing, it should never be taken for granted that fever in a lupus patient is due to lupus activity alone.

PATIENT 14. A 43-year-old woman had had a rocky course with her lupus. A year before the current admission she had been brought to the ER with acute right upper quadrant abdominal pain, nausea, and vomiting. She was admitted with a diagnosis of cholecystitis, but surgeons decided to hydrate and watch her overnight in the medical service. Interestingly, the next morning the team's attending noticed that her neck veins were markedly distended, there was hepatojugular reflux, and the Kussmaul sign was markedly positive. She ended up having pericardial aspiration, which improved her immediately, rather than a cholecystectomy.

This time she came in with severe arthralgias, febrile for 3 to 4 days, and with a prominent facial rash, especially over the bridge of the nose (Figure 13–3). Respiratory sounds were muffled at the bases. The WBC was 18,000/mm³ with 80% polys and 10% bands. Urinalysis showed 2+ protein and leukocytes and granular casts in the sediment. The ESR was 90. A dermatologist consultant felt that the facial rash was erysipelas. Penicillin was administered, and 1 day later, without modifying the 10 mg prednisone dose plus hydroxychloroquine 200 mg she was taking, the rash appeared inactive. Serum complement levels came back very low, and the anti-native DNA was elevated. Upon discharge the hydroxychloroquine dose was doubled, and she did well.

Unusually, fever may be the sole manifestation of SLE. For instance, a patient may present daily spikes from 38° to 39° C going on for weeks. Diagnosis in these cases is based on negative bacteriologic studies; the presence of leukopenia, lymphocytopenia, low levels of CRP, hypocomplementemia, and increased levels of anti-dsDNA; and particularly by the presence of additional manifestations of SLE such as synovitis, oral ulcers, or a pleural or pericardial rub found in the course of compulsive, daily examinations.

On the other hand, corticosteroid-treated SLE patients may be unable to mount a febrile response in the event of

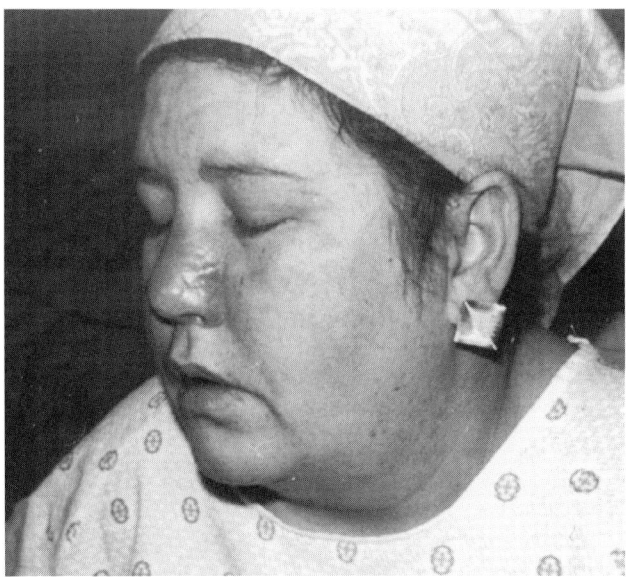

FIGURE 13–3. *Patient 14. Systemic lupus erythematosus.* The rash on her nose was initially thought to be part of her butterfly rash, but the redness and marked tenderness gave the clue to the right diagnosis, erysipelas. She also had active lupus.

overwhelming infection. Apprehension, malaise, asthenia, mental dullness, and hypotension should all be taken as presumptive evidence of sepsis and trigger appropriate action. An inherently difficult differential diagnosis is between SLE and infective endocarditis (IE). Lupus patients share features with IE including a heart murmur, arthralgias, retinal infarctions, splenomegaly, nephritis, small-vessel vasculitis, hypocomplementemia, and a positive rheumatoid factor (latex fixation) test. In IE, however, back pain is often present, there is leukocytosis, and blood cultures are usually positive. This underscores the need to perform ANA (and if this is positive, anti-dsDNA and anti-Sm antibodies) in addition to the routine blood cultures in the evaluation of these patients.

Diagnosis

Summary of Diagnosis

SLE AND FEVER

- Fever is a well-known manifestation of active SLE.
- Fever in inactive SLE suggests infection.
- Leukopenia, lymphopenia, and low levels of CRP suggest lupus fever.
- Shaking chills, leukocytosis, and high levels of CRP strongly indicate microbial infection.
- Concurrent lupus activity must be ruled out in overtly infected SLE patients.
- Corticosteroid-treated patients may be unable to mount a febrile response.
- Fever during immunosuppressive therapy suggests an opportunistic infection.

Natural History

Expected Outcome

Infections are not only more frequent but may also have a more severe course in SLE. This is best exemplified by herpes zoster, which is 2 to 16 times more frequent in lupus patients (particularly in those with advanced renal disease and/or taking immunosuppressant medications) than in the general population, has an increased rate of dissemination, and often serves as portal of entry for a superimposed bacterial infection. In all recent lupus series, infection is the leading cause of death both in early and late disease. A particularly risky scenario is an unrecognized infection in a patient who is adrenal suppressed.

Treatment

Methods

Treatment of infection in SLE includes the appropriate use of antibiotics plus an effective control of lupus activity, even if this implies the use of corticosteroid agents.

When to Refer

Lupus patients with overt or suspected infection should be jointly evaluated by a rheumatologist and an infectious disease specialist.

Key Points

> **SLE AND FEVER**
> - Infection is the leading cause of death in early and late SLE.
> - Infections may trigger lupus activity and active lupus fosters infections.
> - Extricating lupus activity from infection may be a difficult task: Don't hesitate to consult with a rheumatologist and an infectious disease specialist when an SLE patient has fever.
> - Controlling lupus activity is critical in achieving control of the infection.

Suggested Reading

Kahl LE. Herpes zoster infection in systemic lupus erythematosus: Risk factors and outcome. J Rheumatol 21:84–86, 1994.

Manzi S, Kuller LH, Kutzer J, et al. Herpes zoster in systemic lupus erythematosus. J Rheumatol 22:1254–1258, 1995.

Porges AJ, Beattie SL, Ritchlin C, et al. Patients with systemic lupus erythematosus at risk for *Pneumocystis carinii* pneumonia. J Rheumatol 19:1191–1194, 1992.

Watanabe-Duffy KN, Gladman DD. Infection and disease activity in systemic lupus erythematosus: A review of hospitalized patients. J Rheumatol 18:1180–1184, 1991.

Wong DT, Ogra PL. Viral infections in immunocompromised patients. Med Clin North Amer 67:1075–1092, 1983.

Drug-Induced SLE

The age distribution of drug-induced SLE parallels the age distribution of conditions the causative drugs are administered for. Because most of the implicated drugs are used for cardiovascular ailments, drug-induced SLE usually occurs after the age of 50. Different from spontaneous SLE in the elderly, however, drug-induced SLE is mild and readily reversible upon discontinuation of the offending drug.

Presentation and Progression

Cause

Table 13–7 lists most of the drugs capable of triggering a positive ANA and SLE. It is much more frequent, for any given drug, to result in the former than cause the latter. The difference between the two rates, however, varies among drugs. Thus, while chlorpromazine frequently causes an ANA but only exceptionally results in SLE, clinical disease occurs in fully 20% of patients on long-term procainamide treatment. Drugs that cause lupus are widely different chemically, but all seem to yield cytotoxic products when exposed to myeloperoxidase.

Presentation

As mentioned, many drugs cause a positive ANA in the absence of clinical lupus. The usual pattern of nuclear fluorescence is homogeneous, and the specificity of antibodies is against histones. Clinical findings include arthralgias or arthritis in most instances, serositis, usually nonspecific skin rashes, and leukopenia. Only rarely do these patients fulfill classification criteria for SLE.

PATIENT 15. A 74-year-old woman was sent for treatment advice for a poorly responsive case of elderly-onset SLE. One year

TABLE 13–7
DRUGS THAT MAY CAUSE SLE

	Positive ANA (% of Patients)	Clinical SLE (% of Patients)
Procainamide	90	10–30
Hydralazine	20–50	2–20
Isoniazid	20–25	1
Chlorpromazine	20–50	rare
Methyldopa	15	(hemolysis)
Beta blockers	10–30	rare
Captopril	?	very rare
Diphenylhydantoin	?	(true SLE?)
Lithium	?	very rare
Methimazole	?	very rare
Penicillamine	?	very rare
Popylthiouracil	?	very rare
Primidone	?	very rare
Quinidine	?	rare
Sulfasalazine	?	very rare
Trimethadione	?	very rare

before the patient had developed symmetric arthritis in the distal extremities. Her response to choline magnesium salicylate and hydroxychloroquine was poor. She began to lose weight, became depressed, and her ability to manage by herself at home was questioned. Four months before her referral a severe bout of pleuropericarditis, initially thought to be an MI, put her in the hospital. Laboratory studies revealed leukopenia, an ANA on Hep-2 cells of 1:640 (N < 1:80) homogeneous pattern, low C_3, and positive IgM anticardiolipin antibodies. Tests for anti-double-stranded DNA and Sm were negative. Her kidney was spared. She was now taking prednisone 20 mg per day that could not be decreased because the arthritis flared. On taking the history it surfaced that she had been taking quinidine for the past 3 years for the prophylaxis of arrhythmia. The issue of a possible quinidine-induced SLE was raised with her physician and a decision was made to discontinue the quinidine (which the patient did not really need). Slowly, over the course of 3 months, all clinical findings went away. The ANA a year later was 1:40.

Specific lupus antibodies (anti-dsDNA, anti-Sm), as in the case just described, are negative. With some compounds, such as chlorpromazine, antiphospholipid antibodies are quite common.

Diagnosis

Summary of Diagnosis

> **DRUG-INDUCED SLE**
>
> - Positive ANAs are very common with certain medications (procainamide, quinidine, phenothiazines).
> - The pattern of nuclear fluorescence is homogeneous, and antibodies are specific for histone.
> - Clinical manifestations include arthralgias or arthritis, pleuritis, nonspecific rashes, and leukopenia.
> - The required SLE classification criteria are usually not met.
> - Nephritis or a positive anti-Sm or anti-dsDNA antibody test are indicative of idiopathic lupus.

Natural History

Expected Outcome

Persisting disease is to be expected unless the causative drug is discontinued. Complications of drug-induced SLE are rare; pericardial tamponade may occur.

Treatment

Drug-induced lupus is treated by discontinuing the causative drug. If not possible, patients may be treated, as in mild lupus, with a NSAID, hydroxychloroquine, and low-dose prednisone. With drug discontinuation clinical manifestations resolve in 1 to 4 weeks and ANA turns negative in 6 months to 2 years.

When to Refer

Cases that fail to resolve clinically within 6 weeks should be reviewed by a rheumatologist.

Key Points

> **DRUG-INDUCED SLE**
>
> - Drug-induced ANA is much more frequent than clinical SLE.
> - The condition is mild in most patients.
> - Pericardial tamponade may occur.
> - Clinical findings resolve within weeks of discontinuing the offending drug.
> - Resolution of the ANA takes 6 months to 2 years.
> - If drug discontinuation is not possible, cases may be treated like mild SLE.
> - Drugs known to induce ANA/SLE are not contraindicated in spontaneous SLE.

Suggested Reading

Hess E, Mongey A-B. Drug-related lupus: The same as or different from idiopathic disease? In: Lahita RG (ed) Systemic Lupus Erythematosus, 2nd ed. Churchill Livingstone, New York, 893–904, 1992.

Jiang X, Khursigara G, Rubin R. Transformation of lupus-inducing drugs to cytotoxic products by activated neutrophils. Science 266:810–813, 1994.

The Primary and Secondary Antiphospholipid Syndrome (PAPS and SAPS)

This recently described autoimmune entity is best known as a cause of thrombophilia and fetal loss. The condition may occur by itself (PAPS), sometimes simulating SLE, or in association with true SLE (SAPS).

Presentation and Progression

Cause

The cause of PAPS is unknown. Antigen specificity of antiphospholipid antibodies varies among patients. Anticardiolipin activity explains the false positive VDRL often seen in PAPS. Activity against coagulation system phospholipids explains the "lupus anticoagulant"—an obvious misnomer, since the hallmark of the condition is not bleeding but thrombosis—as well as an acquired deficiency of the natural anticoagulants protein S and protein C. As mentioned under the section on laboratory tests, antiphospholipid antibodies may not be directed against phospholipids but against a cofactor, beta-2 glycoprotein 1.

Presentation

Major manifestations of PAPS include recurrent venous and arterial thrombosis and recurrent primarily mid-trimester abortions not necessarily related to placental infarcts. Additional manifestations of the syndrome include thrombocytopenia, hemolytic anemia, livedo reticularis, leg ulcers, cerebral microinfarctions, nephropathy, endocardial vegetations, valvulopathy, retinopathy, pulmonary hemorrhage, and pulmonary arterial hypertension. As expected, SLE patients with SAPS have SLE manifestations plus one or more clinical features of PAPS. It should be stressed that in the absence of major clinical criteria (thrombosis, fetal losses), a positive anticardiolipin test by enzyme-linked immunosorbent assay (ELISA) or a positive lupus anticoagulant test should not be taken as evidence of PAPS or SAPS.

Diagnosis

Summary of Diagnosis

> **PRIMARY ANTIPHOSPHOLIPID ANTIBODY SYNDROME**
> - Consistent clinical findings: recurrent venous or arterial thrombosis, or recurrent mid-trimester abortions.
> - A high-titer IgG or IgM anticardiolipin antibody test by ELISA, or a positive test for the lupus anticoagulant (dilute APTT, kaolin clotting time test, or Russell viper venom time test).
> - Absence of SLE by clinical criteria (a low-titer ANA is present in 30% of PAPS patients).
> - Cardiac echo to determine if vegetations are present.
> - A high-titer anticardiolipin test or lupus anticoagulant test, in the absence of clinical correlates, does not mean PAPS or SAPS.

Natural History

Expected Outcome

The course of PAPS is usually chronic. In the past, the condition has been confused with vasculitis leading to strokes and intestinal infarctions and SLE featuring nephropathy, Libman-Sack's endocarditis, strokes, a false positive VDRL, and a positive ANA.

Complications of PAPS are myriad. Venous thrombosis may occur anywhere including the inferior vena cava, the suprahepatic veins leading to Budd-Chiari's syndrome, mesenteric veins, and the splenic vein. Arterial thrombosis is also ubiquitous, leading, for instance, to cerebral, myocardial, or mesenteric infarction. Valvulopathy occurs in 30% of patients. Some of these patients have thrombotic endocarditis, and multiple cerebral embolic infarctions may occur, leading in rare cases to dementia. Pulmonary hemorrhage clinically similar to lupus pulmonary hemorrhage is well reported. Nephropathy characterized by arterial hypertension and proteinuria, usually mild but occasionally in the nephrotic range, is also common.

Treatment

Methods

Treatment of PAPS is with anticoagulants (Table 13–8). Coumadin anticoagulation with INRs close to 3 is highly effective in preventing venous and arterial thrombosis. In severe cases such as those with stroke or nephropathy, the addition of low-dose ASA may afford an additional prophy-

TABLE 13–8

TREATMENT OF THE ANTIPHOSPHOLIPID SYNDROME

Acute cases of thrombosis treated as routine cases of thrombosis.
Prophylactic oral therapy with anticoagulants (INR at about 3) is advisable.
Low-dose ASA (80 mg/day) may be added.
Thrombolytic therapy is effective to prevent postphlebitic syndrome.
Pregnant patients with a history of pregnancy loss should be treated with low-dose ASA.
Pregnant patients with previous thrombotic events should be treated with low molecular weight heparin plus low-dose ASA.
In severe cases high-dose corticosteroids plus an immunosuppressive agent may be indicated.

lactic effect. Pregnant PAPS patients may be treated with low molecular weight heparin and low-dose ASA through the entire pregnancy, delivery, and the first 3 months postpartum. Some authorities have recommended the use of low- or high-dose prednisone, but a detrimental effect of corticosteroids has been found by others. Intravenous immunoglobulin infusions have also been used with success. In addition to fetal loss, prematurity, intrauterine growth retardation, severe toxemia, maternal renal failure (rare), and peripartum and postpartum maternal thrombotic strokes are important complications of PAPS pregnancies.

Expected Response

The rate of recurrent thrombosis is drastically reduced by high-dose coumadinization. Close obstetrical monitoring and antithrombotic therapy effectively reduce fetal wastage in PAPS pregnancies.

Complications

High-dose coumadin treatment, particularly when associated with ASA, may lead to a massive GI or visceral bleed. However, large studies have shown that bleeding complications are unusual in PAPS patients, with the benefits of treatment far outweighing the risks.

When to Refer

PAPS patients should be followed concurrently with a rheumatologist or hematologist. Pregnancy in PAPS is high risk. Of paramount importance is close follow-up by a rheumatologist and obstetrician. Intrauterine growth retardation and fetal distress may be determined by ultrasonography and fetal heart rate monitoring, respectively. These babies should be delivered as soon as they are viable.

Key Points

> **PRIMARY AND SECONDARY ANTIPHOSPHOLIPID SYNDROME**
> - A positive anticardiolipin or lupus anticoagulant test is insufficient to diagnose PAPS or SAPS. Clinical

> findings such as recurrent arterial or venous thrombosis, or fetal losses must be present for diagnosis.
> - However, a strongly positive anticardiolipin test per se is associated with a twofold increase in fetal loss.
> - Thrombosis prevention in PAPS requires high-dose coumadinization (INR about 3).
> - Moderate heparinization plus low-dose ASA decrease the rate of fetal loss in patients with PAPS.

Suggested Reading

Alarcón-Segovia D, Sánchez-Guerrero J. Primary antiphospholipid syndrome. J Rheumatol 16:482–488, 1989.

Amigo M-C, García-Torres R, Robles M, et al. Renal involvement in primary antiphospholipid syndrome. J Rheumatol 19:1181–1185, 1992.

Lima F, Khamashta MA, Buchanan NMM, et al. A study of sixty pregnancies in patients with the antiphospholipid syndrome. Clin Exper Rheumatol 14:131–136, 1996.

Khamashta MA, Cuadrado MJ, Mujic F, et al. The management of thrombosis in the antiphospholipid antibody syndrome. N Engl J Med 332:993–997, 1995.

Sjögren's Syndrome

Sjögren's syndrome has been aptly described as an autoimmune exocrinopathy. Predominant lacrimal and salivary gland involvement results in dry eyes (keratoconjunctivitis sicca, or KCS) and dry mouth as the salient manifestations of the disease. Involvement of other glands and tissues is less common but still attains prominence in some patients. Inflammation in Sjögren's syndrome is lymphocytic and plasmacytic. Associated findings in lacrimal and salivary tissue include acinar destruction and myoepithelial cell hyperplasia. Sjögren's syndrome may occur per se (primary Sjögren's syndrome) or may represent an association of connective tissue diseases such as RA, SLE, or scleroderma (secondary Sjögren's syndrome). To diagnose primary Sjögren's syndrome as opposed to KCS, minor salivary gland biopsy must show more than one focus of at least 50 lymphocytes/4 mm^2 (score > 1).

Presentation and Progression

The etiology of Sjögren's syndrome remains unknown. Pathogenetically the condition appears to lie between RA and SLE. Similar to other autoimmune diseases, Sjögren's syndrome associates with the histocompatibility antigen HLA-DR3 in Caucasians. The frequency of RA, SLE, and thyroid disease is increased among first-degree relatives of Sjögren's patients. Primary Sjögren's syndrome affects predominantly women with a female to male ratio of 9 to 1. The frequency of the condition increases with advancing age. Secondary Sjögren's parallels demographic features of the underlying connective tissue disease or infection such as HIV or hepatitis C virus infection. Whereas primary Sjögren's syndrome tends to be clinically striking, secondary Sjögren's is usually subtle, an often unidentified complication of the underlying disease.

Initial symptoms involve the eyes, nose, or the oral cavity. Eyes may feel gritty, sandy, or covered with a film. A feeling of eye irritation is exacerbated in a dry environment. Because mucinous secretion is preserved, the question "do you make tears when you cry?" is often answered with a misleading "yes." Corneal ulceration, vascularization, and opacification may occur in late untreated disease. Diagnosis of eye dryness (Table 13–9) requires objective demonstration by the Schirmer's test that can be performed by primary care physicians. Eye dryness may be diagnosed more accurately with a drop of rose Bengal dye followed by inspection with a slit lamp or an ophthalmoscope.

Sjögren's patients have increased staining in the interpalpebral space, which is indicative of small, superficial erosions. Nasal dryness causes rhinitis, crusting, and bloody nasal discharge. Oral symptoms may be subtle. Patients may complain of a metallic taste; burning of the tongue, inner cheeks, or gums; dry mouth; and unusual dental decay. A key question to ask is whether the patient is able to chew and swallow crackers without the help of fluids. The tongue depressor adheres tightly to the mucosal surface.

A distressing but rarely reported symptom (which remains hidden unless asked about) is vaginal dryness. Vaginal dryness may precede other components of the sicca complex.

Spontaneous fluctuation in salivary gland size is frequent. Lacrimal gland enlargement is rare, but parotid gland enlargement is often present on examination. It should be remembered that an enlarged parotid gland bulges behind the lower jaw and elevates the earlobe. Lymphadenopathy, which may fluctuate in size, and thyroid enlargement are common. Spleen may be palpable. Arthralgias or arthritis, usually nonerosive and nondeforming, are present in most Sjögren's patients.

Fibromyalgia is a frequent accompaniment of the disease. Conversely, a sicca syndrome is often present in fibromyalgia as a result of the use of anticholinergic medications or an unusual sensitivity to inhibitory nerve mechanisms (Table 13–10). Autoimmune thyroiditis often develops in Sjögren's syndrome, and the risk is higher in the presence of antithyroglobulin antibodies. If antithyroid antibodies are included, about 75% of primary Sjögren's syndrome have autoimmune thyroid disease or thyroid dysfunction. Clinical hypothyroidism develops in about 20%. Leukopenia occurs in about 30%. Increased serum alanine aminotransferase (ALT) and serum aspartate aminotransferase (AST) may indicate hepatitis or myositis; CPK and aldolase elevation indicates

---

TABLE 13–9

TESTS TO DOCUMENT OCULAR AND ORAL DRYNESS

OCULAR DRYNESS

Schirmer's test: Place a strip of Whatman #41 filter paper under lower lid (avoiding corneal contact) and wait 5 minutes. Remove and measure wet area. Normal wetness: > 15 mm below age 60; > 10 at age 60 or older.

Rose Bengal test: Instill 1 drop of rose Bengal. After 1 minute observe cornea and sclera with ophthalmoscope or slit lamp. Findings in Sjögren's include interpalpebral staining, corneal punctate stain, filamentary strands, abrasions, and erosions.

MOUTH DRYNESS

Tongue depressor test: Apply tongue depressor flat on tongue and remove. In Sjögren's the tongue depressor sticks to the tongue.

Cotton sponge test: Place cotton sponge under tongue for 3 minutes. Compare dry and wet weight.

TABLE 13-10
CAUSES OF DRY EYES AND DRY MOUTH OTHER THAN SJÖGREN'S SYNDROME
Old age
Dehydration (low intake, diabetes,* diuretics)
Use of anticholinergic and antihypertensive medications
Irradiation
Hepatitis C infection*
HIV infection*
Sarcoidosis*
Amyloidosis*
*May cause salivary gland enlargement.

myositis whereas alkaline phosphatase and serum gamma-glutamyl transpeptidase (GGT) elevation indicates hepatitis. Antinuclear antibodies (ANA) with a homogeneous or speckled pattern, rheumatoid factor (RF), and SSA and/or SSB autoantibodies (SS stands for Sjögren's syndrome) are present in most patients. Thyroglobulin antibodies are present in over 50%. Polyclonal elevation of serum immunoglobulins is common. High immunoglobulin elevations associate with polymyositis, hyperglobulinemic purpura, a hyperviscosity syndrome, and renal tubular acidosis. Cryoglobulins and IgM monoclonal immunoglobulins are often present. Sjögren's related cryoglobulinemia, which usually is Type II with a monoclonal IgM rheumatoid factor, associates with vasculitis, glomerulonephritis, pseudolymphoma, and non-Hodgkin's lymphoma.

Less typical presentations of primary Sjögren's include small-vessel vasculitis (palpable purpura, neuropathy, glomerulonephritis), hyperglobulinemic purpura (dependent purpura followed by hyperpigmentation), myositis, which is clinically similar to polymyositis, multiple sclerosis–like CNS disease with multiple areas of demyelination, interstitial pulmonary disease, and tubulointerstitial kidney disease causing renal tubular acidosis.

Diagnosis

Summary of Diagnosis

> **SJÖGREN'S SYNDROME**
>
> - Sicca syndrome (dry eyes, dry mouth).
> - A positive Schirmer's test or punctate and filamentous keratitis as shown by rose Bengal dye and biomicroscopic examination.
> - Minor salivary gland biopsy is confirmatory of primary Sjögren's syndrome. Cases of plain KCS feature minimal salivary gland changes with a score less than 1.
> - Chest x-rays to rule out pseudolymphoma and interstitial pneumonitis.
> - CBC, ESR, serum creatinine, AST, ALT, CPK, aldolase, alkaline phosphatase, GGT, urinalysis, TSH, ANA, RF, SSA, SSB (anti-DNA and anti-Sm if ANA is positive), serum protein electrophoresis, and quantitated IgG and IgM (serum immunoelectrophoresis if an "M" component appears to be present).

Natural History

Expected Outcome

Sjögren's syndrome is in the majority of patients a major nuisance with little functional disability. However, articular symptoms may be prominent and in a few patients myositis, CNS disease, or renal complications develop. Some patients with primary Sjögren's go on to develop manifestations of other connective tissue diseases on follow-up. Patients with primary Sjögren's syndrome may have a massive proliferation of polyclonal B-cells resulting in lymphadenopathy as well as heavy parenchymal infiltration, particularly in the lung. These worrisome benign growths are designated pseudolymphoma. In addition, approximately 10% of cases of primary Sjögren's syndrome go on to develop B-cell lymphoma, often with pseudolymphoma as an antecedent. Because of these uncommon but most interesting transitions, Sjögren's syndrome has come to be viewed as a link between autoimmunity and malignancy. There is no increased risk of lymphoma in patients with plain KCS.

Complications

Decreased saliva production leads to frequent dental caries and periodontitis; it is not unusual to hear from Sjögren's patients that they lost all of their teeth within a few months. Suppurative infections occur frequently as a result of lack of secretions and poor ciliary function. These include acute sinusitis, acute otitis media, suppurative parotitis, and protracted episodes of suppurative bronchitis. Suppurative parotitis is a serious condition that requires early diagnosis and intensive antibiotic treatment. Diagnosis is suggested by fever and the sudden onset of pain, swelling, and severe tenderness in a parotid gland. The parotid duct's aperture is red and swollen, and pus may appear spontaneously or by gently milking the gland. *Staphylococcus aureus* is the usual causative agent.

In a dry environment minor URI episodes tend to be followed by protracted bronchitis, acute sinusitis, and acute otitis media. Oral candidiasis is a complication that should be suspected when oral symptoms suddenly increase or when sore throat or painful swallowing develop. The presence of thrush confirms the diagnosis.

As mentioned, about 20% of patients develop clinical hypothyroidism. Liver involvement is relatively common in Sjögren's. Because there is a two-way association between Sjögren's and primary biliary cirrhosis, antimytochondrial antibodies should be studied if serum alkaline phosphatase is increased. More frequently there is a mild, nonspecific hepatitis. Hepatitis C should be excluded in these patients.

Pseudolymphoma or lymphoma should be suspected in patients with lymphadenopathy when a lymph node or group of lymph nodes starts to grow and also when Sjögren's patients develop pulmonary infiltrates or renal insufficiency. Differentiation between pseudolymphoma (polyclonal B-cell proliferation) and lymphoma (monoclonal B-cell proliferation) may be difficult even by using molecular techniques. A previously positive rheumatoid factor test may turn negative as lymphoma develops. Interestingly, a Sjögren-like syndrome including salivary gland inflammation, positive rheumatoid factor test, polyclonal immunoglobulin elevation, cryoglobulinemia, and transition in some cases to B-cell lymphoma may all appear in hepatitis C virus infection. Indeed, with current knowledge of hepatitis C virus infection, the entire fields of Sjögren's and mixed cryoglobulinemia need to be redefined. Patients with HIV infection may also exhibit a clinically confusing Sjögren's-like condition.

Treatment

Methods

Treatment of Sjögren's syndrome calls for the combined expertise of a rheumatologist, ophthalmologist, and dental medicine specialist. Once the treatment program has been laid down, patients may be followed by the primary care physician. A rheumatologist's input is essential to establish diagnosis and to decide on systemic treatment. Although formal trials have not been conducted, hydroxychloroquine is believed to be highly effective in controlling malaise and articular symptoms as well as reducing ESR, immunoglobulins, and SSA/SSB antibody levels. Prednisone may be added for control of adenopathic, pulmonary, and vasculitic manifestations. An ophthalmologist's input is critical for initial eye assessment, recommendation of topical medications (Table 13–11), advice on measures such as tear duct ligation, treatment of intercurrent lid infections, and the routine control of hydroxychloroquine therapy. A dentist interested in xerosthomia is an important member of the team because frequent dental cleansing, repair of decayed teeth, and use of topical fluoride preparations relieve some of the most distressing Sjögren's symptoms. Recent data suggest that pilocarpine has potential use to increase salivary flow.

The primary care physician should provide routine health maintenance measures; make sure the patient is periodically seen by the consultants just listed; recommend avoiding dry air at work and in the home, in particular a hot air–heated bedroom without proper humidification; treat early bacterial infections as suggested by a lingering URI with purulent secretions, sudden pain and tenderness in a parotid gland, unilateral nasal discharge and blockade, ear pain, or sinus pain; suggest that in the event of surgery, because the operating room air is dry and anticholinergic drugs are likely to be administered, an ocular lubricating ointment and proper occlusion be used to prevent corneal abrasion; check TSH levels at 1 year intervals; and be aware of the possibility of an emerging lymphoma in cases of primary Sjögren's.

Expected Response

On the treatment described here, most patients with Sjögren's syndrome improve. Expert dental care and the routine use of fluorinated mouthwashes relieve distressing oral symptoms. Eye irritation subsides with the appropriate topical treatment. General symptoms and arthralgias improve within 3 to 4 months of initiation of hydroxychloroquine treatment.

When to Refer

Patients suspected of having Sjögren's syndrome should be referred to a rheumatologist for diagnostic confirmation, initial asessment of orificial lesions, and to determine whether systemic involvement is present. Ophthalmologic and oral medicine evaluations should follow. A key issue that cannot be overemphasized is the early institution of dental and ocular prophylaxis.

Resources Available

There are two Sjögren's syndrome associations: the National Sjögren's Syndrome Association and the Sjögren's Syndrome Foundation (see the appendix).

Key Points

SJÖGREN'S SYNDROME

- Primary Sjögren's syndrome is more severe than secondary Sjögren's in terms of salivary and lymphoid tissue growth, visceral involvement, vasculitic

---

TABLE 13–11

LOCAL TREATMENT OF SICCA COMPLEX

DRY EYES MEDICATIONS

1. Preservative-free artificial tears*
Aquasite
Bion tears
Celluvisc
Dry Eye Therapy
Hypo Tears PF
Refresh Plus (50 per box)
Tears Naturale Free

2. Preservative-free ocular ointments†
Duolube
Duratears naturale
Hypo Tears
Refresh PM
Tears Renewed

DRY MOUTH MEDICATIONS

1. Lip balm
Aloe Vera Lip Balm

2. Chewing gums
Biotene Gum
Xylifresh Peppermint Gum
Xylifresh Spearmint Gum

3. Mouthwashes
Biotene Mouthwash

4. Toothpaste
Biotene Toothpaste

5. Oral moisturizers
ORALbalance (gel)
Salivart (spray)

NASAL DRYNESS MEDICATIONS

NaSal (spray)
Nose Better Spray
Ocean

VAGINAL DRYNESS

Replens

*Anticipate use, e.g., 4 times a day, more during dry season or with air pollution.
†At night instill artificial tears first and then apply 1/8 inch of the ointment.

- complications, and the development of pseudolymphoma and lymphoma.
- Autoimmune thyroid disease is quite common in primary Sjögren's syndrome.
- Secondary Sjögren's is often overlooked; it is present in approximately 30% of patients with RA, SLE, and scleroderma. Diagnosis depends on asking the right questions.
- Hepatitis C virus infection and HIV infection may closely resemble Sjögren's.
- Treatment of Sjögren's includes the local care of dry eye and mucosae, prophylaxis and treatment of secondary suppurative and fungal infection, and the use of systemic measures, in particular hydroxychloroquine.

Suggested Reading

Fox RI. Fifth international symposium of Sjögren's syndrome. Arthritis Rheum 39:195–196, 1996.

Fox RI, Kang HI. Sjögren's syndrome. In: Kelley WN, Harris ED Jr, Ruddy S, et al. (eds) Textbook of Rheumatology, 4th ed. W.B. Saunders, Philadelphia, 931–942, 1993.

Jorgensen C, Legouffe M.-C, Perney P, et al. Sicca syndrome associated hepatitis C infection. Arthritis Rheum 39:1166–1171, 1996.

Kruize AA, Hene RJ, van der Heide A, et al. Long-term followup of patients with Sjögren's syndrome. Arthritis Rheum 39:297–303, 1996.

Pérez E-B, Kraus A, López G, et al. Autoimmune thyroid disease in primary Sjögren's syndrome. Am J Med 99:480–484, 1995.

Vitali C, Bombardieri S, Moutsopoulos HM, et al. Preliminary criteria for the classification of Sjögren's syndrome: Results of a prospective concerted action supported by the European community. Arthritis Rheum 36:340–347, 1993.

CHAPTER 14

Inflammatory Conditions of Muscle

There are multiple, interesting, at times puzzling associations between connective tissue diseases and myositis. Rheumatoid arthritis, SLE, Sjögren's syndrome, and scleroderma may feature muscle inflammation. This is usually subclinical, but overt myositis does occur at times.

There are also overlapping conditions (Sharp's mixed connective tissue disease) in which myositis is one of the clinical findings, the others being shared with SLE (rash, alopecia, serositis) and scleroderma (sclerodactily, Raynaud's). Finally, polymyositis and dermatomyositis (the two leading idiopathic inflammatory myopathies) may feature arthritis and pulmonary interstitial disease, an association that could suggest RA. Viewed from another angle, there are conditions such as sarcoidosis in which both myositis and various types of arthritis may be featured. Finally, muscle dystrophies may mimic myositis, and infectious processes such as HIV infection, trichinosis, and Whipple's disease may feature myositis as part of their disease spectrum.

Proximal muscle weakness is the leading finding in the idiopathic inflammatory myopathies (see Chapter 2, on physical examination). Muscle tenderness is relatively uncommon. The clinical suspicion is supported by a characteristic pattern of enzyme elevation as well as consistent EMG changes: muscle irritability as the recording needle is inserted into muscle, also known as increased insertional activity, and low-amplitude, polyphasic motor potentials that show abnormal early recruitment (myopathic triad). Interestingly, there are HLA (DRw52, DRw53) and autoantibodies associations that have helped define clinical and prognostic subgroups. Among the myositis-specific autoantibodies there are aminoacyl-tRNA synthetase antibodies (five and probably more types, the most frequent and best known being the anti-Jo-1 or histidyl transferase antibody); anti-signal recognition particle antibodies; and other antibodies such as the anti-Mi-2 and anti-MAS antibodies. Also, contrary to what could be expected, MRI studies have shown a patchy or regional, rather than a uniform, pattern of muscle involvement in the idiopathic inflammatory myopathies. To this day, muscle biopsy remains the gold standard for a diagnosis of myositis.

Polymyositis (PM)

Presentation and Progression

Cause

Polymyositis affects mainly adults after the second decade of life. Although a viral etiology of PM has long been suspected, results of sophisticated microbiologic studies have so far been negative. Pathologically, predominant findings include endomysial (around individual muscle cells) lymphocytic infiltrates comprised of cytotoxic T-cells and macrophages, muscle cell necrosis and phagocytosis, and basophilic regenerative fibers that can be easily identified on H&E stains. Interestingly, muscle cells in PM express the class I major histocompatibility complex, which is absent in normal muscle, and thus have the potential to present the putative etiologic antigen to cytotoxic T-cells. There is no evidence of autoantibody-mediated injury in PM.

Presentation

The leading finding in PM is a slowly progressive proximal weakness. Patients may report, for instance, difficulties rising from a chair or getting up from bed that require turning to the side and then using the arms to sit. Overhead activities such as replacing a book on a shelf or combing the hair may no longer be possible. Muscle pain and tenderness are uncommon. Additional manifestations may be present. Upper (striate muscle) esophageal involvement may result in dysphagia, regurgitation, and aspiration pneumonia. Respiratory muscle weakness, with or without pulmonary interstitial disease, may cause respiratory failure. Disease onset may be subacute including fever, coarse and fissured skin in the contact area of index and thumb (mechanic's hand), Raynaud's phenomenon, distal and symmetric polyarthritis, and pulmonary interstitial disease, resembling RA. However, prominent muscle weakness, increased muscle enzymes, lack of erosions on x-rays, and negative RF test should suggest PM rather than RA. Interestingly, this clinical cluster almost regularly associates with the presence of anti-Jo-1 or other antisynthetase antibody, which justifies the proposed name "antisynthetase syndrome."

Another emerging clinical syndrome is acute disease usually affecting black women, with palpitations, myalgias, and evidences of carditis. This syndrome associates with the presence of antisignal recognition particle antibodies. There appears to be no association between PM and cancer beyond what could be expected from a detection bias: Because patients with PM are closely scrutinized, the likelihood of detecting cancer is increased. Another, extremely rare form of PM is hyperacute, with a rhabdomyolysis syndrome. Patients present with fever, generalized myalgias, myoglobinuria, and there is a rapid progression to acute renal failure. Polymyositis must be distinguished from other types of myopathy. Among these, inclusion body myopathy, endocrine and metabolic myopathies, and certain types of muscle dystrophy deserve special note and are discussed in a later chapter.

Diagnosis

Summary of Diagnosis

> **POLYMYOSITIS**
>
> - History of muscle weakness, coarse skin on hands, Raynaud's, upper dysphagia, regurgitation, palpitations, dyspnea, arthralgias.
> - Physical examination showing proximal muscle weakness, mechanic's hands, crackling rales, synovitis.
> - Request alkaline phosphatase, AST, ALT, CPK, aldolase; ANA; anti-Jo-1.
> - Request TSH, K, Ca, and Mg.
> - Chest x-rays, PFTs with diffusive capacity.
> - Ba swallow to detect upper esophageal dysfunction.
> - EMG on one side to confirm myopathic changes, determine abnormal muscle, and exclude myasthenia gravis and Eaton-Lambert's syndrome.
> - Document myositis by contralateral muscle biopsy in a muscle homologous to the one showing EMG changes.

Natural History

The natural course of PM varies with the clinical cluster. Cases of "antisynthetase syndrome" tend to have a protracted course with progressive interstitial pulmonary disease if left untreated. Survival at 5 years in this group is 70%. Prognosis is more severe in patients with the unusual "antisignal recognition particle syndrome" owing to myocardial involvement. The 5 year survival rate in this group is 25%. In the remaining cases, which comprise the bulk of PM patients, the condition tends to run a chronic course. There is improvement with medications, and flares often occur when medications are discontinued. Muscle atrophy and contractures are common in long-standing cases. A few cases seem to remit permanently.

Complications of PM include respiratory failure from one or more of the following: respiratory muscle weakness, interstitial pneumonitis, aspiration pneumonia, and opportunistic infection; and cardiac arrhythmias. Poor prognostic factors (in both PM and DM) include delayed onset of treatment, pulmonary interstitial disease, and cardiac disease. In PM, carrying antisynthetase antibodies and antisignal recognition particle antibodies are associated with a poorer prognosis.

Treatment

Methods

Treatment of PM is with high-dose oral prednisone (1–2 mg/kg/day) given in divided doses for the first week or two and then once a day. Full doses of prednisone are continued until the CPK (or the enzyme that was highest in the initial screen) has been normalized for approximately 4 weeks. A slow dose reduction, usually by 10 mg per month, is then undertaken. The addition of immunosuppressives, usually MTX or azathioprine, is considered in two situations: (1) patients who fail to improve on high-dose prednisone, and (2) increasing enzyme levels as corticosteroids are reduced. The latter situation may be also handled by resuming the previous prednisone dose, but the cost in terms of steroid complications may be too high.

Azathioprine (or cyclophosphamide) may be a better choice than MTX in patients with interstitial pneumonitis. Intravenous immunoglobulins have been used with success in refractory PM cases, but cost is high and improvement is usually transient. In addition to medications, PM patients should receive appropriate physical therapy measures. Active-assistive exercises are important during the period of active myositis. Strengthening exercises are started once muscle enzyme levels become normal. Stretching exercises are essential in the treatment of late cases with muscle and tendon contractures. In the rare acute cases associated with rhabdomyolysis, vigorous hydration, mannitol, and sodium bicarbonate may avert development of acute renal failure.

Expected Response

With the treatment just described, most patients may be expected to improve. Typically, enzyme levels normalize first, preceding the clinical improvement by a few weeks to 6 months. A mirror phenomenon occurs in flares: Enzyme levels rise first, followed by weakness weeks to months later. Approximately 50% of cases experience remission. Permanent muscle atrophy and contractures are the unfortunate complications of insufficient or delayed treatment. Polymyositis cases that are unresponsive to therapy should be reevaluated for the possibility of inclusion-body myositis or muscle dystrophy.

Complications

Complications of treatment, mainly toxicities, may cause long-standing disability of their own. Approximately 10% of patients develop osteonecrosis within a 2 year follow-up. Osteoporotic spinal fractures are also frequent. Preventive measures for osteoporosis should be routinely implemented. A particularly difficult situation arises when PM patients with interstitial pneumonitis are given MTX and their condition deteriorates. Although opportunistic infection may be ruled in or out with relative ease, progression of PM pneumonitis may be difficult to sort out from MTX pneumonitis even on open biopsy. Given this potential problem, the author favors azathioprine, or even I.V. cyclophosphamide, in PM patients with interstitial pneumonitis.

When to Refer

Polymyositis is an infrequent condition that is only exceptionally encountered in a general practice. Suspected cases should be refered to a rheumatologist or neurologist for further evaluation and treatment.

Key Points

> **POLYMYOSITIS**
>
> - Polymyositis occurs in several clinical patterns that range from acute rhabdomyolysis to a chronic, indolent disease with wasting and contractures.
> - Complications of PM include acute renal failure from rhabdomyolysis; respiratory failure (from PM-related respiratory muscle weakness, pneumonitis, or aspiration; MTX pneumonitis; or opportunistic infection); and myocarditis.
> - Treatment of PM is with high-dose corticosteroids plus, in severe cases, an immunosuppressant drug.
> - Physical therapy is an integral component of the treatment program.
> - Enzyme normalization occurs within a few weeks of treatment; strength improvement lags behind a few weeks to 6 months.
> - There is no association between PM and cancer (other than detection bias).
> - Long-term course of PM depends on the clinical form. In general, the condition tends to recur following interruption of therapy.

Suggested Reading

Bohan A, Peter JB, Bowman RL, et al. A computer-assisted analysis of 153 patients with polymyositis and dermatomyositis. Medicine (Baltimore) 56:255–286, 1977.
Dalakas M. Polymyositis, dermatomyositis, and inclusion body myositis. N Engl J Med 325:1487–1498, 1991.
Love LA, Leff RL, Fraser DD, et al. A new approach to the classification of idiopathic inflammatory myopathy: Myositis-specific autoantibodies define useful homogeneous patient groups. Medicine (Baltimore) 70:360–374, 1991.
Medsger TA Jr, Oddis CV. Classification and diagnostic criteria for polymyositis and dermatomyositis. J Rheumatol 22:581–585, 1995.
Tanimoto K, Nakano K, Kano S, et al. Classification criteria for polymyositis and dermatomyositis. J Rheumatol 22:668–674, 1995.

Dermatomyositis (DM)

Presentation and Progression

Cause

Dermatomyositis occurs in children as well as in adults. What sets this condition apart from the rest of idiopathic inflammatory myopathies is the striking dermal involvement. Skin findings are so distinctive that even DM without myositis can be diagnosed (amyopathic DM). In adults, particularly over the age of 50, DM often associates with a neoplasm. The neoplasm may be diagnosed prior to, concurrently with, or following the diagnosis of DM. Malignancies tend to cluster around the time of diagnosis of DM plus or minus 2 years. Overall, about 20% of late-adult DM cases are neoplasm related. Ovarian tumors appear to be overrepresented in patients with malignancy-related DM. In children and in nonmalignant adult cases the etiology of DM is unknown.

Histologic findings in DM differ from PM. In DM, the inflammatory infiltrates are perivascular or interfascicular. There is evidence of complement-induced damage in the intramuscular vessels. Frank vasculitis may occur, particularly in pediatric cases. As a result there is focal ischemic muscle damage with groups of necrotic, degenerating, and regenerating cells randomly involving portions of the muscle fascicle. Some cases without an inflammatory infiltrate still show perifascicular atrophy (several layers of atrophic fibers in the peripheral portion of the fascicle).

Presentation

Characteristic of DM is diffuse erythema of exposed skin, often photosensitive, involving the face, neck, and anterior upper chest in the form of a V or a shawl (upper chest and shoulders) (Figure 14–1). Superficial edema is typical of the lesion. Also characteristic is a bluish, "heliotrope" hue of the upper lids. Flat, violaceous papules on the knuckles (MCPs and PIPs) known as Gottron's sign are also typical of DM. Acral scaliness that is particularly prominent over the elbows and knees may closely resemble psoriasis. Subcutaneous and fascial calcification, a frequent late finding in children's DM, is not seen in adults. Another feature that is most unusual in adults is necrotizing vasculitis involving the digits and the gut.

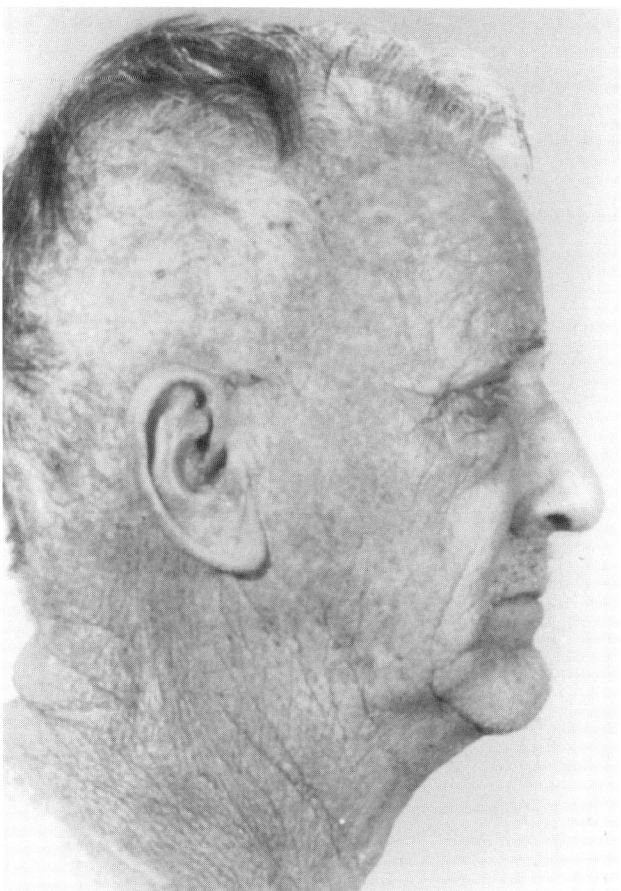

FIGURE 14–1. *Dermatomyositis.* This man presented with an erythematous, edematous rash on his head, neck, and anterior chest. CPK levels were very high, and muscle biopsy showed myositis. He was a heavy smoker. Initial chest x-rays were negative, but 6 months later a right hilar mass was apparent.

Muscle findings in DM range from prominent to none. Proximal muscles are characteristically involved. Patients with DM rash, fatigue, and normal strength may have modest enzyme elevations or may lack laboratory, biopsy, or MRI evidence of muscle involvement (amyopathic DM). A deficit in muscle metabolism that makes these patients unable to normally sustain heavy work is probably caused by ischemia.

Associated findings in DM include polyarthralgias in half of cases, fever in 30%, and less frequently Raynaud's phenomenon. Esophageal, pulmonary, and cardiac manifestations in DM resemble the findings in PM. A variable number of patients, depending on the referral path, have an associated connective tissue disease, usually SLE or scleroderma. Patients with neoplasm-related dermatomyositis tend to have skin and muscle findings only, without overlapping features with other connective tissue diseases. Also, muscle enzymes may be near normal in these patients.

Recommendations for tumor search in patients with PM are as follows: Adult patients, particularly those over 45, should have an initial and then annual routine physical examination including rectal and vaginal examinations, complete blood count, urinalysis, blood chemistry tests, and a chest film. In addition, any clinical lead suggesting a tumor should be investigated. An example would be DM appearing in a heavy smoker; this patient deserves a very critical chest evaluation; a small lung tumor not visible on x-rays but detectable on CT may be present. Also, given the recent evidence of overrepresentation of ovarian cancer, a pelvic ultrasound should be added, in the author's opinion, to the initial and follow-up evaluations of women with DM.

Diagnosis

Summary of Diagnosis

> **DERMATOMYOSITIS**
> - Childhood and adulthood condition.
> - History of proximal muscle weakness.
> - Dermal changes including face, neck, and chest erythema; heliotrope hue in the upper lids; Gottron's papules; and scaly, pseudopsoriasiform acral lesions.
> - Patients may have fever, polyarthralgias, Raynaud's, upper esophageal dysfunction, pneumonitis, and carditis.
> - Increased muscle enzymes in most patients.
> - Myopathic changes on EMG in most patients.
> - Muscle biopsy showing perivascular or interfascicular infiltrates, focal necrotic and regenerative changes, and perifascicular muscle atrophy in most patients.
> - Consider an associated neoplasm in patients in their late middle age (50 or older), particularly in the absence of overlapping features with connective tissue disease and when muscle enzymes are near normal.

Natural History

Expected Outcome

Dermatomyositis and PM are similar in terms of muscle, esophageal, pulmonary, and cardiac involvement. Patients with DM have the added disability from the skin lesions that can be painfully itchy and disfiguring, plus an increased risk of neoplasm. A large nationwide Finnish study showed that DM patients had an overall risk of developing neoplasia of six (six times higher) compared with the general population. The risk was highest in the over-50 age group, especially within the first year following the diagnosis of DM. No association was found between cytotoxic therapy of DM and the risk of developing cancer. Markers of poor prognosis include delay in starting treatment, pulmonary interstitial disease, cardiac involvement, and association with neoplasia.

Treatment

Methods

Treatment of DM is similar to the treatment of PM, plus any treatment deemed necessary for the dermatitis. Sun-blocking agents should be used in photosensitive patients (see appendix). Hydroxychloroquine, as an adjunct, has a beneficial effect on both the dermatitis and the photosensitivity. It has been recommended that malignancy-associated DM be treated with corticosteroids alone.

Expected Response

Treatment response in adult DM is similar to PM. Skin inflammation may be harder to control than muscle inflammation. Prognosis in patients with malignancy-associated DM is poor mainly due to tumor dissemination.

Complications

Complications of therapy were discussed in Chapter 13.

When to Refer

Patients with suspected DM should be referred to a rheumatologist or neurologist for further evaluation and treatment. Cases with an associated neoplasm, depending on the stage, are best followed by the primary care physician and a consultant oncologist.

Key Points

> **DERMATOMYOSITIS**
> - The rash of DM is unmistakable and represents, without question, the most helpful clue to diagnosis.
> - Most patients with DM have clinical and/or biochemical evidence of muscle inflammation. However, some patients don't (amyopathic DM).
> - Cases of DM beginning in late middle age should be suspected of harboring a neoplasm.
> - Neoplasms in DM are usually detectable on routine medical follow-up.
> - Treatment of DM is similar to PM, plus the special care required by the dermal component.

Suggested Reading

Airio A, Pukkala E, Isomäki H. Elevated cancer incidence in patients with dermatomyositis. A population based study. J Rheumatol 22:1300–1303, 1995.

Clarke AN, Bloch DA, Medsger TA Jr, et al. A longitudinal study of functional disability in a national cohort of patients with polymyositis/dermatomyositis. Arthritis Rheum 38:1218–1224, 1995.

Park JH, Olsen NJ, King L Jr, et al. Use of magnetic resonance imaging and P-31 magnetic resonance spectroscopy to detect and quantify muscle dysfunction in the amyopathic and myopathic variants of dermatomyositis. Arthritis Rheum 38:68–77, 1995.

Wortmann RL. Inflammatory diseases of muscle. In: Kelley WN, Harris ED Jr, Ruddy S, et al. (eds) Textbook of Rheumatology. W.B. Saunders, Philadelphia, 1159–1188, 1993.

Inclusion Body Myositis (IBM) and Idiopathic Inflammatory Myopathy Mimickers

IBM is characterized histologically by vacuoles rimmed or lined by basophilic granules, clusters of atrophic fibers, and by electron microscopy cytoplasmic and intranuclear microtubular filaments in muscle cells. The condition must be distinguished from other vacuolar myopathies.

Presentation and Progression

Cause

The differential diagnosis of PM and DM includes IBM, a third member of the idiopathic inflammatory myopathies; connective tissue disorders; endocrine disorders; metabolic myopathies; infections; sarcoidosis; muscle dystrophies; neuromuscular junction disorders; various types of neuropathy; and fibromyalgia.

Onset of IBM is after the age of 50. An incorrect diagnosis of PM is often made, the true nature of the condition being identified during evaluation of steroid-resistant PM. A distinguishing feature of IBM is the presence of distal as well as proximal muscle weakness. Indeed, the insidious onset of painless lower extremity weakness, involvement of foot extensors and finger flexors, and loss of patellar reflex are characteristic of the condition. Focal and asymmetric involvement are additional features of IBM. There may be a predominant involvement of the erector spinae muscles resulting in an inability to maintain the erect posture. Dysphagia is often severe. The serum CPK level is slightly or moderately elevated in 80% of patients. A connective tissue disease often coexists with IBM including SLE, scleroderma, and Sjögren's. Other rheumatic disease associations have also been reported, but some could represent chance associations. There is no relation between IBM and malignancy.

Table 14–1 lists conditions that may mimic an idiopathic inflammatory myopathy. Particularly troublesome are muscle dystrophies featuring increased levels of CPK as well as inflammatory findings on biopsy. A possible diagnosis of muscle dystrophy is suggested by onset in childhood or young age and a positive family history. Limb girdle muscular dystrophy, with onset between the second and fourth decades of life (autosomal recessive), and Becker's dystrophy, which may present findings in late adolescence (X-linked), are the most likely to be confused with PM. Thus, patients with suspected PM with early onset, an unusual pattern of muscle involvement, or with familial cases should be evaluated by a neurologist familiar with the various types of muscle dystrophy. Neuropathies such as diabetic amyotrophy cause muscle weakness and atrophy, but enzyme levels are normal. Fatigability and ocular muscle involvement are hallmarks of myasthenia gravis. Both myasthenia gravis and Eaton-Lambert's disease have characteristic findings on EMG. Infectious myositis should be suspected in the right setting such as exposure to raw pork meat and eosinophilia in trichinosis, and weight loss and risk factors for infection in HIV. Enzyme errors of glycogen metabolism cause muscle weakness and cramps associated with exercise. Certain drugs, such as hydroxychloroquine, administered for years, particularly in patients with some degree of renal failure, are capable of inducing a vacuolar-type myopathy. The presentation may include unexplained cardiac dyastolic failure. Endomyocardial biopsy has been useful to identify these cases. Hypothyroidism, by causing proximal muscle weakness, carpal tunnel syndrome, and increased CPK levels, is a potential cause of diagnostic error. Similarly, hypo- and hyperparathyroidism and hypophosphatemia (particularly tumor induced) may feature prominent myopathic weakness.

Diagnosis

Summary of Diagnosis

> **INCLUSION BODY MYOSITIS AND IDIOPATHIC INFLAMMATORY MYOPATHY MIMICKERS**
>
> - IBM should be suspected (1) when myopathic findings involve both proximal and distal muscles, is spotty, or is asymmetric, (2) when tendon reflexes are lost, and (3) in steroid-resistant PM.
> - A thorough review of muscle biopsy reveals the diagnostic features of IBM.
> - Several conditions may mimic idiopathic inflammatory myopathy, in particular muscle dystrophy, proximal neuropathies (diabetes), neuromuscular transmission disorders, infection (trichinosis, HIV), alcoholic myopathy, enzyme errors of glycogen metabolism (weakness and cramps with exercising), hypothyroidism, and hypophosphatemia.
> - Make sure to include CBC with differential count, TSH, K, Ca, and P determinations in patients with presumed idiopathic inflammatory myopathy.

Natural History

Expected Outcome

Cases of IBM are slowly progressive. Dysphagia may be severe. Involvement of paraspinal muscles may result in camptocormia (a sharply angulated back while standing, a straight back on bed rest; previously considered hysterical). Mimickers of PM each have their own course. Diabetic amyotrophy improves slowly, over months, with control of the diabetes. HIV myositis needs to be distinguished from zidovudine myopathy, which is reversible upon discontinua-

TABLE 14-1
CONDITIONS THAT CAUSE MYOPATHIC SYMPTOMS

CONNECTIVE TISSUE DISEASES
Mixed connective tissue disease
Rheumatoid arthritis
Scleroderma
Sjögren's syndrome
SLE

MUSCLE DYSTROPHIES
Becker's muscular dystrophy
Duchenne's muscular dystrophy
Facioscapulohumeral muscular dystrophy
Limb-girdle muscular dystrophy

DENERVATING CONDITIONS
Amyotrophic lateral sclerosis
Spinal muscular atrophies

NEUROMUSCULAR JUNCTION DISORDERS
Eaton-Lambert's syndrome
Myasthenia gravis

PROXIMAL NEUROPATHIES
Diabetic amyotrophy
Diabetic plexopathy
Guillain-Barré's syndrome
Neoplasia
Porphyria, acute intermittent

DRUG-RELATED CONDITIONS
Alcohol
Chloroquine, hydroxychloroquine
Cocaine
Colchicine
D-penicillamine
Glucocorticoids
Heroin
Hydralazine
Procainamide
Rifampin
Gemfibrozil
Lovastatin
Levodopa

Phenytoin
Valproic acid
Sulfonamides
Zidovudine (AZT)
Ipecac
Cimetidine
L-tryptophan
Vincristine
Danazol

INFECTIONS
Viral
Adenovirus
Coxackievirus
Cytomegalovirus
Echovirus A9
Epstein Barr virus
Hepatitis B virus
Human immunodeficiency virus
Influenza A and B virus
Mumps virus
Parainfluenza virus 4b
Rubella virus
Varicella-zoster virus

Bacterial
Borrelia burgdorferi
Clostridium welchii
Mycobacterium (leprae, tuberculosis)
Mycoplasma pneumoniae
Rickettsia
Staphylococcus
Streptococcus

Fungal
Cryptococcus

Parasitic
Cysticercus
Sarcocystis
Schistosoma

Trichinella
Trypanosoma

METABOLIC

Disordered glycogen metabolism
Myophosphorilase deficiency (McArdle's disease)
Deficiency of acid maltase
Others

Disordered lipid metabolism
Carnitine deficiency
Others

Myoadenilate deaminase deficiency
Mitochondrial myopathies
Nutritional-metabolic
Uremia
Hepatic failure
Malabsorption
Periodic paralysis
Others

Electrolyte disturbances
Hyper Na
Hypo Na
Hyper K
Hypo K
Hyper Ca
Hypo Ca
Hypo P
Hypo Mg

Endocrine
Acromegaly
Hypothyroidism
Hyperthyroidism
Hyperparathyroidism
Cushing's disease
Addison's disease
Hyperaldosteronism
Carcinoid syndrome

tion of the drug. Hypothyroid and hypophosphatemic myopathy also have a slow recovery.

Treatment

Methods

There is evidence that IBM responds, albeit slowly and incompletely, to intense immunosuppressive therapy. Endoscopic division of the cricoesophageal sphincter has been useful in the treatment of severe dysphagia in IBM.

Treatment of each of the PM mimickers, with the possible exception of diabetic amyotrophy (control of diabetes), hypothyroid myopathy (thyroid hormone replacement), and muscle weakness associated with electrolytic disturbances (correction of concentrations), exceeds the scope of this book and should be left in the hands of an appropriate consultant.

When to Refer

Cases of IBM should be referred to a rheumatologist or neurologist. Myositis mimickers, once identified, should be either treated by the primary care physician (e.g., hypothyroid and electrolyte imbalance myopathies) or by the appropriate specialist, usually a neurologist or a rheumatologist.

Key Points

> **INCLUSION BODY MYOSITIS AND IDIOPATHIC INFLAMMATORY MYOPATHY MIMICKERS**
>
> - There are myriad myopathies beyond the familiar PM and DM.
> - Inclusion body myopathy should be looked for in PM cases that fail to respond to standard corticosteroid doses.
> - Consider other types of muscle injury from metabolic errors, through trichinosis, through hypophosphatemia, when assessing patients with myopathic weakness.
> - Don't hesitate to enlist a rheumatologist or neurologist in the evaluation of patients with proximal muscle weakness.

Suggested Reading

Dalakas M. Polymyositis, dermatomyositis, and inclusion body myositis. N Engl J Med 325:1487–1498, 1991.

Lotz BP, Engel AG, Nishino H, et al. Inclusion body myositis: Observations in 40 patients. Brain 112:727–747, 1989.

Wortmann RL. Inflammatory diseases of muscle. In: Kelley WN, Harris ED Jr, Ruddy S, et al. (eds) Textbook of Rheumatology. W.B. Saunders, Philadelphia, 1159–1188, 1993.

CHAPTER 15

Systemic Sclerosis (Scleroderma) and Related Syndromes

Clearly, systemic sclerosis is a heterogeneous condition with subsets that have different prognostic import (Table 15–1). Limited systemic sclerosis (lss), often described with the acronym CREST (C = calcinosis, R = Raynaud's, E = esophageal, S = sclerodactyly, T = telangiectasia), usually follows a benign course, although pulmonary hypertension or significant bleed from internal telangiectases occasionally occur.

Patients with diffuse systemic sclerosis (dss), on the other hand, often have a severe course in terms of skin involvement, hand disability, and renal disease. Primary care physicians should become familiar with the polar forms of scleroderma and learn to distinguish Raynaud's disease, which is a benign condition, from Raynaud's phenomenon, which occurs in scleroderma, other connective tissue diseases, and a miscellany of additional conditions. Finally, there are localized forms of scleroderma such as morphea and linear scleroderma that are separate from systemic sclerosis and pose problems, mainly cosmetic, of their own (Table 15–2).

Presentation and Progression

Cause

A variety of autoantibodies can be found in the serum of patients with systemic sclerosis. Whether they are pathogenic is still unknown. In a scleroderma kidney, for instance, immune complexes are conspicuously absent from the microvascular and glomerular lesions. Scleroderma-related autoantibodies are very useful, however, in patient classification. For instance, antitopoisomerase-I (formerly Sclero-70) antibody identifies almost half of patients with dss whereas anticentromeric antibodies are largely confined to the limited form of the disease. T- and B-cells regulate autoantibody production, but a pathogenetic role of cellular immunity remains speculative. Exposure to environmental factors such as silica dust and certain industrial solvents may have had a triggering role in some cases. In the majority of patients, however, the cause of systemic sclerosis remains unknown.

Presentation

Raynaud's phenomenon, defined as blanching of the digits in response to environmental cold or emotion, is a major finding in systemic sclerosis, being present in over 95% of patients. In lss, Raynaud's phenomenon typically precedes other changes by several years to decades. In dss, however, onset of Raynaud's is concurrent with or precedes diagnosis by only a few months. In both forms of systemic sclerosis, small fingertip infarctions lead to thinning of the pulp and the formation of tiny pitted scars. Polygonal telangiectases are common in the palm and face. Inspection of the capillary loops at the nail fold is an important adjunct in the evaluation of patients with Raynaud's phenomenon and questionable skin findings. The normal pattern consists of a single row of slender, symmetric hairpin capillary loops. In scleroderma, capillary loops are abnormal in that some areas appear devoid of capillaries while individual loops, here and there, are grossly and irregularly dilated. Although these changes are best seen with a wide-angle microscope, with some practice they may also be seen with an ophthalmoscope after placing on the skin a small amount of clear lubricating cream or a drop of microscope oil.

The hallmark of systemic sclerosis is skin hardening (sclerosis) due to dermal and then subcutaneous collagen accretion. In lss, changes first become noticeable in the digits

---

TABLE 15–1

CLASSIFICATION OF SYSTEMIC SCLEROSIS

1. Limited systemic sclerosis (lss), or CREST syndrome (C, calcinosis; R, Raynaud's phenomenon; E, esophageal dysmotility; S, sclerodactyly; T, telangiectasias): upper extremity distal to elbows, lower extremities distal to knees, face, neck.
2. Diffuse systemic sclerosis (dss): trunk, proximal and distal upper and lower extremities, face, neck.
3. Sine scleroderma: visceral, vascular, and serologic involvement of systemic sclerosis without detectable cutaneous findings.
4. Overlap syndromes: 1–3 *plus* features of RA, SLE, or idiopathic inflammatory myopathy. Synonyms: mixed connective tissue disease (MCTD), lupoderma, sclerodermatomyositis.
5. Undifferentiated connective tissue disease (UCTD): Raynaud's phenomenon with clinical or serologic features of systemic sclerosis (digital ulceration, abnormal nail fold capillary loops, serum anticentromeric antibody, finger edema) but without skin thickening and without internal organ abnormalities of systemic sclerosis.

Modified from Seibold JR. Scleroderma. In: Kelley WN, Harris ED Jr, Ruddy S, et al. (eds) Textbook of Rheumatology, 4th ed. W.B. Saunders, Philadelphia, 1113–1143, 1993.

TABLE 15–2

LOCALIZED SCLERODERMA (LINEAR SCLERODERMA AND MORPHEA)

LINEAR SCLERODERMA

Onset in childhood
Sclerotic band on arm, leg, trunk, or head (en coup de sabre)*
May have peripheral blood eosinophilia
Anti-single-stranded DNA antibodies in 30%
Evolution to atrophy and dyschromia in 1–2 years

MORPHEA (a) droplike patches (gutatte morphea); (b) single plaque; (c) generalized

Onset at any age
Ivory colored with surrounding violaceous border in early lesions
May have peripheral blood eosinophilia
Anti-single-stranded DNA antibodies in 30%
Evolution to atrophy and dyschromia in 1–2 years

*An appearance likened to a saber blow.

---

as the initial phase of diffuse hand edema subsides. The adjective *limited* in lss reflects the pattern of skin involvement: digits, sometimes extending proximally in the limbs to the elbow and knee, face, and neck. Skin changes in dss involve the entire upper and lower extremities, face, neck, anterior chest including breasts, and abdomen. Identifying skin thickening may be difficult for the noninitiated. Patients are usually aware of the changes in their skin and can often describe the extent of abnormal skin with great accuracy. A useful maneuver is to press and then glide the skin longitudinally, back and forth, with the pulp of the index finger. The author has found it useful to explore gliding in partially stretched skin. Thus, to examine the skin in the dorsum of the proximal phalanx, both the MCP and the PIP are semiflexed, which creates some stretching. Normal skin can still be glided; no gliding is possible in involved skin. The same principle is applied in the dorsum of the hand (keeping wrist and MCPs flexed), upper forearm over the wrist extensor mass (elbow extended and wrist palmarly flexed), sides and front of the neck (neck bent contralaterally or backward), front of the chest (shoulders brought back), and anterior leg, lateral to the shin (knee in semiflexion and foot plantarly flexed).

Gastrointestinal involvement is very common and is similar in both types of scleroderma. Esophageal involvement caused initially by a disordered cholinergic neural function and later by smooth muscle atrophy and fibrosis occurs in over 90% of patients. Patients present dysphagia for solids, food regurgitation, and reflux esophagitis. Secondary strictures often develop. Recurrent aspiration pneumonias may also occur secondary to the esophageal changes. A secondary Sjögren's syndrome occurs in approximately 30% of scleroderma patients. Small-bowel dysfunction may lead to malabsorption from bacterial overgrowth. Antimesenteric, wide-mouth pseudodiverticula often develop in the large bowel. Pseudointestinal occlusion and pneumatosis cystoides are additional gastrointestinal complications of systemic sclerosis. Primary biliary cirrhosis intriguingly associates with lss. Because early biliary cirrhosis is treatable, patients with lss should have antimitochondrial antibody determination and if positive, in the author's opinion, a liver biopsy.

Arthralgias or mild arthritis, usually with a distal and symmetric pattern, is often seen in both types of scleroderma. Interstitial pulmonary fibrosis expressed clinically by dry cough, progressive dyspnea, and Velcro-like rales develops in 5% to 10% of scleroderma cases irrespective of clinical form. Acute pleuritis is rare.

Heart disease in scleroderma may be caused by several mechanisms. Cardiac failure and arrhythmias are caused by myocardial fibrosis. Acute pericarditis rarely occurs. Another rare manifestation is effusive pericarditis, which has been reported to occur as a prodrome to renal crisis. Pulmonary arterial hypertension is rare in dss but develops in approximately 10% of patients with lss.

Last but not least, renal failure develops in approximately 10% of dss patients; it is almost unheard of in lss. Scleroderma kidney is characterized by myxoid and proliferative changes in the interlobular arteries, fibrinoid necrosis of afferent arterioles, and segmental necrosis of the glomerulus. Clinically, patients become hypertensive (high-renin hypertension) and oliguric, microangiopathic changes and thrombocytopenia develop, and there is a rapid deterioration of glomerular function. Grade 3–4 hypertensive retinopathy, hypertensive encephalopathy, and heart failure are common in this setting.

Diagnosis

Summary of Diagnosis

SYSTEMIC SCLEROSIS

- Raynaud's phenomenon.
- Skin fibrosis, limited or diffuse.
- Dysphagia.
- Arthralgias or arthritis.
- Inspect nail fold capillaries with an opthalmoscope or a wide-angle microscope.
- Obtain chest x-rays.
- Determine CBC, platelet count, reticulocyte count, BUN, creatinine, CPK, aldolase, and urinalysis.
- If limited systemic sclerosis, determine anticentromeric antibodies for diagnostic support and antimitochondrial antibodies to detect early biliary cirrhosis.
- If diffuse systemic sclerosis, determine antitopoisomerase-I antibodies, which are confirmatory if present.

Natural History

Expected Outcome

Systemic sclerosis is a chronic, progressive disease in which, even within clinical groups, there is marked variation in organ involvement and course. Limited systemic sclerosis

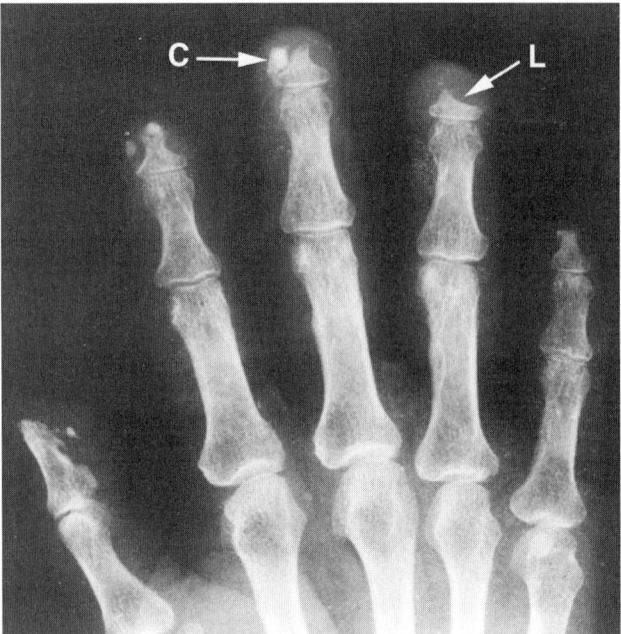

FIGURE 15–1. *Scleroderma.* Hand of a 45-year-old woman with long-standing Raynaud's, sclerodactyly, and prominent angiomas on her lips and face. Reflux esophagitis was her main concern. Hand x-rays showed bone lysis of distal phalanges (L) and calcinosis (C). This form of scleroderma is known as CREST (see text).

often runs a chronic, uneventful course, its main effects being hand dysfunction, acral calcifications with a tendency to ulcerate and become infected (Figure 15–1), and disfiguration from telangiectases and facial fibrosis. However, pulmonary arterial hypertension may develop resulting in intractable cardiac failure, and in a small proportion of cases primary biliary cirrhosis sets in.

The course of dss is much rockier. For starters, skin involvement is far more severe, resulting frequently in hand distortion, disability, and ischemic ulcers at the fingertips and the knuckles. Phalangeal autoamputation may occur. Chronic ischemic neuritic pain is common. Friction rubs presumably caused by fibrin layering in tendon sheaths and bursae are often present in early, rapidly evolving dss and represent a red flag for sclerodermic renal crisis. In these patients, weekly home monitoring of blood pressure (BP) is essential to identify reversible renal involvement. Pulmonary fibrosis leading to respiratory insufficiency is a frequent cause of death in scleroderma patients.

The previously dreaded renal crisis is largely reversible with current antihypertensive medications. Renal ultrasound should be done to rule out obstruction. A renal biopsy is indicated in renal crisis with normal blood pressure, in cases of "sine scleroderma," and in any situation when the diagnosis is in doubt (for instance, when the diagnosis in scleroderma is not firm and there is a possibility of immune complex nephritis). In addition, renal transplantation has been successfully performed in scleroderma patients. Prior to current therapies, patients with scleroderma with myocardial involvement or renal crises lived on the average less than 6 months.

Treatment

Methods

Treatment of scleroderma is aimed at (1) relieving vasospastic disease, (2) suppressing fibrosis, and (3) treating organ involvement. Treatment of Raynaud's phenomenon is critical not only to improve the hands (sometimes the feet, ears, or nose) but also because cold-induced vasospasm also occurs in internal organs such as the heart, the kidney, and the lung. Patients should be advised to dress warmly around the chest and abdomen, preferably with several layers of clothes to raise core temperature and induce peripheral vasodilation. Wool mittens and even electric mittens should be used if being out in the cold is a necessity. Cigarette smoking, both active and passive, and oral, nasal, or percutaneous nicotine administration should be forbidden.

Calcium channel blockers have a measurable beneficial effect in many of these patients. An approach is to administer extended release nifedipine 30 mg once daily, increasing the dose if necessary to 60 mg once daily. An alternative is the use of diltiazem in slow-release capsules 180 mg to 240 mg once daily. Interestingly, there is uncontrolled evidence that the long-term use of diltiazem is associated with regression of calcinosis. No other medication may be needed. Treatment of failures of calcium channel blockers is discussed in the section in this chapter on Raynaud's.

Hand stetching exercises are essential in the prevention and treatment of sclerodermic contractures. In preparation for this exercise, which the author learned at the late National Hansen's Disease Center, Carville, Louisiana, the patient's hand is first soaked in warm water for 10 minutes. Following this and while water is still dripping, the hands are covered with lanolin that will seal the skin moisture. The hands are now ready for the exercise, which is done as follows: (1) The patient stands by a table. (2) The hand is applied flat on the table and, by advancing a foot and tilting the body forward, the MCPs and then the wrist are passively brought into hyperextension. (3) The fully stretched position is held 30 seconds followed by relaxation for 1 to 2 minutes. The exercise is repeated three times on each hand twice a day.

Medications aimed at decreasing fibrosis should be utilized in patients with lss and marked sclerodactyly and patients with dss preferably in an early stage of the disease. The cornerstone of treatment is D-penicillamine (DP), which interferes with the intermolecular cross linking of type I collagen and has a suppressive effect on CD4 cells. Treatment should be started with a low dose, usually 125 or 250 mg once daily, increased every 4 to 6 weeks by 250 mg until an optimal maintenance dose of 1000 mg once daily is reached. The drug should be taken 2 hours before a meal.

Although the first multicenter double-blind trial of low-dose and high-dose DP has not been completed, most experts believe the drug has beneficial effects on skin and visceral sclerodermic involvement. Unfortunately, DP causes significant adverse effects in approximately 30% of patients. Skin rashes, nausea, and anorexia are usually not serious. Myelosuppression, in particular leukopenia and thrombocytopenia, require hematologic evaluation, since they may be a harbinger of marrow aplasia. The nephrotic syndrome is usually dose related and often reverses itself by lowering the dose. Rare but severe adverse effects include pemphigus, myasthenia gravis, a Goodpasture-like syndrome, polymyositis, and SLE. In most cases, however, DP is well tolerated and can be administered indefinitely.

Articular symptoms should be controlled mainly with nonacetylated salicylates to avoid as much as possible gastric irritation and changes in GFR. Low-dose prednisone may be used, albeit with great care, in the treatment of the edema and synovitis of early disease. Prednisone doses greater than 15 mg per day should be avoided because of a possible triggering effect on scleroderma crisis.

All scleroderma patients should be instructed on prophylaxis of reflux esophagitis. This includes elevating the head of the bed by applying 5 inch blocks under the legs, avoiding meals past 6 p.m. and bedtime snacks, ceasing smoking, reducing alcohol consumption, and during symptomatic periods the use of histamine-receptor blockers such as cimetidine 800 mg bid, ranitidine 150 mg bid, or omeprazol 20 mg once daily. Reflux esophagitis may be severe by the time the patient is first seen, including strictures. An early endoscopy is appropriate in scleroderma patients presenting dysphagia. Esophageal dilatations are very effective in this setting. Rapid weight loss should raise the possibility of malabsorption as a result of bacterial overgrowth. Artificial tears should be used if a secondary Sjögren's is present. All patients with scleroderma merit meticulous dental care. A decline in pulmonary function justifies consideration of the use of cyclophosphamide, which on uncontrolled studies appears to stabilize or improve pulmonary function. Antihypertensive agents are the mainstay of treatment in the sclerodermic renal crisis. Angiotensin-converting enzyme inhibitors such as captopril and enalapril are particularly effective in this setting. Other antihypertensive agents such as minoxidil and alpha-methyldopa are also effective. By decreasing the BP, fibrinoid necrosis of renal vessels does not follow, improved perfusion cancels the high-renin state, and any degree of renal insufficiency already present (provided that serum creatinine has not reached 4 mg per dl) either arrests or improves.

When to Refer

Systemic sclerosis is an unusual condition, and most general practitioners will have little if any expertise in its management. Once a diagnosis of systemic sclerosis has been established, the subsequent care of the patient should be a combined effort between a rheumatologist and the primary care physician. Familiarity with the disorder is therefore highly desirable.

Resources Available

There are two scleroderma associations: the Scleroderma Federation and the United Scleroderma Foundation. Their addresses are listed in the appendix.

Key Points

SYSTEMIC SCLEROSIS
- Edematous hands plus Raynaud's are featured by early systemic sclerosis, overlap syndromes, undifferentiated connective tissue disease, and mixed connective tissue disease.
- Limited systemic sclerosis associates with pulmonary arterial hypertension, and diffuse systemic sclerosis with the scleroderma crisis (hypertension and rapidly progressive renal insufficiency).
- Risk factors for scleroderma crisis include early, rapidly evolving diffuse disease; tendon friction rubs; cold exposure; and intermediate or high doses of glucocorticoids.
- Localized lesions such as morphea and linear scleroderma primarily represent a cosmetic problem. They are unrelated to systemic sclerosis.
- Treatment of systemic sclerosis includes vasodilators, D-penicillamine to decrease collagen accretion, and measures aimed at preventing or improving organ damage.
- Prophylaxis of reflux esophagitis is essential in these patients.

Suggested Reading

Abu-Shakra M, Lee P. Mortality in systemic sclerosis: A comparison with the general population. J Rheumatol 22:2100–2102, 1995.

Akeson A, Scheja A, Lundin A, et al. Improved pulmonary dysfunction in systemic sclerosis after treatment with cyclophosphamide. Arthritis Rheum 37:729–735, 1994.

Palmieri G, Sebes JI, Aelion JA, et al. Treatment of calcinosis with diltiazem. Arthritis Rheum 38:1646–1654, 1995.

Pope CE II. Current concepts: Acid-reflux disorders. N Engl J Med 331:656–660, 1994.

Seibold JR. Scleroderma. In: Kelley WN, Harris ED Jr, Ruddy S, et al. (eds) Textbook of Rheumatology, 4th ed. W.B. Saunders, Philadelphia, 1113–1143, 1993.

Mixed Connective Tissue Disease (MCTD), Rhupus, Other Overlap Syndromes, and Undifferentiated Connective Tissue Disease (UCTD)

It has long been observed that there are patients with clinical and laboratory findings of two or more connective tissue diseases, for example, RA/scleroderma, RA/Hashimoto thyroiditis, SLE/RA, SLE/scleroderma/myositis, and so on. This has led to attempts at classifying these patients in named overlaps, such as MCTD or "Rhupus" (for RA/lupus), rather than considering them in one category, for example, SLE adding "with features of" another, for example, scleroderma. There are also patients who have features of scleroderma, including autoantibodies, without skin sclerosis or visceral manifestations of the disease. These patients are said to have UCTD.

Presentation and Progression

Cause

The same considerations apply as in RA, SLE, polymyositis, and scleroderma. Mention should be made of RNP (U1 small nuclear RNP) antibodies, which when present in high titers, as seen in MCTD, associate with the immunogenetic marker HLA-DR4.

Presentation

Mixed connective tissue disease, as defined by Sharp, is a distinct syndrome that includes Raynaud's phenomenon, swollen hands, sclerodactyly, telangiectasia, arthralgia or arthritis, myositis, fibrosing alveolitis, and abnormal distal esophageal motility. Patients with MCTD have high-titer speckled-pattern antinuclear antibodies by immunofluorescence, high titers of RNP antibodies, and no other autoantibodies (Table 15–3). It should be made clear that RNP antibodies occur also in SLE and less frequently in scleroderma and in myositis. Although patients with clinical MCTD as defined by Sharp definitely exist, a similar clinical syndrome has been observed in patients with Sm and other autoantibodies. Rhupus patients combine features of seropositive, erosive RA with malar rash, nephritis, anti-dsDNA antibodies, and hypocomplementemia. Interestingly, the female/male ratio in rhupus is about 7 to 1, which is closer to an SLE rather than an RA sex ratio. Patients with UCTD have Raynaud's, finger edema, fingertip ulcerations, abnormal nail fold capillary loops, and positive anticentromeric antibodies, but no skin sclerosis can be documented and there are no esophageal, pulmonary, or other visceral manifestations of scleroderma. On long-term follow-up some of these patients go on to develop CREST.

Diagnosis

Summary of Diagnosis

MIXED CONNECTIVE TISSUE DISEASE (MCTD), RHUPUS, OTHER OVERLAP SYNDROMES, AND UNDIFFERENTIATED CONNECTIVE TISSUE DISEASE (UCTD)

- Diagnosis of MCTD is suspected clinically (overlap of features of SLE, scleroderma, and myositis).
- Diagnosis of MCTD is confirmed by high-titer RNP antibodies and absence of other autoantibodies.
- Diagnosis of rhupus is suspected clinically by rheumatoid-like arthritis plus clinical features of lupus and confirmed by the presence of radiographic erosions, positive RF, and positive ANA.
- Other overlaps include features of RA/scleroderma, RA/Hashimoto thyroiditis, SLE/scleroderma/myositis, and scleroderma/myositis.
- UCTD is suspected clinically (absence of cutaneous sclerosis), but diagnosis requires ruling out visceral manifestation of scleroderma.

Natural History

Expected Outcome

On a 5 year follow-up of the original MCTD patients described by Sharp, having had the typical arthritis, serositis, and myositis controlled by low-dose corticosteroids, most had predominant sclerodermic features such as dysphagia and sclerodactyly and some had typical SLE. Thus, MCTD appears to be largely a transition syndrome. The long-term course of rhupus patients appears to be closer to lupus than RA. Long-term course of other overlaps is lesser known.

Important complications of MCTD as such include pulmonary hypertension, trigeminal neuritis, and Sjögren's syndrome. Most of the deaths in MCTD are due to pulmonary hypertension.

TABLE 15–3
SUGGESTED DIAGNOSTIC CRITERIA FOR MIXED CONNECTIVE TISSUE DISEASE (MCTD)

SEROLOGIC

Anti-RNP > 1:600 by hemaglutination method

CLINICAL

Hand edema
Synovitis in 1 or more hand joints
Myositis by biopsy or CPK elevation
Raynaud's phenomenon
Acrosclerosis

Requirements for diagnosing MCTD: positive serology *plus* 3 or more of the clinical criteria.

After Alarcón-Segovia D, Cardiel M. Comparison between three diagnostic criteria for mixed connective tissue disease. Study of 593 patients. J Rheumatol 16:328–334, 1989.

Treatment

Methods

Low-dose prednisone treatment was initially recommended for the treatment of MCTD. However, it makes more sense to treat these patients according to their specific involvements, for example, Raynaud's with the usual nonpharmacologic treatment plus nifedipine, arthritis with a nonacetylated salicylate plus hydroxychloroquine, and myositis, if clinically symptomatic, with corticosteroids in the lowest effective dose. This treatment plan would not be additive, but hierarchical. As an example, if corticosteroids are going to be used for myositis, hydroxychloroquine and a nonacetylated salicylate will not be required.

When to Refer

Patients with overlap syndromes, similarly to patients with a well-defined connective tissue disease, should have the benefit of rheumatologic evaluation. Periodic rheumatologic evaluation is important for the early detection of transitions.

Key Points

MIXED CONNECTIVE TISSUE DISEASE (MCTD), RHUPUS, OTHER OVERLAP SYNDROMES, AND UNDIFFERENTIATED CONNECTIVE TISSUE DISEASE (UCTD)

- Connective tissue diseases are classified according to clinical and laboratory findings rather than etiology.

- Thus, it is not surprising that serologically defined syndromes have clinical overlaps, and clinically defined syndromes have serologic overlaps.
- MCTD is, for the most part, a transition-type condition that eventually evolves into scleroderma or SLE.
- While it stays as MCTD, peculiar complications may occur including pulmonary arterial hypertension and trigeminal neuritis.
- The course of rhupus and other overlaps is less well defined.
- UCTD is not a condition with features of two or more conditions, but a condition with features of less than one, scleroderma.

Suggested Reading

Hoffman RW, Sharp GC. Is anti-U1-RNP autoantibody positive connective tissue disease genetically distinct? J Rheumatol 22:586–589, 1995.

Lázaro MA, Maldonado JA, Catoggio LJ, et al. Clinical and serological characteristics of patients with overlap syndrome: Is mixed connective tissue disease a distinct clinical entity? Medicine (Baltimore) 68:58–65, 1989.

Panush RS, Edwards NG, Longley S, et al. "Rhupus syndrome." Arch Intern Med 148:1633–1636, 1988.

Sharp GG, Irvin WS, Tan EM, et al. Mixed connective tissue disease—an apparently distinct rheumatic syndrome associated with a specific antibody to an extractable nuclear antigen. Am J Med 52:148–159, 1972.

Raynaud's Disease and Secondary Raynaud's Phenomenon

Raynaud's disease refers to idiopathic episodic digital ischemia triggered by cold and emotion. In the secondary Raynaud's phenomenon, the same changes are caused by an underlying condition (Table 15-4). A related entity is the so-called vibration white finger. More distantly related are perniosis and acrocyanosis, which are briefly discussed in this chapter.

TABLE 15-4
CLINICAL DIFFERENTIATION BETWEEN PRIMARY RAYNAUD'S (RAYNAUD'S DISEASE) AND SECONDARY RAYNAUD'S

	Primary	Secondary
Sex (F/M)	5–10/1	Variable
Age at onset	Menarche	20 or later
Duration of symptoms at evaluation	Often > 5 years	Usually < 2 years
Number of digits involved	Usually all digits	Usually begins in 1
Frequency of attacks	Many a day	Few a day
Emotion as a precipitant	Yes	Unusual
Ischemic injury (fingertip ulcers or pulp retraction)	No	Yes
Finger edema	Rare	Common
Arthralgia, fever, or other systemic symptom	No	Common

Presentation and Progression

Cause

Raynaud's disease occurs more often in females with a female/male ratio of 5 to 1. The condition is quite frequent, affecting 5% to 10% of women in the general population. Disease onset typically occurs at puberty. There is a loose association with variant angina and migraines. Raynaud's syndrome occurs in both males and females. The various conditions associated with secondary Raynaud's phenomenon, including the vibration white finger, are listed in Table 15-5. It is now established that the pathophysiology of these conditions differs for each category.

Presentation

Raynaud's disease tends to occur in young women who normally have cold hands and feet. Typically, one or more fingers of both hands become dead white with a sensation of numbness or paresthesias on cold exposure. Less frequently, feet, ears, and nose become involved. Upon rewarming, such as returning indoors, the involved digits turn first blue (as capillaries and venules dilate) and then bright red from reactive hyperemia. Episodes are also triggered by emotion. Multiple attacks may occur each day. Patients are otherwise well (except for a possible migraine), and no ischemic fingertip ulcers are noted. Patients usually have symptoms for several years, even decades, before

TABLE 15-5
CLASSIFICATION OF RAYNAUD'S PHENOMENON

VASOSPASTIC

Primary (idiopathic): Raynaud's disease
Drug-induced (beta-adrenergic receptor blockers, ergot derivatives, methysergide)
Variant angina/migraine
Pheochromocytoma
Neurologic disorders (syringomyelia, spinal cord tumors, stroke, polyomyelitis)

STRUCTURAL

Distal limb activity related (vibration injury, hammer hand syndrome, typing, piano playing)
Compressive (crutch walking, thoracic outlet syndrome, carpal tunnel syndrome)
Arterial diseases (arteriosclerosis of peripheral arteries, thromboangiitis obliterans)
Vibration syndrome
Cold injury (frostbite, pernio, immersion foot)
Connective tissue diseases (systemic sclerosis, systemic lupus erythematosus, overlap syndrome, rheumatoid arthritis, poly/dermatomyositis)
Polyvinyl chloride disease
Chemotherapy (bleomycin, vinblastin, cysplatin)

BLOOD DYSCRASIAS

Cold-induced precipitation (cold agglutinins, cryoglobulinemia, cryofibrinogenemia)
Plasma cell dyscrasia (multiple myeloma, Waldenström macroglobulinemia)
Myeloproliferative disorders (essential thrombocytemia, polycytemia vera)

Raynaud's disease is diagnosed. The one underlying condition that features protracted Raynaud's at onset is lss. Abnormal capillary nail fold capillaries and/or a positive ANA with anticentromeric specificity allow an early diagnosis in this condition. With the exception noted, in secondary Raynaud's the time lag between onset of symptoms and diagnosis is usually less than 2 years. Secondary Raynaud's may be unilateral at onset and episodes are often protracted. Ischemic changes are frequent including fingertip infarctions or ulcers, a retracted pulp, pitted fingertip depressions, and sometimes finger gangrene. Associated findings depend on the underlying condition.

Diagnosis

Summary of Diagnosis

> **RAYNAUD'S DISEASE AND SECONDARY RAYNAUD'S PHENOMENON**
> - Episodic blanching of digits in response to cold and emotion.
> - Symmetric, multiple fingers, multiple episodes a day, onset at menarche: Raynaud's disease.
> - Unilateral onset, few fingers, persistent episodes, onset in adulthood: Raynaud's syndrome.
> - Unilateral, adult patient, use of a vibrating tool: vibration white finger.
> - In Raynaud's syndrome, do a historic review of possible causes.
> - In all patients, inspect nail fold capillaries and obtain ANA. If both are negative, scleroderma is most unlikely.
> - Follow the undiagnosed rheumatic syndrome patient at semiannual intervals.

Note: Nail fold capillary loops inspection may be done with a wide-angle biomicroscope or with a regular ophthalmoscope. The author uses the latter, as follows: With the patient's hand flat on the desk surface, after placing a drop of immersion oil or a small amount of clear lubricating cream at the nail fold (the skin fold immediately adjacent to the nail), the skin is closely inspected under progressive magnification. With some practice a front of thin hairpin-like capillary loops arranged side by side will be seen around the nail. In systemic sclerosis there are avascular areas as well as isolated, giant, irregularly dilated capillary loops in random order. Many normal individuals should be inspected to develop a feeling for normal findings.

Natural History

Expected Outcome

Raynaud's disease has a benign course. In 15% to 20% the condition spontaneously improves, in 30% it gets worse, and the remaining patients continue unchanged.

Secondary Raynaud's phenomenon has the prognosis of the underlying disease plus whatever local damage results from ischemia. Complications of secondary Raynaud's include neuritic pain at the fingertips from damaged skin nerves and decreased padding, ischemic ulcers that may secondarily become infected, and digital gangrene.

Treatment

Methods

Treatment of Raynaud's syndrome is along a hierarchy that is applicable to all patients. (1) Removal of an offending cause such as tobacco smoking, ergotism, or a pheochromocytoma may solve the problem. In the hyperviscosity syndrome, plasmapheresis and treatment of the underlying condition may afford transient relief. Patients with the vibration white finger usually improve when exposure to vibration is reduced. Smoking even one cigarette a day should be prohibited. (2) Patients should dress warmly and with several layers of clothing around the trunk to raise core temperature and cause peripheral vasodilation. Avoid wet, cold, and windy climatic conditions. Woolen gloves, sheepskin mittens, and even electric mittens should be used when being outdoors in the cold cannot be avoided. (3) Vasodilator drugs are considered in cases that are resistant to conservative measures. The calcium channel antagonists such as nifedipine in extended-release tablets 30 mg once daily or twice a day, or diltiazem in slow-release capsules 180 mg to 240 mg once daily, are usually well tolerated and at least partially effective. (4) Biofeedback training is sometimes capable of raising skin temperature by several degrees. This and other behavioral treatments should be considered in patients who cannot take, or are unwilling to take, vasodilator drugs. (5) Severe cases in which viability of a digit is in question may require digital or cervical sympathectomy or experimental treatments such as intavenous Iloprost (a stable prostacyclin analog) or tissue plasminogen activator (TPA) infusions.

Expected Response

Raynaud's disease is in most cases a benign condition that can be managed conservatively. In secondary cases, general measures, calcium channel blockers, and treatments aimed at the underlying condition usually ameliorate the Raynaud's. Iloprost infusions under an experimental protocol have healed persistent ulcers. Complications of treatment are the usual for calcium channel antagonists including flushing, dizziness, headaches, and nasal stuffiness. Cases of vibration white finger that persist upon exposure reduction may benefit from diltiazem.

When to Refer

Patients with Raynaud's disease should be treated by primary care physicians. Referral to a rheumatologist or an expert in peripheral vascular conditions is warranted in patients with suspected secondary Raynaud's phenomenon.

Key Points

> **RAYNAUD'S DISEASE AND SECONDARY RAYNAUD'S PHENOMENON**
> - Raynaud's disease is a benign condition that often does not require specific therapy.

- Workup in Raynaud's disease should be limited to obtaining an ANA and inspecting the nail fold capillaries with an ophthalmoscope or wide-angle microscope.
- Secondary Raynaud's phenomenon is an important red flag for a number of conditions that may be in need of treatment; most of these conditions can be diagnosed by a careful history. Laboratory evaluation should be based on the clinical leads (don't do a blind workup!).
- Treatment of Raynaud's includes stopping smoking, dressing warmly, and, if required, the use of vasodilator measures ranging from biofeedback to calcium channel blockers to digital or cervical sympathectomy.

Suggested Reading

Coffman JD. Raynaud's Phenomenon. Oxford, New York, 1989.

Dowd PM, Goldsmith PC, Bull HA, et al. Raynaud's phenomenon. Lancet 346:283–290, 1995.

Kahaleh B, Matucci-Cerinic M. Raynaud's phenomenon and scleroderma. Dysregulated neuroendothelial control of vascular tone. Arthritis Rheum 38:1–4, 1995.

Eosinophilic Fasciitis (Shulman's Disease) and Eosinophilia-Myalgia Syndrome (EMS)

These interesting conditions present overlapping features. Indeed, prior to understanding the true nature of EMS, many cases were misdiagnosed as eosinophilic fasciitis.

Presentation and Progression

Cause

The cause of eosinophilic fasciitis is unknown. Many cases appear to follow overexercise or trauma. EMS represents a drug reaction to an altered L-tryptophan dietary supplement. A few months after the relationship between L-tryptophan and EMS was identified in 1989, the sale of L-tryptophan was banned, after which no new cases were reported. Eosinophilia myalgia syndrome, in turn, resembles the toxic oil syndrome, a condition that affected thousands of people in Spain in 1981 following ingestion of a tainted rapeseed oil. No new cases of toxic oil syndrome have occurred since the initial cluster of cases. These and other conditions have been recently discussed under the designation of "fasciitis-panniculitis syndromes" (Table 15–6).

Presentation

Eosinophilic fasciitis appears abruptly with diffuse pain and nonpitting edema in the upper extremities, lower extremities, and sometimes the trunk. Fingers are not involved. There is no synovitis. Carpal tunnel syndrome is often present. In late stages, the superficial skin is tethered to woody deeper tissues. The groove sign, or depressions along the veins' paths when the limb is elevated (Figure 15–2), is pathognomonic of eosinophilic fasciitis because EMS is no longer seen. In EMS, initial symptoms included severe myalgias, fatigue, fever, various rashes, nonproductive cough, dyspnea, arthralgias, and cognitive involvement. After several weeks to months these symptoms subsided, giving way to skin induration in about 50%, in all respects similar to eosinophilic fasciitis. Another important development in about one-third of the cases was peripheral neuropathy. In the toxic oil syndrome acute manifestations included fever, rashes, myalgias, arthralgias, muscle cramping, intense peripheral eosinophilia, and pulmonary infiltrates on chest x-rays. Severe muscle cramps, various types of neuropathy, sclerodermatous skin induration, and pulmonary arterial hypertension were common in the intermediate and late phases of the disease. Laboratory findings in eosinophilic fasciitis include leukocytosis with intense eosinophilia, thrombocytosis, often an elevated aldolase level (with normal CPK), and a polyclonal increase in immunoglobulins. Findings in the EMS and the toxic oil syndrome were similar, with the addition of increased liver enzymes in some of the cases.

Diagnosis

Summary of Diagnosis

TABLE 15–6

DISORDERS THAT MAY BE CONFUSED WITH SCLERODERMA: TOPOGRAPHY OF LESIONS, PRESENCE OR ABSENCE OF RAYNAUD'S, AND ASSOCIATED FINDINGS

Trichloroethylene exposure (D, R)
Vinyl chloride exposure (D, R)
Bleomycin treatment (D, R)
Diabetic cheiroarthropathy (D); diabetes
Chronic sympathetic dystrophy (D); chronic pain
Porphyria cutanea tarda (D); bullae formation, photosensitivity
Silicone or paraffin implantation (D)*
Cutaneous amyloidosis (G); firm papules or nodules usually present; M component
Scleromyxedema (P or D); M component
Generalized morphea (P)
Scleredema (P)
Carcinoid syndrome (lower limbs, R); facial flushing, telangiectases
Eosinophilic fasciitis (P); eosinophilia
Eosinophilia-myalgia syndrome (EMS) (P); eosinophilia; ingestion of contaminated L-tryptophan
Toxic oil syndrome (P); ingestion of tainted rapeseed oil

*Controverted association.
D = Distal fibrosis (hands including fingers)
G = Generalized
P = Proximal fibrosis (face, trunk, limbs sparing hands)
R = Raynaud's phenomenon

EOSINOPHILIC FASCIITIS AND EOSINOPHILIA-MYALGIA SYNDROME (EMS)

- Eosinophilic fasciitis presents abruptly, often after undue exercise, with myalgias and nonpitting edema of the extremities and sometimes the trunk.

- In EMS there is an initial nonspecific febrile phase prior to developing skin findings similar to eosinophilic fasciitis.
- The main lead to diagnosis is peripheral eosinophilia.
- A full thickness biopsy including skin, subcutaneous tissue, fascia, and muscle is key to the diagnosis of eosinophilic fasciitis.

Natural History

Expected Outcome

Eosinophilic fasciitis runs a chronic but eventually self-limited course. Two to 3 years may elapse before the condition arrests. Approximately 30% of cases have diffuse changes involving the limbs and trunk. Residual flexor deformities are frequent. About 5% of cases of eosinophilic fasciitis are complicated by a blood condition, particularly aplastic anemia and myeloproliferative syndromes. Long-term follow-up EMS has shown regression of all findings with the exception of neuropathy, which has persisted, and cognitive changes, which have become accentuated over the years. In the toxic oil syndrome, residual symptoms after 12 years include muscle cramping, fatigue, arthralgias, subjective cognitive impairment, psychiatric disease, and soft tissue tenderness. Sclerodermatous findings and pulmonary hypertension were not detected on follow-up.

Treatment

Methods

Treatment of eosinophilic fasciitis has traditionally included moderate doses of glucocorticoids. Cimetidine is often added. Some cases have been treated with hydroxychloroquine, apparently with success. Stretching exercises (see appendix) are important in the prevention and treatment of flexor deformities. Corticosteroids were also symptomatically effective in the treatment of EMS. Whether corticosteroids only improve symptoms or shorten disease duration in these conditions is not known.

When to Refer

Eosinophilic fasciitis is a rare disease that is seldom encountered in a primary care practice. Suspected cases should be referred to a rheumatologist.

Key Points

EOSINOPHILIC FASCIITIS AND EOSINOPHILIA-MYALGIA SYNDROME (EMS)
- There is a close resemblance between eosinophilic fasciitis and the late stages of the EMS and toxic oil syndrome.
- No new cases of EMS have been reported since L-tryptophan was removed from the market in 1989.
- No new cases of toxic oil syndrome occurred after the tainted rapeseed oil was removed from the Spanish market in 1981.
- Eosinophilic fasciitis is clinically characterized by painful woody induration of the limbs. Fingers are spared, superficial skin is normal, and the pathognomonic "groove sign" is present.
- Eosinophilic fasciitis arrests spontaneously in approximately 3 years; residual contractures are common.
- Treatment of eosinophilic fasciitis is empirical. Intermediate-dose prednisone plus cimetidine and also hydroxychloroquine have been used with apparent success.
- Aplastic anemia or a myelodysplastic syndrome complicate approximately 5% of cases of eosinophilic fasciitis.

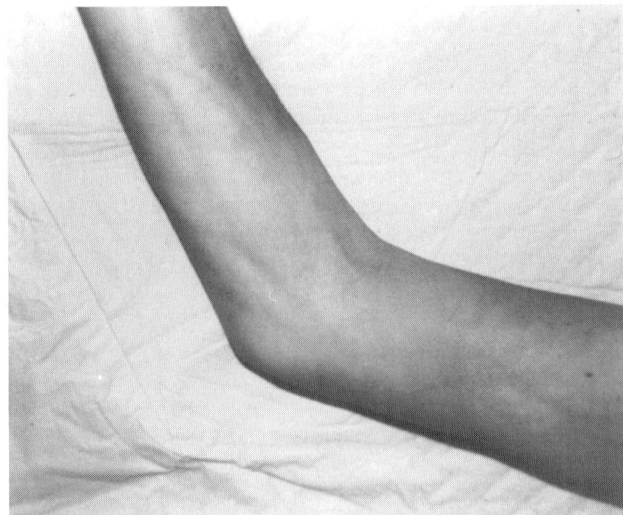

FIGURE 15-2. *Eosinophilic fasciitis.* This 29-year-old butcher had to stop working because of generalized painful induration of his skin. Fingers were spared. As he raised his forearms the collapsed veins appeared as grooves (the "groove sign"), which is pathognomonic of eosinophilic fasciitis. Four years later his condition subsided, leaving joint contractures.

Suggested Reading

Hertzman PA, Clauw DJ, Kauffman LD, et al. The eosinophilia-myalgia syndrome: Status of 205 patients and results of treatment 2 years after onset. Ann Intern Med 122:851–855, 1995.

Kaufman LD, Izquierdo Martínez M, Serrano JM, et al. 12-year followup study of epidemic Spanish toxic oil syndrome. J Rheumatol 22:282–288, 1995.

Naschitz JE, Boss JH, Misselevich I, et al. The fasciitis-panniculitis syndromes. Medicine (Baltimore) 75:6–16, 1996.

Shulman LE. Diffuse fasciitis with eosinophilia: A new syndrome? Trans Assoc Am Physicians 88:70–76, 1975.

Adjuvant Disease or Connective Tissue Disease (CTD) Following Breast Implants

A bitter controversy goes on regarding the very existence of adjuvant disease. This is a prime example of the need to base court decisions on scientific evidence rather than opinions.

Presentation and Progression

Cause

An ill-defined CTD appearing in women who received paraffin injection cosmetic augmentation was described by Japanese investigators in the mid-1960s. A resemblance with adjuvant arthritis in rats was noted, hence the name "adjuvant disease." More recently, cases of CTD in silicone-filled breast implant patients appeared in the literature, receiving by extension the label of adjuvant disease. Although a random association of CTD could not be excluded, an overrepresentation of scleroderma and sclerodermalike illness suggested a causal association. Pathogenetically, a granulomatous reaction around leaked silicone gel is believed to result in autoantibody formation and clinical disease. In support of this view there is a known increased incidence of scleroderma in miners exposed to silica dust as well as a high prevalence of autoantibodies, particularly ANA, in patients with silicosis. Understandably, enormous public anxiety was created, a class action suit against the manufacturers followed, and as a result large sums of money were adjudicated to patients before any solid epidemiologic data supported the claim.

Presentation

Patients with adjuvant disease complain of general malaise, marked tiredness, achiness in muscles and joints, and muscle weakness. Physical examination is negative in most patients with the exception of a cognitive disturbance that can frequently be demonstrated by standardized psychologic testing. Additional manifestations of the condition are mainly neurologic, with vague symptoms and findings that are not easily categorized in standard nosology. Laboratory studies are generally normal including ESR and muscle enzymes. A variable proportion of patients exhibit low titer, speckled, homogeneous, or nucleolar pattern positive ANA. As expected, given the large number of women who have implants, some of the patients indeed have symptoms and physical and laboratory findings of CTD that may have preceded or followed the implant.

Diagnosis

Summary of Diagnosis

> **ADJUVANT DISEASE OR CONNECTIVE TISSUE DISEASE (CTD) FOLLOWING BREAST IMPLANTS**
> - The condition is diagnosed clinically by (1) the presence of breast implants, and (2) the appearance of musculoskeletal symptoms, neurologic symptoms, or both in combination.
> - Laboratory studies are largely negative including ESR.
> - Antinuclear antibodies are demonstrable in 20% to 30% of patients, frequently with a nucleolar pattern (unconfirmed in some studies).

Natural History

Expected Outcome

It is still uncertain whether silicone-induced adjuvant disease exists as such or if the condition represents coincidental fibromyalgia or chronic fatigue syndrome appearing in women with breast implants. Definitely, the incidence of clear-cut connective tissue diseases such as scleroderma and SLE is not increased in women who have breast implants.

Treatment

Methods

Empirically, and based on the resemblance of adjuvant disease with chronic fatigue syndrome and fibromyalgia, the condition should be treated along the lines of fibromyalgia. However, the issue usually raised by patients is whether the implants should be removed or not. According to data from the literature and recent recommendations from the American College of Rheumatology, patients should not be encouraged to have the implants removed unless painful granuloma makes removal desirable. Even among proponents of the syndrome, the rate of improvement after implant removal is believed to be not more than 35%.

Expected Response

If the condition is indeed chronic fatigue or fibromyalgia, only a partial response to medications and physical measures can be expected.

When to Refer

If deemed necessary, patients with breast implants and musculoskeletal symptoms may be referred to rheumatologists, and those with predominantly neurologic symptoms should be referred to neurologists. In the author's opinion, patients should be told that available epidemiologic evidence indicates that breast implants do not lead to known connective tissue diseases, that the claim that implants cause a vague condition which defies classification has not been substantiated by valid epidemiologic research, that their condition is likely to be coincidental fibromyalgia (or connective tissue disease), that removal of the implants will most likely fail in improving their symptoms, and that treatment of their condition should be on its merits, irrespective of whether or not they have breast implants.

Guidelines for the Disorder

As of August 1996, the American College of Rheumatology Board of Directors stand on silicone breast implants is as follows: "A revision of the American College of Rheumatology Statement on Silicone Breast Implants was issued in 1995. Since then additional data on the breast implant issue have been published (JAMA 275:616–621, 1996, and others). To date, there continues to be no clear and consistent association of a defined connective tissue disease with silicone breast implant. Continued unbiased reporting of scientifically valid information will ultimately allow a more comprehensive assessment of this problem." (Source: ACR News 15:2, 1996.)

Key Points

ADJUVANT DISEASE OR CONNECTIVE TISSUE DISEASE (CTD) FOLLOWING BREAST IMPLANTS

- An association of connective tissue diseases such as scleroderma and SLE has not been shown in large, well-conducted epidemiologic studies.
- Fibromyalgia or chronic fatigue syndrome symptoms in implant recipients most likely represent the background in the general population, plus the possibility that patients with the psychologic makeup of fibromyalgia and chronic fatigue syndrome may be more likely to seek a breast implant.
- A recent cohort study has shown a slightly increased relative risk of "other connective tissue disease" in breast implant recipients. However, some of the data were collected after publicity regarding the possible health hazards of breast implants had surfaced.
- Removal of the implant has resulted in symptom improvement in only a minority of patients.
- The validity of the concept of silicone-induced adjuvant disease has not been scientifically proven.

Suggested Reading

Gabriel SE, O'Fallon WM, Kurland LT, et al. N Engl J Med 330:1697–1702, 1994.

Hennekens CH, Lee I-M, Cook NR, et al. Self-reported breast implants and connective tissue diseases in female health professionals. JAMA 275:616–621, 1996.

Sánchez-Guerrero J, Colditz GA, Karlson EW, et al. Silicone breast implants and the risk of connective tissue diseases and symptoms. N Engl J Med 332:1666–1670, 1995.

Spiera RF, Gibofsky A, Spiera H. Silicone gel filled breast implants and connective tissue disease: An overview. J Rheumatol 21:239–245, 1994.

CHAPTER 16

The Vasculitides

This heterogeneous group of conditions has, as a common denominator, inflammation of the vessel wall (Figure 16–1, Table 16–1). The predominantly involved vessels are high-caliber arteries in Takayasu arteritis (small vessels are also involved in a minority of cases) and giant cell arteritis; medium and small-size arteries (less commonly arterioles and venules) in polyarteritis nodosa and Churg-Strauss syndrome; small arteries and veins (sometimes larger arteries) in Wegener's granulomatosis; and arterioles and venules (often small arteries and veins) in hypersensitivity angiitis and Henoch-Schönlein purpura.

Thus, a strict classification of arteritis based on caliber of vessel involvement is not possible. Vascular deposition of immune complexes appears to be pathogenic in the necrotizing and small-vessel vasculitides. Cytokines such as tumor necrosis factor alpha may also be involved by initiating inflammation at postcapillary venules' endothelial cells. Some of the vasculitides are idiopathic (cause unknown); others are either idiopathic or secondary to infection, neoplasia, or drug sensitization. There is also a group of nonvasculitic entities that closely resemble vasculitis clinically. The many "pseudovasculitides" are listed in Table 16–2. Thus, the clinician facing a patient with possible vasculitis must (1) exclude pseudovasculitis, (2) confirm anatomically the diagnosis of vasculitis, and (3) exclude underlying conditions that may cause vasculitis. The following case summary illustrates the need of considering pseudovasculitis in patients with presumed vasculitis.

TABLE 16–1

CLASSIFICATION OF VASCULITIS

A. Involving large, medium-sized, and small blood vessels
  1. Takayasu arteritis (ES)
  2. Giant cell (granulomatous) arteritis (ES)
     a. Temporal arteritis
     b. Disseminated granulomatous angiitis
     c. Primary angiitis of the nervous system
  3. Aortitis (SP)
B. Involving predominantly medium-sized and small blood vessels
  1. Thromboangiitis obliterans (Buerger's disease) (ES)
  2. Polyarteritis nodosa (PAN) group (ES, I)
     a. Classic PAN
     b. Microscopic PAN (ANCA) (I)
     c. Infantile PAN (Kawasaki's disease vasculitis)
  3. Pathergic-allergic granulomatosis and angiitis (ES)
     a. Wegener's granulomatosis (ANCA, I)
     b. Churg-Strauss syndrome (ANCA)
C. Involving predominantly small blood vessels (hypersensitivity angiitis, leukocytoclastic vasculitis)
  1. Hypersensitivity angiitis (CTD, D/V, ES, I, NEO)
  2. Henoch-Schönlein syndrome (anaphylactoid purpura) (I)
  3. Mixed cryoglobulinemia (CTD, ES, I, NEO)
  4. Hypocomplementemic urticarial vasculitis (ES)

ANCA = Anti-neutrophil cytoplasmic antibodies. CTD = Connective tissue disease. D/V = Drug or vaccine induced. ES = Essential (none). I = Infectious. NEO = Neoplastic. SP = Spondyloarthropathy.

Modified from Lie JT. Nomenclature and classification of vasculitis: Plus ça change, plus c'est la même chose. Arthritis Rheum 37:181–186, 1994.

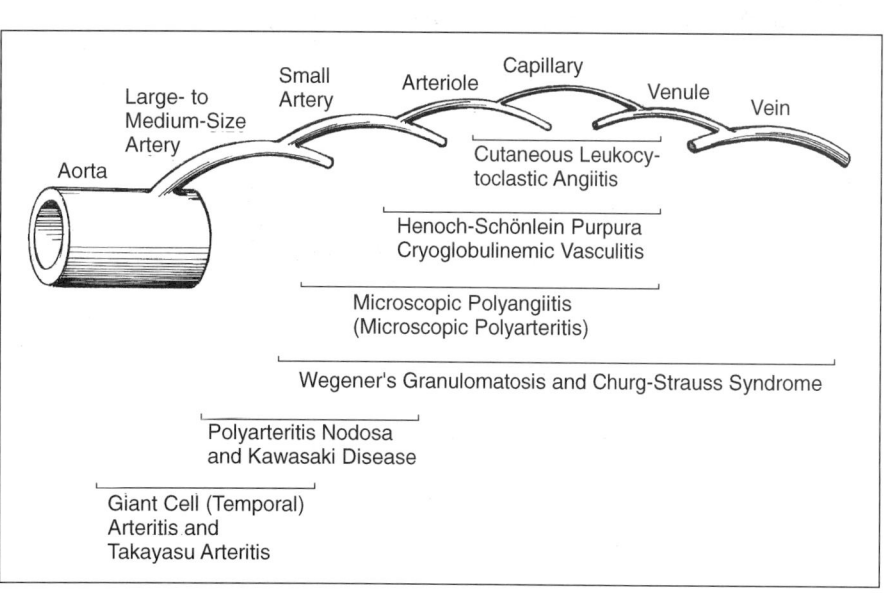

FIGURE 16–1. *Vasculitis.* Caliber of vessel(s) involved by the various vasculitides according to the Chapel Hill Consensus conference. There are overlaps among most types of vasculitis. (After Jennette JC, Falk RJ, Andrassy K, et al. Nomenclature of systemic vasculitis. Arthritis Rheum 37:187–192, 1994.)

TABLE 16-2
PSEUDOVASCULITIS SYNDROMES

Atheromatous embolization	Pernio (chilblains)
Atrial myxoma*	Thrombotic thrombocytopenic
Cancer	purpura*
Metastatic disease involving the	Spontaneous dissection of arteries*
peritoneum*	Fibromuscular dysplasia
Mucin and fat emboli in mucinous	Goodpasture's syndrome
carcinomas†	Sweet's syndrome
Calciphylaxis	Stevens-Johnson's syndrome
Infection	Weber-Christian disease and
Gonococcemia	systemic pancreatic steaton-
Infective endocarditis*	ecrosis
Meningococcemia	Oxalosis (renal failure treated with
Pheochromocytoma	hemodialysis, primary)
Primary antiphospholipid syndrome	Ergotism
Sneddon's syndrome	

*May have the angiographic appearance of PAN.
†Usually cerebral emboli.

PATIENT 16. A 51-year-old woman, a heavy smoker, was seen in consultation for a possible giant cell vasculitis involving the popliteal arteries. During a cruise 8 months before, left calf claudication and permanent numbness of the great toe developed. Four months later similar symptoms appeared in the right leg. There had been wide fluctuations in ischemic pain. Peaks, such as after a brisk walk, had been consistently associated with watery diarrhea and rectal pain. Recently, ischemic pain was triggered by minimal efforts and the pulp of all left toes became hyperesthetic. There was no fever, but a significant weight loss had been noticed, recovering partially during the last month. Of six physicians who had examined her during her illness, two, including the ship physician, had found missing pulses in the left foot; four had stated that pulses were normal. Upon further questioning she denied polymyalgic symptoms. She had had headaches, but they were no different from the usual ones she had experienced for the past 20 years. There was no upper extremity claudication, history of Raynaud's, or other features of connective tissue disease. Admission temperature was 36.6° C and BP was 120/80. There were no ulcers or other ischemic lesions. Temporal arteries were normal on palpation. The Allen's test revealed excellent radial and ulnar artery flow in both hands. Pulses were missing in both lower extremities below femorals. An arteriogram obtained the morning of admission (Figure 16–2A and B) showed occlusion of the popliteal artery on the left with some irregular collateral circulation and marked narrowing on the same artery on the right. Laboratory results included Hct 38, WBC 7400 with normal differential, platelet count 244,000, and ESR 23. Serum creatinine, alkaline phosphatase, ALT, AST, and urinalysis were all normal. As a more detailed history of the headaches was obtained, however, it turned out that the patient had been taking an average of 15 mg of ergotamine tartrate per week for the previous 5 years. She was informed of the strong possibility that her arterial disease was due to ergotism plus nicotine use. Late on the day of admission, pulses were felt in the right foot, and by the next morning, popliteal and pedal pulses had appeared on the left. Numbness resolved within days. On a 4 month follow-up she has been entirely asymptomatic.

The difficult issue of classifying vasculitic conditions was tackled by the American College of Rheumatology (ACR) (then the American Rheumatism Association) in the early 1980s, and as a result of those efforts, classification criteria for the major types of vasculitis were published in 1990. It should be understood that the ACR vasculitis criteria were created to distinguish the various categories of vasculitis from each other rather than to differentiate vasculitis from nonvasculitic processes.

The recommendations of an international consensus conference on the nomenclature of vasculitis published in 1994 are also of great interest (see guidelines in the appendix). The aim of the conference was to agree on the definition of terms commonly used in vasculitis. Unfortunately, differences in the interpretation of small-vessel involvement in polyarteritis nodosa precludes the complementary use of the two sets of recommendations. There is much to be learned from review-

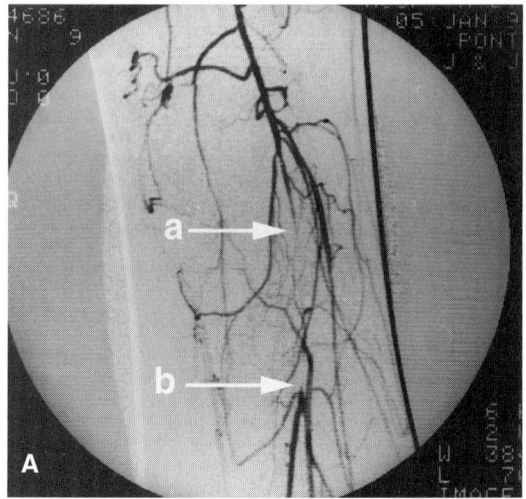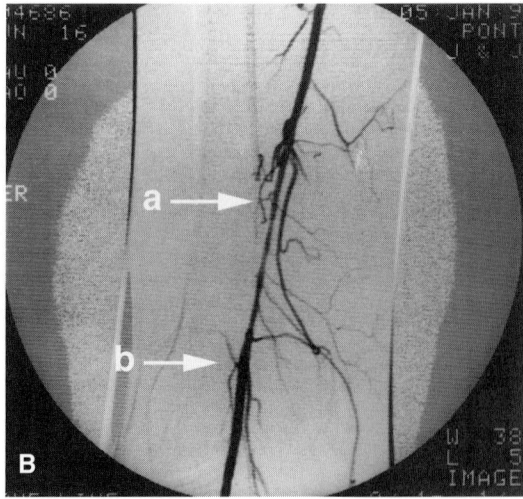

FIGURE 16–2. *Patient 16. Pseudovasculitis.* This woman presented with bilateral lower extremity ischemia and turned out to have ergotism (see text). A, Left popliteal artery occlusion (segment a–b). B, Right popliteal artery narrowing (segment a–b).

ing both sets of criteria. An attempt is made here to reconcile the two as each of the major forms of vasculitis are discussed.

Hypersensitivity Vasculitis

Hypersensitivity vasculitis (HV; Table 16–3) closely resembles Henoch-Shönlein's syndrome (HSS) in terms of the elemental vascular lesion. However, HV affects adults instead of children and lacks the peculiar IgA deposition that characterizes the vascular and renal lesion in HSS. Related entities include (1) urticarial vasculitis, which is a stubborn condition of young women presenting mainly with urticaria, acquired angioedema, and arthralgias, and (2) mixed cryoglobulinemia, a condition characterized by recurrent HV in a patient with liver enlargement, hypocomplementemia, and a positive rheumatoid factor test. Hepatitis C is a prominent cause of mixed cryoglobulinemia.

Presentation and Progression

Cause

Several causes of HV should be considered: drug or vaccine (serum sickness) exposure; infections such as bacterial endocarditis, gonococcemia, meningococcemia, types A, B, and C hepatitis, and HIV infection; cryoglobulinemia; connective tissue diseases, particularly SLE and Sjögren's syndrome; and malignancy.

Hypersensitivity vasculitis develops abruptly with a purpuric rash, malaise, fever, and often arthralgias. The typical lesion, a slightly raised purpuric rash that does not blanch with pressure, is known as palpable purpura. Characteristically, all purpuric lesions are the same age. Papules, vesicles, and ulcers may be present and "splinter hemorrhages" may be found at the nailbed. The HV rash predominates in dependent areas such as the legs and hands in ambulatory patients, and legs, buttocks, and back in bedridden patients. A commmon mistake on ward rounds is not to ask the patient to turn to one side and inspect the back side when a few questionable lesions are seen on the legs.

Diagnosis

Summary of Diagnosis

> **HYPERSENSITIVITY VASCULITIS**
> - Palpable purpura; often fever and arthralgias. Rarely hepatitis, nephritis, carditis, pneumonitis.
> - Review medications and recent history of vaccination.
> - Consider infection (fever, heart murmur, presence of pustulas or extensive skin hemorrhage, exposure to hepatitis, blood transfusion, parenteral drug use, and other risk factors for HIV).
> - Consider urticarial vasculitis (chronic urticaria, angioneurotic edema, arthralgias) and cryoglobulinemia (history of hepatitis, abnormal liver function tests, high-titer rheumatoid factor).
> - Consider SLE and Sjögren's (appropriate questions).
> - Consider malignancy (weight loss and other findings).
> - Obtain skin biopsy and additional studies as clinically indicated.

Natural History

In drug-induced HV, which comprises the majority of cases, the condition usually fades over several days following removal of the offending agent. There are also relapsing cases and chronic cases. In rare instances HV is complicated by hepatitis, interstitial nephritis, myocarditis, or pneumonitis.

Treatment

Treatment of drug-induced HV is with removal of the offending agent and local skin care. Corticosteroids are indicated in patients with extensive disease or severe systemic symptoms (prednisone about 20 mg per day) and when visceral involvement is present (prednisone about 60 mg per day). Treatment of infection cures infection-related cases, and control of connective tissue disease takes care of HV in SLE and Sjögren's.

Expected Response

With treatment expect gradual clearing of lesions in drug-induced and infection-related cases, control of systemic symptoms, and reversal of visceral involvement.

When to Refer

Most cases of HV should be handled by the primary care physician. Recurring cases, chronic cases, and cases in which an underlying cause may be playing a role should be referred to a rheumatologist for further evaluation and treatment.

TABLE 16–3

1990 ACR CRITERIA FOR THE CLASSIFICATION OF HYPERSENSITIVITY VASCULITIS

Criterion	Definition
1. Age at disease onset > 16 years	Development of symptoms after age 16
2. Medication at disease onset	Medication was taken at onset of symptoms that may have been a precipitating factor
3. Palpable purpura	Slightly elevated purpuric rash over one or more areas of the skin; does not blanch with pressure and is not related to thrombocytopenia
4. Maculopapular rash	Flat and raised lesions of various sizes over one or more areas of skin
5. Biopsy including arteriole and venule	Histologic changes showing granulocytes in a perivascular or extravascular location

For purposes of classification, a patient shall be said to have hypersensitivity vasculitis if at least 3 of these 5 criteria are present. The presence of any 3 or more criteria yields a sensitivity of 71.0% and a specificity of 83.9%.

ACR = American College of Rheumatology.
From Calabrese LH, Michel BA, Bloch DA, et al. American College of Rheumatology 1990 criteria for the classification of hypersensitivity vasculitis. Arthritis Rheum 33:1108–1113, 1990.

Key Points

> **HYPERSENSITIVITY VASCULITIS**
>
> - The most common of the vasculitides.
> - Palpable purpura is the characteristic finding on examination.
> - It may be drug or vaccine induced or secondary to a variety of conditions, particularly infections and neoplasms.
> - Course may be a single crop of lesions, recurring crops, or chronic disease.
> - Visceral involvement in drug-related cases is both uncommon and mild.
> - Mild drug-induced HV is treated with removal of the offending drug. Extensive lesions, severe systemic symptoms, and visceral involvement are indications for the use of corticosteroids.
> - Treatment of the underlying condition leads to resolution in secondary HV.

Suggested Reading

Mader R, Narendran A, Letwas J, et al. Systemic vasculitis following influenza vaccination. Report of 3 cases and literature review. J Rheumatol 20:1429–1431, 1993.

Chronic Urticaria and Urticarial Vasculitis

Chronic urticaria is fairly common in clinical practice. Urticarial vasculitis is relatively rare, although some cases may be misclassified as SLE. Although treatment may be frustrating and call for the expertise of a dermatologist, allergist, or rheumatologist, a working knowledge of diagnosis and treatment may solve many of the milder cases.

Presentation and Progression

Cause

An immune reaction is assumed to be responsible for both conditions. However, an actual cause cannot be determined in 80% to 90% of cases. Aspirin and NSAIDs are known to trigger or aggravate urticarial vasculitis in approximately 30% of patients.

Presentation

Both chronic urticaria and urticarial vasculitis feature urticarial wheals and angioedema (Table 16–4). An urticarial wheal is an itchy, slightly raised papule or plaque that expands by the edge, often clears in the center, and disappears leaving no trace. Angioedema is a circumscribed, raised patch that originates deeply in the subcutaneous tissue or the submucosa, hurts rather than itches, moves slowly in the affected area, and fades without residuals.

Whereas in chronic urticaria single urticarial lesions fade within 24 hours, they usually last up to 3 to 4 days in vasculitic urticaria. Fever, purpura, arthralgias, obstructive pulmonary disease, eye inflammation, abdominal pain, hypocomplementemia, and occasionally glomerulonephritis suggest urticarial vasculitis. Hereditary angioedema does not feature urticaria, the larynx is frequently involved, bowel wall edema causes severe abdominal pain, a positive family history is often present, and complement studies show low C_4 as well as deficiency of C_1 esterase inhibitor.

Diagnosis

Summary of Diagnosis

TABLE 16–4

DIFFERENTIATION BETWEEN CHRONIC URTICARIA AND URTICARIAL VASCULITIS

	Chronic Urticaria	Urticarial Vasculitis
Duration of wheals	< 24 hours	> 24 hours
Purpura	No	Yes
Pain	No	Yes
Arthralgias	No	Yes
Fever	No	Yes
Abdominal pain	No	Yes
Nephritis	No	Yes
Elevated ESR	No	Yes
Decreased C_3	No	Maybe
Leukocytoclastic vasculitis	No	Yes
C_3/immunoglobulin deposits	No	Yes

Modified from Greaves MW. Chronic urticaria. N Engl J Med 22:1767–1772, 1995.

> **CHRONIC URTICARIA AND URTICARIAL VASCULITIS**
>
> - Both conditions feature urticarial lesions and angioedema.
> - In cases without urticaria, hereditary (autosomal dominant) deficiency of C_1 esterase inhibitor must be ruled out.
> - Individual urticarial lesions last longer in urticarial vasculitis.
> - Variants of chronic urticaria include cold-induced urticaria, solar urticaria, and cholinergic urticaria in which lesions appear, for instance, during exercise or taking a hot shower.
> - Fever, arthralgias, abdominal pain, purpura, glomerulonephritis, increased ESR, and depressed complement are features of urticarial vasculitis.
> - Differential diagnosis of urticarial vasculitis includes SLE and Sjögren's syndrome.
> - Laboratory evaluation should include CBC, ESR, ANA, complement levels C_3 and C_4, and urinalysis. A low C1q and presence of C1q antibodies are diagnostic of urticarial vasculitis.
> - Presence of peripheral blood eosinophilia suggests parasitic disease.
> - Diagnosis of urticarial vasculitis should be confirmed with a skin biopsy obtained at the edge of the lesion.

Natural History

Expected Outcome

Both are chronic conditions amenable only to suppressive therapy.

Treatment

Methods

A physical causation (cold, sun, pressure, heat) should be excluded in all cases. Aspirin, NSAIDs, and angiotensin-converting enzyme inhibitors are to be proscribed. An H_1 antihistaminic such as astemizole or terfenadine 60 mg bid per se fails in many patients. It is useful to add an H_2 antihistaminic such as cimetidine 600 mg bid. Brief courses of corticosteroids such as prednisone 30 mg daily tapered over 3 weeks may be used when antihistaminics fail to control the urticaria.

When to Refer

Patients with chronic urticaria often improve on simple measures. Failures of treatment, as well as patients with urticarial vasculitis, should be referred to an allergist or rheumatologist for evaluation and treatment advice.

Key Points

CHRONIC URTICARIA AND URTICARIAL VASCULITIS

- Urticarial lesions and angioedema are featured by both conditions. When only angioedema is present, hereditary angioedema must be ruled out.
- Urticarial vasculitis has distinctive systemic features: ocular inflammation, arthralgias or arthritis, obstructive pulmonary disease, and glomerulonephritis.
- Peripheral blood eosinophilia suggests parasitic disease. Examine stools for ova and parasites.
- Treatment in both conditions begins with the use of H_1 and H_2 blockers.
- Patients who fail to improve should be treated with a short corticosteroid course.
- Resistant cases should be referred to an allergist.

Suggested Reading

Agostoni A, Cicardi M. Hereditary and acquired C1-inhibitor deficiency: Biological and clinical characteristics in 235 patients. Medicine (Baltimore) 71:206–215, 1992.

Greaves MW. Chronic urticaria. N Engl J Med 332:1767–1772, 1995.

Wisniewski JJ, Baer AN, Christensen J, et al. Hypocomplementemic urticarial vasculitis syndrome. Medicine (Baltimore) 74:24–41, 1995.

Henoch-Schönlein Purpura

Henoch-Schönlein purpura (HSP; Table 16–5) is the most common form of small-vessel vasculitis in the pediatric group. Typically, skin, gut, and kidney are involved. Characteristically, IgA-, C_3-, and properdin-containing deposits are present in glomeruli and dermal capillaries, arterioles, and venules, and serum IgA levels are increased in over 50% of patients. The kidney lesion of HSP is similar clinically and pathologically to Berger's disease.

TABLE 16–5

THE 1990 AMERICAN COLLEGE OF RHEUMATOLOGY CRITERIA FOR CLASSIFICATION OF HENOCH-SCHÖNLEIN PURPURA

Criterion	Definition
1. Palpable purpura	Slightly raised "palpable" hemorrhagic skin lesions not related to thrombocytopenia
2. Age < 20 at disease onset	Patient 20 years or younger at onset of first symptoms
3. Bowel angina	Diffuse abdominal pain worse after meals, or the diagnosis of bowel ischemia, usually including bloody diarrhea
4. Wall granulocytes on biopsy	Histologic changes showing granulocytes in the walls of arterioles or venules

For purposes of classification, a patient shall be said to have Henoch-Schönlein purpura if at least 2 of these 4 criteria are present. The presence of any 2 or more criteria yields a sensitivity of 87.1% and a specificity of 87.7%.

From Mills JA, Michel BA, Bloch DA, et al. American College of Rheumatology 1990 criteria for the classification of Henoch-Schönlein purpura. Arthritis Rheum 33:1114–1121, 1990.

Presentation and Progression

Cause

HSP has a seasonal pattern; it peaks in spring, fall, and winter and affects predominantly children between the ages of 5 and 15. Epidemiologic and immunologic considerations suggest an IgA-mediated immune response with alternate complement system activation. Half of cases are preceded by URI. The causing agent(s) remains unknown.

The condition begins abruptly with malaise, arthralgias, or arthritis involving predominantly the knees and ankles, low-grade fever, and an urticarial and then palpable purpuric rash that is most prominent on the extremities and buttocks. Edema involving scalp or other areas is often present. A few days later colicky abdominal pain appears with or without features of abdominal angina along with occult or overt intestinal bleeding. Renal involvement featuring hematuria and proteinuria occurs in 25% to 40% of cases.

Diagnosis

Summary of Diagnosis

HENOCH-SCHÖNLEIN PURPURA

- Antecedent URI in 50%.
- Palpable purpura.

- Arthralgia or arthritis involving knees and ankles.
- Scalp or other edema.
- Abdominal pain.
- Blood in stool.
- Hematuria, proteinuria.
- Skin biopsy showing leukocytoclastic vasculitis with IgA, C_3, and properdin deposits in the vessel wall.

Natural History

Expected Outcome

In over 80% of cases the condition spontaneously goes away within 2 weeks. Abdominal pain is usually of short duration (1 to 3 days). In 10% to 20% of cases there are one or more relapses of purpura, arthralgia, abdominal pain, and glomerulitis. Poor prognostic factors in HSP include persistent rash over 2 to 3 months, melena, hematuria with proteinuria more than 1 g/24 hours, nephrotic syndrome with renal insufficiency, and more than 50% crescents on renal biopsy.

There are two serious complications of the condition, an acute abdomen from intestinal intussusception (< 5% of cases) and progression of glomerulitis to serious renal disease and renal insufficiency (10% of pediatric cases with renal involvement or 2% to 4% of the total group).

Adult cases of HSP do occur and differ from the pediatric cases in a much higher rate of progressive renal disease. Also, Berger's disease has been considered an adult, monosymptomatic form of HSP. Interestingly, Berger's disease is a known complication of ankylosing spondylitis and other spondyloarthropathies that feature elevated levels of serum IgA.

Treatment

Methods

Treatment of HSP depends on the severity of systemic and abdominal symptoms. Mild cases require supportive therapy only, including acetaminophen for analgesia. Corticosteroids do not change the ultimate course of the disease and should only be used for the treatment of severe systemic symptoms such as severe abdominal pain, melena, and massive bleeding. Cyclophosphamide and cyclosporine have been used empirically in HSP associated with progressive renal disease, but a clear beneficial effect has not been shown. High-dose immunoglobulin therapy appears to halt renal disease progression in some patients.

Expected Response

Corticosteroids lead to rapid improvement of malaise, fever, skin lesions, articular symptoms, and abdominal pain. Hematuria and proteinuria remain unaffected. Intravenous immunoglobulins may stabilize renal function, decrease renal IgA and C_3 deposits, and decrease the activity index of the renal lesion.

Complications

Expect the usual complications of corticosteroid therapy.

Key Points

HENOCH-SCHÖNLEIN PURPURA

- Most frequent in children.
- Small-vessel leukocytoclastic vasculitis involving skin, joints, gut, and kidney.
- Lesional deposition of IgA, C_3, and properdin.
- Complications include intussusception and progressive renal disease (2% to 4% of pediatric patients; a higher proportion of adult cases).
- Poor prognostic factors include melena, persisting rash, heavy proteinuria, renal insufficiency, and more than 50% crescents on renal biopsy.
- Corticosteroids and immunosuppressives should be considered when poor prognostic factors are present.
- Intravenous immunoglobulins appear to halt disease progression in severe HSP renal disease.

Suggested Reading

Cassidy JT, Petty RE. Vasculitis. In: Textbook of Pediatric Rheumatology, 3rd ed. W. B. Saunders, Philadelphia, 365–422, 1995.

Niaudet P, Murcia I, Beaufils H, Broyer M, Habib R. Primary IgA nephropathy in children. Prognosis and treatment. Adv Nephrol 22:121–140, 1993.

Rostoker G, Desvaux-Belghiti D, Pilatte Y, et al. High-dose immunoglobulin therapy for severe IgA nephropathy and Henoch-Schönlein purpura. Ann Intern Med 120:476–484, 1994.

Thromboangiitis Obliterans (Buerger's Disease)

Thromboangiitis obliterans (TAO) is an occlusive vasculitis involving small- and medium-sized arteries and veins. Almost exclusively seen in heavy smokers, unchecked TAO results in excruciatingly painful distal ulcerations and multiple limb amputations.

Presentation and Progression

Cause

Tobacco smoking is clearly implicated in the pathogenesis of TAO. Formerly the male/female ratio was 9 to 1. An increased prevalence of female smoking in recent years has resulted in an increased rate of TAO among women.

Presentation

The typical TAO patient is a young male or female smoker presenting with distal (for example, thenar) intermittent claudication and upper and/or lower extremity ischemic ulcerations. Raynaud's phenomenon and thrombophlebitis are often present. Pedal pulses are usually absent, and the Allen's test shows disturbed perfusion in the hands and fingers, that is, fair or good perfusion through the radial artery and no perfusion through the ulnar.

Diagnosis

Summary of Diagnosis

> **THROMBOANGIITIS OBLITERANS (TAO)**
> - A condition confined to young tobacco smokers.
> - Embolic disease, other vasculitides, scleroderma, and thrombotic conditions such as the primary antiphospholipid syndrome must be ruled out.
> - Distal ischemic ulcers and intermittent claudication in upper and/or lower extremities; Raynaud's phenomenon; thrombophlebitis.
> - Distal arterial occlusions with normal proximal pulses.
> - The Allen's test is usually positive.
> - Pulse volume recordings document distal disease.
> - Arteriography shows occlusion of infrapopliteal arteries or arteries distal to the elbow and normal proximal arteries. Sites of occlusion are multiple with corkscrew collaterals around the occlusions.
> - Histologic diagnosis should be an exception (as it is usually performed in amputated specimens).

Natural History

Expected Outcome

Complete cessation of smoking halts disease progression. Unfortunately, many patients continue to smoke, and multiple upper and lower extremity amputations are the sad result.

Treatment

Methods

The key issue in TAO is to quit smoking. Iloprost, a prostacyclin analog, has shown effectiveness in promoting ulcer healing and improving rest pain. Sympathectomy may be used in resistant cases and may afford temporary relief.

When to Refer

Patients in whom TAO is suspected should be fully evaluated for embolic disease (including a transesophageal cardiac echo), vasculitis, scleroderma, and thrombotic conditions including the antiphospholipid syndrome. Peripheral vascular diseases experts are in the best position to care for TAO patients.

Key Points

> **THROMBOANGIITIS OBLITERANS (TAO)**
> - Cessation of smoking is essential to halt the disease.
> - Iloprost infusions promote ulcer healing and reduce rest pain.
> - Sympathectomy may be used for the treatment of nonhealing ulcers.
> - Bypass surgery is not applicable in this condition.

Suggested Reading

Olin JW. Thromboangiitis obliterans (Buerger's disease). Current Opin Rheumatol 6:44–49, 1994.

Olin JW, Young JR, Graor RA, et al. The changing clinical spectrum of thromboangiitis obliterans (Buerger's disease). Circulation (suppl IV) 82:3–8, 1990.

Yorukogly Y, Ilgit E, Zengin M, et al. Thromboangiitis obliterans (Buerger's disease) in women. A reevaluation. Angiology 44:527–532, 1993.

Polyarteritis Nodosa

Polyarteritis nodosa (PAN; Table 16–6) is a necrotizing vasculitis affecting predominantly middle-sized and small muscular arteries. Arterioles and venules are less prominently involved. Vessel involvement is focal and segmental, and new (necrotic) and old (sclerotic) lesions coexist in the same or different tissues. Focal weakening in arterial wall causes microaneurysm formation. Thrombosis and endothelial proliferation results in skin, visceral, and nervous system infarctions.

Presentation and Progression

Cause

In 10% to 50% of cases there is evidence of hepatitis B virus infection. In one study hepatitis C virus antibodies were present in 20% of patients. Some instances apparently caused by the HIV virus are also on record. A variable proportion of cases in the earlier literature had an antecedent of intravenous drug use; whether or not these cases had an associated viral infection is not known. Some cases appear to follow serous otitis media. Occasional cases follow vaccination, such as influenza vaccination. In children, typical lesions of PAN occur in the coronary vessels late in the course of Kawasaki disease. There is an interesting but little understood association between polyarteritis nodosa and hairy cell leukemia. A vasculitis clinically similar to PAN may occur in Sjögren's syndrome, RA, and certain malignancies. Finally, there is an ever-shrinking proportion of PAN cases in which no predisposing condition is found. Arteriographic changes similar to PAN may occur in Wegener's granulomatosis, SLE, plus the pseudovasculitic conditions listed in Table 16–2.

Polyarteritis nodosa is more common in males (male/female ratio is 2 to 1), and most cases occur in the fourth and fifth decades of life. Patients develop, usually within a few weeks, profound fatigue, fever, myalgias, and weight loss. Abdominal pain, sometimes with the characteristic of abdominal angina, is frequent. Acute abdomen from bowel or mesenteric infarction or bowel perforation may occur, as well as massive GI bleeding. Renal involvement may be clinically detected in 70%. Gross hematuria may result from kidney infarction; proteinuria and microhematuria usually indicate segmental necrotizing glomerulonephritis. Arterial hypertension from renal arterial involvement or

TABLE 16–6

THE 1990 AMERICAN COLLEGE OF RHEUMATOLOGY CRITERIA FOR THE CLASSIFICATION OF POLYARTERITIS NODOSA

Criterion	Definition
1. Weight loss > 4 kg	Since illness began, not due to dieting or other factors
2. Livedo reticularis	Mottled reticular pattern over the skin of portions of the extremities or torso
3. Testicular pain or tenderness	Not due to infection, trauma, or other causes
4. Myalgias, weakness, or leg tenderness	Diffuse myalgias (excluding shoulder and hip girdle) or weakness of muscles or tenderness of leg muscles
5. Mononeuropathy or polyneuropathy	Development of mononeuropathy, multiple mononeuropathies, or polyneuropathy
6. Diastolic BP > 90 mm	Development of hypertension
7. Elevated BUN or creatinine	BUN > 40 mg/dl or creatinine > 1.5 mg/dl
8. Hepatitis B virus	Presence of hepatitis B surface antigen or antibody in the serum
9. Arteriographic abnormality	Aneurysms or occlusions of the visceral arteries, not due to arteriosclerosis, fibromuscular dysplasia, or other noninflammatory causes
10. Biopsy of small or medium-size artery containing PMN	Histologic changes showing the presence of granulocytes or granulocytes and mononuclear leukocytes in the artery wall

For purposes of classification, a patient shall be said to have polyarteritis nodosa if at least 3 of these 10 criteria are present. The presence of any 3 or more criteria yields a sensitivity of 82.2% and a specificity of 86.6%.

BP = blood pressure; BUN = blood urea nitrogen; PMN = polymorphonuclear neutrophils.
From Lightfoot RW Jr, Michel BA, Bloch DA, et al. American College of Rheumatology 1990 criteria for the classification of polyarteritis nodosa. Arthritis Rheum 33:1088–1093, 1990.

glomerulitis occurs in 25%. Skin manifestations include palpable purpura, painful nodules, ulcers, livedo reticularis, and necrosis of fingertips. The onset of mononeuritis (60% to 70%), usually multiplex, is often marked by sudden foot or wrist drop. Peripheral neuropathy may also occur. Strokes and seizures are uncommon. Arthralgias or frank arthritis, which resembles RA but is nonerosive, are frequently present. Arteritis in muscular arteries results in calf pain and tenderness and intermittent claudication. Cardiac involvement, present in 30%, may result from myocardial infarction (usually silent) or arterial hypertension. Retinal hemorrhages and exudates are common. Testicular pain and swelling may occur from vasculitis of the testicular or epididimal arteries. It should be realized that there are cases with limited involvement: isolated involvement of the appendix or the gallbladder and cutaneous polyarteritis nodosa in which changes are limited to skin arteries. This form of arteritis is seen in association with Crohn's disease and ulcerative colitis.

Laboratory findings present in most cases include chronic disease anemia, leukocytosis, thrombocytosis, increased ESR, proteinuria (rarely in the nephrotic range), and urine sediment abnormalities such as hematuria and red blood cell casts. Liver enzymes levels are often abnormal, particularly the serum alkaline phosphatase, in cases due to hepatitis B or C infection. Rheumatoid factor tests are positive in about half the cases. Hypocomplementemia and cryoglobulinemia are present in about 20% and associate with evidence of hepatitis C infection.

Diagnosis

Summary of Diagnosis

POLYARTERITIS NODOSA

- Clinical cluster with malaise, fever, weight loss, abdominal pain, mononeuritis or mononeuritis multiplex, arterial hypertension, abnormalities in urinalysis.
- Blood cultures to exclude infective endocarditis.
- CBC, platelet count, ESR.
- BUN and creatinine determination.
- Urinalysis.
- Hepatitis B antigen and antibody and hepatitis C antibody.
- Biopsy of an involved site (skin, sural nerve, muscle, kidney, testes).
- Angiography to visualize kidney vessels and mesenteric angiography when there is evidence of intraabdominal involvement. Characteristic features include saccular or fusiform aneurysms and tapering of arteries.

Natural History

Expected Outcome

The course of PAN is highly variable. In a few patients the disease seems to die out after the first bout. The course in other patients is fulminant with death occurring within a few months. Indeed, most deaths occur within the first year of illness. Renal involvement (by histology and/or elevated creatinine) and/or cardiac involvement are poor prognostic factors with survival at 6 months 55% with, and 91% without, these factors. In most patients the disease has a chronic relapsing course. Residual organ damage is quite common. Untreated, the 5 year survival in PAN is less than 20%. With current treatment the survival at 5 years has improved to 80%.

Complications

Persistent sensory and motor deficits occur in most patients as a result of neuropathy. Paresis from stroke and residual renal insufficiency are also common. Early deaths in PAN occur from relentless vasculitis, in particular intestinal perforation, or complications of corticosteroid or immunosuppressive treatment. Late deaths are from stroke or myocardial infarction. Poor prognostic factors include renal involvement and severe GI manifestations.

Treatment

Methods

Treatment of PAN is with high-dose corticosteroids such as prednisone 60 to 100 mg per day, initially in divided doses. Cyclophosphamide in monthly boluses or in daily oral doses should be added in unresponsive cases. Plasma exchanges do not add any benefit to the combination of prednisone/cyclophosphamide.

Expected Response

Response to treatment is slow, occurring over months. In the majority of patients multiple treatment courses are required.

Complications of therapy are common from the use of high-dose corticosteroids and immunosuppressant agents.

When to Refer

Patients with suspected PAN should be evaluated by a rheumatologist and if the diagnosis is proven, followed by a rheumatologist.

Key Points

> **POLYARTERITIS NODOSA**
>
> - Febrile, catabolic multisystem disease caused by necrotizing vasculitis of medium-sized and small muscular arteries and smaller vessels.
> - In at least 60% of cases there is evidence of hepatitis B or C infection.
> - Peripheral nerve involvement causes stepwise incapacitation.
> - Catastrophic events are associated with renal, cerebral, cardiac, and mesenteric vessels.
> - Treatment is with high-dose corticosteroids plus cyclophosphamide in uncontrolled cases.
> - Survival at 5 years has improved from 20% to 80%.
> - Poor prognostic factors include renal involvement and cardiac involvement.
> - Neurologic sequelae and residual arterial hypertension are common in successfully treated patients.

Suggested Reading

Carson CW, Conn DL, Czaja AJ, et al. Frequency and significance of antibodies to hepatitis C virus in polyarteritis nodosa. J Rheumatol 20:304–309, 1993.

Fortin PR, Larson MG, Watters AK, et al. Prognostic factors in systemic necrotizing vasculitis of the polyarteritis nodosa group—A review of 45 cases. J Rheumatol 22:78–84, 1995.

Gherardi R, Belec L, Mhiri C, et al. The spectrum of vasculitis in human immunodeficiency virus-infected patients. Arthritis Rheum 36:1164–1174, 1993.

Guillevin L, Lhote F, Gayraud M, et al. Prognostic factors in polyarteritis nodosa and Churg-Strauss syndrome. A prospective study of 342 patients. Medicine (Baltimore) 75:17–28, 1996.

Churg-Strauss Syndrome

Churg-Strauss syndrome (CSS; Table 16–7), also known as allergic granulomatosis and angiitis, is an uncommon vasculitic disease characterized by asthma, pulmonary infiltrates, intense peripheral blood eosinophilia, and pathologic findings that include small- and medium-vessel necrotizing vasculitis, extravascular necrotizing granulomas, and tissue eosinophilia.

Presentation and Progression

Cause

The cause of CSS is unknown. Both clinically and pathologically the condition exhibits overlapping features with polyarteritis nodosa (necrotizing vasculitis, mononeuritis multiplex) and Wegener's granulomatosis (extravascular necrotizing granulomas, frequent involvement of the upper airway).

CSS affects young and middle-age adults. Allergic rhinitis complicated by polyposis and recurrent sinusitis is a frequent antecedent of the disease. The initial manifestation is asthma. Several months to several years later, systemic vasculitis develops including fever; transient, migratory, or fixed pulmonary

TABLE 16–7

THE 1990 AMERICAN COLLEGE OF RHEUMATOLOGY CRITERIA FOR THE CLASSIFICATION OF CHURG-STRAUSS SYNDROME

Criterion	Definition
1. Asthma	History of wheezing or diffuse high-pitched rales on expiration
2. Eosinophilia	Eosinophilia > 10% on white blood cell differential count
3. Mononeuropathy or polyneuropathy	Development of mononeuropathy, multiple mononeuropathies, or polyneuropathy (e.g., glove/stocking distribution attributable to a systemic vasculitis)
4. Pulmonary infiltrates, nonfixed	Migratory or transitory pulmonary infiltrates on radiographs (not including fixed infiltrates)
5. Paranasal sinus abnormalities	History of acute or chronic paranasal sinus pain or tenderness or radiographic opacification of the paranasal sinuses
6. Extravascular eosinophils	Biopsy including artery, arteriole, or venule, showing accumulations of eosinophils in extravascular areas

For purposes of classification, a patient shall be said to have Churg-Strauss syndrome if at least 4 of these 6 criteria are positive. The presence of any 4 or more of the 6 criteria yields a sensitivity of 85% and a specificity of 99.7%.

From Masi AT, Hunder GG, Michel BA, et al. American College of Rheumatology 1990 criteria for the classification of Churg-Strauss syndrome. Arthritis Rheum 33:1094–1100, 1990.

infiltrates; mononeuritis, mononeuritis multiplex, or peripheral neuropathy (present in the aggregate in most patients); skin lesions (palpable purpura, urticaria, subcutaneous nodules); arthralgias or arthritis; and myopericarditis. A characteristic finding is intense peripheral blood eosinophilia.

Diagnosis

Summary of Diagnosis

CHURG-STRAUSS SYNDROME
- Recent-onset asthma in an adult.
- Intense peripheral blood eosinophilia.
- Pulmonary infiltrates.
- Neuropathy.
- Skin lesions.
- Biopsy of skin lesion, sural nerve, lung.

Natural History

Expected Outcome

The condition has a chronic course; in untreated patients frequent causes of death included myopericarditis and cerebral hemorrhage. Poor prognostic factors include renal involvement and severe GI manifestations.

Treatment

Methods

Treatment of CSS is primarily with corticosteroids as used in Wegener's granulomatosis. Immunosuppressives may be added in severely ill patients.

Expected Response

Remissions are obtained in virtually all patients. Half of the remissions are permanent. Survival rate at 5 years is 80%.

Complications

Expect the complications of corticosteroids and immunosuppressives (see complications of corticosteroids, cyclophosphamide, methotrexate, azathioprine).

When to Refer

Patients suspected of having CSS should be referred to a pulmonary specialist for assessment and treatment.

Key Points

CHURG-STRAUSS SYNDROME
- Asthma in the adult followed by systemic vasculitis.
- Systemic involvement includes pulmonary infiltrates, upper respiratory lesions, mononeuritis multiplex or other neuropathy, skin lesions, and myopericardial lesions.
- Renal involvement, hypertension, and GI vasculitis are rare in CSS.
- Response to corticosteroids is excellent with virtually all cases undergoing remission.
- Remission is permanent in about 50%.

Suggested Reading

Abu-Shakra, Smythe H, Lewtas J, et al. Outcome of polyarteritis nodosa and Churg-Strauss syndrome. An analysis of twenty-five patients. Arthritis Rheum 37:1798–1803, 1994.

Guillevin L, Lhote F, Gayraud M, et al. Prognostic factors in polyarteritis nodosa and Churg-Strauss syndrome. A prospective study of 342 patients. Medicine (Baltimore) 75:17–28, 1996.

Lanham JG, Elkon KB, Pusey CD, et al. Systemic vasculitis with asthma and eosinophilia: A clinical approach to the Churg-Strauss syndrome. Medicine (Baltimore) 63:65–79, 1984.

Wegener's Granulomatosis

Wegener granulomatosis (WG; Table 16–8) is characterized by necrotizing granulomas of the upper and lower airway; small-vessel (arteries and veins) necrotizing or granulomatous vasculitis; and focal, segmental necrotizing glomerulonephritis. Diffuse proliferative, necrotizing, and crescentic glomerulonephritis is present in patients with severe renal disease. Wegener's lesions are ubiquitous, which makes the clinical spectrum of the disease seemingly endless.

Presentation and Progression

Cause

The cause of WG is unknown. Upper respiratory *Staphylococcus aureus* colonization is believed by some to trigger flares of the condition. A recent epidemiologic study has identified several small communities with seemingly excessive cases of WG. Cytoplasmic antineutrophil antibodies (c-ANCA), which are found in the overwhelming majority of patients, appear to play a pathogenetic role in WG. C-ANCA in Wegener's granulomatosis has antigen specificity for proteinase 3 and casts diffuse cytoplasmic fluorescence when studied by indirect immunofluorescence. In contrast, ANCA with antigen specificity for myeloperoxidase results in a perinuclear fluorescence pattern and occurs in a variety of conditions in addition to some cases of Wegener's granulomatosis.

The mean age of cases is in the sixth decade. The condition is equally frequent in men and women. Most patients with Wegener's granulomatosis first develop malaise, weight loss, and proximal airway symptoms including severe chronic sinusitis or obstructive rhinitis. Bloody rhinorrhea is common. Septal ulceration may lead to a saddle nose. Patients may have otitis with local pain and serous or bloody middle ear discharge. Eye involvement eventually occurs in one-half of patients. Lesions include episcleritis, scleritis, granulomatous uveitis, and proptosis caused by retrobulbar granulomas. Oral ulcers are frequent. Lower respiratory symptoms are present at onset in about one-half of patients and in most patients during disease course. A nonresolving

TABLE 16–8

THE 1990 AMERICAN COLLEGE OF RHEUMATOLOGY CRITERIA FOR THE CLASSIFICATION OF WEGENER'S GRANULOMATOSIS

Criterion	Definition
1. Nasal or oral inflammation	Development of painful or painless oral ulcers or purulent or bloody nasal discharge
2. Abnormal chest radiograph	Chest radiograph showing the presence of nodules, fixed infiltrates, or cavities
3. Urinary sediment abnormalities	Microhematuria (> 5 red blood cells per high power field) or red cell casts in urine sediment
4. Granulomatous inflammation on biopsy	Histologic changes showing granulomatous inflammation within the wall of an artery or in the perivascular or extravascular area (artery or arteriole)

For purposes of classification, a patient shall be said to have Wegener's granulomatosis if at least 2 of these 4 criteria are present. The presence of any 2 or more criteria yields a sensitivity of 88.2% and a specificity of 92.0%.

From Leavitt RY, Fauci AS, Bloch DA, et al. American College of Rheumatology 1990 criteria for the classification of Wegener's granulomatosis. Arthritis Rheum 33:1101–1107, 1990.

pneumonia, hemoptysis, or pleurisy may be the first indicator of the disease. Glomerulonephritis is present at onset in less than one-quarter of patients and later in the course in three-fourths of patients. Early renal involvement is asymptomatic and is usually identified by the presence of red cell casts in the urinary sediment (Table 16–9). Skin findings include palpable purpura, ulcers, and subcutaneous nodules. Arthralgias, oligoarticular arthritis, or rheumatoid-like arthritis is present in about two-third of patients. Finally, pericarditis (about 6% of patients), peripheral neuropathy of the mononeuritis multiplex type (about 15% of patients), and central nervous system disease (about 8% of patients) may occur in WG.

Laboratory abnormalities in active disease include chronic disease anemia, leukocytosis, thrombocytosis, and high elevations of ESR. Rheumatoid factor tests are positive in over one-half of cases. As mentioned, c-ANCA are present in the majority of cases of Wegener's granulomatosis.

Chest x-rays are usually abnormal, showing multiple nodules often with cavitation or pneumonitis that may also cavitate. Cases without clinical kidney involvement are often categorized as "limited WG." Because generalized disease may later develop in these patients, so-called limited WG may in fact represent early disease. The differential diagnosis between WG and midline granuloma is frequently brought up in patients with severe upper airway disease. The distinction can be readily made by using simple clinical criteria, as shown in Table 16–10.

Diagnosis

Summary of Diagnosis

WEGENER'S GRANULOMATOSIS

- Upper airway lesions (rhinitis, sinusitis, otitis media).
- Ocular lesions (sclera, uveal tract, orbit).
- Mouth ulcers, skin nodules or ulcers, arthritis.
- Chest x-ray abnormalities (nodules, pneumonitis, with or without cavitation).
- Urine sediment abnormalities; progression to severe glomerulonephritis.
- Anemia, leukocytosis, thrombocytosis.
- Low-titer positive rheumatoid factor in over 50% of patients.
- c-ANCA positivity.

TABLE 16–9

PULMONARY-RENAL VASCULITIC SYNDROMES

Little or no immune deposits (often associated with ANCA)
    Wegener's granulomatosis
    Microscopic polyangiitis (microscopic polyarteritis)
    Churg-Strauss syndrome*
Immune complex deposits
    Cryoglobulinemic vasculitis
    Henoch-Schönlein purpura
    Other immune complex small-vessel vasculitis (e.g., serum sickness, lupus)
Anti–basement membrane antibody deposits
    Goodpasture's syndrome

Types of small-vessel vasculitis that can manifest as concurrent pulmonary vasculitis and glomerulonephritis, categorized on the basis of immunopathologic findings. These vasculitides may also manifest as pulmonary involvement without glomerulonephritis.

*Only rarely is there severe nephritis.
ANCA = antineutrophil cytoplasmic autoantibodies.
From Jennette JC, Falk RJ, Andrassy K, et al. Nomenclature of systemic vasculitis. Proposal of an international consensus conference. Arthritis Rheum 37:187–192, 1994.

TABLE 16–10

CLINICOPATHOLOGIC CRITERIA TO DISTINGUISH MIDLINE GRANULOMA FROM WEGENER'S GRANULOMATOSIS

Midline Granuloma	Wegener's Granulomatosis
1. Destructive upper airway lesions with characteristic extension through palate	1. Inflammatory upper airway disease predominantly of sinuses and nasal mucosa
2. Lungs not involved	2. Characteristic pulmonary infiltrates
3. Kidneys not involved	3. Characteristic early focal glomerulitis, progressing to fulminant glomerulonephritis
4. Disseminated vasculitis very rare	4. Characteristic disseminated vasculitis

Modified from Fauci AS, Johnson RE, Wolff SM. Radiation therapy for midline granuloma. Ann Intern Med 84:140–147, 1976.

Natural History

Prior to cytostatic treatment, WG had a uniformly fatal course, with death occurring within a few months from renal insufficiency, microangiopathic anemia, and cardiopulmonary failure.

Complications of WG include suppurative upper airway infections, hearing loss, saddle nose deformity from nasal septum perforation, upper airway stenosis from chronic epiglotitis, massive hemoptysis, and bacterial pneumonia.

Treatment

Methods

Corticosteroids alone only ameliorate symptoms and at best postpone death by a few months. Current treatment of WG, as developed at the NIH by Drs. A. Fauci and the late S. Wolff, has as its mainstay the use of cyclophosphamide (CYC). Oral CYC is probably more effective in WG than I.V. boluses. Initial treatment includes CYC 2 mg/kg per day plus prednisone 1 mg/kg per day in 3 to 4 divided doses for 7 to 10 days, then converted to a single morning dose by the second or third week. The CYC is continued for 1 year after remission and is then tapered by 25 mg decrements every 2 to 3 months until discontinuation or resumption of a higher dose in the event of flare. Prednisone is continued at full dose for a month, then gradually changed over to an every-other-day schedule over 1 to 3 months, and finally tapered to discontinuation with a total duration of treatment of about 1 year. The same schedule of CYC and prednisone is used in subsequent disease flares. Higher doses of both agents may be used in severely ill patients. Methotrexate (MTX) in weekly oral doses may be used instead of CYC in mild flares and when there is intolerance to CYC. Opportunistic infections appear to be more frequent in patients treated with MTX than in those treated with CYC. Indeed, concurrent prophylactic treatment with low-dose T/S (trimethoprim 160 mg/sulfamethoxazole 800 mg, 3 times weekly) or monthly inhaled pentamidine has been recommended in MTX-treated patients. There is also evidence that T/S itself is useful in limited WG and in the prevention of relapses in patients whose WG is in remission.

Expected Response

Most WG patients improve on therapy, and true remission is achieved in about 75%. Remission occurs within the first year of therapy in 50% and within the second year in an additional 20%. The condition has a tendency to relapse, usually after several months to several years, and additional treatment courses are thus required. Because of the protracted and relapsing nature of the condition, WG patients are at a high risk of treatment complications (see corticosteroids, CYC, and MTX in antirheumatic agents section).

When to Refer

Patients with WG should be followed primarily by an experienced physician, usually a rheumatologist or a pulmonary specialist. A nephrologist's input is essential in cases with renal insufficiency, for kidney biopsy, and in seemingly limited WG prior to T/S treatment.

Key Points

WEGENER'S GRANULOMATOSIS

- Upper and lower airway necrotizing granulomas, necrotizing and granulomatous vasculitis, and focal segmental necrotizing glomerulonephritis with progression to diffuse, crescentic disease characterize the condition.
- Treatment of severe cases is with cyclophosphamide and glucocorticoids. Methotrexate may be substituted for the cyclophosphamide in mild or limited cases or when there is intolerance to cyclophosphamide. Trimethoprim/sulfamethoxazole may be effective in limited disease.
- Complete remission is seen in about 75% of cases.
- Relapses are frequent and usually involve previously affected areas.
- Trimethoprim/sulfamethoxazole is effective in preventing relapses in patients with WG in remission.

Suggested Reading

Cotch MF, Hoffman GS, Yerg DE, et al. The epidemiology of Wegener's granulomatosis. Arthritis Rheum 39:87–92, 1996.

Hoffman GS, Kerr GS, Leavitt RY, et al. Wegener granulomatosis: An analysis of 158 patients. Ann Intern Med 116:488–498, 1992.

Sneller MC, Hoffman GS, Talar-Williams C, et al. An analysis of forty-two Wegener's granulomatosis patients treated with methotrexate and prednisone. Arthritis Rheum 38:608–613, 1995.

Stegeman CA, Cohen Tervaert JW, de Jong PE, et al. Trimethoprim-sulfamethoxazole (Co-trimoxazole) for the prevention of relapses of Wegener's granulomatosis. N Engl J Med 335:16–20, 1996.

Giant Cell Arteritis

Giant cell arteritis (GCA; Table 16–11), also known as temporal arteritis, particularly affects branches of the external carotid artery, less frequently the carotid, axillary, and vertebral arteries, and the aorta. There is chronic focal and segmental inflammation near the internal elastic lamina, which becomes disrupted, and giant cell formation in approximately 50% of cases. The incidence of GCA increases with age, and the condition is most common over the age of 70. Studied over time there appears to be a cyclic pattern of incidence rates with peaks every 7 years that last about 3 years.

Presentation and Progression

Cause

The cause of GCA is unknown. The reported cyclic change in incidence rates is in support of a microbial etiology.

The usual patient is an elderly individual (female/male ratio is 4 to 1) complaining of a new-onset headache that is usually lateralized, malaise, and fever. Branches of the tempo-

TABLE 16–11

THE 1990 AMERICAN COLLEGE OF RHEUMATOLOGY CRITERIA FOR THE CLASSIFICATION OF GIANT CELL ARTERITIS

Criterion	Definition
1. Age at disease onset > 50 years	Development of symptoms or findings beginning at age 50 or older
2. New headache	New onset of or new type of localized pain in the head
3. Temporal artery abnormality	Temporal artery tenderness to palpation or decreased pulsation, unrelated to arteriosclerosis of cervical arteries
4. Elevated ESR	ESR > 50 mm/hour by the Westergren method
5. Abnormal artery on biopsy	Artery showing vasculitis characterized by a predominance of mononuclear cell infiltration or granulomatous inflammation, usually with multinucleated giant cells

For purposes of classification, a patient shall be said to have giant cell (temporal) arteritis if at least 3 of these 5 criteria are present. The presence of any 3 or more criteria yields a sensitivity of 93.5% and a specificity of 91.2%.

ESR = erythrocyte sedimentation rate.
From Hunder GG, Bloch DA, Michel BA, et al. American College of Rheumatology 1990 criteria for the classification of giant cell arteritis. Arthritis Rheum 33:1122–1128, 1990.

ral artery are often tender and thickened. In some patients other branches of the external carotid are involved, such as the facial artery as it bends over the mandible, and the occipital artery. Fever is common, usually spiking to 38° C, and there may be pallor and wasting in patients with protracted disease. About 30% of patients have, in addition, polymyalgia rheumatica (PMR), a condition characterized by severe aching pain and stiffness about the shoulders, hips, neck, and lower back. Symptoms of PMR are severe at night and in the early morning hours. Laboratory abnormalities in GCA are usually striking and include anemia, leukocytosis, and pronounced thrombocytosis. Serum alkaline phosphatase and other liver enzymes are frequently elevated.

There are many atypical presentations of GCA. Bizarre additional cephalic findings may occur such as jaw claudication due to masseter muscle ischemia, tongue ischemia that may lead to necrosis, and prolonged gum pain with multiple negative dental evaluations. Yet other patients have no cephalic symptoms at all, and the main findings are fever, wasting, and progressive chronic disease anemia. There are typical cases of biopsy-proven giant cell arteritis with normal ESR and cases of temporal artery involvement in vasculitis of other types, particularly PAN, Wegener's granulomatosis, and Churg-Strauss syndrome. It has been found that patients without abnormal findings in the temporal arteries, without claudication (jaw or tongue) symptoms, with a minimally elevated ESR, and with synovitis usually have a negative temporal artery biopsy (> 95% probability). In these patients, a search for alternative diagnoses should take precedence over the temporal artery biopsy.

Diagnosis

Summary of Diagnosis

GIANT CELL ARTERITIS

- GCA should be considered any time elderly patients have transient or permanent visual loss; new headache, facial pain, occipital pain, chewing pain, unexplained gum pain, or tongue pain/paresthesia; unexplained malaise, weight loss, or anemia; PMR; or limb claudication.
- A tender, thickened temporal artery is characteristic of the condition.
- ESR and/or CRP are increased.
- Leukocytosis and thrombocytosis are frequent.
- Diagnosis should be confirmed by temporal artery biopsy.
- A positive biopsy shows chronic granulomatous inflammation and giant cell formation near the elastic lamina (50%) or a panarteritis with a predominantly lymphomononuclear infiltrate (50%).*

*Biopsy results are little changed by corticosteroid treatment of less than 2 weeks' duration.

Natural History

Expected Outcome

Giant cell arteritis runs a self-limited course, burning out after 1 to 2 years. Some patients, especially those with aortic involvement, may have a smoldering course over several years. Relapses are not uncommon. It is not unusual to encounter patients who had symptoms for several months prior to diagnosis. This is more likely to occur in patients without typical temporal artery symptoms. In patients with cephalic complaints, several erroneous diagnoses may have been made prior to someone's thinking about the condition. The condition may have been labeled "cluster headaches," "spondylosis," "apical tooth infections," and "carotidynia." Untreated patients have anorexia and night sweats, and they become anemic and wasted as one would expect in a disseminated neoplastic disease.

A dire complication of GCA is blindness, unilateral or bilateral, which occurs in approximately 15% of patients (previously in 30%–40% of untreated cases). Rather than simultaneously, bilateral visual loss tends to involve one eye first and after 1 to 3 weeks the contralateral eye. Other ocular findings include diplopia, ptosis, and ischemic optic neuropathy. Mononeuropathy, polyneuropathy, TIA, or stroke occur during the course of GCA in approximately 30% of patients. Dementia and depression are known to occur in debilitated untreated patients. Bruits over large peripheral arteries and claudication of the extremities occur in about 10%. GCA patients are 17.3 times more likely to develop thoracic aortic aneurysm and 2.4 times more likely to develop abdominal aneurysms than controls. Interestingly, in a large study the life expectancy of GCA was the same as that in the general population.

Treatment

Methods

Once GCA is diagnosed based on symptoms plus thickened and tender temporal arteries, high-dose oral corticosteroids should be started at once. A commonly used schedule is prednisone 60 mg per day in divided doses for a week and then as a single morning dose to complete 1 month. Patients with visual symptoms should be given an initial 1000 mg I.V. methylprednisolone bolus and perhaps another the next day followed by the regular corticosteroid schedule. In less clear cases treatment should be started as soon as an elevated ESR (> 40 mm in 1 hour) is reported. Arrangements should promptly be made to obtain a temporal artery biopsy in all cases. A failure to improve on the regime just described is an indication to use higher corticosteroid doses. After 1 month on high-dose prednisone a slow dose reduction should be undertaken, usually by 10% every 2 weeks. It is often found that as the prednisone is reduced, the ESR rises. This ESR elevation may or not be significant. Normal ESR values increase with age, and ESRs between 20 and 30 mm are normal in the elderly population. Thus, achieving an ESR of 10 is an unrealistic goal in an 80-year-old patient. But if the ESR elevation clearly falls into the abnormal range, the prednisone should be increased to the last effective dose to be followed by a slower taper.

Another dilemma the clinician may encounter is a rising ESR in a proven GCA patient who, as a result of the corticosteroid treatment, has been rendered diabetic, psychotic, or has suffered vertebral fractures. The addition of methotrexate, azathioprine, or cyclophosphamide should be considered in this patient. There are also patients in whom a temporal artery biopsy was not deemed necessary because the treating physician relied on the clinical findings and an elevated ESR. If in such a patient complications of corticosteroid treatment arise, the natural temptation is to reconsider the initial diagnosis, attribute the initial findings to some other condition(s), and discontinue treatment. This is a situation that could have been fully prevented by a positive temporal artery biopsy. But what about patients with a negative temporal artery biopsy? Remember that because GCA is a segmental condition, an abnormal portion could have been missed. The highest yield is obtained when the resected segment is 2 to 3 cm long, frozen sections are obtained, and the contralateral artery is biopsied if findings in the initial biopsy are normal.

Expected Response

Malaise and headache usually subside within 1 week. The ESR and the thrombocytosis normalize in 2 to 4 weeks.

Complications

As would be expected in an elderly population exposed to high-dose corticosteroids for several months, complications of treatment are commonplace. The most frequent are arterial hypertension, diabetes, cataracts, myopathy, and osteoporotic fractures. Twenty-six percent to 56% of patients develop major complications of corticosteroid therapy during the treatment of GCA. Patients should be checked every 2 to 4 weeks, and a prophylactic treatment for steroid-induced osteoporosis should be instituted at onset of treatment (see Chapter 22).

When to Refer

Ideally, all patients with GCA should be followed primarily by a rheumatologist, and if this is not feasible, by the primary care physician in close contact with a rheumatologist. Temporal artery biopsies are performed by ophthalmologists or by vascular or general surgeons. The procedure is simple, rapid, and safely performed in an office.

Key Points

> **GIANT CELL ARTERITIS**
>
> - GCA affects predominantly ascending branches of the aorta, particularly the external carotid, but may involve major arteries elsewhere and even the aorta.
> - Clinical manifestations include a febrile and catabolic syndrome; cephalic, facial, or visual symptoms; and limb claudication.
> - Some patients present with just malaise, fever, weight loss, and anemia.
> - Visual loss is the most serious complication of GCA.
> - An early diagnosis (prior to catastrophe) requires that the possibility of GCA be raised in the clinician's mind.
> - Treatment of GCA is with high-dose corticosteroids for at least 1 month followed by a taper over 1–3 years.
> - A positive temporal artery biopsy helps withstand unavoidable corticosteroid side effects.
> - Parameters to follow include symptoms, hematocrit, platelet count, and ESR.
> - Normal ESR values increase with age.
> - Life expectancy in GCA is the same as that of the general population.

Suggested Reading

Achkar AA, Lie JT, Hunder GG, et al. How does previous corticosteroid treatment affect the biopsy findings in giant cell (temporal) arteritis? Ann Intern Med 120:987–992, 1994.

Evans JM, O'Fallon WM, Hunder GG. Increased incidence of aortic aneurysm and dissection in giant cell (temporal) arteritis. Ann Intern Med 122:502–507, 1995.

Gabriel SE, O'Fallon WM, Achkar AA, et al. The use of clinical characteristics to predict the results of temporal artery biopsy among patients with suspected giant cell arteritis. J Rheumatol 22:93–96, 1995.

Jundt JW, Mock D. Temporal arteritis with normal erythrocyte sedimentation rates presenting as occipital neuralgia. Arthritis Rheum 34:217–223, 1991.

Matteson L, Gold KN, Bloch DA, et al. Long-term survival of patients with giant cell arteritis in the American College of Rheumatology giant cell arteritis classification criteria cohort. Am J Med 100:193–196, 1996.

Nishino H, DeRemee RA, Rubino FA, et al. Wegener's granulomatosis associated with vasculitis of the temporal artery: Report of five cases. Mayo Clin Proc 68:115–121, 1993.

Salvarani C, Gabriel SE, O'Fallon WM, et al. The incidence of giant cell arteritis in Olmsted County, Minnesota: Apparent fluctuations in a cyclic pattern. Ann Intern Med 123:192–194, 1995.

Takayasu Arteritis

Takayasu arteritis (Table 16–12) has pathologic similarities with GCA. Differences include a younger age of the patients (usually less than 25 years old); a high prevalence in Orientals and Mexicans, in whom GCA is rare; a predominant involvement of the aorta and its main branches; and the association of small-vessel vasculitis expressed as erythema nodosum and occasionally glomerulitis in early cases of Takayasu arteritis. In a Caucasian North American population, Takayasu arteritis has about one-thirtieth the incidence of GCA. The reverse is probably true in the Mexican population. Whereas pathologic changes in early or active arterial disease include lymphoplasmacytic infiltrates and giant cell formation, late and inactive cases show chiefly fibrosis with interspersed residual mononuclear aggregates.

Presentation and Progression

Cause

The cause of Takayasu arteritis is unknown. The possibility of a delayed-type hypersensitivity reaction to an infectious process such as *M. tuberculosis* has been considered by several investigators.

TABLE 16–12

THE 1990 AMERICAN COLLEGE OF RHEUMATOLOGY CRITERIA FOR THE CLASSIFICATION OF TAKAYASU ARTERITIS

Criterion	Definition
1. Age at disease onset < 40 years	Development of symptoms or findings related to Takayasu arteritis at age < 40 years
2. Claudication of extremities	Development and worsening of fatigue and discomfort in muscles of 1 or more extremity while in use, especially the upper extremities
3. Decreased brachial artery pulse	Decreased pulsation of 1 or both brachial arteries
4. BP difference > 10 mm Hg	Difference of > 10 mm Hg in systolic blood pressure between arms
5. Bruit over subclavian arteries or aorta	Bruit audible on auscultation over 1 or both subclavian arteries or abdominal aorta
6. Arteriogram abnormality	Narrowing or occlusion of the entire aorta, its primary branches, or large arteries in the proximal upper or lower extremities, not due to arteriosclerosis, fibromuscular dysplasia, or similar causes; changes usually focal or segmental

For purposes of classification, a patient shall be said to have Takayasu arteritis if at least 3 of these 6 criteria are present. The presence of any 3 or more criteria yields a sensitivity of 90.5% and a specificity of 97.8%.

BP = blood pressure (systolic; difference between arms).
From Arend WP, Michel BA, Bloch DA, et al. American College of Rheumatology 1990 criteria for the classification of Takayasu arteritis. Arthritis Rheum 33:1129–1134, 1990. © American College of Rheumatology.

Usual Symptoms and Signs

The condition is more frequent in females with a female/male ratio of 9 to 1. About 75% of patients feature at onset nonspecific inflammatory manifestations including malaise, anorexia, weight loss, low-grade fever, myalgias, arthralgias or arthritis, erythema nodosum–like lesions in the lower extremities, and anemia. Urinary sediment abnormalities from glomerulitis rarely occur. Concurrently or after a variable period of time, the typical ischemic manifestations of the condition emerge. Findings depend on location and degree of arterial narrowing.

Four types of Takayasu arteritis are recognized based on the topography of lesions. In type I (8%) the involvement is localized to the aortic arch and its branches; in type II (11%), also known as "atypical coarctation of the aorta," only the descending thoracic aorta and the abdominal aorta are involved; in type III (65%) there are features of both type I and type II; and in type IV (16%) there is pulmonary artery involvement in addition to types I, II, or III aortic involvement. Findings include arm or leg claudication, a carotid steal syndrome, postural dizziness, headaches, seizures, episodic amaurosis, or rarely a stroke or a coronary event. Patients often describe increased ischemic symptoms while taking a hot bath. Physical examination reveals audible and palpable bruits over the subclavian arteries and the aorta (90%), wide BP differences between extremities (90%), arterial hypertension (70%), absent pulses, and aortic regurgitation (7%). As expected, arterial hypertension predominates in type III and right heart strain in type IV. Ocular manifestations in Takayasu arteritis include hypertensive retinopathy and rarely iritis, scleritis, and arteriovenous communications around the papilla. The latter, which only occur in patients with partial or complete carotid occlusion, led the Japanese ophthalmologist Takayasu to recognize the condition that bears his name. Laboratory findings are meager except for anemia, thrombocytosis, and ERS elevation in early disease as well as in arteritis flares, with the caveat that vascular lesions may sometimes progress in the face of a normal ESR.

PATIENT 17. A 19-year-old woman was admitted to the hospital for evaluation of bilateral arm claudication and abdominal pain. Four months before she had become febrile after falling in a cave during an archeological expedition, at which time she swallowed some still water. Severe headaches and abdominal pain followed. Approximately 4 weeks after the onset of this illness, arthralgias and typical erythema nodosum lesions appeared on her legs. Laboratory evaluation revealed leukocytosis, a high ESR, and high-titer *S. typhi* antibodies. Blood and stool cultures were negative. The patient was treated with ciprofloxacin for 2 weeks, and all findings disappeared.

I first saw the patient during her second admission after fever and abdominal pain had recurred followed by forearm cramps and numbness upon minimal activities. Both brachial pulses were absent, forearms and hands were cold, and skin capillaries filled slowly after releasing digital pressure. Leg pulses and perfusion were normal. Abdomen was tender in the lower quadrants. An arteriogram (Figure 16–3) revealed occlusion of the left subclavian, stenosis of the right subclavian, and a questionable left renal artery. The night of admission she had pressure-type precordial pain and hypotension. Preadmission laboratory studies once again revealed raised *S. typhi* antibody titers and negative stool and blood culture results. With a diagnosis of type III Takayasu arteritis with probable coronary involvement, the patient was treated with a bolus of intravenous methylprednisolone along with ciprofloxacin. She improved dramatically overnight. Two days later the right brachial pulse had reappeared. After the initial corticosteroid bolus she was placed on prednisone 60 mg per day to which methotrexate was added 3 weeks later as a steroid-sparing agent. Three months later she is on prednisone 20 mg per day plus methotrexate 15 mg per week. The patient is back to school and leads an almost normal life. Left arm claudication is still present.

While *S. typhi* endarteritis cannot be definitely excluded in this patient, typical clinical findings plus negative bacteriologic studies indicate Takayasu arteritis as the most likely diagnosis. The positive S. typhi serology is most likely nonspecific, as false positives are known to occur in autoimmune conditions. This case exemplifies the ambiguity that may surround a diagnosis of vasculitis. Diagnosing Takayasu arteritis is difficult in early disease when arterial findings may be lacking. Once ischemic findings set in (making the diagnosis obvious), it is incumbent on the physician to exclude thrombotic disease (i.e., the antiphospholipid syndrome), endocarditis, as well as the large artery involvement that is rarely seen in other vasculitides and connective tissue diseases.

Diagnosis

Summary of Diagnosis

> **TAKAYASU ARTERITIS**
> - Young age of the patient, usually a woman.
> - Systemic symptoms including malaise, fever, and arthralgias in early disease.
> - Symptoms and findings of major artery insufficiency.
> - BP difference between upper extremities more than 10 mm Hg.
> - Bruits over sublavian(s) or abdominal aorta.
> - ESR elevated in early disease and in phases of active arteritis; ESR normal in quiescent disease.
> - Arteriography allows both diagnosis and classification. Findings include aortic or major branch narrowing, poststenotic dilatation, saccular aneurysms, and occlusion.

Natural History

Expected Outcome

Untreated, Takayasu arteritis has a high morbidity and mortality from arterial stenosis and organ ischemia including extremity claudication, renovascular arterial hypertension,

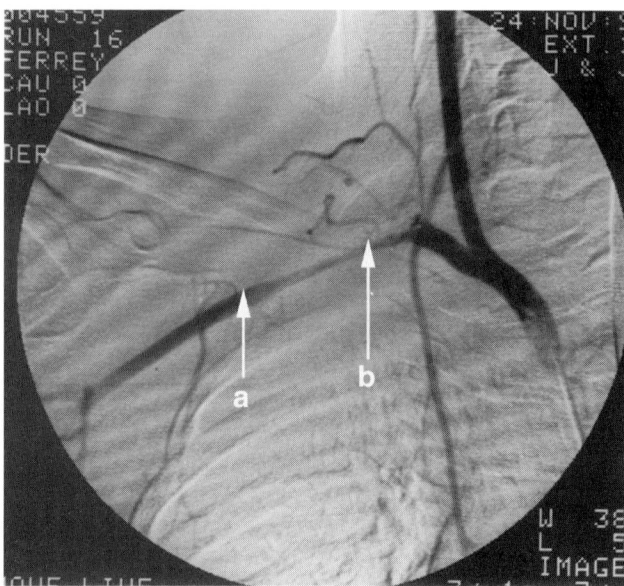

FIGURE 16–3. *Patient 17. Takayasu arteritis.* Right subclavian artery narrowing (a–b). An occlusive lesion was present on the left. On treatment, full restoration of flow was achieved on the right. The left artery remains occluded.

aortic insufficiency, myocardial infarction, stroke, and mesenteric ischemia.

Treatment

Methods

Takayasu's patients may be treated for the systemic symptoms of early disease, active arteritis, and ischemia from active or inactive arterial disease. Early disease without gross arterial compromise is seldom diagnosed with accuracy. Active arteritis (progressive narrowing, carotid artery tenderness, arthralgias or myalgias, fever, high ESR) should be treated with high-dose oral corticosteroids and the patient closely followed for the ensuing 1 to 3 months. Lack of improvement or an inability to lower the steroids past the initial month are indications to add cyclophosphamide, such as in Wegener's granulomatosis, or methotrexate, such as in rheumatoid arthritis. The ESR is excellent to monitor disease activity and treatment response in early disease, but chronic arterial lesions may progress in spite of a normal ESR. Impending ischemic disease, severe aortic regurgitation, and aneurysm formation are indications for surgical or angioplastic treatment. Vascular surgeons prefer to operate in inactive lesions; however, emergency vascular surgery may be required in early disease when there is critical ischemia.

Expected Response

Systemic findings improve within days or weeks. Absent pulses often return with high-dose corticosteroid therapy (50%). Transluminal angioplasty and vascular surgical procedures are usually successful in Takayasu arteritis. Modern treatment has also led to a substantial reduction in mortality. For example, in the NIH series of 20 cases, no deaths occurred during an average follow-up of 4.6 years.

Key Points

> **TAKAYASU ARTERITIS**
>
> - Takayasu arteritis predominates in young women.
> - The initial phase of the disease is usually not recognized.
> - Predominant involvement is in the aorta, its main branches, and the proximal pulmonary artery.
> - Active arteritis is recognized by progressive narrowing and an elevated ESR.
> - Prognosis used to be poor and is now good to excellent.
> - Treatment of active arteritis is with prednisone alone or in conjunction with cyclophosphamide or methotrexate.
> - Impending ischemic damage, significant aortic regurgitation, and aneurysm formation are indications for angioplasty or vascular surgery.

Suggested Reading

Hall S, Barr W, Lie JT, et al. Takayasu arteritis. A study of 32 North American patients. Medicine (Baltimore) 64:89–99, 1985.

Hoffman GS, Leavitt RY, Kerr GS, et al. Treatment of glucocorticoid-resistant or relapsing Takayasu arteritis with methotrexate. Arthritis Rheum 37:578–582, 1994.

Lupi-Herrera E, Sánchez-Torres G, Marcushamer J, et al. Takayasu's arteritis. Clinical study of 107 cases. Am Heart J 93:94–103, 1977.

Numano F, Kakuta T (eds.) Takayasu arteritis II. Int J Cardiol 54 (Suppl):S1–S202, 1996.

Cryoglobulinemia and Cryofibrinogenemia

Cryoglobulins are immunoglobulins that precipitate in the cold in their monomeric form or bound to an antigen as an immune complex. Based on biochemical characteristics, cryoglobulinemias are classified in type I, II, and III (Table 6–3). In type I the cryoglobulins are monoclonal immunoglobulins that lack rheumatoid factor activity and precipitate in the cold as an inherent property of the molecule. In types II and type III cryoglobulinemia, also known as mixed cryoglobulinemias, the cold-precipitating molecules (monoclonal IgG, IgM, or IgA in type II; polyclonal IgG in type III) exhibit rheumatoid factor activity and precipitate in the cold bound to polyclonal IgG. Vessel and organ involvement in the cryoglobulinemias may be due in part to crystallization in vessel walls and tissues. Also, complement activation by cryoglobulins may occur in cold areas of the body, resulting in leukocytoclastic vasculitis and purpura. Cryofibrinogens also precipitate in the cold and may result in microvascular changes that overlap with cryoglobulinemia.

Presentation and Progression

Cause

Type I cryoglobulinemia occurs in individuals with multiple myeloma, Waldenström's macroglobulinemia, sometimes lymphomas B or T, or a monoclonal gammopathy of undetermined significance (MGUS). Cryoglobulinemias types II and III may be caused by viral infection (hepatitis virus B or C, EB virus, cytomegalovirus); infective endocarditis; beta-hemolytic streptococcal infection; leprosy; syphilis; connective tissue diseases such as SLE and Sjögren's; lymphoma; and solid tumors. The designation *essential* is applied to cases in which an underlying etiology, after a thorough search, does not surface. Thus, as the hepatitis C virus story unfolded, most of the formerly "essential" cryoglobulinemias became hepatitis C virus–induced type II or type III cryoglobulinemias. The immune aberrations triggered by hepatitis C virus need to be stressed. In a recently reported series of hepatitis C–induced chronic hepatitis, 36% of patients had cryoglobulinemia, 71% had rheumatoid factor, and 22% had a positive ANA. In addition, minor salivary gland biopsies revealed that 49% had lymphocytic capillaritis and 14% lymphocytic sialadenitis such as seen in Sjögren's syndrome. Cryoglobulinemias are to be distinguished from the cryofibrinogenemias. Cryofibrinogenemias are rare; they may occur in patients with malignancy, or be essential. Cryofibrinogens are detected in plasma rather than in serum.

Presentation

The clinician should suspect cryoglobulinemia when one or more of the following manifestations are present: (1) *skin involvement* including dependent purpura that is often palpable, livedo reticularis, Raynaud's phenomenon, acrocyanosis, and acral necrosis with ulceration in extreme cases; (2) *peripheral nerve lesions* including peripheral neuropathy, mononeuritis, and mononeuritis multiplex; and (3) *kidney involvement,* which is rare in type I cryoglobulinemia, frequent and often severe in type II cryoglobulinemia (proliferative GN with or without crescents), and varied in its morphology and significance in type III cryoglobulinemia, reflecting the heterogeneity of underlying disorders to this syndrome. Cryoglobulinemic purpura is usually a leukocytoclastic palpable purpura, but a *hyperglobulinemic purpura* may also occur, particularly in cases of Sjögren's syndrome with a massive load of polyclonal IgG. Typically, hyperglobulinemic purpura is heralded by a burning, stingy sensation that precedes the hemorrhagic suffusion. Recurring purpuric episodes cause residual hyperpimentation. Local superficial nerves may become involved and result in a patch of residual numbness. Patients with type I and II cryoglobulinemia may also manifest a *hyperviscosity syndrome.* Findings include lethargy; confusion; muscle weakness; and visual disturbances in association with engorgement of retinal veins, retinal hemorrhages, and blurring of the disc.

Clues to an underlying condition are often present. Bone tenderness, lymphadenopathies, and splenomegaly (multiple myeloma, lymphoma) are frequent in type I cryoglobulinemia. Frequently associated findings in types II and III cryoglobulinemia include hepatomegaly and abnormal serum liver enzyme levels (hepatitis B or C); heart murmur, fever, and splenomegaly (infective endocarditis); skin and other features of various infections (syphilis, leprosy, etc.); sicca syndrome (Sjögren's); multisystem disease (SLE); or signs of local or metastatic disease (lymphomas and other malignancies). Cryofibrinogens may cause cutaneous findings similar to cryoglobulinemia.

Diagnosis

Summary of Diagnosis

> **CRYOGLOBULINEMIA AND CRYOFIBRINOGENEMIA**
>
> - Cryoglobulins cause palpable purpura, neuropathy, renal disease, and Raynaud's phenomenon. Possible associations include hyperglobulinemic purpura and a hyperviscosity syndrome.
> - Pursue any evidence of an underlying disease (infectious, autoimmune, neoplasic).
> - For cryoglobulin determination blood is allowed to clot at 37° C and the serum is placed in the refrigerator at 1° C for 7 days; precipitation indicates a cryoglobulin; centrifuge the specimen to obtain cryocrit; perform immunoelectrophoresis in the precipitate.
> - Analysis of the cryoglobulin is seldom indicated in the clinical setting.
> - Perform serum protein electrophoresis; if an M component appears to be present, serum immunoelectrophoresis should be requested for confirmation.
> - Classify the patient as having type I, II, or III cryoglobulinemia and according to underlying condition.
> - Cryofibrinogenemia results in livedo reticularis, skin ulcers, gangrene, and thrombosis.
> - Cryofibrinogens are determined in EDTA plasma obtained at 37° C; place the sample at 1° C. The test is read as positive or negative.

Natural History

Expected Outcome

Outcome entirely depends on the underlying condition. Type I cryoglobulinemia has the prognosis of the hematologic condition that causes the monoclonal spike. Types II and III cryoglobulinemia parallel the course of the underlying infectious, autoimmune, or neoplastic disease. Cases due to hepatitis B and C and those associated with connective tissue disease typically run a fluctuating course. Hepatitis C infection may cause hepatoma and non-Hodgkin's lymphoma years down the line. Cryofibrinogenemia resembles cryoglobulinemia but may feature arterial and venous thrombosis.

Treatment

Methods

Treatment of cryoglobulinemia includes the rapid removal of cryoglobulins by apheresis as well as measures directed to the underlying process causing the cryoglobulinemia, if one is identified. Thus, patients may respond to the treatment of multiple myeloma or to the treatment of an autoimmune condition such as Sjögren's syndrome or SLE. However, no better example can be given than the treatment of chronic hepatitis C with interferon-alpha, where improvement of hepatitis is followed by resolution of cryoglobulinemia. The anabolic steroid stanozolol has been found useful in leg ulcers caused by cryofibrinogenemia.

When to Refer

The cryoglobulinemias are rare conditions except in the experience of rheumatologists, oncologists, and hepatologists. Suspected cases should be referred to a rheumatologist for initial evaluation. Once the condition is diagnosed, patients should have specialized care as needed for the underlying condition.

Key Points

> **CRYOGLOBULINEMIA AND CRYOFIBRINOGENEMIA**
>
> - A heterogeneous group of conditions unified by immunoglobulin precipitation in the cold.
> - Biochemically, cryoglobulinemias are classified as types I, II, and III according to the composition of the precipitate.
> - Skin, peripheral nervous system, and kidney are often involved.
> - The clinician's task is to identify the underlying condition (infective, autoimmune, neoplasic, "essential").
> - Treatment includes (1) corticosteroids for the treatment of cryoglobulin-caused leucocytoklastic vasculitis, (2) removal of the cryoglobulin if clinically indicated, and (3) treatment of the underlying condition, for example, interferon treatment of hepatitis C if clinically indicated.
> - Cryofibrinogenemia exhibits the cutaneous features of cryoglobulinemia, plus thrombosis.

Suggested Reading

Agnello V, Chung RT, Kaplan LM. A role for hepatitis C virus infection in Type II cryoglobulinemia. N Engl J Med 327:1490–1495, 1992.

Brouet JC, Clauvel JP, Danon F, et al. Biologic and clinical significance of cryoglobulins. A report of 86 cases. Am J Med 57:775–788, 1974.

Burruss JB, Fabre VC, Callen JP. Painful acral purpuric nodules. Arthritis Rheum 37:1812–1815, 1994.

Gumber SC, Chopra S. Hepatitis C: A multifaceted disease. Ann Intern Med 123:615–620, 1995.

Muñoz-Fernández S, Barbado FJ, Martín Mola E, et al. Evidence of hepatitis C virus antibodies in the cryoprecipitate of patients with mixed cryoglobulinemia. J Rheumatol 21:229–233, 1994.

Wener MH, Johnson RJ, Sasso EH, Gretch DR. Hepatitis C virus and rheumatic disease. J Rheumatol 23:953–959, 1996.

CHAPTER 17

The Spondyloarthropathies

This group of clinically, pathologically, and genetically intertwined conditions includes ankylosing spondylitis (AS), reactive arthritis including Reiter's syndrome as a subset, inflammatory bowel disease–related arthritis, psoriatic arthritis, as well as rare conditions such as Behçet's disease and Whipple's disease. Characteristic of spondyloarthropathies is primary inflammation at the entheses (sites of tendon and ligament attachment into bone), rather than diarthrodial joints. A great deal of attention is being focused today on this group of conditions because of the distinct possibility that infectious agents are involved in causation. Primary physicians should be aware that antibiotic treatment is indicated in some cases of these conditions in addition to the routine use of physical therapy and anti-inflammatory and other antirheumatic agents.

Suggested Reading

Sieper J, Braun J. Review: Pathogenesis of the spondyloarthropathies: Persistent bacterial antigen, autoimmunity, or both? Arthritis Rheum 38:1547–1554, 1995.

Ankylosing Spondylitis

Ankylosing spondylitis (AS; Table 17–1) represents one end in the spectrum of the spondyloarthropathies, the other end being represented by reactive arthritis.

Presentation and Progression

Cause

Ankylosing spondylitis, which has a prevalence in the general population of 1 in 1000, occurs three to four times more frequently in males than in females. In females, because of prominent peripheral joint symptoms and usually subtle spinal rigidity, the process is often misdiagnosed as "seronegative RA." About 95% of white AS patients and 50% of black AS patients are HLA-B27 positive compared with 5% and 1% in the general population, respectively. A similar association with the HLA-B27 antigen in reactive arthritis has raised the possibility that AS represents the cummulative effect of many episodes of reactive arthritis. However, the majority of AS patients do not have a history of such episodes. It is more likely that both reactive arthritis and AS represent independent associations of the HLA-B27 antigen, or that additional genes are necessary to express one or the other of these conditions. Interestingly, up to 50% of AS patients have subclinical Crohn's-like chronic distal ileal inflammation as detected by ileocolonoscopy. Similar findings in reactive arthritis and less frequently in psoriatic arthritis with axial involvement suggest shared pathogenetic mechanisms.

Presentation

Ankylosing spondylitis usually begins in adolescence or early adulthood. Chronic inflammation affects symmetrically the sacroiliac joints (initially in the capsule and ligaments that bind the sacrum and the iliac bone together) and ascends along the spine causing postinflammatory ossification in the outer layers of the annulus fibrosus (syndesmophytes). Thus, the condition features variable degrees of spinal and thoracic cage rigidity.

Ankylosing spondylitis patients have inflammatory-type low back pain, for example, insidious onset, chronic course, prolonged morning stiffness (hours), and improvement with activities. Typically involved entheses include the Achilles tendon near its insertion and the plantar fascia near the medial plantar calcaneal tubercle. Shoulders and hips become involved in half of the patients. Findings in these joints tend to be subacute or chronic in nature, for example, nocturnal pain, protracted morning stiffness. Other peripheral joints are less frequently involved. Dactylitis (sausage

---

TABLE 17–1

MODIFIED NEW YORK CRITERIA FOR ANKYLOSING SPONDYLITIS, 1984

1. Low back pain of at least 3 months' duration improved by exercise and not relieved by rest
2. Limitation of motion of lumbar spine in the sagittal and frontal planes
3. Chest expansion decreased relative to normal values for age and sex
4. Bilateral sacroiliitis grade 2 to 4
5. Unilateral sacroiliitis grade 3 to 4.

Definite ankylosing spondylitis: Unilateral grade 3 to 4 or bilateral 2 to 4 sacroiliitis and at least 1 of the 3 clinical criteria.

Grade 2 sacroiliitis: Definite early changes. Pseudowidening with erosion or sclerosis in both sides of the joint.
Grade 3 sacroiliitis: Unequivocal abnormality. Erosions, sclerosis, widening, narrowing, or partial ankylosis.
Grade 4 sacroiliitis: Severe abnormalities. Narrowed joint space, ankylosis.

From van der Linden SM, Valkenburg HA, Cats A. Evaluation of diagnostic criteria for ankylosing spondylitis. A proposal for modification of the New York criteria. Arthritis Rheum 27:361, 1984.

toe) may be present. Effusions are uncommon and restriction from postinflammatory capsular thickening is more frequent than erosions. Laboratory findings in AS include mild normocytic anemia in about half of patients; increased ESR, CRP, and IgA, particularly in cases with peripheral joint involvement; and occasionally a slight elevation of CPK and alkaline phosphatase. A diagnosis of AS is suggested by inflammatory back complaints, is strengthened by an abnormal Schober test and reduced chest expansion, and is proven by sacroiliitis shown on x-rays.

Diagnosis

Summary of Diagnosis

ANKYLOSING SPONDYLITIS

- Male predominance.
- Inflammatory-type low back pain.
- Absence of features of other spondyloarthropathies.
- A positive Schober test; decreased chest expansion.
- Evaluation of sacroiliac joints with an AP of the pelvis with 30 degrees cephalic inclination, or oblique films; if sacroiliitis is present, no other imaging studies are needed.
- Bone scans yield many false positives and false negatives.
- CT and MRI are excellent to prove sacroiliitis; the former is less expensive and is therefore the choice.
- HLA-B27 determination is unnecessary if clinical and radiographic criteria are met. The test is important in pregnant patients.
- CBC, platelet count, ESR, alkaline phosphatase, ALT, serum creatinine, and urinalysis are useful to determine baseline for therapy and disease complications.

Natural History

Some cases of AS remain subclinical and are diagnosed serendipitously during evaluation, for instance, of recurrent anterior uveitis, aortic insufficiency, or SAA amyloidosis. In the majority of cases AS follows a slowly progressive path with an almost imperceptible progression of spinal rigidity and restrictive joint changes. Disabling hip limitation may follow. Here and there flares of spinal inflammation occur, particularly in early disease. With completion of fusion, inflammation can no longer take place in the fused segment, for example, the SI joints.

Untreated or with poor advice, AS patients tend to develop flexor deformity in the neck, hips, and knees. Vision field may become restricted, and considerable gait instability may result. In about 10% of AS cases extraarticular manifestations are preeminent. They may precede clinical axial and peripheral joint symptoms, be present at diagnosis, or occur late in the disease. Extraarticular manifestations include recurrent anterior uveitis in 10%, aortic insufficiency in 5%, SAA-type amyloidosis in 2%, and cauda equina syndrome (from obscure dural cysts) and apical pulmonary fibrosis in 1% each. Apical pulmonary fibrosis occurs in individuals with an unmoving thoracic cage and therefore with poor apical ventilation. The fibrotic process may be colonized by mycobacterias and fungi.

Spinal fractures, but not fractures in the peripheral skeleton, are more frequent in AS than in matched controls (RR 7.6). Spinal osteoporosis, a frequent concomitant of AS, contributes to spinal fragility. Fractures in a fused spine may be subtle. Because the fracture line may be the only moving site, the end result may be a pseudoarthrosis with exuberant bone formation (Andersson lesion). These lesions are often confused with osteomyelitis. A differential point is that in AS the lucent line of pseudoarthrosis traverses posteriorly across the fused facet joints.

Expected Outcome

There is a large pool in the community of patients with advanced, deforming AS. These are late cases from the past. The expected outcome in optimally treated AS includes disease arrest, minimal spinal and lower extremity deformities, and hopefully arrest or prevention of extraarticular involvement. Unfortunately, there is no conclusive evidence that with optimal treatment the extraarticular manifestations of AS can be prevented. Prognostic factors in AS are still to be defined. In a retrospective study of spondyloarthropathy patients, of which the majority had AS, presence within the first 2 years of disease of one or more of the following features conferred a worse prognosis: hip arthritis, ESR more than 30 mm, poor response to NSAIDs, limited lumbar motion, a sausage-like finger or toe, oligoarthritis, and disease onset below the age of 16.

Treatment

Methods

Goals of therapy in AS include suppressing pain and inflammation with NSAIDs plus sulfasalazine; keeping the patient active; strengthening diaphragm and thoracic cage muscles; exercising, through range of motion as well as isometrically, frequently involved joints such as the hips and shoulders; watching for the development of complications such as acute anterior uveitis, aortic insufficiency, and amyloidosis; and maintaining an acceptable posture in cases in which the spine fuses. Exercises useful in AS can be found in the appendix. Basic recommendations include eliminating the pillow or using the lowest pillow possible, strengthening spinal extensors to prevent kyphosis, and performing respiratory exercises to strengthen both diaphragmatic and thoracic cage breathing.

Swimming is excellent for AS patients; however, the style has to be adapted to existing spinal deformities and shoulder and hip limitations. For instance, breast style encourages neck and dorsal spine extension and increases hip motion. On the other hand, a marked flexor deformity of the neck precludes the crawl style but allows overhand and back stroke. Patients should be told that the higher the level of their exercising, the better their prognosis. Patients with a fused spine should be made aware that sudden jerks may cause a spinal fracture. Contact sports are therefore forbidden in these patients. Similarly, jogging poses undue trauma to an unyielding spine and increases the risk of destructive hip changes.

Although all NSAIDs (other than ASA and derivatives) appear to have beneficial effects in AS, indomethacin works best. Doses of 50 mg q 6 to 8 hours are initially used. Once inflammatory symptoms are improved (less pain, a brief or nil a.m. stiffness), a single dose of slow-release indomethacin 75 mg capsule used at night may suffice. Sulfasalazine has been shown to be effective in many cases of AS, reactive arthritis, and psoriatic arthritis. It therefore makes sense to initiate this medication early in the disease course, along with full doses of a NSAID, unless the patient has a history of sulfa intolerance. The starting sulfasalazine dose is 500 mg qid. The dose may be increased by 500 mg every 3 weeks to a maximal dose of 4000 mg per day, which is seldom required. Once improvement has been achieved the indomethacin should be reduced to the lowest possible effective dose. The sulfasalazine should be slowly reduced to a maintenance dose. The sulfasalazine should be continued indefinitely, adding brief courses of indomethacin to control flares. Because of possible hematologic complications (anemia from NSAID-induced GI bleed, bone marrow arrest from the sulfa moiety of sulfasalazine), this treatment program requires monthly CBC determination. Serum creatinine should be checked biweekly for the first 2 months (possible renal insufficiency from the NSAIDs) and then bimonthly. Urinalysis to detect renal amyloidosis and IgA nephrophathy should be checked every 6 months. Finally, methotrexate has been used anecdotally in refractory cases of AS with encouraging results. This should be considered an experimental therapy in AS, and its use should be restricted to specialized settings.

Expected Response

With the program just described, and provided a strongly motivated patient as most AS patients are, a good to excellent treatment response may be expected.

Complications

Complications of therapy are those expected from high-dose, prolonged NSAIDs courses plus the possible side effects, mainly hemocytopenias from the sulfasalazine.

When to Refer

Patients with AS or suspected AS should be referred to a rheumatologist for evaluation and therapeutic advice. Patients may subsequently be followed by a primary care physician; however, there should be a low threshold for referral. To decrease the likelihood of suffering the dire consequences of advanced disease, patients with AS must have the best possible treatment program implemented early in their disease course.

Resources Available

The Spondylitis Association of America (see appendix) provides excellent instructional material for patients. The author has found particularly helpful a booklet entitled "Straight Talk."

Key Points

ANKYLOSING SPONDYLITIS

- Ankylosing spondylitis affects predominantly the SI joints and the spine, particularly at the thoracolumbar junction, and from there spreads up and down the spine.
- Additional frequently involved joints include the manubriosternal, the sternoclavicular, shoulders, and hips.
- Early identification (within 2 years of onset) of hip arthritis, high ESR, lack or response to NSAIDs, and limitation of lumbar motion are indicators of a poor prognosis in AS.
- Local complications include bony fusion and an increased risk of fractures from early osteoporosis and increased brittleness of the spine.
- Fractures through an ossified intervertebral space (Andersson's fractures) may mimic spinal osteomyelitis.
- Extraarticular complications include relapsing anterior uveitis, aortic insufficiency, A-V conduction defects, apical pulmonary fibrosis, amyloidosis, and cauda equina syndrome (as a result of dural cysts).
- Treatment of AS includes stringent PT to prevent flexor deformity of spine and hips, anti-inflammatory medications, and sulfasalazine.
- Prognosis in intensively treated AS is excellent. Severe complications of the disease such as cardiac valvular disease or amyloidosis are fortunately rare.

Suggested Reading

Amor B, Silva Santos R, Nahal R, et al. Predictive factors for the longterm outcome of spondyloarthropathies. J Rheumatol 21:1883–1887, 1994.

Cooper C, Carbone L, Michet CJ, et al. Fracture risk in patients with ankylosing spondylitis: A population based study. J Rheumatol 21:1877–1882, 1994.

Creemers MCW, Franssen MJAM, van de Putte LBA, et al. Methotrexate in severe ankylosing spondylitis: An open study. J Rheumatol 22:1104–1107, 1995.

Dougados M, van der Linden S, Leirisalo-Repo M, et al. Sulfasalazine in the treatment of spondyloarthropathy. Arthritis Rheum 38:618–627, 1995.

Wollheim FA. Ankylosing spondylitis. In: Kelley WN, Harris ED, Ruddy S, et al. (eds) Textbook of Rheumatology, 4th ed. W.B. Saunders, Philadelphia, 943–960, 1993.

Reactive Arthritis and Undifferentiated Spondyloarthropathy

Reactive arthritis is a sterile chronic synovitis that follows documented enteric, urogenital, or pharyngeal infection. Enteric and urogenital reactive arthritis, of which Reiter's syndrome is the best known subset, strongly associates with the HLA-B27 and B7 antigens. Acute rheumatic fever, a multisystem reactive disease that follows group A streptococcal pharyngeal infection, is discussed separately because of its peculiar features: younger age of patients, lack of association with the HLA-B27 antigen, characteristic cardiac sequelae, plus effective measures available for prophylaxis. Undifferentiated spondyloarthropathy is clinically similar to reactive arthritis and keeps the same association with the HLA-B27 antigen, the difference being that an antecedent infection cannot be shown.

Presentation and Progression

Cause

Agents involved in enteric reactive arthritis (Table 17–2) include *Shigella flexneri,* certain salmonellas, *Campylobacter jejuni, yersinia enterocolitica and pseudotuberculosis* (yersinia-induced reactive arthritis is common in Scandinavia but rare in the United States), and a number of less common conditions. *Chlamydia trachomatis* causes most instances of urogenital reactive arthritis. In contrast with previous assumptions, microbial antigens can be shown in affected joints in chlamydia, shigella, salmonella, and yersinia reactive arthritis. Although transient bacteremia may have left poorly digestible bacterial products trapped in the synovium, it is more likely, as shown in chlamydia reactive arthritis, that a modified but still viable agent remains in the synovial membrane, sustaining the inflammatory reaction.

As mentioned, in a significant proportion of reactive arthritis (arthritis, enthesitis), no antecedent infection can be identified. These cases have also been labeled as undifferentiated spondyloarthropathy. It may or not be fair to lump these cases together with proven enteropathic and urogenital reactive arthritis. However, other than the inciting event, both conditions behave similarly.

Early in the HIV epidemics investigators believed that the HIV infection was in the background of many severe cases of Reiter's-type reactive arthritis. Few of these cases are now seen, probably due to avoidance of high-risk sexual behavior that resulted in the HIV infection in the first place, plus high rates of chlamydial infection with the attendant risk of reactive arthritis.

Presentation

Reactive arthritis should be suspected (1) when an oligoarthritis (knees, ankles) follows acute diarrheal illness or urogenital infection, (2) in a weight-bearing joint oligoarthritis that features Achilles tendinitis or plantar fasciitis, (3) in patients with palindromic rheumatism, and (4) when dactylitis is present. Both oligoarthritis and dactylitis are also seen in a close relative, psoriatic arthritis. Another condition that features dactylitis is sarcoidosis.

The usual interval between onset of bowel or urethral symptoms and onset of arthritis is 2 to 3 weeks. Patients may be febrile and on occasion a frankly catabolic state ensues. One or a few joints become swollen and very painful and with involvement of the knee pronounced atrophy of the quadriceps muscle follows. One or a few toes may swell diffusely (dactylitis, or "sausage toes"), sometimes becoming twice as thick as the neighboring toes as a result of arthritis, tenosynovitis, and periostitis (Figure 17–1). Characteristically, sausage toes become cyanotic in the dependent position. Sausage toes are seen in reactive arthritis and also in the closely related psoriatic arthritis. Achilles tendinitis, which may be uni- or bilateral, is characterized by pain, swelling, and tenderness near the calcaneal insertion. The retrocalcaneal bursa is frequently involved. Plantar fasciitis causes heel pain upon weight bearing as well as tenderness on palpation at the medial calcaneal tubercle. Achilles tendinitis and plantar fasciitis frequently coexist. Sacroiliitis featuring buttock and posterior thigh pain, interspinous ligament enthesitis causing pain and local tenderness in the upper dorsal spine, and inflammation at the manubriosternal, sternoclavicular, and costochondral joints are frequent in reactive arthritis.

An important differential diagnosis is Achilles tendinitis caused by fluoroquinolones such as ciprofloxacin and ofloxacin, agents that are frequently used in the treatment of chlamydial urogenital infections. This is a curious situation in which the very agent used to treat chlamydia causes toxic effects that overlap with the condition one is trying to prevent.

PATIENT 18. A 30-year-old man was referred for evaluation of possible chlamydia-induced Reiter's syndrome. Three months prior he had a documented episode of chlamydial urethritis treated with a 7 day course of doxycycline. A few weeks after this treatment there was another documented episode of chlamydial urethritis and a 2 week course of ciprofloxacin was prescribed. One week into this treatment, the patient developed bilateral Achilles tendinitis, which was considered a manifestation of postvenereal

---

TABLE 17–2
MICROORGANISMS INVOLVED IN REACTIVE ARTHRITIS

UROGENITAL PATHOGENS

Chlamydia trachomatis
Chlamydia psittaci
Ureaplasma urealyticum

INTESTINAL PATHOGENS

Shigella disenteriae
Shigella flexneri
Salmonella typhimurium
Salmonella enteritidis
Yersinia enterocolitica
Yersinia pseudotuberculosis
Campylobacter jejuni
Campylobacter fetus
Salmonella paratyphi B
Salmonella paratyphi C

UNCOMMON AND POSSIBLE ASSOCIATIONS

S. pyogenes
C. difficile
Corynebacterium acnes
Propionibacterium acnes
S. aureus (toxic shock arthritis)
Borrelia burgdorferi
M. tuberculosis (Poncet's disease)
M. leprae
Giardia lamblia
Cryptosporidium
Strongyloides stercoralis
Schistosomiasis

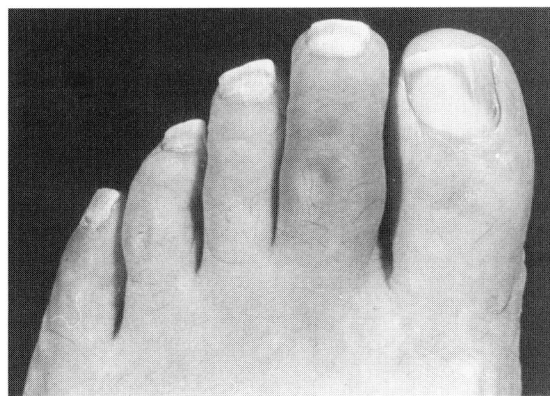

FIGURE 17–1. *"Sausage toe," also known as dactylitis.* However, in this patient, a drinking man, the lesion corresponded to a fracture.

Reiter's. The recommendation was to continue the ciprofloxacin to complete a 2 month course. To everyone's surprise, the patient's symptoms got worse. Pain extended to his knees, elbows, and shoulders and resulted in invalidation. The ESR was repeatedly normal. On examination the patient had a great deal of pain on attempted motions. Both Achilles tendons were thickened and tender in their middle third. There was pain and tenderness at the patellar insertion of the quadriceps tendons, the wrist extensor insertion at the lateral epicondyles, and the rotator cuffs. The lack of joint findings, the unusual location of Achilles tendinitis, and the normal ESR suggested an untoward reaction to ciprofloxacin rather than a reactive arthritis, and the drug was discontinued. A few weeks later the patient was minimally symptomatic.

Ocular involvement (conjunctivitis, acute anterior uveitis) is frequent in reactive arthritis. Patients with nonspecific urethritis followed by conjunctivitis and arthritis are said to have "Reiter's syndrome." Because acute anterior uveitis may be concurrent with, or may be misdiagnosed as, conjunctivitis, a slit-lamp examination is warranted in patients with a red eye.

Painless, discrete erythematous oral lesions, usually involving the palate but sometimes in the tongue, are frequent in reactive arthritis. Another frequent lesion is a well-demarcated erythematous-papular, sometimes hyperkeratotic rash in the glans penis known as "balanitis circinata." This lesion, and also pseudopustular, hyperkeratotic plantar or palmar lesions known as "keratoderma blennorrhagica" (Figure 17–2), resemble psoriasis clinically and pathologically. Interestingly, as in AS, asymptomatic chronic distal ileal inflammation is found on ileocolonoscopy in 50% of reactive arthritis and undifferentiated spondyloarthropathy patients. Myocarditis and acute valvular insufficiency are rare manifestations of reactive arthritis.

Laboratory findings include some degree of normocytic anemia in protracted cases, leukocytosis in acute cases, frequent thrombocytosis in the 500,000 to 600,000/mm^3 range, and a high ESR and CRP. Urinalysis may show pyuria from urethritis or prostatitis, and every effort to identify chlamydia should be made in these patients.

HIV determination is obviously important in patients with severe catabolic disease. Because the HLA-B27 antigen is present in 50% to 70% of reactive arthritis patients, HLA-B27 determination is useful in suspected cases without antecedent infection, in the assessment of rheumatoid factor negative palindromic arthritis, and in patients with low back stiffness

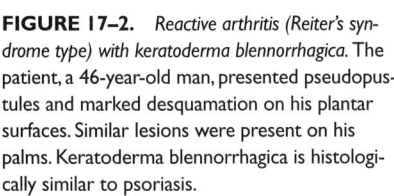

FIGURE 17–2. *Reactive arthritis (Reiter's syndrome type) with keratoderma blennorrhagica.* The patient, a 46-year-old man, presented pseudopustules and marked desquamation on his plantar surfaces. Similar lesions were present on his palms. Keratoderma blennorrhagica is histologically similar to psoriasis.

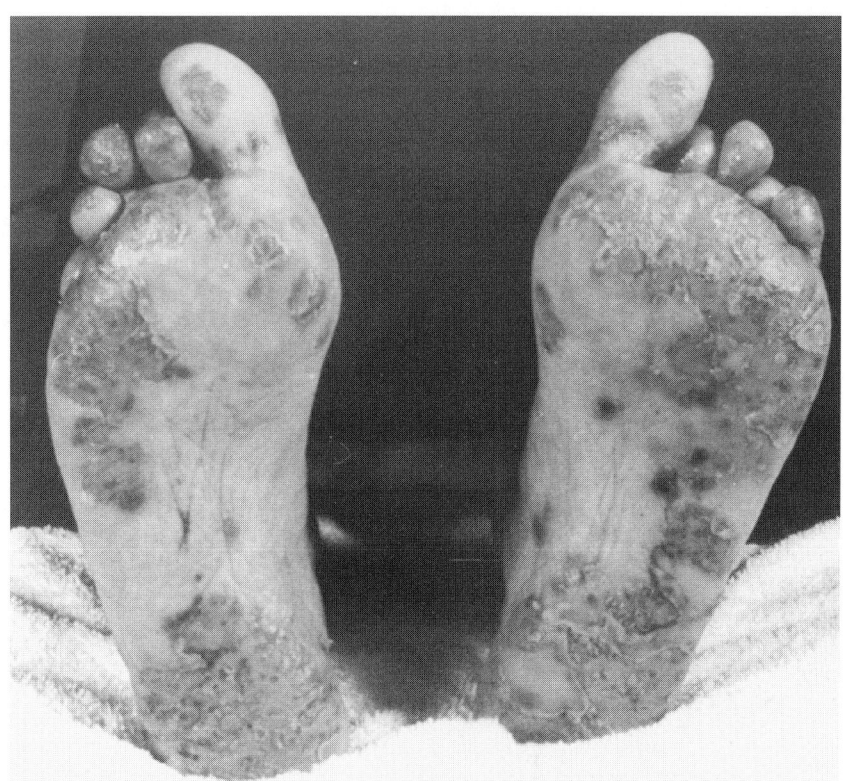

who are unwilling or cannot have (such as in pregnant women) sacroiliac joint films. Early radiographic changes are nonspecific including periarticular or sausagelike soft tissue swelling. However, it is relatively common to find, on initial evaluation, evidence of previous, sometimes remote, reactive arthritis.

PATIENT 19. A 60-year-old woman had a bout of campylobacter diarrhea and 3 weeks later came down with left knee arthritis and left shoulder pain, which on examination corresponded to an inflamed AC joint. Additional findings included tenderness at several interspinous ligaments in the upper dorsal spine and a left Achilles tendonitis. Laboratory abnormalities included a platelet count of 520,000/mm^3 and an ESR of 80 mm. Surprisingly, given the short duration of arthritis, a pelvic film showed sclerosis on both sides of the symphysis pubis and a left-sided sacroiliitis with pronounced sclerosis in the iliac side of the joint. Interestingly, the patient recalled having been febrile for 1 month while in college, with an ESR of about 100 that persisted a full year. Obviously, this woman who appeared to have a first bout of reactive arthritis already had late radiographic features of spondyloarthropathy. The fever of unknown origin (FUO) while in college probably represented a first bout of reactive arthritis leading to sacroiliitis and pubic symphysitis.

Returning to the radiographic changes in reactive arthritis, punched-out articular erosions and periostitis, unilateral sacroiliitis that rarely leads to fusion, and massive paravertebral osteophytes at the thoracolumbar junction characterize protracted or recurrent disease. Ankylosing spondylitis with bilateral, high-grade sacroiliitis and syndesmophytes, sometimes asymptomatic, is occasionally present (Figure 17–3A and B). Since AS is expected to occur in approximately 2% of HLA-B27 positive individuals, the association between reactive arthritis and AS could be a chance event.

Diagnosis

Summary of Diagnosis

> **REACTIVE ARTHRITIS AND UNDIFFERENTIATED SPONDYLOARTHROPATHY**
>
> - Oligoarthritis involving lower extremity joints.
> - Sausage toes.
> - Enthesitis (Achilles tendon, plantar fascia).
> - Sometimes conjunctivitis or uveitis, mucosal lesions, balanitis (balanitis circinata), palmar and plantar pseudopustules (keratoderma blennorrhagica).
> - Sometimes an intense catabolic state (consider HIV in this clinical setting).
> - Preceding enteric or genitourinary infection in reactive arthritis.
> - Anemia, thrombocytosis, increased ESR.
> - Positive HLA-B27 or B7 in 5—70% of cases (not required for diagnosis).

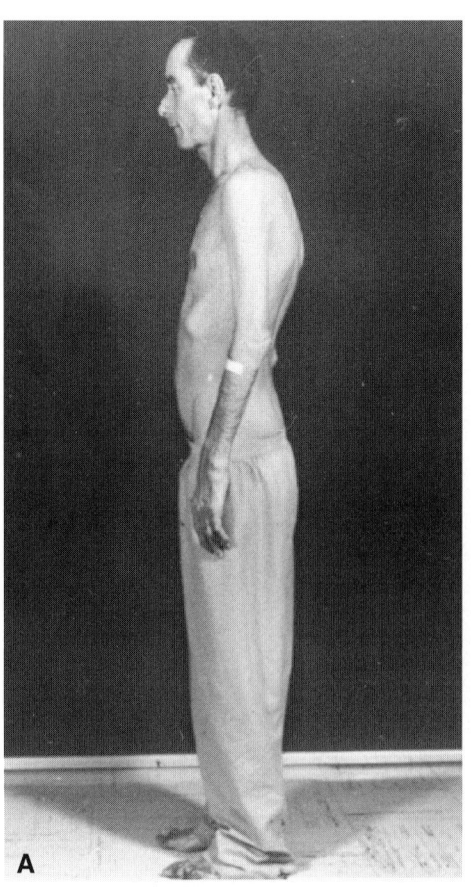

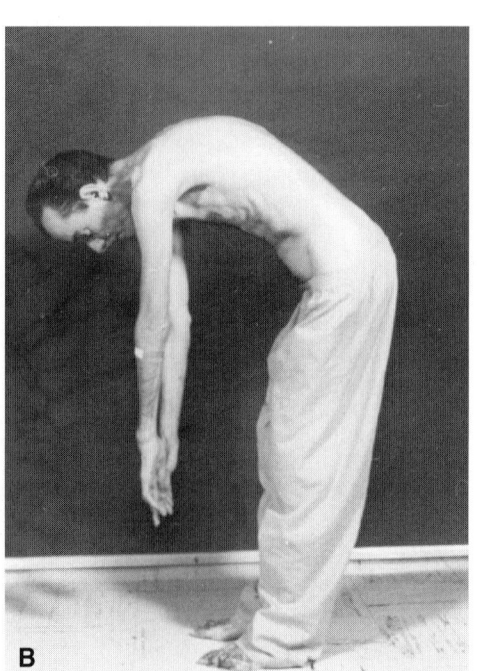

FIGURE 17–3. *Reactive arthritis.* This is the patient whose feet are shown in Figure 17–2. *A*, Erect, there is some dorsal kyphosis. *B*, As he bends forward, the lumbar segment barely rectifies. He had bilateral sacroiliitis and gross nonmarginal syndesmophytes (see text).

Natural History

Expected Outcome

Even in dramatic cases with a high fever and a pronounced weight loss (e.g., 10 kg), reactive arthritis undergoes spontaneous improvement within 2 weeks to 2 years. During this period of inflammation and general debilitation patients may be temporarily invalidated. Permanent peripheral joint damage is rare, but erosion of SI joints and sclerosis as well as ragged ossification at tendon attachments are common in protracted or recurrent disease. Skin lesions may be dramatic. An extension of keratoderma blennorhagica to full-blown, extensive psoriasis, albeit rare, may occur. Inflammatory bowel disease may also become apparent. Long-term follow-up studies of reactive arthritis have shown persistent or intermittent symptoms in 10% to 50% of cases. There is some indication that the rate of chronicity varies with the inciting agent. As an example, over 50% of patients with postsalmonella reactive arthritis, but only 10% of patients with postchlamydial reactive arthritis, have symptoms 5 years after the initial event.

Treatment

Methods

Treatment of reactive arthritis includes the antibiotic treatment of chlamydial urethritis or cervicitis in urogenital cases, physiotherapy, and anti-inflammatory and antirheumatic agents. Because asymptomatic chlamydial infections may trigger reactive arthritis, patients with apparently idiopathic cases should be investigated with the appropriate urethral and cervical studies. Immunofluorescence and enzyme-linked immunosorbent assay (ELISA) tests have a low false negative rate and should be used in the investigation of these patients.

Antibiotic treatment of bowel infection in enteropathic cases is not warranted except in rare cases due to salmonella or yersinia infection. In geographic areas in which a high prevalence of HLA-B27 coincides with a high incidence of chlamydial infections, such as in Iceland, and also in sporadic cases in sexually promiscuous individuals, protracted antibiotic prophylaxis with tetracycline or doxycycline may reduce the tendency to relapse. A recently noted decline in urogenital reactive arthritis has been attributed to an increased awareness of the risks involved in unsafe sex.

Most cases of reactive arthritis respond dramatically to indomethacin 50 mg qid, reduced to 50 mg tid after 1 to 2 weeks. Subsequent dose reductions are usually possible, and in most patients a single 75 mg dose of slow-release indomethacin taken at night may suffice. Other nonsteroidal anti-inflammatories appear to have lesser efficacy but may still be used in patients who are intolerant to indomethacin. Intraarticular corticosteroids should be considered in joints that fail to improve on high-dose NSAID therapy. Corticosteroid infiltrations are quite effective in refractory cases of arthritis, plantar fasciitis, retrocalcaneal bursitis concurrent with Achilles tendinitis, and interspinous ligament enthesitis. Technical aspects of these injections may be found in the appendix. Patients with only a partial response to indomethacin should be offered sulfasalazine, a drug that in controlled trials has been found effective in various spondyloarthropathies at a dose of 2 to 3 g/day (see section on ankylosing spondylitis). Methotrexate should be considered in extreme cases. In the author's experience some cases of reactive arthritis are refractory to all forms of therapy including intravenous boluses of methylprednisolone, plus phenylbutazone (now withdrawn from the market because of its bone marrow toxicity), plus sulfasalazine, plus MTX. Even in these cases the condition eventually improves or subsides, leaving little permanent damage, sometimes after 6 months to 1 year of relentless disease.

Expected Response

Mild cases respond promptly, within 1 to 2 weeks, to indomethacin or other NSAID. Severe cases that require sulfasalazine and/or methotrexate respond gradually, over several months. As mentioned, there are refractory cases that may take a year to improve.

When to Refer

Straightforward reactive arthritis, once diagnosis has been confirmed, may be treated by primary care physicians. Over half of the cases are problematic and should be treated primarily by a rheumatologist.

Key Points

REACTIVE ARTHRITIS AND UNDIFFERENTIATED SPONDYLOARTHROPATHY

- From a concept of aseptic joint and enthesial inflammation following enteric or urogenital infection, the pendulum has swung to either persistent infection or a reaction to bacterial products lodged at articular and possibly enthesial sites.
- Associations between reactive arthritis and ankylosing spondylitis, rather than causal, appear to result from the link that both have with HLA-B27.
- Reactive arthritis may be dramatic and lead to wasting; however, sooner or later the condition improves or goes away.
- Treatment of reactive arthritis includes (1) eradication of the pathogen if still present; (2) a NSAID, particularly indomethacin; and (3) the use of sulfasalazine or methotrexate in resilient cases.
- In certain locales with high rates of reinfection with *C. trachomatis*, antibiotic prophylaxis has succeeded in decreasing the rate of recurrence of reactive arthritis.

Suggested Reading

Iliopoulos A, Karras D, Ioakimidis D, et al. Change in the epidemiology of Reiter's syndrome (reactive arthritis) in the post-AIDS era? An analysis of cases appearing in the Greek Army. J Rheumatol 22:252–254, 1995.

Lauhio A, Leirisalo-Repo M, Lahdevirta J, et al. Double-blind, placebo-controlled study of three-month treatment with lymecycline in reactive arthritis, with special reference to chlamydia arthritis. Arthritis Rheum 34:6–14, 1991.

Nanagara R, Li F, Beutler A, et al. Alteration of *Chlamydia trachomatis* biologic behavior in synovial membranes: Suppression of surface antigen production in reactive arthritis and Reiter's syndrome. Arthritis Rheum 38:1410–1417, 1995.

Thomson GTD, DeRubeis DA, et al. Post-salmonella reactive arthritis: Late clinical sequelae in a point-source cohort. Am J Med 98:13–21, 1995.

Inflammatory Bowel Disease (IBD)–Related Arthritis

Bowel conditions and arthritis are intimately related. Best known is the association of IBD with axial and peripheral arthritis. Another striking finding is the already mentioned high prevalence of subclinical distal ileal inflammation in patients with ankylosing spondylitis (AS), undifferentiated spondyloarthropathy, and psoriatic arthritis. Also, obese patients treated with the ill-fated jejunocolic and jejunoileal bypasses often developed arthritis, cutaneous lesions, and other systemic features that could be corrected by undoing the bypass. Lesser known associations include the arthritis described in patients with collagenous colitis and gluten-sensitive enteropathy.

From an opposite perspective the gastrointestinal tract becomes involved in an array of rheumatologic disorders including SLE, scleroderma, mixed connective tissue disease, dermatomyositis, and the vasculitides. Finally, gastrointestinal lesions represent the most frequent and serious toxicities in rheumatic disease treatment. This brief section discusses IBD-related arthritis, Whipple's disease, and Behçet's disease.

Presentation and Progression

Cause

In a startling experimental model of spondyloarthropathy, transgenic rats expressing the human B27 antigen spontaneously develop a characteristic disease complex including psoriasis-like skin lesions, chronic inflammatory bowel changes, and peripheral and axial arthritis that resembles early ankylosing spondylitis. Interestingly, if these rats are kept in a germ-free environment, neither the bowel inflammation nor the arthritic changes take place. This experimental model highlights a basic interaction between bowel bacteria and the B27 antigen. In patients with spondyloarthropathy and gut inflammation, clinical remission is always associated with normal gut histology, and active synovitis is usually associated with gut inflammation.

Presentation

There are two types of arthritis in IBD patients, the axial and the peripheral. Axial arthritis is identical to ankylosing spondylitis (AS) except that (1) the frequency of AS in the general population is about 1 in 1000, whereas in IBD it is 3% to 5%, and (2) in Caucasian patients with IBD-related AS, only a 50% prevalence of HLA-B27 is found as compared with 95% in idiopathic AS and 5% to 8% in the general Caucasian population. There seems to be little relation between the course of the axial arthritis and bowel disease activity. Indeed, spondylitis usually precedes for years the clinical onset of bowel disease, may remain stationary in the face of severe bowel symptoms, or may slowly progress after colectomy. An additional 15% of patients have silent sacroiliitis, which does not portend progression to a more diffuse spinal disease.

The second type of arthritis is the peripheral, which affects preferentially lower extremity joints, in particular ankles and knees. In UC there is a parallelism between peripheral arthritis and bloody diarrhea. This is less clear in Crohn's disease in which frank bleeding is uncommon and granulomatous bowel inflammation may result in persistent arthritis, abdominal pain, and nutritional disturbances. At any rate, peripheral IBD arthritis tends to be relapsing and subacute. There are instances of angry inflammation in which septic arthritis and gout must be ruled out, as well as large effusions with minimal pain. As expected, synovial fluid findings in IBD arthritis range from mildly to severely inflammatory. Synovial granulomas have been reported in some patients with Crohn's disease.

Additional musculoskeletal manifestations of IBD include hypertrophic osteoarthropathy, granulomatous osteitis, and granulomatous muscle infiltration. Fistula and abscess formation in Crohn's disease has resulted in septic arthritis of the hip. There is also an array of extraintestinal manifestations of IBD that may lead to diagnostic confusion (Table 17–3). Pyoderma gangrenosum, an ulcerated lesion with irregular and raised border, may be difficult to distinguish, without biopsy, from a vasculitic or an antiphospholipid-related ulcer. Livedo reticularis may also be present in IBD, further suggesting vasculitis or an antiphospholipid syndrome. Ocular inflammation, aphthous ulcers, superficial phlebitis, and leg ulcers may all suggest Behçet's disease. Diagnosis of IBD in these cases is based on colonic radiographic findings and the results of ileocolonoscopy. Uveitis, arthritis, and erythema nodosum may suggest sarcoidosis, but there are no pulmonary lesions in Crohn's disease and the bowel is spared in sarcoidosis. Pericarditis may occur in UC and in association with arthritis may suggest SLE. Leucocytosis, thrombocytosis, and a negative ANA help exclude SLE in these patients. Finally, secondary amyloidosis may complicate the course of IBD, particularly Crohn's disease.

Diagnosis

Summary of Diagnosis

> **INFLAMMATORY BOWEL DISEASE (IBD) ARTHRITIS**
>
> - Lower extremity arthritis occurs in 20% of cases of IBD.
> - Spondylitis similar to AS occurs in 3% to 5% of cases of IBD.
> - There is a 50% rate of HLA-B27 in IBD patients with spondylitis.
> - HLA-B27 determination in these patients has no practical value and is therefore not indicated.
> - There is no association between IBD peripheral arthritis and the HLA-B27.

- Review the SI joints in scout abdominal films; AS may present subclinically.
- Erosive changes in peripheral arthritis are rare. X-rays of peripheral joints are therefore not indicated.
- It is important to aspirate the inflamed peripheral joints (1) when symptoms are acute raising the possibility of septic arthritis, and (2) to rule out crystal-induced arthritis.

Natural History

Expected Outcome

Recurrent peripheral arthritis is a nuisance in IBD but has little consequence on the joints. Active peripheral arthritis should be taken as an indicator of IBD activity and may therefore dictate a step up in therapy. Ankylosing spondylitis in IBD, as in essential AS, generally has a slow progressive course.

Treatment

Peripheral IBD Arthritis: If there seems to be little reason, other than the arthritis, for stepping up IBD therapy (such as starting steroids or adding an immunosuppressant), adding a NSAID or increasing the sulfasalazine dose should be tried first. On the other hand, arthritis is an additional evidence of bowel disease activity and may tilt the balance toward starting or increasing corticosteroids, or adding an immunosuppressive agent. Intraarticular corticosteroids are highly effective in IBD arthritis.

Axial Arthritis: Treatment of AS in IBD is similar to the treatment of primary AS. There may be problems with the chronic use of NSAIDs, and emphasis should therefore be placed on sulphasalazine. Methotrexate may have a beneficial effect on IBD, the associated peripheral arthritis, and possibly in IBD-related AS.

Expected Response

Response to NSAIDs is prompt, within days. Response to increased doses of sulfasalazine is slow, taking weeks. Corticosteroids have a prompt beneficial effect on both bowel and articular symptoms.

TABLE 17–3

EXTRAINTESTINAL MANIFESTATIONS OF CROHN'S DISEASE AND ULCERATIVE COLITIS

Peripheral arthritis	Erythema nodosum
Sacroiliitis	Erythema multiforme
Ankylosing spondylitis	Pyoderma gangrenosum
Clubbing	Vasculitis
Conjunctivitis	Sclerosing cholangitis
Episcleritis	Chronic active hepatitis
Uveitis	Cirrhosis
Aphthous ulceration	Amyloidosis

When to Refer

Cases of IBD-related peripheral arthritis should have rheumatologic evaluation to rule out mimicking conditions. Similarly, patients with IBD-related AS should be assessed rheumatologically mainly to coordinate the multidisciplinary treatment these patients require.

Key Points

INFLAMMATORY BOWEL DISEASE (IBD) ARTHRITIS

- Peripheral joint arthritis in IBD, present in 20% of patients, must be distinguished from septic arthritis, gout, and pseudogout.
- Ankylosing spondylitis in IBD, present in 3% to 5% of cases, is similar to idiopathic AS.
- An additional 15% of patients with IBD have silent sacroiliitis, which does not portend progression to AS.
- Hypertrophic osteoarthropathy is an uncommon association of IBD.
- Behçet's disease and SLE may be mimicked.
- Treatment of bowel inflammation suppresses peripheral arthritis but is said to have no bearing on AS course.

Suggested Reading

Hammer RE, Maika SD, Richardson JA, et al. Spontaneous inflammatory disease in transgenic rats expressing HLA-B27 and human beta 2 microglobulin: An animal model of HLA-B27 associated human disorders. Cell 63:109–112, 1990.

Leff RD, Aldo-Benson MA, Maoura JA. The effect of revision of the intestinal bypass on post-intestinal bypass arthritis. Arthritis Rheum 26:678–681, 1983.

Mielants H, Veys EM, Cuvelier C, et al. The evolution of spondyloarthropathies in relation to gut histology. III. Relation between gut and joint. J Rheumatol 22:2279–2284, 1995.

Mielants H, Veys EM, de Vos M, et al. The evolution of spondyloarthropathies in relation to gut histology. I. Clinical aspects. J Rheumatol 22:2266–2272, 1995.

Wright V. Seronegative polyarthritis. A unified concept. Arthritis Rheum 21:619–633, 1978.

Whipple's Disease

Whipple's disease is a rare but potentially curable infection that should be kept in mind in clinical situations involving fever of unknown origin, arthritis, gastrointestinal symptoms with wasting, opthalmologic findings, and CNS disease. The gastroenterologic representation of Whipple's disease as a febrile, massive steatorrhea leading to catastrophic weight loss represents a limited view of late disease.

Presentation and Progression

Cause

The etiologic agent of Whipple's disease, *Tropheryma whippelii* (an actinomycete), has not been cultured but is detectable by

PCR on biopsy and blood samples. For unknown reasons the condition affects with predilection white men.

Presentation

Whipple's disease is a chronic infection with multisystemic manifestations that include fever, lymphadenopathy, arthritis, serositis, pneumonitis, endocarditis, myositis, neurologic findings, opthalmologic findings, weight loss, and steatorrhea. Rheumatic manifestations occur in 75% of patients and may precede, sometimes by decades, the clinical onset of bowel disease. Patients have arthralgias, palindromic-type arthritis, RA-like arthritis, or spondyloarthropathy. Indeed, the frequency of sacroiliitis and AS in Whipple's disease is the same as in IBD. Opthalmologic and neurologic manifestations include posterior uveitis, vitritis, supranuclear ocular palsies, and myoclonus; hypothalamic findings including insomnia, hyperphagia, and polydipsia; and dementia. The association of convergent nystagmus and oculomasticatory myorhythmia (palatal, tongue, and mandibular movements) appears to be pathognomonic of CNS Whipple's. In patients with rheumatoid factor negative arthritis and palindromic rheumatism, the presence of any of the findings just described should raise the possibility of Whipple's disease. Until recently, diagnosis of Whipple's was based on duodenal, lymph nodes, brain, or any available tissue biopsy upon which staining with PAS-diastase reveals diastase-resistant, PAS-positive material within macrophages. In addition, intra- and extracellular bacteria are seen by light and electron microscopy. This pathologic picture is similar to the gastrointestinal lesion seen in *M. avium* infection in patients with AIDS. Differentiation between the two rests on acid-fast staining that is positive in *M. avium* and negative in Whipple's disease. Interestingly, sarcoid-like granulomas have been found in a number of patients with Whipple's disease leading to a wrong diagnosis of sarcoidosis.

Diagnosis

Summary of Diagnosis

> **WHIPPLE'S DISEASE**
> - A rare condition seen predominantly in middle-aged men.
> - Diagnosis is suggested by fever, arthritis, lymphadenopathy, serositis, neurologic and ophthalmologic findings, wasting, and steatorrhea.
> - Tissue biopsies show macrophages laden with PAS-positive, diastase-resistant material.
> - Intra- and extracellular acid-fast negative bacteria are shown by light and electron microscopy.
> - The agent, *T. whippelii*, cannot be cultured but may be identified in tissue samples and blood by PCR.

Natural History

Expected Outcome

Undiagnosed, Whipple's disease is a progressive and eventually lethal condition. Complications of untreated disease include severe wasting, profound dementia, and death from cardiac arrhythmia.

Treatment

Methods

Several antibiotics are useful in Whipple's disease. Unfortunately, secondary resistance appears in some cases. A tested regime is the administration of intravenous penicillin G (24 million units per day) for 2 weeks, plus I.M. streptomycin 1 g per day, followed by trimetoprim-sulfamethoxazole that should be continued indefinitely. The use of agents that cross the blood-brain barrier is recommended.

Expected Response

Response to antibiotic treatment is slow, with articular and bowel symptoms improving first.

Complications

A Jarish-Herxheimer reaction may occur a few hours after initiation of intravenous penicillin.

When to Refer

Cases of suspected Whipple's disease should be referred to the appropriate specialist for patient evaluation and treatment. In patients with steatorrhea the diagnostic procedure of choice is endoscopy and duodenal biopsy.

Key Points

> **WHIPPLE'S DISEASE**
> - Whipple's disease may present as a seronegative arthritis, a wasting steatorrhea, a sarcoidlike multisystem disease, or an obscure neuro-opthalmologic disease including dementia, convergent nystagmus, and masticatory movements.
> - Diagnosis depends on knowledge of disease spectrum and the use of appropriate stains (PAS-diastase, acid-fast) on tissue biopsy.
> - Bacteriologic confirmation may be obtained by PCR.
> - Antibiotic treatment should be lifelong, since brain involvement has surfaced in presumably cured individuals. Secondary resistance to antibiotics may develop.

Suggested Reading

Dobbins WO. The diagnosis of Whipple's disease. N Engl J Med 332:390–392, 1995.

Relman DA, Schmidt TM, MacDermott RP, et al. Identification of the uncultured bacillus of Whipple's disease. N Engl J Med 327:293–301, 1992.

Psoriatic Arthritis

The nosologic validity of psoriatic arthritis, beyond a chance association of psoriasis and some form of arthritis, has been questioned in the past. However, not only have statistics borne an association between both conditions, but the articular findings are often diagnostic in their own right.

Presentation and Progression

Cause

Psoriasis affects 1% to 3% of the population. Among psoriatic patients, 20% to 30% develop arthritis. The mechanisms underlying this association, which appears to be more frequent in patients with early-onset psoriasis, are unknown. There is familial aggregation not only with psoriasis but with other spondyloarthropathies as well. Some researchers believe that bacteria lodged in the psoriatic plaques trigger an immune reaction. Interestingly, as in other spondyloarthropathies, gut inflammation is present in 20% of psoriatic patients with oligoarthritis and 30% of psoriatic patients with spondylitis. Characteristic of psoriatic arthritis is a role of trauma in determining joint involvement, which resembles the Koebner phenomenon observed in the skin (striking normal skin in a psoriatic patient results in a psoriatic plaque). Thus, genetic factors, possibly environmental factors, and gut inflammation all appear to be involved in psoriatic arthritis pathogenesis. Sudden onset of psoriasis and psoriatic arthritis should lead to investigation of HIV status.

Presentation

Several types of psoriatic arthritis have been described.

1. *RA-like* with negative rheumatoid factor is a common form of psoriatic arthritis. In addition to symmetrical distal arthritis, proliferative tenosynovitis is common particularly around wrists and ankles (Figure 17–4).
2. *Asymmetric oligoarthritis* is perhaps the best known type. One or a few joints are involved such as an elbow, a knee, and a toe. Inflammation is protracted and joint erosion minimal and late (Figure 17–5A and B).
3. Psoriatic *spondylitis* often has little spinal rigidity and radiographically there is asymmetric or unilateral sacroiliitis, resembling the findings in reactive arthritis. In contrast, sacroiliitis is symmetric in ankylosing spondylitis and chronic inflammatory bowel disease.
4. *"Mutilans" arthritis* is a fortunately rare form of psoriatic arthritis. There is resorption of phalanges, telescoping of digits (if you pull from the distal phalanx you extend the finger almost to its original length), and tendons are usually preserved. The condition causes little pain and the dwarfed finger(s) curiously exhibit full active motion.
5. The well-known but rare *distal IP arthritis* occurs as a transition from or as an accompaniment to other types of psoriatic arthritis. Given its location, DIP psoriatic arthritis must be distinguished from DIP osteoarthritis. A recently described variant of distal toe and finger psoriatic arthritis is the psoriatic onycho-pachydermo-periostitis in which the DIP is spared but there is exuberant periostitis under the nail plate.
6. A common finding in psoriasis is *enthesitis,* such as Achilles tendinitis and plantar fasciitis, which usually occurs in a context of psoriatic arthritis but may occasionally occur by itself.
7. Still another finding is *psoriatic dactylitis* in which a toe or a finger becomes diffusely inflamed (joints, flexor sheath, and periosteum) resulting in a cylindrical enlargement known as a "sausage" toe or finger. Psoriatic dactylitis may occur by itself but is more commonly seen in association with other types of psoriatic arthritis, mainly oligoarthritis.
8. Finally, psoriatic arthritis patients may present bone changes similar to those seen in the SAPHO syndrome (see anterior chest wall pain).

Although in the majority of patients psoriatic plaques

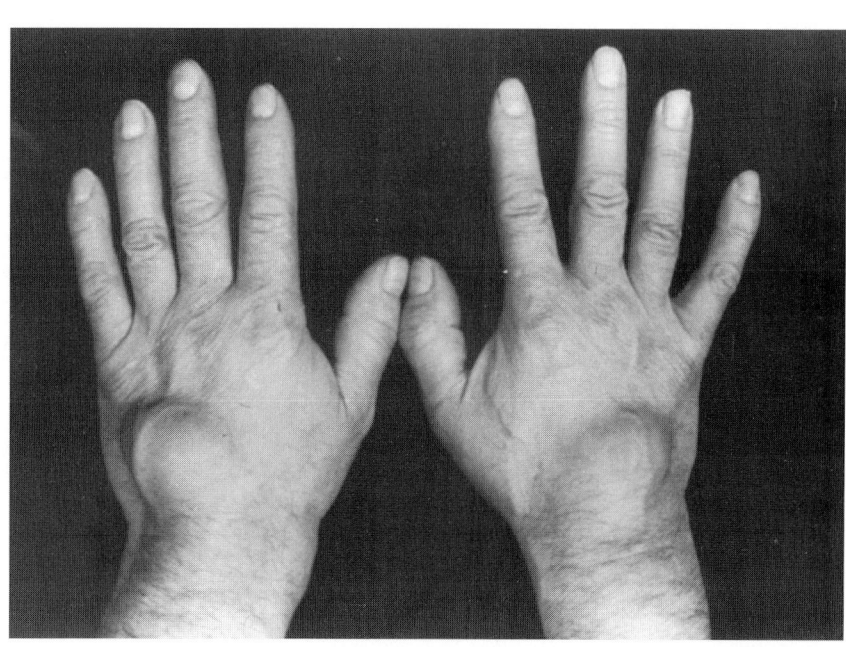

FIGURE 17–4. *Psoriatic arthritis, pseudorheumatoid type.* The patient had peripheral symmetric arthritis with marked dorsal tenosynovitis in his wrists. He had psoriasis on extensor surface of elbows, anterior knees, and lower back, and rheumatoid factor titers were repeatedly negative.

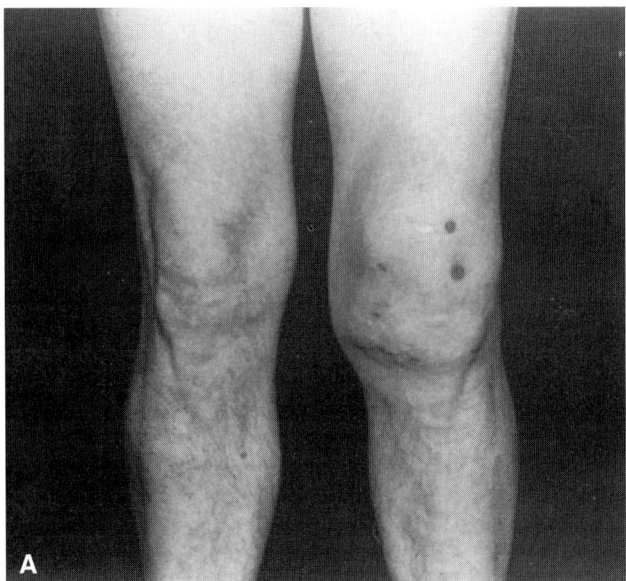

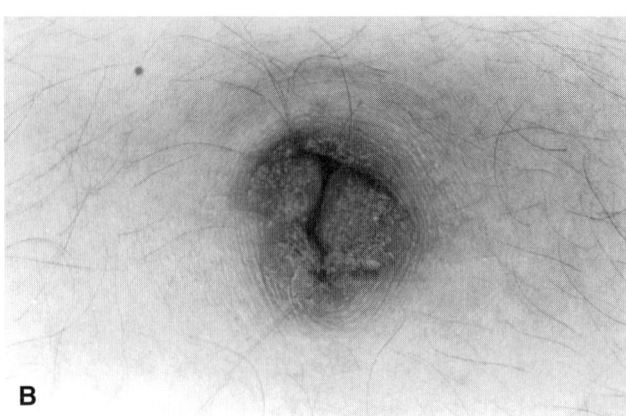

FIGURE 17–5. *Psoriatic arthritis.* The clue to the etiology of this patient's chronic knee monoarthritis (A) was a psoriatic lesion in his umbilicus (B).

precede the arthritis sometimes for years, in about 5% of cases arthritis appears first. Awareness of the peculiar features of psoriatic arthritis allows diagnosis in these patients. A family history of psoriasis is particularly helpful in diagnosing prepsoriatic psoriatic arthritis. In some of the cases, psoriasis remains occult. "Occult" psoriasis may be present in the scalp, umbilicus, behind the ears, or in the intergluteal groove. In the latter two locations psoriasis appears as a well-demarcated intertriginous plaque with little hyperkeratosis. Candidiasis must be excluded in these lesions.

PATIENT 20. A 35-year-old woman was admitted for treatment of severe oligoarthritis involving the right knee, proximal and distal interfalangeal joints of the right middle finger, and the left ankle. The condition had been present for 2 years. Recently, the right knee had flared and the patient was no longer able to walk. Psoriatic arthritis had long been suspected based on the pattern of joint involvement plus extensive psoriasis in her mother. However, no one was comfortable with this diagnosis in the absence of psoriasis. On detailed skin examination, including the "occult" areas, no lesions were found. A pilonidal sinus was found in the coccygeal area. The case was presented to the consulting attending who reexamined the patient and concurred with the findings, except that he opened the pilonidal fistula and found psoriasis (later confirmed by a dermatologist). A photograph of this lesion was not obtained, but Figure 17–6 shows a psoriatic intertriginous lesion in the intergluteal groove in a young woman whose polyarthritis and sacroiliitis went undiagnosed for 5 years prior to this examination.

Diagnosis

Summary of Diagnosis

> **PSORIATIC ARTHRITIS**
> - There are at least eight clinical patterns of psoriatic arthritis.
> - Some of the patterns are highly suggestive of the disease: chronic oligoarthritis, DIP arthritis, "mutilans arthritis," and the sausage digit.
> - Presence of psoriasis (review overt and "occult" areas).
> - Often psoriasis in the immediate family.
> - Often spondyloarthropathy in the immediate family.
> - Laboratory findings are nonspecific (increased ESR, increased CRP, sometimes elevation of liver enzymes from concurrent alcoholism).
> - X-rays are characteristic in late stages of the disease.

Natural History

Expected Outcome

The clinical course of psoriatic arthritis varies according to the type. The pseudorheumatoid type behaves as a mild case

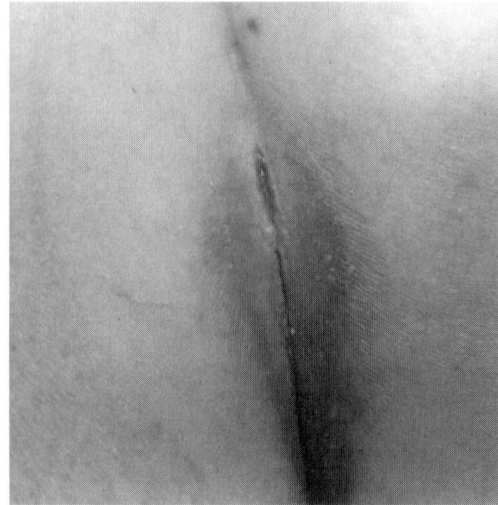

FIGURE 17–6. *Psoriatic arthritis.* This is the lesion mentioned apropos of Patient 20. Fissured intertriginous psoriatic lesion in the intergluteal groove. Candida infection was ruled out.

of RA. Psoriatic oligoarthritis is quite indolent and shows little erosive potential over the years. Psoriatic spondylitis may progress to a functionally fused spine with little in the way of syndesmophyte formation, as the limitation appears to reflect postinflammatory fibrosis at the facet joints. Mutilans psoriatic arthritis has a destructive course in the involved joints, but extension to new joints may not happen on prolonged follow-up. The author has been impressed by the restricted joint involvement in this form of the disease. The cosmetic repercussions of mutilans arthritis, which involves most frequently the hand, are staggering. DIP arthritis may also be quite disfiguring, resulting in flexion deformity of DIPs. Functionally, it has little effect except when normal DIP function is required.

PATIENT 21. A 19-year-old boy was preparing for a career as a classical violinist. Unfortunately, as he turned 18, psoriasis appeared on his nails and 4 months prior to his referral DIP arthritis appeared in the 2 through 5 digits of his left hand, the very fingers that pressed the violin strings. In the right hand the nails were involved but the DIPs were spared. His arthritis improved on indomethacin and methotrexate, but he never recovered the dexterity he once had.

Psoriatic enthesitis tends to respond well to systemic therapy. Dactylitis, in contrast, has an indolent course, often persisting far beyond other manifestations of the disease. There are few predictors of progression in psoriatic arthritis. It has been found that a high number of joint effusions and a history of multiple medications predict progressive damage, while a low ESR appears to be "protective."

Complications of psoriatic arthritis are mainly local and relate to location and degree of joint damage. Given the effects of trauma, joints that are needed the most are the ones that deteriorate the most. Systemic complications of psoriatic arthritis are few. Acute anterior uveitis is seen in 10% to 20% of patients with psoriatic spondyloarthropathy. Sjögren's is rare. There are no pleuropulmonary changes or vasculitis. Amyloidosis of the AA type rarely develops.

Treatment

Methods

In patients with psoriatic arthritis there are two areas to worry about, the skin and the joints. The DIP form of the condition often responds exquisitely to NSAIDs, particularly indomethacin. The remaining forms usually improve with the combination of a NSAID plus sulfasalazine. Neither of these agents improves the skin, which needs separate treatment with topical medications. In cases with severe skin involvement and also when psoriatic arthritis fails to improve with a NSAID plus sulfasalazine, methotrexate (MTX) may be used. Interestingly, doses of MTX that improve the arthritis may be insufficient to improve the skin. This is one of the reasons why high MTX doses are often required. There is the impression that MTX has greater liver toxicity in psoriatic patients than in RA. For instance, cirrhosis is said to develop in 3% of psoriatic patients given MTX, which is 10-fold higher than the rate found in MTX-treated RA patients. This increased rate may reflect an adverse effect of psoriasis on the liver or a higher rate of alcoholism in psoriasis than in RA.

Corticosteroid infiltrations are very helpful in psoriatic arthritis, tenosynovitis, and dactylitis, but great care must be exerted to avoid infection. Structures should be entered through normal skin and only after exacting antisepsis. As in RA, orthopedic surgery plays a major role in the treatment of psoriatic arthritis. Because psoriatic plaques are known to harbor staphylococci, skin lesions must be cleared prior to arthroplasty.

Expected Response

Response to treatment in psoriatic arthritis depends to some extent on the clinical type. Improvement is easier to detect in the RA-like, oligoarticular, and DIP types of arthritis. Treatment response in spondylitic and mutilans types is very difficult to determine.

When to Refer

Psoriatic arthritis is best cared for by a rheumatologist working in close association with a dermatologist. Mild cases, or already stabilized cases, may be handled by primary care physicians as long as close contact is kept with consultants.

Resources Available

The National Psoriasis Foundation (see appendix for address) provides sound advice to patients.

Key Points

PSORIATIC ARTHRITIS

- Arthritis occurs in about 20% to 30% of psoriatic patients, a 10-fold increase compared with the general population.
- Eight patterns of articular involvement are recognized. Several of these patterns (oligoarthritis, enthesitis, spondylitis, DIP arthritis, dactylitis) are also seen in reactive arthritis.
- Extraarticular manifestations are uncommon except uveitis in cases with spondylitis.
- Treatment of psoriatic arthritis includes NSAIDs, sulfasalazine, and, in severe or unresponsive cases, methotrexate.
- Methotrexate treatment of psoriasis is said to cause cirrhosis in about 3% of patients, a 10-fold increase over the rate observed in similarly treated RA.

Suggested Reading

Boiseau-Garsaud A-M, Beylot-Barry M, Doutre M-S, et al. Psoriatic onycho-pachydermo-periostitis. Arch Dermatol 132:176–180, 1996.

Dougados M, van der Linden S, Leirisalo-Repo M, et al. Sulfasalazine in the treatment of spondyloarthropathy. A randomized, multicenter, double-blind, placebo-controlled study. Arthritis Rheum 38:618–627, 1995.

Gladman DD, Farewell VT, Nadeau C. Clinical indicators of progression in psoriatic arthritis: Multivariate relative risk model. J Rheumatol 22:675–679, 1995.

Greaves MW, Weinstein GD. Treatment of psoriasis. N Engl J Med 332:581–588, 1995.

Gupta AK, Grober JS, Hamilton TA, et al. Sulfasalazine therapy for psoriatic arthritis: A double blind, placebo controlled trial. J Rheumatol 22:894–898, 1995.

Salvarani C, Lo Scocco G, Macchioni P, et al. Prevalence of psoriatic arthritis in Italian psoriatic patients. J Rheumatol 22:1499–1503, 1995.

Schatteman L, Mielants H, Veys EM, et al. Gut inflammation in psoriatic arthritis: A prospective ileocolonoscopic study. J Rheumatol 22:680–683, 1995.

Behçet's Disease (BD)

Early descriptions portrayed BD as a triad: oral ulcers, genital ulcers, and uveitis. However, astute clinical and pathologic observations over the past five decades have greatly expanded the spectrum of BD. Pathologically, BD is a systemic vasculitis involving veins, arteries, and capillaries. Clinical manifestations are mucocutaneous, ophthalmic, cardiovascular, gastrointestinal, urogenital, musculoskeletal, and neurologic.

Presentation and Progression

Cause

The etiology of BD remains unknown. The condition appears to have two phenotypes. One is observed in Japan, Korea, Middle Eastern countries, in particular Turkey, and the Mediterranean basin. The other phenotype is encountered in the United States and Europe. An association with the HLA-B51 (a subset of HLA-B5) is present in the Middle East but not in U.S. or English patients.

Presentation

Initially there are recurrent, slow-healing, very painful oral and genital ulcers (Figures 17–7 and 17–8). Later in the course of the disease painless anterior and/or posterior uveitis or retinal vasculitis develops with the potential to

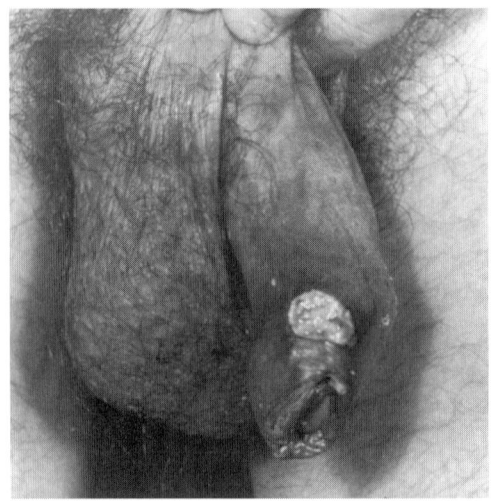

FIGURE 17–8. *Behçet's syndrome.* Painful prepuceal ulcer in a male with superficial thrombophlebitis, oral ulcers, and bowel vasculitis.

result in blindness. Behçet's ulcers differ from the common variety of aphthous ulcers in that they are large (few to 10 mm) and involve unusual sites such as the pharynx, the shaft of the penis, the scrotum, the vagina, and the cervix. A curious phenomenon seen in 25% to 75% of Middle Eastern patients is the pathergy response: a nodule or pustule developing within 24 to 48 hours at the site of a sterile puncture with a #20 needle. The pathergy response is rarely seen in the United States and Europe. Additional manifestations of Behçet's include superficial or deep (leg veins, vena cava, hepatic veins) thrombophlebitis, erythema nodosum or papulopustules, colitis, oligoarthritis, and meningoencephalitis or cerebral vasculitis. Occlusive or aneurysmal large-artery lesions complicate 5% to 7% of cases. Sites of occlusion include the axillary, femoral, popliteal, tibial, and coronary arteries. Aneurysms may occur in the aorta, the iliac, the femoral, and the pulmonary arteries.

Diagnosis

Summary of Diagnosis

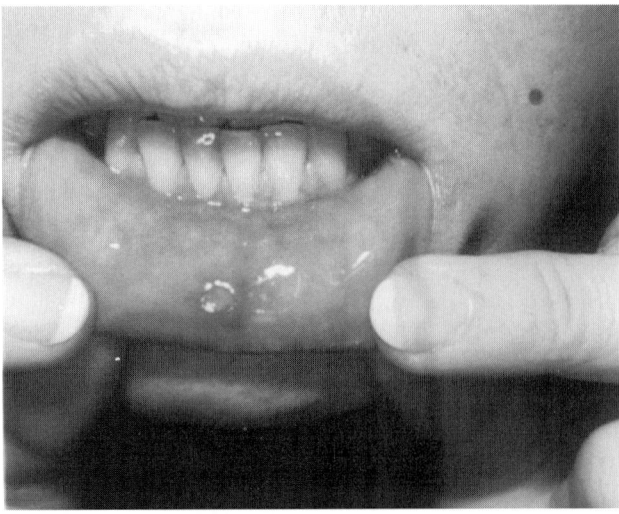

FIGURE 17–7. *Behçet's syndrome.* Painful aphthous inner lower lip ulcer in a 30-year-old Chinese woman with relapsing oral and genital ulcers and uveitis. She did well on low-dose prednisone plus colchicine.

BEHÇET'S DISEASE

- Classic triad: recurrent painful oral aphthae, genital aphthae, and anterior and/or posterior uveitis.
- Systemic involvement includes erythema nodosum and other skin lesions, superficial and deep phlebitis, colitis, oligoarthritis, and meningoencephalitis or cerebral vasculitis.
- Ophthalmologic consultation is in order to detect uveitis.
- LP if meningismus is present.
- Leukocytosis; neutrophilia, thrombocytosis. Negative ANA, negative ANCA.
- Colonoscopy if colitis is present to rule out ulcerative colitis and Crohn's disease.

Natural History

Expected Outcome

The condition has unpredictable remissions and exacerbations. Serious complications include blindness from vasculitic occlusions, stroke from cerebral vasculitis, limb ischemia from arterial occlusions, bowel perforations from colonic vasculitis, and massive bleeding from bowel or aneurysmal bleed. Pulmonary embolism is said to be rare in patients with major vein thrombosis.

Treatment

Methods

Oral and genital ulcers benefit from triamcynolone pastes or gels. Oral colchicine appears to prevent recurrences in some cases. Dapsone and thalidomide (this one if available, under research protocol, and with the appropriate precautions) can be used to treat mucocutaneous lesions. Systemic vasculitis and meningoencephalitis respond poorly to corticosteroids but are highly responsive to alkylating agents such as chlorambucil and cyclophosphamide. Corticosteroids may be administered in conjunction with the latter to treat cerebral lesions, followed by a rapid tapering. Eye lesions respond well to chlorambucil and to cyclosporine. Arterial occlusions may be treated with autologous or prosthetic grafts, but there is a high rate of reocclusion. Aneurysms in BD are unusually prone to rupture, warranting early surgery.

Expected Response

Chlorambucil is the treatment of choice in severe Behçet's cases. Treatment is usually discontinued 1 year after remission was obtained. Minor manifestations of BD can be treated with topical steroids plus colchicine or dapsone.

When to Refer

BD is unusual in the United States, and few primary care physicians will see more than one or two cases in their professional lives. Behçet's patients should be followed jointly by a rheumatologist and an ophthalmologist.

Resources Available

Behçet's patients should contact the American Behçet's Association for useful information (see the appendix).

Key Points

> **BEHÇET'S DISEASE**
> - Diagnosis of Behçet's disease is clinical.
> - Suspected cases should be referred to a rheumatologist and an ophthalmologist.
> - The risk of blindness is higher in Middle East countries; the risk of meningoencephalitis is higher in the United States.
> - Oral and genital ulcers respond to local corticosteroids plus either oral colchicine or dapsone.
> - Ocular inflammation may be treated with chlorambucil, cyclophosphamide, or cyclosporine.
> - CNS inflammation or vasculitis responds best to cyclophosphamide.

Suggested Reading

Huong DLT, Wechsler B, Papo T, et al. Arterial lesions in Behçet's disease. A study in 25 patients. J Rheumatol 22:2103–2113, 1995.

Acute Rheumatic Fever (ARF) and Streptococcal Reactive Arthritis

Acute rheumatic fever has had worldwide, and still has in developing countries, a tremendous impact on public health. Although under a different paradigm from the one that prevails today, ARF focused researchers' attention on nonmicrobial rheumatic disease triggered by infection, setting the ground for the emerging concept of reactive arthritis. Interestingly, since the 1950s, the incidence of acute rheumatic fever has dramatically decreased, which was taken as a triumph of penicillin over streptococcal disease. However, as streptococcal infections have been on the rise since the 1980s, pockets of ARF have reappeared even in the affluent population.

Presentation and Progression

Cause

Acute rheumatic fever follows a group A streptococcus (*S. pyogenes*) pharyngeal infection. Interestingly, skin and soft tissue streptococcal infections do not cause ARF. In approximately one-third of cases the triggering infection is silent but still demonstrable serologically. The condition has a predilection for lower strata of the population reflecting overcrowding, late access to treatment of pharyngitis, and poor treatment compliance. In addition, there is a genetic predisposition to ARF that can be determined by histocompatibility factors. The incubation period between onset of streptococcal pharyngitis and onset of arthritis varies from 1 to 5 weeks (usually 2 to 3 weeks). At the time of onset of ARF, high (peak) titers of streptococcal antibodies are regularly demonstrable in the serum. These antibodies are not protective against reinfection. Recurrences of ARF are similarly triggered by apparent or silent pharyngeal group A streptococcal infection. Prompt penicillin treatment of *S. pyogenes* pharyngitis eliminates the risk of developing ARF, and effective penicillin prophylaxis prevents recurrences of ARF and progression to serious heart disease.

Presentation

The patient with ARF is usually a child or an adolescent. There are adult cases, however, that because of the unusual age of onset tend to be misdiagnosed. Acute rheumatic fever debuts with an extremely painful additive arthritis that affects large joints such as knees, ankles, elbows, and wrists. Large effusions are rare. Acute symptoms persist up to 1 week in each joint after which the joint becomes normal.

The hallmark of ARF is cardiac involvement. Although all layers of the heart may be affected, isolated myocarditis or pericarditis in the absence of a murmur would suggest an etiology other than ARF. Cardiac involvement usually occurs within 6 months from the initial attack. Most patients have no cardiovascular symptoms. To be diagnosed, rheumatic carditis must be intentionally sought. Solid evidence of carditis is afforded by mitral or (rarely) aortic regurgitation murmurs. Myocarditis features tachycardia, cardiac enlargement, and in severe cases congestive failure. Findings in pericarditis include a rub, chest pain, and rarely tamponade. Chest x-rays show cardiomegaly. Pericardial effusion is best confirmed by echocardiogrphy.

Two types of skin lesions may appear in ARF, both in association with rheumatic carditis: an evanescent, nonpruritic serpiginous rash (erythema marginatum), and small subcutaneous nodules in pressure areas such as the back and the occiput in bedridden patients. Another striking presentations of ARF is chorea, which characteristically occurs in an afebrile child who suddenly develops emotional instability and purposeless motions in the extremities and face. It is important to remember that chorea may be a manifestation of SLE, the antiphospholipid syndrome, and pregnancy (chorea gravidarum). Fever (at least 39° C) is constant and prominent in cases with arthritis, is often present in isolated carditis, and is absent in isolated chorea.

There are several unusual manifestations of ARF. Jaccoud's arthritis refers to a rare deforming, nonerosive form of arthritis that occurs after many episodes of ARF. The very rare rheumatic pneumonitis and encephalitis appear in gravely ill patients and have dismal prognoses. An association with poststreptococcal glomerulonephritis is exceptional. Acute rheumatic fever in the adult is not only uncommon, but it features a more symmetric arthritis, tenosynovitis is often present, and the rate of carditis is definitively lower than in children. Poststreptococcal reactive arthritis is a controversial condition. Reported patients were very ill and had arthritis and periarthritis, sometimes with additional manifestations such as glomerulonephritis or vasculitis following streptococcal pharyngitis. Carditis was not present in these patients either initially or in follow-up. There is some danger in diagnosing this condition because carditis in ARF may appear late in disease course and a premature diagnosis of reactive arthritis may lead to withholding antibiotic prophylaxis.

Laboratory abnormalities in ARF include leukocytosis, neutrophilia, high ESR, and high CRP. Very important diagnostically, high titers of streptococcal antibodies are regularly present in the serum. Most patients have antistreptolysin-O antibodies. About 20% have other antistreptococcal antibodies. In the Streptozyme test, sheep red blood cells covered with a mixture of streptococcal antigens are mixed with the patient's serum. Because streptococcal antibodies tend to decline after 2 months, patients with isolated carditis or isolated chorea may have borderline or negative titers at the time of diagnosis. In contrast, ARF arthritis is virtually always associated with positive antibody tests. Diagnosis of ARF is established following the time-honored Jones's criteria (Table 17–4). Although these criteria are very useful in field work and in cardiology settings where mimicking rheumatic conditions are infrequent, they are problematic in rheumatologic use. Thus, a number of rheumatic conditions unrelated to ARF have recently been listed that may fulfill Jones's criteria. This should not surprise nor discourage physicians. The key element is to know how to recognize mimicking conditions and ruling them out. The author has had the opportunity of practicing rheumatology in the United States and in Mexico. Given a patient with rheumatic fever, a Mexican rheumatologist might say: "The patient looks as though he has ARF. However, conditions A, B, and C must be ruled out." Seeing the same patient, an American rheumatologist might say: "The patient does not seem to have conditions A, B, and C. Jones's criteria are fulfilled; he may therefore have ARF."

Diagnosis

Summary of Diagnosis

TABLE 17–4

GUIDELINES FOR THE DIAGNOSIS OF RHEUMATIC FEVER. JONES'S CRITERIA, 1992 UPDATE*

MAJOR MANIFESTATIONS

  Carditis
  Polyarthritis
  Chorea
  Erythema marginatum
  Subcutaneous nodules

MINOR MANIFESTATIONS

Clinical findings

  a. Arthralgia
  b. Fever

Laboratory findings

  a. Elevated acute-phase reactants
     1. Erythrocyte sedimentation rate
     2. Prolonged PR interval

SUPPORTING EVIDENCE OF ANTECEDENT GROUP A STREPTOCOCCAL INFECTION

  Positive throat culture or rapid streptococcal antigen test
  Elevated or rising antibody titer

*If supported by evidence of preceding group A streptococcal infection, the presence of two major manifestations or one major and two minor manifestations indicates a high probability of acute rheumatic fever.
Committee of the American Heart Association, JAMA, 268:2069–2073, 1992.

ACUTE RHEUMATIC FEVER (ARF)

- Usually a child or an adolescent; sometimes an adult.
- Severe febrile illness with very painful, additive, fully reversible arthritis.
- Is there evidence of carditis? Is there a mitral or aortic regurgitation murmur present?
- Examine purposefully the skin for the rare erythema marginatum and pebbly subcutaneous nodules.
- Other patients present with isolated Sydenham's chorea.

- Laboratory studies: CBC, ESR, CRP, urinalysis.
- A positive pharyngeal culture (about 20%) has little diagnostic value because it may only indicate a chronic carrier state.
- Streptococcal antibody tests are critical.
- Chest x-rays, EKG, cardiac echo.
- Rule out SBE, JRA, Lyme disease, SLE, primary antiphospholipid syndrome, and so on.

Natural History

Expected Outcome

Untreated, arthritis in ARF lasts approximately 1 month. Joint symptoms are dramatically improved (within 48 hours) with salicylates. Isolated mitral regurgitation may disappear as the flare is brought under control, but it may also progress, leading to early heart surgery. Different from mitral insufficiency, which has an early presentation, mitral stenosis may appear after years of disease. There are cases of chronic carditis that go on for several months and even years. Each recurrence of ARF adds to the risk of serious valvulopathy. Erythema marginatum, subcutaneous nodules, pneumonitis, and the very rare encephalitis are manifestations of severe disease. In contrast, chorea has a benign, albeit protacted (it may last years) course.

Treatment

Methods

Treatment of ARF includes anti-inflammatory therapy for the various manifestations of the disease, antibiotic therapy for eradication of streptococcal pharyngitis, and antibiotic prophylaxis for recurrence prevention. In very ill patients cardiac involvement requires specific cardiovascular therapy. Likewise, Sydenham's chorea calls for specific treatment of the movement disorder.

1. *Anti-inflammatory therapy.* The preferred anti-inflammatory in ARF is aspirin, given in doses to attain serum concentrations of 20 mg/dl. Aspirin is not only effective for the fever and the arthritis, but also in mild forms of carditis. Severe cases of carditis are treated with parenteral or oral corticosteroids at an average dose of 1 to 2 mg/kg until improvement has occurred and the ESR is normal. The steroid is then decreased and phased out over several weeks.
2. *Eradication of streptococcal pharingitis.* This is best achieved with intramuscular procaine penicillin 600,000 units per day for 10 days, or a single injection of benzatinic penicillin 1.2 million units. The single injection treatment is the choice because compliance is 100%. There is no demonstrated resistance to this form of therapy.
3. *Antibiotic prophylaxis.* The safest method is the tri-weekly intramuscular administration of benzatinic penicillin 1.2 million units. The previously used monthly schedule leaves some patients uncovered for up to a week. An alternative is oral sulfadiazine 1 g per day in a single dose. Prophylaxis should be indefinite.
4. *Sydenham's chorea.* It may be treated with haloperidol or diazepam. There is also some successful experience with the use of hydroxychloroquine.

Needless to say, it is essential that the patient's parents, or the immediate family, become aware of the importance of strict adherence to penicillin prophylaxis. Lapses should not be allowed to occur.

Complications

Other than the occasional allergic patient, there are no known complications of initial and prophylactic penicillin.

When to Refer

Patients with suspected ARF should be evaluated jointly with an adult rheumatologist or pediatric rheumatologist depending on the age of the patient.

Guidelines for the Disorder

Diagnostic guidelines for ARF are given in Table 17–4.

Key Points

ACUTE RHEUMATIC FEVER (ARF)

- Acute rheumatic fever follows pharyngeal (not other location) streptococcal infection.
- Mitral regurgitation appears during the ARF episode.
- Mitral stenosis is a late development, sometimes appearing decades after mitral insufficiency, even without clear relapses of the condition.
- Prompt and adequate treatment of streptococcal pharyngitis prevents ARF.
- Secondary prevention is achieved with I.M. benzatinic PNC every 3 weeks.
- There have been some foci of ARF in the United States over the past 10 years.
- Different from classic ARF, the condition has not been limited to the lower strata of the population.

Suggested Reading

American Heart Association. Guidelines for the diagnosis of rheumatic fever. JAMA 268:2069–2073, 1992.

Amigo M-C, Martínez-Lavín M, Reyes PA. Acute rheumatic fever. Clin Rheum Dis 19:333–350, 1993.

Gutiérrez-Ureña S, Molina J, García CO, et al. Poststreptococcal Re A, clinical course, and outcome in 6 adult patients. J Rheumatol 22:1710–1713, 1995.

Marcus RH, Sareli P, Pocock WA, et al. The spectrum of severe rheumatic mitral valve disease in a developing country. Ann Intern Med 120:177–183, 1994.

CHAPTER 18

Crystal-Induced Arthritides

The crystal-induced arthritides include gout or monosodium urate (MSU) crystal deposition disease; pseudogout or calcium pyrophosphate dihydrate (CPPD) crystal deposition disease; calcific tendinitis and bursitis or basic calcium phosphate (BCP) crystal deposition disease; oxalate synovitis and bursitis; corticosteroid-induced synovitis; and arguably synovitis induced by foreign bodies having a crystalline structure. There is a trend, which the author suscribes to, of categorizing the crystal-induced arthritides using a Lynnaean genus and species system, for example, *genus gout* (crystal-induced synovitis) followed by the *crystal species* identified (urate or MSU, pyrophosphate or CPPD, apatite or BCC, oxalate, etc.). Following this nomenclature, crystal conditions include urate gout, pyrophosphate gout, apatite gout, cholesterol gout, and oxalate gout, each in their corresponding acute, subacute, and chronic varieties. However, not to generate confusion, the commonly used terminology is followed in the remainder of this discussion.

Gout

Gout is the clinical condition that results from serum UA levels chronically exceeding saturation (above 7.5–8 mg/dl with most automated methods), resulting in crystal precipitation in tissues. Is a diagnosis of hyperuricemia tantamount to a diagnosis of gout? Definitely not; uric acid levels are often elevated in the population at large, there are no known ill effects caused by high-serum uric acid levels, and only a minority of hyperuricemic individuals eventually develop gout.

On the other hand, documentation of hyperuricemia should lead the physician to consider the presence of concomitants such as overweight, hypertriglyceridemia, heavy alcohol consumption, arterial hypertension, use of diuretics, and so on (Table 18–1). There are two sides to the gout issue: One has to do with the acute synovial inflammation triggered by MSU crystals and the other relates to tissue deposition of MSU crystals in aggregates (tophi), granulomatous inflammation around tophi, bone erosion, fibrosis, and organ dysfunction.

Three clinical stages are recognized in gout: stage I, or asymptomatic hyperuricemia; stage II, or recurrent acute gout without permanent joint damage ("intercritical gout"); and stage III, or chronic tophaceous gout. This is a useful classification for treatment decisions. However, by the time a patient first develops acute gout, microtophi are already present in the synovium, and recurrent acute gout often continues over a background of chronic articular gout.

Presentation and Progression

Cause

Gout may result from increased UA production, decreased UA renal excretion, or both mechanisms combined (Table 18–1). Increased UA production may be caused by genetic factors, chronic hemolysis, myeloproliferative disorders, or exogenous mechanisms, in particular obesity, excessive alcohol consumption, and a high purine intake. It is estimated that 10% of primary gout patients are uric acid hyperproducers. Decreased UA renal excretion may result from decreased GFR in arterial hypertension, thiazides, and loop diuretics; a raised threshold of tubular excretion in acute alcohol consumption; chronic renal insufficiency of any etiology, in particular polycystic disease and lead intoxication; and obesity by unclear mechanisms. Also, 90% of primary gout patients have a decreased uric acid clearance. In these patients normal uric acid excretion values are achieved with serum urate levels that are 2 to 3 mg higher than in normal individuals.

Presentation

Clinical aspects of acute gout are so well known that little descriptive efforts appear warranted. However, experience

---

TABLE 18–1

CLASSIFICATION OF HYPERURICEMIA

URIC ACID HYPERPRODUCTION

Primary gout (10% of cases)
Genetic factors (HGPRT deficiency, hyperactive PRPP)
Overweight
Diet rich in purine
Excessive alcohol use
Psoriasis
Hemolysis
Myeloproliferative disease
Lymphoma

DECREASED EXCRETION

Primary gout (90%)
Renal insufficiency
Arterial hypertension
Overweight
Lead intoxication
Hyperparathyroidism

Hypothyroidism
Toxemia of pregnancy
Down syndrome
Acidosis
Drug ingestion:
  Alcohol
  Diuretics
  Low-dose salicylates (< 2 g/day)
  Cyclosporine
  Levodopa

COMBINATION OF HYPER-PRODUCTION AND HYPO-EXCRETION

Primary gout
Overweight
Excessive alcohol use (usually increased production; decreased excretion with lactacidosis)

has taught the author that many cases which appear to be gout are not, and vice versa. There is an ingrained concept that raised UA levels indicate a patient's articular symptoms are due to gout, but in fact they don't. This is understood if one considers that in the older population hyperuricemia occurs in about 10% while musculoskeletal symptoms appear in as many as 50% (including the 2% who have gout). As a result most cases of arthritis with hyperuricemia will not be gout.

Conversely, about 30% of patients with acute gout have normal uric acid levels at least in the vicinity of the attack. Crystal demonstration of gout is highly desirable, but diagnostic certainty may not be required in early disease when a lifelong commitment to uric acid lowering agents is not under consideration. While acute first MPT arthritis in a middle-age male who takes diuretics usually means gout, primary care physicians should be aware of a substantial list of conditions that cause podagra in addition to gout. In these conditions, collectively known as "pseudopodagra" (Table 18–2), a wrong diagnosis of gout may not only lead to uncalled for treatments, but the actual causative condition may go untreated. A classic example is the patient with hallux rigidus (see hallux rigidus) who has recurrent first MTP joint pain for which he may receive colchicine and even allopurinol, whereas an appropriate treatment would be an orthosis or a simple surgical procedure.

Certain clinical characteristics are highly suggestive of gout: (1) podagra beginning during the night or in the early morning hours; (2) pain bad enough to make unbearable the weight of a sheath on the painful toe; (3) a peculiar pink color to the inflamed joint with prominence of regional veins; and (4) absence of symptoms between attacks, a characteristic that is lost as accretion of MSU crystals leads to chronic destructive tophaceous arthritis.

A relevant question is, is it necessary to add the agony of a joint aspiration to the agony of a gout attack? No; treat the patient as if he or she had gout. If crystal documentation is needed the MTP joint can be aspirated a few days later after the acute inflammation has subsided; the procedure will be easier, less painful, and crystals will still be there for a firm diagnosis to be made. Underlying this leniency is the notion that septic arthritis of the first MTP joint is extremely uncommon. It would be different if the podagra had followed a puncture wound or if a plantar ulcer was present beneath the joint. On the other hand, failure to respond to a standard treatment of acute gout should make one consider alternative diagnoses including bacterial infection. The first MTP joint should only be aspirated if the results are likely to impact on patient management. The following is a typical example.

PATIENT 22. A previously well 56-year-old man had a string of episodes of severe podagra within the course of a year. Each had responded well to NSAIDs, but the patient's lifestyle was disrupted by unpredictable attacks. Serum uric acid levels were minimally elevated, and no tophi were present on examination. Several treatment options were considered: (1) the chronic use of a NSAID, (2) colchicine prophylaxis (vide infra), and (3) long-term allopurinol treatment with prn treatment of podagra or colchicine prophylaxis during the initial 6 months of therapy.

Approach 1 would suppress acute gout as well as several forms of pseudopodagra at a risk of causing NSAID gastropathy. Approach 2 would only suppress gout. Neither of these approaches would address the chronic hyperuricemic state or prevent its consequences. On the other hand, approach 3 would control the hyperuricemia and its consequences at the risk of inducing recurrent acute attacks in 10% to 20% of patients. This risk could be reduced by the prophylactic use of colchicine 0.6 mg once or twice daily or the individual attacks could be treated with colchicine, a NSAID, ACTH, or a glucocorticoid. In assessing such a patient, joint aspiration becomes essential. If MSU crystals were present, plausible options would be approach 2 with periodic surveillance for the appearance of tophaceous gout or approach 3, which is the one preferred by the author. If no crystals were found, option 1 would be preferable while further evaluation takes place.

Other frequently involved joints in gout are the knee, the ankle, the wrist, and the elbow. Joint aspiration is usually required in these settings to confirm gout (if gout is suspected) but mainly to exclude alternative diagnoses, particularly bacterial infection.

Certain joints are curiously immune to acute gout. The hip, for instance, is very rarely involved in absence of acute symptoms in other joints (the author has seen only one such case), although "a touch" of hip synovitis may occur in the context of polyarticular gout and improve in concert with the rest of joints. Similar considerations apply to the shoulder.

Nodal gout represents gout superimposed on one or more Heberden's nodes. The condition has a predilection for older women who take diuretics. This is one situation in which visible tophi may precede gout attacks. Nodal gout should be suspected when acute inflammation supervenes on an already burned-out Heberden's node.

Polyarticular gout is a particularly distressing syndrome that appears late in disease course. A polyarticular onset is most frequent in women, patients with myeloproliferative disorders, and in cyclosporine-induced gout. Fever and leukocytosis go hand in hand with number of involved joints, and they may be prominent to the point of suggesting

---

TABLE 18–2
CAUSES OF PSEUDOPODAGRA

Cellulitis
Septic arthritis
Bunion bursitis
Hallux rigidus
Hallux valgus with bursitis or DJD
Sesamoiditis
Stress fracture
Basic calcium phosphate crystal deposition
Calcium pyrophosphate crystal deposition disease
Reactive arthritis
Psoriatic arthritis
Inflammatory bowel disease arthritis
Palindromic rheumatism
Morton's neuroma
Tarsal tunnel syndrome

infection. Blood and synovial fluid Gram stain and cultures are critical in these cases to rule out concurrent infection.

Acute cervical and lumbar spine gout is not only rare but cannot be crystal proven. A presumptive diagnosis of spinal gout can only be made if gout is proven by aspiration in a concurrently involved joint and if both this joint and the back pain improve on colchicine, which is a gout-specific agent. The use of a NSAID would not allow such a diagnosis to be made.

Early-onset gout calls for evaluation of a possible genetic disorder such as PRPP (phosphoribosylpyrophosphate) synthetase hyperactivity or a partial deficiency of HGPRT (hypoxanthine-guanine phosphoribosyltransferase). In the Lesch-Nyhan syndrome there is a complete deficiency of HGPRT in addition to the devastating neurologic syndrome that appears in infancy or early childhood. Gross uric acid hyperexcretion is present in both conditions on a 24 hour urine collection. Diagnosis requires specific enzyme determination in red cells or fibroblasts at specialized centers.

To diagnose gout definitely, any joint fluid present or any nodule that could represent a tophus should be aspirated and the specimen examined under the polarizing microscope. Techniques of joint aspiration are discussed in the appendix, and routine synovial fluid analysis and crystal identification are explained in detail in the introduction.

Nodule aspiration is a simple and virtually painless procedure: Without anesthesia insert a #20 needle attached to a 10 to 20 mL syringe in the center of the nodule and pull the embolus as hard as you can. Maintain the aspiration for about 1 minute (nothing will come into the syringe). Then gently release the suction, disconnect the needle, aspirate some air in the syringe, reconnect the needle, and push hard on the embolus, squirting the needle contents, a tiny amount of chalky material or serous fluid, onto a clean microscope slide that should be rapidly covered with a clean coverslide (Figure 18–1A and B). If a rheumatologist is not available to inspect the slide, seal the edges of the coverslide with nail polish (to prevent the specimen from drying up) and place the slide in a refrigerator until inspection. A tophus will yield a chalky material with myriad free needle-shaped crystals, the largest about the size of three red cell diameters. If the aspirated nodule turns out to be a rheumatoid nodule, the aspirated material may contain cholesterol crystals that appear as huge (about 10–20 red cells long) rectangular plates.

The basic laboratory evaluation used by the author in documented gout includes a complete blood cell count; determination of serum creatinine, uric acid, triglycerides, and cholesterol; urinalysis; and uric acid and creatinine determination in a 24 hour urine collection. The CBC will uncover the rare associations of thalassemia and hemolytic anemias, but its main use is to serve as a baseline, since NSAIDs, colchicine, and allopurinol have untoward effects that impact on this test. Serum creatinine will identify cases of gout secondary to chronic renal insufficiency and is an important parameter to follow in patients using NSAIDs, colchicine, and allopurinol. Serum uric acid levels are used to monitor the effectiveness of (and compliance with) allopurinol and probenecid treatment. Serum triglycerides and to some extent cholesterol are often elevated in gout. Urinalysis is abnormal in patients with nephropathy and will show hematuria in intercurrent urolithiasis (uric acid stones may be small and quite difficult to diagnose).

The 24 hour uric acid excretion deserves special note. Normal individuals placed on a purine-free diet excrete less than 600 mg of uric acid in 24 hours. A regular diet adds 200 mg to the excretion. Thus, an 800 mg uric acid excretion in a 24 hour urine sample (completeness being assessed by concurrent creatinine excretion) represents the upper limit in normals.

Identification of hyperexcretors is important, particularly if probenecid use is under consideration. Since probenecid decreases uric acid tubular resorption, the added load in the urine may result in recurrent stone formation in a hyperexcretor patient. Functionally, a 24 hour uric acid excretion above 800 mg is definitely abnormal and represents the cutoff used by the author to separate patients who cannot take probenecid from those who can (800 mg or less of uric acid in 24 hour urine).

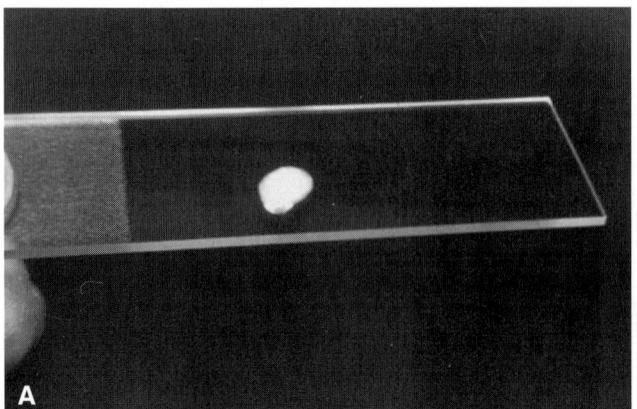 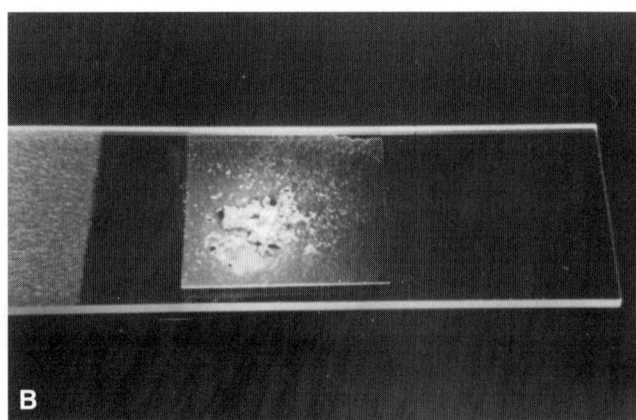

FIGURE 18–1. *Gout. Tophus aspirate.* A, A drop of the chalky aspirate is placed onto a microscope slide. B, Typical appearance after the coverslide is placed prior to inspection under the polarizing microscope.

Diagnosis

Summary of Diagnosis

> **GOUT, ACUTE AND CHRONIC**
>
> - Clinical features of acute gout: Important subsets include podagra; acute gout involving large joints; nodal gout; polyarticular gout; gout in rarely affected joints such as the hip, shoulder, and spine; and early-onset gout.
> - Serum uric acid is normal in 30% of gout patients at the time of an acute attack.
> - Clinical features of chronic tophaceous gout (cutaneous deposits, chronic arthritis or x-ray changes, visceral).
> - Crystal documentation by joint fluid analysis or tophus aspiration.
> - Identification of risk factors: overweight, excessive purine consumption, alcohol abuse, arterial hypertension, diuretic use.
> - CBC, serum creatinine, serum uric acid, serum triglyceride and cholesterol.
> - Uric acid and creatinine excretion in 24 hour urine.
> - X-rays may provide diagnostic features in chronic tophaceous gout but have little value in early gout.

Natural History

Expected Outcome

Acute Gout. It is well known that 30% to 40% of patients with a first episode of podagra will not present another episode within a year, and half of these will escape recurrence during the second year. In the remaining 60% to 70% of patients, recurrences of acute gout pose significant morbidity from the outset. Attacks of gout are fully preventable with the use of suppressive medications or the prolonged use of uric acid lowering drugs.

Tophaceous Deposits. Patients with acute gout may or may not have tophi detectable on examination. Tophi tend to appear after years of recurrences of articular gout, with the notable exception of nodal gout in which tophi are usually present by the first attack. Current prevalence of tophi is 10% to 15%, down from a high of 50% in older series doubtlessly as a result of the widespread use of uric acid lowering drugs. The usual tophus is a hard nodule that appears in cold areas such as the olecranon region, the vicinity of the first MTP, Heberden's nodes, or the pinnae of the ears. The predilection of tophi for colder areas is explained by temperature-dependent solubility changes, for example, a solubility limit of 7 mg/dl at 37° C as compared to 4.5 mg/dl at 30° C. Most tophi are subcutaneous, periosteal attached, or paraarticular. Superficial tophi, which tend to involve the ear and the skin overlying Heberden's nodes (nodal gout), appear as clusters of small yellowish or whitish areas that stand out by tensing the skin. Tophaceous deposits are fully preventable with the use of uric acid lowering drugs.

Chronic Gouty Arthritis. The condition results from tophaceous deposits in the synovial membrane, paraarticular bone, and periarticular soft tissues. These tophi must be viewed as potentially destructive lesions as a result of the pressure they exert, plus lytic enzymes released by the surrounding granuloma. The author has been impressed by the change in symptoms that occurs when relapsing gout gives way to chronic, tophaceous, polyarticular gouty synovitis. Morning stiffness appears, joints assume rheumatoid-like deformities such as ulnar deviation of digits, and smoldering pain replaces the acute seizures of early gout. Are these findings reflecting a granulomatous disease of known (MSU crystals) origin that comes to replace the violent neutrophil influx that characterizes acute gout? Chronic gouty arthritis is vastly improved by uric acid lowering agents.

PATIENT 23. A 70-year-old patient was seen for evaluation of chronic arthritis. At age 50 he began to experience recurrent acute arthritis in his ankles, knees, forefeet, and more recently in his wrists and elbows. A diagnosis of gout was made clinically, and individual attacks were treated with p.o. colchicine or NSAIDs. Within the past 10 years joint symptoms have become widespread and persistent, and residual limitation has appeared in his ankles, knees, and wrists. Five years prior to evaluation, subcutaneous nodules were noted in both elbows, joint pain became permanent, and morning stiffness lasting hours developed. Physical examination revealed flexor deformities of MCPs, flexible and fixed swan-neck deformities, marked ulnar deviation of digits (Figure 18–2), hard subcutaneous nodules in the olecranon regions, and effusion, synovial proliferation, and limitation of passive motion at MCPs, wrists, elbows, knees, and ankles. Knees were aspirated at the initial visit, yielding an inflammatory fluid with myriad intra- and extracellular MSU crystals. A small amount of chalky material aspirated from one of the nodules represented a dense suspension of extracellular MSU crystals (Figure 18–1A and B). Hand x-rays revealed cystic changes in carpal bones and metacarpal heads, dense periarticular soft tissues, and a striking lack of periarticular osteopenia. Laboratory results included Hct 36%, ESR 60 mm/1 hour, serum uric acid 10 mg/dl, and serum creatinine 1.3 mg/dl. Urinalysis was normal and a rheumatoid factor test was negative. A diagnosis of chronic tophaceous arthritis was made, and the patient was treated with allopurinol 300 mg per day plus colchicine prophylaxis during the first year. Improvement was slow but steady; within 2 years joint pain was minimal, he no longer felt stiff, and subcutaneous tophi and synovial bulk had drastically decreased.

This case exemplifies chronic tophaceous gout mimicking RA, a situation the author has encountered repeatedly over the years. Rheumatoid-like tophaceous gout should be suspected, along with some rarer conditions, in patients with nodular "RA" and a negative RF test. Chronic tophaceous arthritis can either be prevented or improved with the use of uric acid lowering agents.

Urinary Stones. It is estimated that approximately 40% of gout patients have an associated (preceding or concurrent) urolithiasis. Calcium oxalate stones outnumber uric acid stones by a 4 to 1 ratio. Remember that oxalate stones are radioopaque and uric acid stones are radiolucent. Although

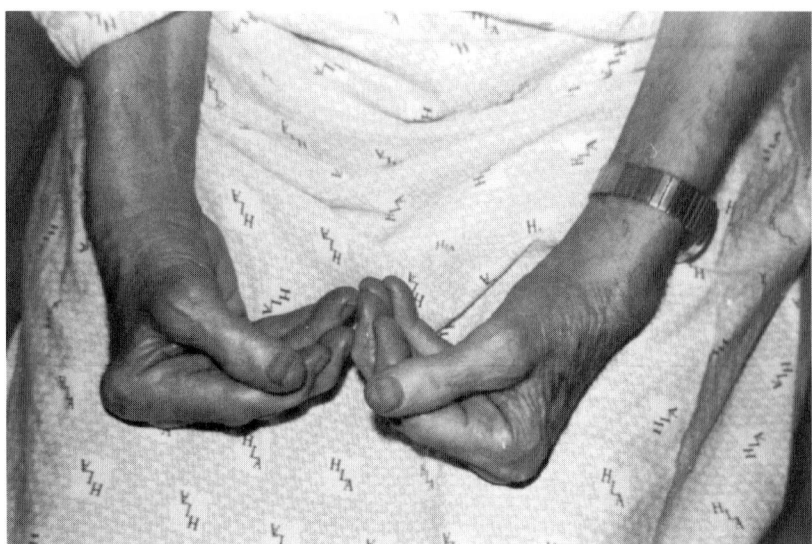

FIGURE 18–2. *Patient 23. Gout.* Pseudorheumatoid deformities. Older patients like this may have a positive rheumatoid factor test on the basis of advanced age. Add to this a subcutaneous tophus (masquerading as a rheumatoid nodule) and the stage is set for a major diagnostic error.

both uric acid hyperexcretors and normoexcretors are at an increased risk of developing calcium oxalate stones, uric acid stones occur predominantly in the hyperexcretor group. Allopurinol is highly effective in preventing urolithiasis in gout patients.

Gouty Nephropathy. Gouty nephropathy is nowadays exceptional, being seen only in late, undiagnosed cases of tophaceous gout. The condition features arterial hypertension, mild proteinuria, and the very slow progression of renal insufficiency. Gouty nephropathy is probably multifactorial including hypertensive nephrosclerosis, urate crystal deposition in the renal medulla leading to chronic inflammation and fibrosis, plus complications of nephrolithiasis. Effective antihypertensive agents and the use of uric acid lowering agents prevent renal damage in gouty patients.

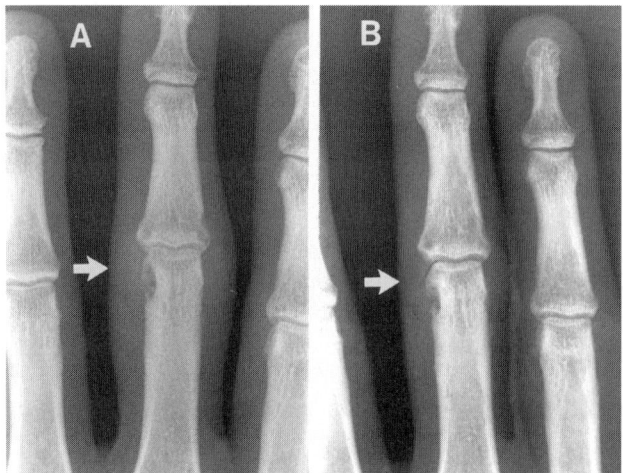

FIGURE 18–3. *Patient 24. Gout.* A, Notice, in the right long finger, high-density paraarticular swelling and a nonmarginal erosion with an overhanging edge (arrow). B, Same digit 2 years after initiation of allopurinol. The paraarticular high-density swelling is gone and the erosion has started to fill.

Cardiovascular Risk. Gout and hyperuricemia associate with an increased risk of coronary artery disease. The association is not causal, that is, excess uric acid damaging the coronary arteries, but represents the added risk of metabolic and cardiovascular concomitants of gout including overweight, excessive alcohol consumption, hyperlipidemia, and arterial hypertension.

Treatment

Methods

Treatment of gout includes two separate issues: the treatment of acute attacks and the treatment of the chronic hyperuricemic state that ultimately terminates recurrent attacks, prevents tophus formation and articular damage, and eliminates the risk of gouty nephropathy.

Treatment of Acute Gout. Host factors such as age and comorbid diseases largely dictate the treatment of acute gout. Principles that apply to all patients, including the oldest and sickest, are be discussed first as follows: (1) Crystal-induced inflammation is dose dependent. Joint aspiration, by removing crystals, fosters recovery. (2) Joint motion aggravates crystal synovitis and joint rest is anti-inflammatory. Consider the use of temporary rest. Bed rest for a day or two is essential in lower extremity gout, and a wrist splint works wonders in wrist gout. (3) Heating the joint increases crystal-induced inflammation and decreasing joint temperature is anti-inflammatory. Consider the use of cold packs. (4) Acute gout is a self-limited condition that fades in a few days to 2 weeks. Trust that the attack will at some point cease. Summing up, if medications cannot be used in a particular patient, aspirate (which will also serve to exclude infection), immobilize, and cool the joint and wait for spontaneous resolution. (5) Acute gout responds dramatically to colchicine; NSAIDs with the exception of aspirin and other salicylates; ACTH; and parenteral or oral corticosteroids. All of these treatment modalities are highly effective in an individual patient.

Colchicine given p.o. 1.2 mg initially and then 0.6 mg each hour until improvement; side effects such as nausea, vomiting, or diarrhea; or a count of 10 pills (total 6 mg) is a time-honored and highly effective treatment of acute gout except it produces diarrhea in over 75% of patients. Nonsteroidal anti-inflammatory agents such as indomethacin 50 mg qid, ibuprofen 800 mg qid, naproxen 500 mg tid, or diclofenac 75 mg bid given for 2 to 3 days and tapered to discontinuation in 3 to 4 additional days are as effective as oral colchicine in acute gout without causing diarrhea.

ACTH 40 units given I.M. or triamcinolone acetonide 60 mg given I.M. repeated the next day if less than 50% improvement occurred are as effective as oral colchicine and NSAIDs and can be given when gastric, renal, cardiac, or hepatic problems or anticoagulation preclude the use of NSAIDs or colchicine. Many clinicians believe that polyarticular gout responds better to ACTH than to other agents. Two or three daily injections may be required until significant improvement is reached. Patients treated with ACTH or glucocorticoids should additionally receive colchicine 0.6 mg bid for 1 month or longer to prevent relapse. Gout in critically ill patients may be treated with conservative measures 1 through 4, plus, if judged safe, ACTH or triamcinolone acetonide as just described, or prednisone 10 mg p.o. per day until termination of the attack.

It may appear odd that I.V. colchicine is being discussed at the end. Intravenous colchicine, which rarely produces diarrhea, when administered imprudently, that is, in too high a dose, in the face of marrow suppression, or in patients with liver or kidney failure, may cause death. In the author's opinion I.V. colchicine treatment is only acceptable when the drug is administered by the physician. The risk of human error is increased when the injection is delegated to others.

With this proviso and given to low-risk patients, the intravenous administration of 2 mg of colchicine diluted in 20 mL of saline through an established intravenous catheter (to avert serious tissue burn) plus 1 mg the next day if response is incomplete to maximum total dose for the attack of 3 mg is an effective way of treating gout. However, I.M. ACTH or triamcinolone acetonide provide the same superior results at a substantially lower risk and should be preferred to I.V. colchicine.

Another modality of treatment purposefully left to the end is the intraarticular injection of corticosteroids. Although in the right setting (a sterile joint) the procedure works well, it is not possible to be *absolutely sure* at the time of injection that the joint is indeed sterile simply because such certainty requires a negative culture result. In the author's opinion, using intraarticular corticosteroids to treat gout is a gamble in which sooner or later the patient (and therefore the physician) will lose. Suppression of recurrent acute gout in an individual without tophi, residual joint inflammation, or findings on x-rays (intercritical gout) may be conveniently achieved with the chronic use of colchicine 0.6 to 1.2 mg per day or maintenance doses of a NSAID. The latter are particularly useful when the patient has a concurrent painful joint condition, such as osteoarthritis of the hip or knee. Chronic acute gout prophylaxis, by eliminating a dramatic clinical indicator of the underlying hyperuricemic state, may create problems of its own as shown in the next case summary.

PATIENT 24. A 45-year-old man was referred for evaluation of possible psoriatic arthritis. Psoriasis had developed at age 32 and was extensive in the extremities. An almost painless joint swelling developed at age 43 involving most MCPs and PIPs. Recently, his right Achilles tendon became thickened and a few episodes of minimally painful posterior tibialis tenosynovitis occurred following intensive tennis playing. Interestingly, the patient had a history of familial Mediterranean fever (FMF) diagnosed at age 20, and he was one of the first patients in the United States to receive colchicine prophylaxis. The FMF was fully suppressed with colchicine 1.2 mg/day, which was continued to the present. Physical examination confirmed the hand and Achilles tendon findings and there was, in addition, painless diffuse thickening at the roof of the left olecranon bursa. It was suspected that the patient had, rather than psoriatic arthritis, silent (suppressed) tophaceous gout. Gout was proven by aspiration of the olecranon bursa. Hand x-rays revealed punched-out erosions overlaid by high-density soft tissue thickening, findings characteristic of gout (Figure 18–3A). Serum uric acid was 10.2 mg/dl. Allopurinol 300 mg per day was added to the colchicine prophylaxis and the psoriasis was treated topically. In the ensuing 4 years all physical findings resolved and there was some filling in of the bone erosions (Figure 18–3B).

Treatment of the Hyperuricemic State (Table 18–3). Similar to the treatment of acute gout there are general measures applicable to all hyperuricemic patients, as follows: (1) Reduce weight to the ideal weight. With successful weight reduction uric acid levels will decrease an average 1 mg/dl. Concurrent hypertriglyceridemia and arterial hypertension will also respond to weight control. Beware of drastic weight reduction programs that result in ketosis and therefore acute hyperuricemia, since wild variations in uric acid levels (such as those induced by ketosis) are a known cause of recurrent gout. (2) Cut down on alcohol consumption. (3) Avoid high-purine foodstuffs such as herring, meat extracts, anchovies, smelts, sweetbreads, liver, and kidneys. Although rarely included in a standard American diet, some of these items may be heavily consumed by certain ethnic groups. Make sure you ask. (4) Discontinue diuretics, if at all possible.

TABLE 18–3

TREATMENT OF INTERVAL GOUT

Identification and correction of predisposing factors
    Elimination of drugs causing hyperuricemia, e.g., thiazides
    Control of alcohol intake
    Gradual weight reduction for obese patients
Restriction of purine-rich food, e.g., liver, kidneys, brains, meat extracts, shellfish
Treatment of individual gout attacks
Colchicine prophylaxis*
    0.6 mg once daily or bid
Serum uric acid lowering therapy
    Those with significant sustained hyperuricemia (> 9 mg/dl) and/or significant hyperuricosuria (> 1000 mg on a regular diet), and gout attacks that interfere with lifestyle
    All patients with interval gout?

*Patients so treated need periodic surveillance for possible silent tophaceous gout.
Modified from Fam AG. Should patients with interval gout be treated with urate lowering drugs? J Rheumatol 22:1621–1623, 1995.

Indications for the use of uric acid lowering agents include frequent attacks of podagra that interfere with the patient's lifestyle, tophaceous gout in the assumption that there are additional joint and visceral tophi that may be inflicting silent damage, persistent joint changes that unchecked lead to bone erosion, and a history of urolithiasis. Serum uric acid levels should be brought well below the saturation point so urate crystals will no longer deposit in tissues. In addition, if allopurinol is used, the urinary uric acid output will be reduced, averting the risk of recurrent urolithiasis.

Basically, two types of uric acid lowering agents are used: uricosurics, such as probenecid and sulfinpyrazone, and allopurinol, an inhibitor of uric acid production. Because probenecid has been used for over 45 years and allopurinol for over 30 years, their relative merits and risks are well known. Probenecid is a weak acid that administered orally twice a day interferes with distal tubular uric acid resorption, causes uricosuria, and decreases serum uric acid levels. To exert its action probenecid requires a nearly normal kidney function. With creatinine levels in excess of 2 mg/dl, or the concomitant use of salicylates, probenecid will not work. Finally, twice a day administration increases the risk of noncompliance. Owing to one or more of these reasons, one in four patients on probenecid fails to achieve the treatment goals. Side effects of probenecid include skin rashes, gastrointestinal intolerance, nephrolithiasis, and rarely hepatic necrosis and proteinuria. As mentioned, because probenecid enhances uric acid excretion, it cannot be used in uric acid hyperexcretors or in patients with a history of kidney stones. Forced hydration and urine alkalinization with sodium bicarbonate 1 g three to four times a day are important in the initial weeks of uricosuric therapy to decrease the chances of precipitating nephrolithiasis. Probenecid is usually started at 250 mg (½ tablet) twice a day, increasing the dose by 500 mg every 2 weeks until uric acid levels are consistently below 6 mg/dl. In some patients this goal will be reached with 1 g per day; others will require 3 g per day. Most patients require 1.5 to 2 g of probenecid per day.

Allopurinol, on the other hand, works as a potent competitive inhibitor of xanthine oxydase, thereby blocking the transformation of hypoxanthine into xanthine, and xanthine into uric acid. Allopurinol halts uric acid production, and at the same time results in a plethora of hypoxanthine and xanthine, which surprisingly have few ill effects. Allopurinol can be used in normoexcretors and hyperexcretors and arguably represents the uric acid lowering agent of choice. Maculopapular rashes develop in about 10% of patients. Allopurinol has the potential to induce, in about 1 per 1000 cases, epidermal necrolysis, exfoliative dermatitis, vasculitis, severe hepatotoxicity, interstitial nephritis, and renal failure. Patients in renal failure or taking ampicillin are particularly prone to developing cutaneous toxicity. Desensitization treatment may be used in patients who develop rashes on allopurinol. The drug should not be tried again in patients who developed more serious side effects.

Remember that both 6-mercaptopurine and azathioprine are metabolized by xanthine oxydase. The half-life of these drugs is prolonged by allopurinol, which enhances both their therapeutic and toxic effects. Thus, patients receiving allopurinol should only receive one-fourth of the 6-mercaptopurine or azathioprine usual dose.

In average risk patients, allopurinol should be started at a reduced dose of 100 mg (single dose) per day reaching the usual 300 mg per day dose by 3 to 4 weeks. Lower doses are used in patients with renal insufficiency, for example, 100 mg/day if the glomerular filtration rate is 30 mL per minute, 200 mg per day if the glomerular filtration rate is about 60 mL per minute, and 300 mg per day if kidney function is normal. Probenecid should be considered in patients who are normoexcretors, have normal or near normal kidney function, and have a negative history for urolithiasis. Allopurinol is the first choice in uric acid hyperexcretors, patients with a history of urinary stones, and with the appropriate dose adjustments in patients with more than mild renal insufficiency.

Since both probenecid and allopurinol are relatively safe, cost and convenience considerations may favor the use of allopurinol over probenecid in the generality of patients. Patients receiving uric acid lowering agents should receive 0.6 to 1.2 mg of p.o. colchicine for about 6 months. Colchicine prophylaxis, even if using reduced doses, is probably unwise in patients with a compromised renal function.

Expected Response

Acute gout responds to treatment within a few hours to 2 days. Response is usually dramatic. Polyarticular gout and gout in severely compromised individuals (such as organ transplant recipients) responds slowly. With allopurinol, uric acid levels decrease within 24 hours and reach a lowest value within 4 to 14 days. Response to probenecid is slow, reaching normal or low uric acid levels in the course of weeks if not months. The concurrent use of allopurinol and probenecid is sometimes needed in truly refractory cases of hyperuricemia. Before adding agents discuss once again compliance, alcohol intake, weight reduction, and reconsider the need of diuretics.

Complications

Complications of therapy occur frequently in the treatment of gout. Untoward effects of colchicine, NSAIDs, allopurinol, and probenecid have already been discussed. Oral colchicine given for long periods of time in patients with some degree of renal failure may be a cause of neuropathy or myopathy. Particularly difficult is the treatment of hyperuricemia in a patient in renal failure who has developed an allergic reaction to allopurinol. Maximal doses of uricosurics may be tried in these patients, in addition to avoiding diuretics and correcting exogenous factors that may be contributing to the hyperuricemia.

When to Refer

It is the rare gout patient who needs rheumatologic referral. There are specific situations when referral is justified: documentation of gout in difficult to aspirate joints, gout with onset below the age of 30, therapeutic guidance in patients with organ failure, treatment of polyarticular gout, and treatment of refractory gout, among others.

Key Points

> **GOUT**
> - Hyperuricemia, acute gout, and chronic tophaceous gout should be clearly distinguished because their health implications differ.
> - Asymptomatic hyperuricemia (except in individuals with a history of urolithiasis) does not require specific evaluation or treatment above and beyond advice on weight reduction, decrease in alcohol intake, and possibly a change in antihypertensive medications.
> - Acute gout may be treated in many different ways. The choice of treatment depends on the patient's age and comorbidity.
> - Medications are not necessarily required for the treatment of acute gout; remember this in situations of multiple organ failures and when severe complications of therapy have already occurred. Nonpharmacologic treatment includes joint aspiration, immobilization, cold packs, and time.
> - Uric acid lowering drugs are considered in patients with frequent acute gout, tophaceous gout (including persistent joint inflammation and bone erosion), and urolithiasis.
> - The choice between probenecid and allopurinol is based on the 24 hour uric acid excretion, adequacy of kidney function, presence or absence of urolithiasis, and cost.
> - Realistically, allopurinol is a more practical drug to use (single dose) and may have far better compliance than uricosurics.
> - After 6 months or 1 year of using a uric acid lowering drug, gout attacks should cease and gross urate deposits should at least partially regress.

Suggested Reading

Axelrod D, Preston S. Comparison of parenteral adrenocorticotropic hormone with oral indomethacin in the treatment of acute gout. Arthritis Rheum 31:803–805, 1988.

Emmerson BT. The management of gout. N Engl J Med 334:445–451, 1996.

Fam AG. Should patients with interval gout be treated with urate lowering drugs? J Rheumatol 22:1621–1623, 1995.

Ferraz MB, O'Brien B. A cost effectiveness analysis of urate lowering drugs in nontophaceous recurrent gouty arthritis. J Rheumatol 22:908–914, 1995.

McCarty DJ. Gout without hyperuricemia. JAMA 271:302–303, 1994.

Siegel LB, Alloway JA, Nashel DJ. Comparison of ACTH and triamcinolone acetonide in the treatment of acute gouty arthritis. J Rheumatol 21:1325–1327, 1994.

Calcium Pyrophosphate Dihydrate (CPPD) Crystal Deposition Disease; Calcium Pyrophosphate Deposition Disease (CPDD)

This condition is characterized by acute attacks of pseudogout, unusual degenerative joint changes, plus the presence of systemic chondrocalcinosis on x-rays (Figure 18–4).

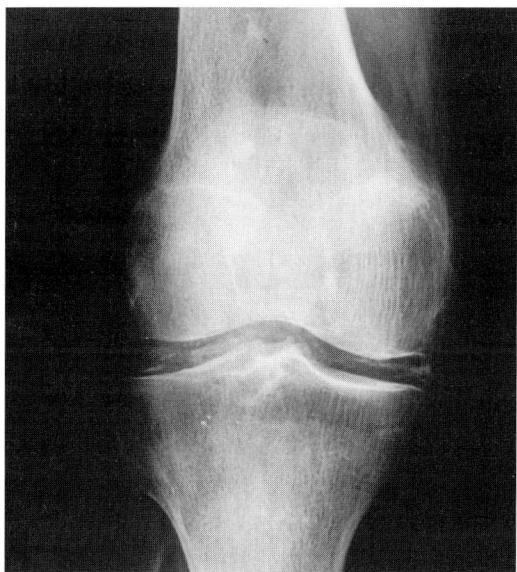

FIGURE 18–4. *CPPD deposition disease.* Right knee of a patient with chondrocalcinosis and recurrent pseudogout attacks. Both menisci are calcified. (Courtesy of Dr. Carlos Pineda, México City.)

Presentation and Progression

Cause

The cause of CPPD crystal deposition in cartilage is in most cases unknown. There are familial forms of the disease that may occur in isolation or with epiphysial dysplasia. An association has been described with osteoarthritis, diabetes, hyperparathyroidism, hypothyroidism (not confirmed epidemiologically), hemochromatosis, renal insufficiency, as well as rare disorders such as Bartter's syndrome and hypophosphatasia (Table 18–4).

Presentation

Calcium pyrophosphate deposition disease may be encountered serendipitously in asymptomatic chondrocalcinosis or may appear under various clinical patterns: acute joint

TABLE 18–4
CONDITIONS ASSOCIATED WITH CALCIUM PYROPHOSPHATE DEPOSITION DISEASE (CPDD)
Aging
Familial/epiphyseal dysplasia
Osteoarthritis
Diabetes
Hyperparathyroidism
Hypothyroidism
Hemochromatosis
Hemosiderosis
Hypomagnesemia
Hypophosphatasia
Bartter's syndrome
Familial hypocalciuric hypercalcemia
Neuropathic joints

inflammation resembling gout (pseudogout); an unusual form of osteoarthritis (OA); a distal chronic polyarthritis mimicking rheumatoid arthritis (RA); a predominantly axial arthropathy resembling ankylosing spondylitis (AS); a rapidly destructive arthropathy, the so-called pseudoneuropathic form of CPPD deposition disease; and in the form of tophaceous deposits, usually in association with articular manifestations of the disease. The prevalence of silent chondrocalcinosis increases with age to a high of 30% in individuals over 75 years old. Fibrocartilage including the knee menisci, the triangular ligament of the wrist, the AC joint meniscus, and the symphysis pubis are most frequently involved. It is believed that chondrocalcinosis alters biomechanical properties of cartilage explaining the accelerated OA seen in some of the patients.

Interestingly, pieces of degenerating calcified cartilage may be released free in the joint cavity closely resembling synovial chondromatosis. However, in the latter there are no evidences of OA or chondrocalcinosis in the involved joint.

Pseudogout attacks resemble gout (hence the name) except that knees, wrists, and elbows are preferentially involved. The first MTP joint is only rarely affected. Also, pseudogout tends to occur in older individuals (usually over 60) whereas gout usually strikes in the 40s. Only about 1 in 5 individuals with chondrocalcinosis ever develops pseudogout. A peculiar pattern of OA associates with chondrocalcinosis. Findings include wrist and hand involvement with narrowing of radiocarpal joints and MCPs 2,3 similar to the changes seen in hemochromatosis. Elbows are often involved, limiting extension. Knee changes in the medial compartment result in genu varum. Calcified menisci degenerate, fissure, and meniscal cysts usually involving the lateral meniscus may occur. The distal, RA-like pattern of CPPD crystal deposition disease may be confusing.

PATIENT 25. A 48-year-old man, a physical education professor, was referred for a second opinion on his rheumatoid arthritis. Two years before, bilateral wrist and MCP synovitis developed followed by painful swelling in both knees. The patient became progressively limited and got around with crutches with difficulty. He had been treated with NSAIDs, most recently indomethacin 200 mg per day, with minimal improvement. Methotrexate treatment was being considered. In the clinic, the patient was unable to climb on the examining table and was therefore examined sitting in his wheelchair. He had florid synovitis in PIPs, MCPs, wrists, elbows, and shoulders with marked limitation of motion in each segment. His neck hurt in all directions of motion, and each motion was limited 50%. Lumbar spine motion appeared normal. Hips adducted and abducted without pain. He had major difficulties in his knees and ankles where pain was so severe that the slightest attempt at weight bearing was impossible. X-rays were reviewed and faint chondrocalcinosis was noted in wrists and knees. With the patient in the sitting position one of his knees was aspirated yielding 10 mL of turbid fluid, which on examination in the polarizing microscope was loaded with intra- and extracellular CPPD crystals. The patient was admitted to the hospital, and 10 mg of prednisone daily plus colchicine 0.6 mg tid were added to the indomethacin. Improvement was slow. By the third day range of motion and isometric exercises were added and the colchicine was reduced to 0.6 mg bid. The patient was discharged home on day 7. The prednisone was phased out over 2 months. The indomethacin was continued at 200 mg per day for 1 month and then reduced by 25 mg per week to 100 mg per day. The colchicine was continued. One year after discharge the patient was working full time as director of a physical education college department.

The pseudospondylitic form of CPDD is rare in the United States, but the author had the privilege of seeing some of Dr. Antonio Reginato's patients in southern Chile. The resemblance with late AS is striking. However, the presence of chondrocalcinosis and evidences of epiphysial dysplasia set these cases apart from AS. The pseudoneuropathic form of CPDD features internal collapse of a joint within a few weeks. This rare form of CPDD resembles fully a Charcot's joint. Tophi composed of CPPD crystals are rarely encountered in CPDD. When they occur, however, the resemblance with gout or RA, depending on the associated arthropathy, gets even closer.

Diagnosis

Summary of Diagnosis

> **CALCIUM PYROPHOSPHATE DEPOSITION DISEASE (CPPD)**
>
> - The condition may be asymptomatic (chondrocalcinosis) or present clinically as acute arthritis (pseudogout), unusual osteoarthritis, rheumatoid-like arthritis, pseudo AS, and a pseudoneuropathic arthropathy. CPPD tophi are rarely present.
> - Chondrocalcinosis is a descriptive radiologic diagnosis that is not confined to the presence of CPPD crystals. Other crystal species, such as basic calcium phosphate and Ca oxalate, may cast similar radiographic findings.
> - Best areas to x-ray include hands (wrists), knees, and pelvis (symphysis pubis).
> - CPPD crystals are short, weakly birefringent, and positively birefringent in contradistinction to MSU crystals that are longer, strongly birefringent, and negatively birefringent.
> - CPPD with onset below age 50 should prompt a metabolic/endocrine evaluation including serum glucose, Fe, ferritin, alkaline phosphatase, Ca, P, Mg, and TSH; between ages 50 and 70, Ca, P, and TSH. Above age 70, none.

Natural History

Expected Outcome

The natural history of CPDD varies with the clinical form. Pseudogout attacks are self-limited. In some patients attacks recur in the same or other joints causing significant morbidity. In most cases, however, CPDD behaves as a slowly progressive degenerative joint condition. Whether acute flares accelerate joint deterioration has not been determined. In the rare pseudoneuropathic form, joint destruction is abrupt.

Treatment

Methods

There is no curative treatment for CPPD crystal chondrocalcinosis. Even in cases secondary to metabolic or endocrine disease (hemochromatosis, hyperparathyroidism), correction of the underlying disorder is not followed by resorption of CPPD deposits. Indeed, parathyroidectomy may be followed by a string of pseudogout attacks. Pseudogout responds well to all treatments that are effective in acute gout. Joint aspiration per se often arrests the inflammatory process, further suggesting that crystal-induced inflammation is a dose-dependent phenomenon. Joint rest, joint aspiration, joint cooling, passage of time, oral colchicine, NSAIDs, ACTH, and parenteral and oral corticosteroids are all efficacious in pseudogout. The first four measures may be used in severely compromised hosts; any of the pharmacologic treatments may be used barring contraindications.

Of the anti-inflammatory agents the author prefers using I.M. ACTH or a NSAID. In addition, clinical experience and the results of a controlled trial have shown that the long-term administration of oral colchicine 0.6 to 1.2 mg per day effectively decreases the frequency of recurrent pseudogout. The same results, with the added benefit of improving osteoarthritic pain, may be obtained with the long-term administration of a NSAID. Different from gout, however, there is no way to deal with the long-term effects of CPPD crystals on cartilage properties and joint biomechanics. Refractory synovitis may be treated successfully by arthroscopic synovectomy. Similarly, meniscal cysts, large crystalline deposits, obstructive osteophytosis, and free cartilaginous bodies may be handled arthroscopically. Prosthetic joint replacements can be successfully inserted in badly damaged joints.

Expected Response

Treatment response in pseudogout is usually rapid, a matter of 1 to 2 days. Suppression of recurrent pseudogout is not an all-or-nothing phenomenon. In the author's experience there is only a decreased frequency of attacks, rather than a halt. Treatment of CPPD crystal-related OA or RA-like illness is along guidelines discussed in the OA chapters, plus the chronic suppression of pseudogout with colchicine and/or a NSAID.

When to Refer

Chondrocalcinosis found serendipitously in an older individual, clinical OA associated with chondrocalcinosis, and pseudogout should be handled by the primary care physician. Early chondrocalcinosis and cases of recurrent pseudogout, OA with osteochondral bodies, pseudo RA, pseudo AS, and the rare destructive arthropathy should have rheumatologic evaluation.

Key Points

CALCIUM PYROPHOSPHATE DIHYDRATE DEPOSITION DISEASE (CPDD)

- CPDD may be primary (older people's condition) or secondary to genetic, metabolic, or endocrine disease.
- Correction of an underlying metabolic/endocrine condition does not help established chondrocalcinosis.
- Parathyroidectomy may be followed by an increased rate of recurrent pseudogout; colchicine prophylaxis should be used in this setting.
- No laboratory marker has been identified in primary CPDD.
- Pseudogout and gout are treated similarly.
- Chronic colchicine or NSAID administration is effective in decreasing the frequency of recurrent pseudogout.
- Arthroscopic synovectomy and debridement should be considered in severely osteoarthritic knees.
- Joint replacement is an effective treatment in end-stage CPPD crystal arthropathy.

Suggested Reading

Doherty M, Dieppe P, Watt I. Pyrophosphate arthropathy: A prospective study. Br J Rheumatol 32:189–196, 1993.

Reginato AJ, Reginato AM, Fernández-Dapica MP, et al. Familial calcium pyrophosphate crystal deposition disease or calcium pyrophosphate gout. Rev Rheum 62:376–391, 1995.

Ryan LM, McCarty DJ. Calcium pyrophosphate crystal deposition disease; pseudogout; articular chondrocalcinosis. In: McCarty DJ, Koopman WJ (eds) Arthritis and Allied Conditions. Lea & Febiger, Philadelphia, 1835–1855, 1993.

Ryan LM, McCarty DJ. Understanding inorganic pyrophosphate metabolism: Toward prevention of calcium pyrophosphate dihydrate crystal deposition. Ann Rheum Dis 54:939–941, 1995.

Sanmarti R, Kanterewicz E, Pladevall M, et al. Analysis of the association between chondrocalcinosis and osteoarthritis: A community based study. Ann Rheum Dis 55:30–33, 1996.

Basic Calcium Phosphate (BCP) Crystal Deposition Disease

For some unknown reason, apatite BCP crystal deposits have a predilection for tendons, ligaments, and fasciae. The crystal species involved are heterogeneous including carbonated-substituted apatite, octacalcium phosphate, tricalcium phosphate or whitlockite, and dicalcium phosphate dihydrate (brushite).

Presentation and Progression

Cause

The cause of BCP crystal deposition is of course unknown. Trauma and overuse may set the ground for calcification. An additional cause may be ischemia, since BCP crystals deposit in a relatively avascular, hypoperfused tendon (see rotator cuff structure in Chapter 25, Shoulder Pain). Presumably, inflammation occurs from crystal phagocytosis and PMN enzyme release. In cases with cortical bone erosion, mononuclear cell phagocytosis of apatite crystals may have resulted in prostaglandin and metalloproteinases release, causing bone resorption.

Presentation

Acute tendinitis is the usual presentation of BCP crystal deposition disease. Typically involved areas include the rotator cuff, the extensor carpi ulnaris and flexor carpi radialis at the wrist, the iliopsoas tendon as it inserts in the lesser tuberosity, and toe tendons (young women's podagra). Paradiaphyseal deposits occur near the linea aspera of the femur and at the lips of the bicipital groove. Free BCP crystals are present in synovial fluid in cases of rotator cuff arthropathy (Milwaukee shoulder) and sometimes in fluids aspirated from OA joints undergoing flare. Finally, BCP crystals cause the capsular calcifications that follow MCP and PIP corticosteroid infiltrations, the subcutaneous and tendon sheath calcifications seen in CREST, and the subcutaneous and fascial calcifications that complicate juvenile dermatomyositis.

Clinically, acute calcific tendinitis causes excruciating pain and transient function loss. Swelling, redness, and exquisite tenderness are characteristically present in acute calcific digital flexor tenosynovitis and over the affected tendons at the wrist. In the shoulder, acute calcific tendinitis causes abrupt, excruciating pain and function loss that depends on the tendon involved. In the hip, acute tendinitis in the iliopsoas tendon may be confused with iliopsoas bursitis and acute arthritis of the coxofemoral joint (maneuvers to differentiate these conditions are discussed under iliopsoas bursitis). A baffling posterior hip pain characterizes acute calcifications at the gluteus magnus insertion in the linea aspera, and upper arm pain in insertional calcifications at the edge of the bicipital groove. In both situations cortical bone erosion may occur, raising the suspicion of malignancy. As mentioned, podagra in a premenopausal woman is usually caused by acute BCP deposition in the soft tissues around the first MTP joint. Radiographically, there is amorphous calcification at the involved tendon or site, and effusion, with or without calcium spillage, may be noted in an adjacent bursa. An unusual condition once in a while encountered is the so-called multicentric calcific tendinitis in which recurrent episodes of calcific periarthritis occur at various sites. Some of these cases are familial. Interestingly, the small BCP crystals do not cast birefringence (remain dark) when the specimen is inspected under polarized light.

Diagnosis

Summary of Diagnosis

> **BASIC CALCIUM PHOSPHATE (BCP) CRYSTAL DEPOSITION DISEASE**
> - The condition may occur in tendons, ligaments, and fasciae.
> - Crystal spillage and inflammation in adjacent bursae is common.
> - Symptoms are acute with severe pain and pain-induced paralysis.
> - Shoulder, wrist, hip, and the great toe are the most frequently involved sites.
> - Podagra in a premenopausal woman is usually due to BCP deposits.
> - X-ray findings include amorphous calcification within a tendon, with or without bursal spillage, or along a ligament or fascia. Bone erosion may occur in paradiaphyseal calcifications.
> - Laboratory findings (except variable leukocytosis and slightly increased ESR) are normal.
> - Polarizing microscopy does not identify BCP crystals. With the Alizarin red stain, BCP crystals may be identified in synovial fluid with the ordinary microscope.

Natural History

Expected Outcome

The process is self-limited, but several days or weeks may elapse before symptoms subside. Rapid control can be achieved with anti-inflammatory agents. Within months to years most amorphous calcifications spontaneously dissolve. Bone erosions adjacent to paradiaphyseal calcifications eventually fill in. Unusually large deposits may persist and chronically obstruct tendon function (such as subacromial impingement). Some cases of acute calcific tendinitis keep recurring, affecting different sites.

Treatment

Methods

Treatment of acute BCP tendinitis is along the lines of the treatment of gout and pseudogout. A temporary sling in supraspinatus calcific tendinitis or a wrist splint in wrist tendinitis afford instant analgesia and favor the effect of anti-inflammatory medications. NSAIDs and ACTH are highly effective medications in BCP tendinitis and should be administered as in acute gout. Colchicine has received little use. Large obstructive calcific masses are less likely to reabsorb spontaneously, and aspiration under fluoroscopic or echographic control may be indicated for pain relief and recovery of function. The aspirated material is thick, resembling toothpaste. Additional instructions for shoulder calcific tendinitis can be found in the section on shoulder tendinitis. Also similar to gout and recurrent pseudogout, recurrent calcific tendinitis may be suppressed with the long-term use of low-dose colchicine or a NSAID.

Expected Response

Response of BCP tendinitis is rapid, usually 1 to 2 days. Disappearance of calcifications takes months to 2 years.

When to Refer

Calcific tendinitis is rarely a reason for referral. The rare multicentric cases should be evaluated by a rheumatologist and a decision should be arrived at regarding chronic colchicine prophylaxis. Large calcific masses should be evaluated by a rheumatologist or an orthopedist for possible aspiration or surgical drainage.

Key Points

> **BASIC CALCIUM PHOSPHATE (BCP) CRYSTAL DEPOSITION DISEASE**
>
> - No underlying metabolic or endocrine problem has been identified.
> - Some recurrent cases are familial.
> - The course of amorphous calcific deposits is to spontaneous resorption in most instances.
> - Large deposits may persist and cause tendon obstruction.
> - Treatment of acute calcific tendinitis is similar to gout.
> - Large deposits may be treated by thick needle aspiration or surgical removal.
> - Recurrent cases may be suppressed with prophylactic doses of colchicine or a NSAID.

Suggested Reading

Fam AG, Rubenstein J. Hydroxyapatite pseudopodagra. Arthritis Rheum 32:741–747, 1989.

Fritz P, Bardin T, Laredo J-D, et al. Paradiaphyseal calcific tendinitis with cortical joint erosion. Arthritis Rheum 37:718–723, 1994.

Halverson PB, McCarty DJ. Basic calcium phosphate (apatite octacalcium phosphate, tricalcium phosphate) crystal deposition diseases. In: McCarty DJ, Koopman WJ (eds) Arthritis and Allied Conditions, 12th ed. Lea & Febiger, Philadelphia, 1857–1872, 1993.

Reginato AJ, Schumacher HR. Apatite crystals in joint fluid; clinical relevance and the search for a simple and accurate diagnostic test. Rheum Rev 3:9–20, 1994.

CHAPTER 19

Infectious Arthritis

In addition to causing the reactive arthritides, microbial agents, whether viruses, bacterias, mycobacterias, fungi, or spirochetes, may directly involve joints.

HIV Infection and Musculoskeletal Disease

Soon after the acquired immunodeficiency syndrome (AIDS) was recognized in 1981, it became apparent that musculoskeletal manifestations of the condition were common (Table 19–1). Another early finding was what appeared to be an increased incidence of reactive arthritis, psoriasis, and psoriatic arthritis. HIV infection shares clinical manifestations with several connective tissue diseases, and many of the initial patients were thought to have SLE or polymyositis. Another confounding feature was the presence of IgG anticardiolipin antibodies in 80% of AIDS patients. Interestingly, both HIV infection and zidovudine treatment may be complicated by myositis. AIDS patients are prone to developing musculoskeletal infections, particularly pyomyositis and musculoskeletal tuberculosis. *M. avium intracellulare* infection resembles Whipple's disease clinically and pathologically. Finally, HIV-infected patients may have coincidental rheumatic disease.

Presentation and Progression

Cause

Arthralgias and myalgias are prominent symptoms in about 20% of symptomatic patients with primary HIV infection. Arthritis, acute articular or bone pain, myositis, Sjögren's syndrome, chronic fatigue, and possibly fibromyalgia may also be caused by HIV infection. It is believed that the increased incidence of reactive arthritis noted in HIV infection is due to a high rate of enteric or chlamydial infections in these patients. Zidovudine causes myositis directly, via a toxic effect. Pyomyositis is more likely to develop in patients who contracted AIDS from parenteral drug use. In contast to the high rate of reactive arthritis (and perhaps psoriatic arthritis) in HIV infection, an amelioration of disease activity was noted in rheumatoid arthritis (RA) patients who subsequently developed AIDS. This finding came in support of the generally accepted view that CD4 cells are prominently involved in RA synovitis and implied that RA and reactive arthritis could involve different disease mechanisms. As further observations accrued, however, the RA-ameliorating effect of HIV infection has been questioned.

Presentation

Patients with HIV infection may present self-limited lower extremities arthritis without additional features of reactive arthritis. Myositis quite similar to polymyositis may appear in patients with AIDS. There is a poorly understood syndrome in which abrupt pain develops in a long bone or a joint that spontaneously resolves in a few hours to 2 days. Laboratory and imaging studies are characteristically normal in these patients. HIV infection may feature Sjögren's syndrome with prominent salivary gland enlargement and extraglandular infiltrates. Different from routine cases of Sjögren's, the condition predominates in males, joints are uninvolved, and anti-Ro/La antibodies are absent. Reactive arthritis, usually preceded by enteric infection and sometimes featuring the Reiter's triad (arthritis, urethritis, conjunctivi-

TABLE 19–1
RHEUMATIC CONDITIONS ASSOCIATED WITH AIDS

CAUSED BY THE HIV INFECTION

Fibromyalgia
Chronic fatigue
Arthritis
Acute arthralgia
Acute long bone pain
Osteonecrosis
Myalgias
Polymyositis
Sjögren's
Vasculitis
Anticardiolipin antibodies

FAVORED BY THE HIV INFECTION

Reactive arthritis (including Reiter's)
Psoriatic arthritis

CAUSED BY THE IMMUNOSUPPRESSION

Septic bursitis
Pyomyositis (usually *S. aureus*)
Septic arthritis
Musculoskeletal tuberculosis
Pseudo-Whipple's (*M. avium*)
Hypertrophic osteoarthropathy (with *P. carinii* pneumonia)

CAUSED BY THE TREATMENT OF THE HIV INFECTION

Zidovudine-associated myopathy

tis), is relatively common in HIV infection. Patients have disabling lower extremities oligoarthritis, Achilles tendinitis, and palmar-plantar keratoderma with pseudopustules and gross desquamation. Close to 80% of Caucasian HIV-infected reactive arthritis patients are HLA-B27 positive. Psoriasis appears to be more frequent in patients with AIDS than in the general population, and the rate of psoriatic arthritis in some series reaches 30%. Psoriasis in HIV infection has an abrupt onset, and disease spectrum ranges from mild plaques to pustular hyperkeratotic disease. It is often difficult in a patient with AIDS to distinguish reactive arthritis with keratoderma from psoriatic arthritis. Zidovudine myositis may be asymptomatic or may cause weakness and enzyme elevation similar to HIV-associated myositis. Sorting out one from the other is at times difficult, and muscle biopsy may be required. HIV- and zidovudine-related myositis may coexist. Pyomyositis features low-grade fever and muscle induration that evolves to suppuration (see soft tissue infections chapter). Musculoskeletal tuberculosis should be suspected any time an HIV-infected patient develops focal spinal pain, protracted pain in an extremity, persistent monoarthritis, or indolent tenosynovitis. Pseudo-Whipple's from *M. avium intracellulare* features encephalitis, chronic diarrhea, and muscle wasting. Intestinal biopsies are identical to Whipple's on light microscopy.

Diagnosis

Summary of Diagnosis

HIV-RELATED MUSCULOSKELETAL CONDITIONS

- A variety of musculoskeletal conditions may occur in HIV infection either caused by the virus itself, the resulting immunosuppression, enteric or genital infections that trigger reactive arthritis, the treatment used, or by chance association.
- Underlying HIV infection should be considered in (1) individuals who are at a greater risk; (2) patients presenting reactive arthritis, abrupt-onset psoriatic arthritis, undiagnosed synovitis, the syndrome of acute bone or articular pain, and male Sjögren's without arthritis or anti-Ro/La; and (3) the presence of findings that could be indicative of AIDS including fever, fatigue, weight loss, and diarrhea; lymphadenopathy; unexplained oral thrush; mollusca contagiosa; unexplained leukopenia or thrombocytopenia; and so on.
- AIDS-related rheumatic disease should be suspected when a known AIDS patient presents pain, synovitis, myopathic weakness, sicca syndrome, mononeuritis multiplex, or leg ulcers.
- Diagnosis of rheumatic disease in HIV-infected patients requires rheumatologic skills plus an informed use of available microbiologic techniques.
- Accuracy in diagnosis is essential to target appropriate treatment, for example, distinguishing HIV-associated polymyositis from zidovudine-induced myopathy.

Natural History

Expected Outcome

Some of the reviewed entities such as HIV-related arthritis and the acute articular or bone pain syndrome are self-limited. The course of reactive arthritis may be self-limited but is often progresive, leading to severe disability.

Treatment

Methods

HIV arthritis may be treated with NSAIDs. Treatment of reactive arthritis is based on the use of a NSAID plus sulfasalazine, leaving methotrexate for the most serious forms as well as for severe psoriatic arthritis. Intraarticular corticosteroid injections should only be used after excluding microbial etiology of arthritis. HIV polymyositis may be treated with prednisone and, if necessary, methotrexate. All potentially immunosuppressive medications should be used in combination with full antiretroviral therapy plus appropriate antibiotic prophylaxis.

Expected Response

Response in HIV-related musculoskeletal conditions varies and is often blurred by progression of the underlying disease.

When to Refer

Rheumatologic consultation should be requested whenever diagnosis is unclear or when response to therapy is less than satisfactory.

Key Points

AIDS-RELATED MUSCULOSKELETAL CONDITIONS

- The AIDS epidemic affects millions of people and a chance association with all of the rheumatic diseases is to be expected.
- Several rheumatic conditions are caused by the HIV virus. There is also an increased rate of reactive arthritis probably as a result of increased exposure to enteric pathogens and chlamydia.
- The immune suppression that goes along with HIV infection makes patients prone to musculoskeletal infections, particularly pyomyositis and tuberculosis.
- Finally, treatment of AIDS with zidovudine is a known cause of myopathy.
- The rate of rheumatic manifestations of HIV has been declining with the generalized use of antiretroviral agents and the practice of safer sex.
- An often mentioned RA-suppressing effect of HIV infection is probably untrue. Aggressive RA often continues in the face of AIDS, implying that CD4 lymphocytes are not essential to produce erosive RA.

Suggested Reading

Calabrese LH. Human immunodeficiency virus (HIV) infection and arthritis. Clin Rheum Dis 19:477–488, 1993.

Espinosa LR. Retrovirus-associated rheumatic syndromes. In: McCarty DJ, Koopman WJ (eds) Arthritis and Allied Conditions. Lea & Febiger, Philadelphia, 2087–2100, 1993.

Viral Arthritis (Other Than HIV)

There are a number of viral arthritides. The condition is usually suspected from the association of an evanescent rash, which may be suggestive of one or another of the known viral exanthemata, plus a transient arthritis. There are, however, viral arthritides that last several weeks or months, and occasionally years. Internal organ involvement is very uncommon.

Presentation and Progression

Cause

Best known viruses causing arthritis include hepatitis B virus, rubella virus and vaccine, parvovirus B-19, occasionally mumps, varicella-zoster virus, Epstein-Barr virus, herpes simplex virus, cytomegalovirus, and hepatitis A virus. In addition, there is the well-known association between hepatitic C virus and Sjögren's syndrome and mixed cryoglobulinemia. Interestingly, in parvovirus B-19 arthritis, HLA-DR4 positive patients tend to have persistent joint symptoms.

Presentation

Hepatitis B arthritis is symmetric or migratory, associates with an urticarial rash, and ceases in 1 to 3 weeks as jaundice develops. Rubella arthritis occurs most commonly in young women following vaccination with attenuated live rubella virus. The arthritis is symmetric, polyarticular, and goes away in a few days to a month. Diagnosis is suggested by the history of recent vaccination, a maculopapular rash initially on the forehead, then spreading to the face and the extremities within the initial 24 hours, and retroauricular and posterior cervical adenopathy first noted in the prodrome. Exceptional cases have been followed by chronic arthritis. Parvovirus arthritis also tends to occur in adults, and the macular rash is indistinct and occurs anywhere, as opposed to the "slapped cheeks" rash seen in children. The arthritis is acute in onset and symmetric, affecting peripheral joints. An acute bilateral carpal tunnel syndrome accompanied by fever and arthralgias is another musculoskeletal manifestation of parvovirus B-19 infection. Acute symptoms improve in about 2 weeks, but arthralgias may continue for a few months. Cases of arthritis that last several years and have a rheumatoid-like appearance have been reported.

Diagnosis

Summary of Diagnosis

> **VIRAL ARTHRITIS**
>
> - Hepatitis B arthritis is usually diagnosed retrospectively once the patient develops jaundice. The condition should be suspected in patients who develop arthritis in association with urticaria.
> - Rubella arthritis is diagnosed based on a history of recent vaccination, the characteristic rash, and the adenopathy.
> - Parvovirus arthritis should be suspected from the association of a rash and RA-like findings. The condition may be confirmed, if needed, by finding anti-parvovirus B19 IgM antibodies.
> - Other viruses only rarely cause arthritis, and diagnosis is made based on the associated findings.

Natural History

Expected Outcome

Most viral arthritides resolve in days or weeks, with the exception of some cases of rubella arthritis and parvovirus arthritis that may go on for years.

Treatment

Methods

Treatment of the viral arthritides is symptomatic.

When to Refer

Most of the viral synovitides are self-limiting, and there is no need or opportunity to refer the patients to a rheumatologist. An exception are cases of prolonged rubella or parvovirus arthritis that occasionally require protracted anti-inflammatory treatment.

Key Points

> **VIRAL ARTHRITIS**
>
> - The condition seldom attains clinical significance.
> - Rubella arthritis and parvovirus arthritis occasionally become chronic.
> - HLA-DR4 positive patients with parvovirus arthritis tend to have protracted symptoms.
> - Treatment of viral arthritis is symptomatic.

Suggested Reading

Fawaz-Estrup F. Human parvovirus infection: Rheumatic manifestations, angioedema, C_1 esterase inhibitor deficiency, ANA positivity, and possible onset of SLE. J Rheumatol 23:1180–1185, 1996.

Gendi NST, Gibson K, Wordsworth BP. Effect of HLA type and hypocomplementemia on the expression of parvovirus arthritis: One year followup of an outbreak. Ann Rheum Dis 55:63–65, 1996.

Naides SJ. Parvovirus B19 infection. Clin Rheum Dis 19:457–475, 1993.

Parsons ME, Russo GG, Millikan LE. Dermatologic disorders associated with viral hepatitis infections. Int J Dermatol 35:77–81, 1996.

Samii K, Cassinotti P, de Freudenreich J, et al. Acute bilateral carpal tunnel syndrome associated with human parvovirus B-19 infection. Clin Infect Dis 22:162–164, 1996.

Bacterial Arthritis

There is a varied clinical presentation to septic involvement of joints. Differences are explained by intrinsic characteristics of the bacteria, mode of infection (hematogenous vs. direct innoculation), anatomy of the joint involved, age of the patient, and presence or absence of immunosuppression.

Presentation and Progression

Cause

Most cases of septic arthritis are infected hematogenously. With some agents, such as *S. aureus, S. pyogenes, S. pneumoniae,* gram negative agents, and anaerobes, only one joint is usually involved. Polyarticular involvement is more likely to occur, with these and other agents, in debilitated or otherwise immunosuppressed individuals. *H. influenzae, meningococcus,* and *N. gonorrhea* infections tend to be polyarticular. Direct innoculation may occur following open trauma including a puncture wound, joint surgery, arthroscopy, intraarticular steroid injection particularly in rheumatoid arthritis patients, or be self-inflicted. Some cases represent extension from nearby infections such as osteomyelitis, abscesses, tenosynovitis, and rarely septic subcutaneous bursitis. In addition, joint prostheses may become infected at the time of insertion or, less frequently, hematogenously. Frequent pathogens involved in prosthetic joint infections include *S. epidermidis, S. aureus,* streptococci, and enteric bacteria. Risk factors for the development of septic arthritis among patients with joint diseases include age over 80, diabetes, rheumatoid arthritis, hip or knee joint replacement, joint surgery, and skin infection.

Presentation

A patient with septic arthritis may or not look septic. Fever is usually present but varies from a mild temperature elevation to a septic fever with shaking chills. In the conscious individual, septic joints are extremely painful. Also, an automatic position is adopted that varies with the joint. Thus, a septic wrist is held in neutral, an elbow in semiflexion, a shoulder in slight abduction, a hip in semiflexion and external rotation, a knee in semiflexion, and an ankle in neutral. Any attempt at changing this position, in which the joint attains its greatest capacity, is met by severe pain. In addition, the joint is swollen, sometimes erythematous, and has an increased temperature on palpation. These external inflammatory signs cannot be demonstrated in the hip or the sacroiliac joint. In a rheumatoid patient, a deteriorating joint while other joints are improving, particularly if this particular joint has been recently infiltrated with corticosteroids, should be considered septic unless proven otherwise by aspiration, gram stain, and culture.

A high index of suspicion is required to diagnose septic arthritis in joints such as the acromioclavicular, sternoclavicular, sacroiliac, manubriosternal, and symphysis pubis. These joints are frequently the target of infection in intravenous drug users (Table 19–2). In this population the risk of HIV infection is high so that unusual agents such as tuberculosis, other mycobacteria, and fungi may be expected. Acromioclavicular and sternoclavicular infection are also more likely to occur in individuals with indwelling subclavian venous catheters. Sternoclavicular joint sepsis occurs predominantly in immunosuppressed individuals including alcoholics, cirrhotics, and patients on chronic hemodialysis. Septic arthritis of the AC joint may have a torpid course; a tender soft tissue bump is usually present, and an AP radiograph is likely to show cortical erosions in both sides of the joint. Sternoclavicular septic arthritis is a treacherous condition because abscess formation is frequent plus the abscesses tend to grow into the superior mediastinum. The author has seen a case in which the abscess reached the pericardium. Also, sternal and clavicular osteomyelitis are almost the rule in sternoclavicular joint septic arthritis.

Sacroiliac septic arthritis characteristically produces buttock and posterior thigh pain. This is a situation in which maneuvers to elicit SI pain really work! The reader is reminded of one: Place the patient on the side, painless side down, and apply firm downward pressure on the iliac crest. Acute SI pain will be elicited.

Needless to say, any patient with an acutely painful joint should have a directed general examination with particular attention to fundi, skin, oral cavity, heart, and genitalia. Any red, raised lesion should be closely looked at for vesicle or pustule formation, which if present would make the case suspicious of gonococcal arthritis. Ecchymoses and palpable purpura are frequent in meningococcemia (which may not feature meningitis) (Table 19–3). Concurrent tenosynovitis usually indicates gonococcal, meningococcal, and *H. influenzae* infection.

TABLE 19–2

MUSCULOSKELETAL MICROBIAL INFECTION IN INTRAVENOUS DRUG USERS

Coexistence with HIV infection in many cases
Soft tissues
   Septic bursitis: protracted course
   Necrotizing fasciitis (group A streptococci; *S. aureus*): acute, severe disease (see soft tissue infections)
   Pyomyositis (*S. aureus*)
Joints and bones
   Gram negative bacterial arthritis (often polyarticular; involvement of unusual joints such as acromioclavicular, sternoclavicular, manubriosternal, sacroiliac, symphysis pubis); *S. aureus;* group A streptococci.

PATIENT 26. A 34-year-old woman came to the emergency room complaining of fever, rash, and arthritis. Three days before she had a transient sore throat. Since then she felt poorly, developed a fever, and had two shaking chills. Temperature was 39° C and BP 130/80. No pustular lesions were present, and the patient was sexually inactive. Her throat was red. There was an erythematous/hemorrhagic rash with single elements from 5 mm to 2 cm and partial coalescence on her knees and ankles. Knees and right wrist were swollen and painful, and there was angry tenosynovitis in her right wrist and both ankles. Left knee and right wrist aspirates contained 10,000 and 8,500 WBC/mm^3, respectively, with high neutrofilia and a negative gram stain. Right knee yielded purulent fluid with intracellular gram negative diplococci on gram stain. The clinical suspicion of meningococcemia with septic arthritis was proven by throat culture, blood culture, and right knee SF culture. The patient had uneventful recovery with intravenous ceftriaxone and serial joint aspirations.

It should be reemphasized that gonococcal and meningococcal arthritis may be quite similar. Look for petechial and ecchymotic lesions that would make a diagnosis of meningococcemia more likely.

Diagnosis of septic arthritis requires aspiration of the joint and adequate handling of the specimen. Treating presumed septic arthritis (based on a positive blood culture) without aspiration or other form of joint drainage is a serious mistake. Technical aspects of joint aspiration are given in the appendix. Attempts at obtaining joint fluid should not be timid. A large-bore needle, #18 or larger, should be used because purulent fluid may clog a narrower needle. Dry taps are not acceptable except when intraarticular placement of the needle has been proven. In some joints such as the hip, shoulder, and sacroiliac joint, such an assurance may require fluoroscopy and the instillation of a nonbacteriostatic solution which, if drawn back, provides proof of intraarticular location as well as a sample for study. Alternatively, a small amount of urografin may be instilled in the joint. Fluid obtained should be submitted for cell count and differential, aerobic and anaerobic culture, and crystal analysis. A request for fungal and *M. tuberculosis* cultures should be added in immunosuppressed individuals.

Blood cultures should be obtained in all suspected cases of septic arthritis; occasionally SF cultures will be negative and blood cultures positive, allowing a targeted treatment. Synovial fluid glucose and lactate determination have limited value and are not worth requesting. In suspected cases of gonococcal infection, SF should be directly plated on agar chocolate and the dish hand-carried to the laboratory. In all other instances the needle should be discarded, the syringe capped with a sterile rubber cap, and the specimen promptly brought to the laboratory for aerobic and anaerobic culture. Therapeutic decisions can often be made based on the results of a gram stain. Needless to say, the staining procedure should be flawless, and an experienced observer, and preferably more than one if the initial reading is negative, should read the slide.

Joint prosthesis infection has become less frequent as a result of a more careful preoperative evaluation, improved operating room discipline, and a more rapid performance of the procedures. However, there is still a 1% rate of deep infections. Postoperative infections are classified as stage I infections, which include the classic fulminant postoperative infection, the infected hematoma, and the superficial infection that will progress to a deep infection; stage II infections occur between 6 and 24 months after the arthroplasty; and stage III infections, which occur hematogenously 2 or more years after the surgical procedure.

Postoperative infection is suggested by mounting pain and a raising ESR or CRP. In aseptic loosening the ESR and the CRP are normal in patients without concurrent inflammatory disease such as RA or neoplasia. Faced with a patient with pain at the site of a prosthesis, x-rays, ESR, and CRP should be obtained. If the ESR or the CRP are increased and the x-rays show periosteal elevation, infection is virtually diagnosed. If the ESR or the CRP are elevated and the x-rays only show loosening, an indium-111-labeled autologous WBC scintigraphy should be obtained. A positive scan is diagnostic of infection. The next step is to identify the agent. This may be achieved by arthrography and aspiration using both aerobic and anaerobic media, or by a limited open biopsy. Currently most infections are due to *S. epidermidis*, followed by *S. aureus*, a variety of gram positive and gram negative bacterias, anaerobes, and very rarely fungi and mycobacterias.

Diagnosis

Summary of Diagnosis

TABLE 19–3
MENINGOCOCCAL ARTHRITIS

1. Purulent arthritis*†
   Monoarthritis, purulent SF; positive SF culture
2. Gonococcal-like arthritis*†
   Polyarthritis
   Tenosynovitis
   Rash: maculopapular, petechial, or purpuric
   Variable SF; culture positive or negative
3. Chronic meningococcemia†
   Palpable purpura
   Migratory oligo- or polyarthritis
   Episcleritis
   Leg edema
   Blood cultures positive

*Abrupt onset.
†In patients over 24 years old, associated immune defect is common (complement deficiency, HIV, SLE, corticosteroid use, etc.).

SEPTIC ARTHRITIS

- Joint sepsis may be suspected from the acuteness of the arthritis, the circumstances of development, and associated findings.
- A history of exposure and a possible portal of entry (such as a skin infection) add some weight to the hypothesis, but a negative history should not detract from considering septic arthritis.
- The patient should be thoroughly examined with particular attention paid to skin (pustular lesions, petechiae, needle marks) and genitalia.
- Suspicion of septic arthritis implies aspiration of the joint for WBC and differential, gram stain, and appropriate cultures.
- Blood cultures should be routinely obtained.
- Dry taps are not acceptable in the investigation of septic arthritis.
- Initial x-rays will show articular and periarticular swelling plus any preexistent joint changes.
- Infected arthroplasties increase the ESR and/or CRP. If one or both of these tests were abnormal, perform an indium-111-labeled WBC scan. If this test is positive, proceed with arthrography and aspiration or, as a last resort, a limited bone biopsy.

Natural History

Expected Outcome

Left untreated, septic arthritis has a well-known destructive course. Within 1 to 2 weeks joint cartilage will be totally degraded and lost forever. This is why it makes such a big difference to begin treatment as soon as possible. Bone infection will next occur, initially in pockets, leading to total destruction of the joint. Cases that go on to ankylosis may attain a spontaneous cure. Infected prostheses produce unbearable pain and are a source of septicemia. Even with current treatment the estimated fatality rate of nongonococcal septic arthritis reaches 10% to 25%.

Treatment

Methods

Therapy of septic arthritis involves the already discussed measures to arrive at a bacteriologic diagnosis, joint drainage, the administration of parenteral antibiotics, and physical measures that will help in fighting infection and minimizing muscle atrophy.

Joint Drainage: The reasons why joint drainage is essential in septic arthritis are many. Drainage removes proteolytic enzymes released by leukocytes, viable and dying PMNs capable of eliciting further enzymatic damage, cytokines, and bacterias. In addition, joint drainage decreases intraarticular pressure, thus improving synovial microcirculation, enhancing antibiotic penetration, allowing further range of motion to the joint, and decreasing muscle inhibition.

Joint drainage may be achieved by needle aspiration, a distension-irrigation apparatus, a cannula inserted under echo or CT guidance, arthroscopy, or arthrotomy. Each of these procedures has advantages and disadvantages. There are advocates of one or another of these techniques, but no formal comparative studies have been done of needle aspiration versus other methods to assess their relative worth. However, there is general agreement that knee infections which are recent and not loculated should be drained daily or twice daily by needle aspiration.

Needle drainage is simple, inexpensive, and provides a sample that may be studied with cell counts and serial cultures, allowing an ongoing assessment of treatment. On the other hand, neglected infections, suspected loculation, and cases that for one or another reason do not appear to be responding to needle aspirations should be lavaged through a large-bore needle (tidal lavage), arthroscoped, or subject to arthrotomy. Again, there are no formal studies comparing tidal lavage with the much more expensive arthroscopy, or arthroscopy with open drainage. Of the latter two, arthroscopy makes better sense because a lesser incision will interfere less with joint rehabilitation. There are joints that by virtue of their anatomy are not amenable to needle or tidal drainage. These include hip, shoulder, acromioclavicular, sternoclavicular, and sacroiliac joints.

Although the author is aware that pediatric cases of hip septic arthritis have responded well to catheter drainage placed under fluoroscopic or echo control, it appears safer to go ahead with surgical drainage. Infected prosthetic joints should be debrided including removal of the prosthesis.

Parenteral Antibiotic Treatment: In addition to drainage, patients should be placed immediately on parenteral antibiotics according to the most likely pathogen. This is of course facilitated by the findings on gram stain and if this showed no bacteria, by the likely source of infection. For instance, in a patient who recently had sexual intercourse with an unknown partner, has some pustular lesions on the skin, and does not appear to have another reason to get a joint infection, treatment for disseminated gonococcal infection alone is appropriate. In contrast, in a parenteral drug user (and therefore a likely HIV carrier), a variety of agents causing septic arthritis must be considered, in particular *S. aureus,* streptococci, and pseudomonas infection, and antibiotic coverage should address these possibilities. An interesting setting is the patient who has had recurrent joint and soft tissue infections with a variety of agents. A factitious infection must be considered with repeated self-injection of the joint using saliva, feces, or other contaminated material.

An issue frequently raised when dealing with a joint infection is the adequacy of synovial penetration of the antibiotic at hand. Indeed, all antibiotics attain excellent synovial fluid levels. The intraarticular administration of antibiotics is totally out of fashion. It is generally agreed that, with the exception of gonococcal arthritis, at least 3 weeks of parenteral antibiotics is needed.

Physical Measures: A joint splint is initially necessary to relieve pain. In the knee and elbow joints, which when acutely inflamed spontaneously adopt a flexed position, placing too much emphasis early on on extension may so increase intraarticular pressures as to result in ischemic damage and suboptimal antibiotic penetration. Of course, as inflammation decreases and some extension can be gained, the splint should be modified to parallel this gain. In joints such as the wrist and ankle (or subtalar), a splint in neutral is optimal.

Joint splintage is not synonymous with 24 hour immobility. The splint should be removed two to three times daily for passive range of motion exercises within the limits of tolerable pain. This motion is essential to allow cartilage to pick up nutrients and get rid of waste products (remember that cartilage nourishes itself by diffusion from SF and that the squeezing provided by joint motion moves fluid in and out the collagen/proteoglycan cushion meshwork). The use of a continuous passive motion machine, which helps in experimental septic arthritis, has not been formally tested in humans, but its use makes sense. As soon as volume of effusion is less and the joint (the knee in this case) can be extended, isometric quadriceps exercises should be started. Isometric contractions may be poor initially, for the vastus medialis becomes quite feeble within a week. However, with supervision, stronger and stronger contractions will be achieved and rehabilitation of the joint will be less troublesome. Once the acute findings have subsided (it may take 1 to 2 weeks), the exercise program may be stepped up.

Treatment of an Infected Prosthesis: There are three possible avenues to handle this problem. One is a two-stage procedure in which the prosthesis is resected, the patient is treated at least 4 weeks with an appropriate antibiotic, and another prosthesis is inserted a year later. The second is to resect the original prosthesis and reinsert a new prosthesis during the same procedure using an antibiotic-impregnated cement. The third is not to remove the prosthesis, but to treat with suppressive antibiotics, usually rifampin plus a fluoroquinolone, for a minimum of 6 months.

Expected Response

With the outlined program, assuming proper identification of the bacteria and antibiotic sensitivity, a nonimmunosuppressed host, and initiation of therapy within a few days of onset, an excellent treatment response can be anticipated. Response to treatment in septic arthritis is slow. Sterilization of SF is usually achieved in 3 to 5 days. Sometime during this period the SF WBC count will start to decrease, and if glucose has been measured, an steady increase in SF glucose will be noted. As the joint improves, effusion will decrease, reflex muscle inhibition will be less, and further motion will be gained. If, as treatment proceeds, difficulties are noted in fully draining the joint, fevers recur, WBCs become erratic, and SF cultures remain positive for more than 5 days, a failure of needle drainage should be declared and another mode of drainage should be tried.

The standard procedure at this time would be to go ahead with arthroscopic debridement. Others would use open surgery. Tidal lavage deserves a trial before arthroscopy is performed. Delayed improvement in septic arthritis risks permanent cartilage damage and the prospect of postinfectious osteoarthritis. Most patients with an infected prosthesis can be handled well with either the two-stage or the one-stage procedure using antibiotic-impregnated cement. The former procedure, which is over 90% successful, is the one most frequently used in the United States. However, it is extremely inconvenient to patients, who have to be on crutches for 1 year between procedures. The one-stage procedure has gained acceptance in Europe and has a success rate of close to 90%. The third procedure may be used in patients who cannot sustain another surgical procedure; early results are encouraging.

When to Refer

Septic arthritis, or the possibility of septic arthritis, is handled infrequently by primary care physicians; it is a relatively frequent problem in a rheumatology, orthopedic, or infectious disease practice. With the exception of cases of gonococcal arthritis, which rarely presents logistic problems, these patients should be transferred to specialized care. Needless to say, all patients with suspected septic arthritis should be hospitalized for evaluation and treatment. Septic arthritis in accessible joints that can be effectively drained, knee, ankle, and elbow, should be handled by rheumatologists with an input from infectious diseases. Infections in other joints—shoulder, wrist, AC, sternoclavicular, sacroiliac, and hip—should definitely be handled by an orthopedist with input from an infectious disease specialist.

Key Points

> **SEPTIC ARTHRITIS**
>
> - Risk factors for septic arthritis include age greater than 80, diabetes mellitus, rheumatoid arthritis, a prosthetic hip or knee, joint surgery, and skin infection.
> - Untreated, septic arthritis destroys the joint. Treated late (5 days or more after onset of symptoms), it frequently causes postinfectious DJD. The rate of joint damage after nongonococcal septic arthritis is 25% to 50%.
> - The estimated mortality rate of nongonococcal septic arthritis is 10% to 25%.
> - Thus, be thorough but move fast, implementing treatment early.
> - An infected joint must be effectively drained by needle aspiration, tidal lavage, arthroscopy, or arthrotomy.
> - All antibiotics have an excellent joint penetration.
> - Septic joints should be both rested and exercised to decrease pain, improve cartilage nutrition, and decrease long-term disability.
> - Infection complicates about 1% of hip or knee prostheses. Microbiologic documentation is cumbersome but essential for good results.
> - Treatment of prosthetic joint infection is difficult, implying in most cases removal of the hardware and insertion of another prosthesis either in two stages 1 year apart or in one stage using antibiotic-impregnated cement.

Suggested Reading

Fitzgerald RH Jr. Infected total hip arthroplasty: Diagnosis and treatment. J Am Acad Orthop Surg 3:249–262, 1995.

Goldenberg D. Bacterial arthritis. In: Kelley WN, Harris ED, Ruddy S, et al. (eds) Textbook of Rheumatology, 4th ed. W.B. Saunders, Philadelphia, 1449–1466, 1993.

Kaandorp CJE, van Schaardenburg, Krijnen P, et al. Risk factors for septic arthritis in patients with joint disease. Arthritis Rheum 38:1819–1825, 1995.

Mikhail IS, Alarcón G. Nongonococcal bacterial arthritis. Clin Rheum Dis 19:311–329, 1993.

Stephens DS, Hajjeh RA, Baughman WS, et al. Sporadic meningococcal disease in adults: Results of a 5-year population-based study. Ann Intern Med 123:937–940, 1995.

Gonococcal Arthritis

Gonococcal arthritis differs from all other etiologies of septic arthritis in that its course is rapidly halted by antibiotic treatment. Two forms of presentation of gonococcal arthritis are often mentioned: a purulent monoarthritis and the dermatitis/arthritis syndrome. In the light of recent molecular studies, these clinical forms clearly represent the extremes of a continuum rather than different entities.

Presentation and Progression

Cause

Gonococcal arthritis results from hematogenous seeding of one or more joints from a primary site in the urethra, pharynx, or rectum. In patients with purulent gonococcal monoarthritis, synovial fluid (SF) cultures often grow *N. gonorrhoeae* and blood cultures are usually negative. In contrast, in patients with the dermatitis/arthritis syndrome, blood cultures are often positive whereas SF cultures are almost regularly negative. The recent finding of gonococcal DNA in SF of patients with dermatitis/arthritis syndrome supports the view that synovial infection rather than immune complex disease accounts for the joint findings in the dermatitis/arthritis syndrome.

Presentation

Gonococcal arthritis is an acute condition of sexually active young adults that features fever, malaise, and articular and tenosynovial inflammation. Clinical evidence of urethral, cervix, rectal, or pharyngeal gonorrhea is present in a minority of patients. In women the condition tends to develop in the perimenstrual period. On examination, a few pustular lesions may be present in the skin of the extremities and/or trunk, strongly supporting the diagnosis. Florid tenosynovitis occurs in over 75% of patients, and one or more of the painful joints may contain an effusion. Joint aspirates vary from an almost normal SF to a frankly purulent effusion in which intracellular gram negative cocci may be found.

Diagnosis

Summary of Diagnosis

> **GONOCOCCAL ARTHRITIS**
> - Usually in a young adult; close proximity to menses in women.
> - Arthritis, tenosynovitis, pustular skin lesions.
> - Differential diagnosis includes meningococcemia, reactive arthritis, secondary syphilis, hepatitis B prodrome, acute rheumatic fever, and microbial endocarditis.
> - Obtain blood, urethral, cervical, anal, and throat cultures.
> - Aspirate effused joints. Synovial fluid varies from mildly inflammatory to purulent.
> - Purulent fluids are likely to show *N. gonorrhoeae* on gram stain and culture.
> - Consider chlamydial coinfection in all cases.

Natural History

Expected Outcome

Untreated gonococcal arthritis may lead to joint destruction.

Treatment

Methods

Patients with a significantly joint effusion, particularly if SF is purulent and bacteria are not visualized on gram stain, should be admitted to the hospital to assess early response to therapy and also because some of the cases will be meningococcal. Milder cases may be treated on an outpatient basis. Treatment response is so rapid in gonococcal arthritis that additional measures such as serial splints, daily joint aspirations, and physiotherapy seldom apply. Exceptions include rare cases that have a slow resolution and cases with an associated reactive arthritis. The treatment of choice in gonococcal arthritis is ceftriaxone 1 g I.M. daily until symptoms improve followed by ciprofloxacin 500 mg p.o. bid to complete 1 week of therapy. Doxycycline 100 mg p.o. bid for 1 week or azithromycin 1 g orally once should be added for the treatment of possible concomitant chlamydial infection.

Expected Response

Response of gonococcal arthritis is rapid, usually within 48 hours. Very rarely, purulent gonococcal arthritis follows a very slow resolution. If cultures are negative and no features of reactive arthritis are present, such as mucosal, cutaneous, or enthesitic changes, these effusions represent postinfectious synovitis triggered by residual bacterial products. These effusions are self-limited but may take several weeks to go away. The extremely rare cases with persistent infection may require arthroscopic or surgical drainage.

When to Refer

Routine cases of gonococcal arthritis may be treated by primary care physicians. Rheumatology consultation should be sought in cases that tend to linger as well as in cases developing additional manifestations which suggest reactive arthritis.

Key Points

> **GONOCOCCAL ARTHRITIS**
> - The most common form of arthritis in sexually active young males and females.
> - Diagnosis is suggested by the association of arthritis, tenosynovitis, and pustular skin lesions.
> - Coexistent *Chlamydia trachomatis* infection may result in a superimposed or subsequent reactive arthritis.
> - Gonococcal arthritis dramatically improves within 48 hours of initiation of therapy. Different from other etiologies of bacterial arthritis, only 1 week of antibiotics is required.
> - Treatment of possible coexistent chlamydial infection is indicated.
> - Persistent synovitis may indicate postinfectious synovitis, an associated reactive arthritis, or persistent infection.

Suggested Reading

Brandt KD, Cathcart ES, Cohen AS. Gonococcal arthritis: Clinical features correlated with blood, synovial fluid and genitourinary cultures. Arthritis Rheum 17:503–510, 1974.

Liebling MR, Arkfeld DG, Michelini GA, et al. Identification of Neisseria gonorrhoeae in synovial fluid using the polymerase chain reaction. Arthritis Rheum 37:710–717, 1994.

Scopelitis E, Martínez-Osuna P. Gonococcal arthritis. Clin Rheum Dis 19:363–377, 1993.

Mycobacterial and Fungal Arthritis

Both mycobacterial and fungal synovitis may present as a chronic destructive monoarthritis or as a chronic proliferative tenosynovitis. In addition, *M. tuberculosis* causes a particularly destructive form of spinal osteomyelitis. Finally, certain fungal conditions are close mimickers of acute sarcoidosis.

Presentation and Progression

Cause

Tuberculous synovitis, whether affecting a joint or a tendon sheath, occurs by hematogenous seeding. Caseating granulomas seen on biopsy are characteristic but not pathognomonic for this agent because a similar lesion may be caused by atypical mycobacterias and fungal agents such as *H. capsulatum*, *C. immitis*, blastomyces, and *Sporotrix schenkii*.

Presentation

Tuberculous infection is a leading cause of chronic monoarthritis. There is a long differential to this condition. Fever and weight loss are frequent concomitants. Different from other forms of septic arthritis, radiographic studies are helpful in articular tuberculosis. Findings include soft tissue swelling with little in the way of periosteal reaction, joint space narrowing, subchondral erosions in both sides of the joint, and paraarticular bone cysts. Synovial fluid findings in tuberculous arthritis are inflammatory but otherwise nonspecific. Gram stains and routine cultures are negative. The fluorochrome stain (auramine-rhodamine) is a simple and sensitive method to detect acid-fast organisms under a 100 × dry objective and can be readily used in SF. The nite blue stain is similarly useful to locate acid-fast material on joint biopsies but, like the fluorochrome, is not specific for *M. tuberculosis*. The classic Ziehl-Neelsen stain is subject to many variables, and small numbers of bacteria may not be readily identified. Cultures for *M. tuberculosis* in the Lowenstein-Jensen medium take about 2 weeks to grow, although at 1 week mycobacteria may be identified using nucleic acid probe/gas-liquid chromatography. A positive fluorochrome or nite blue stain is sufficient evidence to start treatment, however, pending culture results. The rare cases of fungal synovitis will not be missed if fungal cultures on a Sabouraud agar slant are requested as well. A negative reading for tuberculosis requires 60 days and for fungi 45 days.

Proliferative tenosynovitis is another leading manifestation of infection by *M. tuberculosis*, atypical mycobacterias, in particular *M. marinum*, and fungi such as *Sporotrix schenkii*. Additional cases of chronic tenosynovitis are discussed Part IV. Diagnosis in proliferative tenosynovitis is at the time of tenosynovectomy, which is often done without previous knowledge of the etiology of the process, leading to the appropriate antiinfectious treatment.

Spinal tuberculosis is the third great syndrome in musculoskeletal tuberculosis. The most frequently affected segment is the upper lumbar, in which one vertebra or several contiguous vertebrae may be involved. Bone rarefaction is a key finding and usually involves an anterosuperior or anteroinferior wedge. Rarefaction of vertebral endplates is followed by loss of intervertebral disc height. Granulomatous and caseous material beneath the anterior longitudinal ligament, in the soft tissues anterior and lateral to the spine in a fusiform fashion, or under the iliopsoas fascia emerging in the groin (cold abscesses) are characteristic features of the condition. Multiple vertebrae may be involved. Late in spinal tuberculosis the collapsing wedge results in kyphosis.

Diagnosis

Summary of Diagnosis

> **MYCOBACTERIAL AND FUNGAL MUSCULOSKELETAL INFECTIONS**
>
> - *M. tuberculosis* causes chronic monoarthritis, chronic proliferative tenosynovitis, and spinal osteomyelitis. Atypical mycobacteria and fungal infection may cause chronic arthritis and proliferative tenosynovitis.
> - The PPD is usually positive in musculoskeletal tuberculosis including 75% of cases that occur in HIV-infected patients. Malnutrition is a contributing cause of a false negative PPD in these patients.
> - Lytic bone lesions present on initial x-rays should raise the possibility of *M. tuberculosis* infection.
> - SF is inflammatory but otherwise nonspecific in *M. tuberculosis* and fungal infection.
> - Diagnosis of tuberculous and fungal arthritis is based on fluorochrome and other stains of joint aspirate plus arthroscopic synovial biopsy for histology, nite blue stain, PAS stain, and mycobacterial and fungal culture. Identification of acid-fast bacteria with a fluorochrome technique is quite useful in the tentative diagnosis of mycobacterial infection.
> - Diagnosis of mycobacterial (usually atypical mycobacterias) and fungal tenosynovitis is usually post hoc during evaluation of a tenosynovectomy specimen.
> - Diagnosis of tuberculous spinal osteomyelitis requires spinal needle biopsy for histology, nite blue stain, and mycobacterial culture.

Natural History

Expected Outcome

Musculoskeletal infection with *M. tuberculosis* and fungi is highly destructive long term. In spinal osteomyelitis, vertebral collapse typically leads to sharp thoracolumbar kyphosis.

Treatment

Methods

Treatment of musculoskeletal tuberculosis includes chemotherapy, a complex subject beyond the scope of this book, plus local measures that depend on the involved structure. In peripheral joint synovitis, as in other causes of microbial arthritis, drainage may be performed by needle aspiration, but extensive proliferation is best treated by arthroscopy or surgical synovectomy. Proliferative tenosynovitis usually requires tenosynovectomy. In spinal tuberculosis, treatment is conservative except in the following: marked neurologic deficit or neurologic deficit progressing despite adequate chemotherapy; progression of kyphosis or instability despite adequate chemotherapy; and large abscesses interfering with respiration. If an operation is needed, decompression should be combined with arthrodesis. Similar considerations on systemic and local treatment apply to fungal arthritis and tenosynovitis.

When to Refer

Suspected cases of tuberculosis or fungal arthritis should be referred to a rheumatologist, who in conjunction with an infectious disease specialist and an orthopedic surgeon will plan subsequent evaluation and therapy.

Key Points

> **MYCOBACTERIAL AND FUNGAL MUSCULOSKELETAL INFECTION**
> - Chronic knee or hip arthritis and proliferative tenosynovitis, particularly if bone erosion is present, should raise the suspicion of mycobacterial (usually *M. tuberculosis*) or fungal infection.
> - Protracted back pain and stiffness, anterior erosive changes in one or more adjacent vertebrae, plus evidence of perivertebral or psoas abscess formation strongly suggests tuberculous osteomyelitis.
> - Identification of the etiologic agent and treatment decisions require specialized advice.
> - A positive fluorochrome stain is very useful to initiate treatment pending culture results.
> - If the diagnosis is correct, chemotherapy is tailored to the case, and required orthopedic measures are implemented. Treatment results in musculoskeletal mycobacterial and fungal infections are satisfactory.

Suggested Reading

Medical Research Council of the United Kingdom. Ninth Report of the Working Party on Tuberculosis of the Spine. A 10 year assessment of controlled trials of inpatient and outpatient treatment and of plaster-of-Paris jackets for tuberculosis of the spine in children on standard chemotherapy. J Bone Joint Surg 67B:103–110, 1985.

Mondal A. Cytological diagnosis of vertebral tuberculosis with fine-needle aspiration biopsy. J Bone Joint Surg 76A:181–184, 1994.

Watts HG, Lifeso RM. Tuberculosis of bones and joints. J Bone Joint Surg 78A:288–298, 1996.

Lyme Borreliosis

Few conditions have generated the concern and controversy of Lyme borreliosis. Main issues have been the prevalence of seronegative disease and optimal duration of therapy. Primary care physicians are often asked by patients or patients' parents to obtain Lyme serologies that are unwarranted both on clinical and epidemiologic grounds. Under these circumstances only false positives may be expected. Because a positive enzyme-linked immunosorbent assay (ELISA) test or an immunofluorescence test are hard to argue against, patients with all sorts of conditions, particularly fibromyalgia, will solicit and end up receiving one or more antibiotic courses. These patients obviously fail to improve, and the usual reaction is to put the blame on insufficient, rather than inappropriate, treatment.

Presentation and Progression

Cause

Lyme borreliosis is a tick-borne disease caused by *B. burgdorferi*, a spirochete. Transmission of *B. burgdorferi* requires a suitable tick vector (Ixodes scapularis in the eastern and central United States and Ixodes pacificus in the Pacific Northwest) and a reservoir animal host. Because the infected larva molts into a nymph in the spring and the nymph is the most likely tick stage to attack humans, most early cases of Lyme borreliosis occur in May through July. Geographically, Lyme borreliosis parallels the distribution of the preferred reservoir for adult ticks, the white-tail deer population. In the United States, Lyme borreliosis risk is highest along natural wooded, brushy, or grassy areas in Massachusetts, Connecticut, Rhode Island, New York, New Jersey, Pennsylvania, Maryland, Delaware, Wisconsin, Minnesota, Michigan, and Northern California. There are also wide endemic areas in Europe and Asia as well as sporadic reports from Australia, Africa, Mexico, Brazil, and Chile. In the last three countries, however, *B. burgdorferi* has not yet been isolated.

Presentation

It is useful to divide *B. burgdorferi* infection into three stages: early localized infection, or stage 1; early disseminated infection, or stage 2; and late persistent infection, or stage 3 (Table 19–4). In stage 1 erythema migrans (EM) occurring in the summer months in a known endemic area for Lyme borreliosis is diagnostic. The CDC description of EM cannot be improved on:

> Erythema migrans is defined as a skin lesion that typically begins as a red macule or papule and expands over a period of days to weeks to form a large round lesion, often with partial central clearing. A solitary lesion must reach at least 5 cm in size. Secondary lesions may also occur. Annular erythematous lesions occurring within several hours of a tick bite represent hypersensitivity reactions and do not qualify as erythema migrans. In most patients EM is accompanied by other acute symptoms, particularly fatigue, fever, headache, mild stiff neck, arthralgia, or myalgia. These symptoms are intermittent.

Erythema migrans develops 3 to 32 days (mean, 7 days) after the tick bite. Untreated, EM resolves in several weeks. Patients with EM may be treated so early in the disease that serologic tests are and will remain negative. Interestingly, borrelia may persist in protected niches and result years later in seronegative CNS disease or arthritis. In the generality of cases, however, serologic tests are or will become positive weeks after treatment. It is important to stress that EM is missing, but not the general symptoms, in 25% of patients with early disease.

Stage 2 occurs a few days to weeks after the onset of EM as spirochetes disseminate to multiple organ systems. As a result there are general symptoms as well as skin, central and peripheral nervous system, heart, and joint manifestations. Dissemination causes a flu-like syndrome that includes malaise, fever, chills, arthralgias, myalgias, headaches, photophobia, a stiff neck, anorexia, epigastric pain, and nausea. Secondary skin lesions, which appear in 50% of patients, include evanescent maculae, urticarial rashes, a malar rash, and the rare lymphocytoma, which is a brown or violaceous nodule in the nipple or earlobe. Early neurologic manifestations, present in 15% to 20%, include meningitis, encephalitis, facial palsy, or radiculoneuropathy. Lyme meningitis may wax and wane over several months featuring lymphocytic pleocytosis. Encephalitis is usually subtle. Facial palsy, the most frequent cranial neuropathy, is bilateral in about 25% of cases. The peripheral neuropathy is an asymmetric motor, sensory, or mixed radiculoneuropathy. A peripheral neuropathy may be present as well. Cardiac manifestations occur in 4% to 8% of patients with stage 2 disease. A self-limited fluctuating atrioventricular block is the most frequent manifestation. Even complete heart block seldom lasts more than 1 week. Severe carditis is very rare. Articular manifestations in stage 2 disease consist of a palindromic arthritis that lasts hours to a few days in a given joint and migrates from joint to joint without leaving residuals. Joint effusions or marked swelling are rare. Manifestations of stage 2 disease subside, even in untreated patients, over a period of several weeks to months.

Stage 3 disease may feature arthritis, neurologic disease, and cutaneous manifestations a mean of 6 months after disease onset. Lyme arthritis is typically an intermittent oligoarthritis affecting with predilection the knee. Episodes last days to several weeks, and large effusions are frequent. With each passing year, 10% to 20% of patients cease having arthritis. In 10% of stage 3 patients with joint manifestations, chronic Lyme arthritis develops. The synovium is highly inflammatory, and joint erosions may develop leading to permanent joint damage. Even in these long-term cases arthritis eventually subsides.

Neurologic findings in stage 3 disease may be quite disturbing. Peripheral neuropathy is predominantly sensory with waxing and waning paresthesias or subtle dysesthesias and only rarely muscle weakness. By EMG the findings are consistent with an axonal sensorimotor polyradiculoneuropathy. Patients may also feature a subacute encephalopathy featuring irritability, sleep disturbance, depression, subtle language abnormalities, selective memory impairment, and hearing loss. Fibromyalgia may occur as an unusual manifestation of neuroborreliosis. CSF findings include mild elevation of protein and evidence of intrathecal production of Lyme-specific antibodies. MRI studies sometimes show small hyperintense areas. Documentation of intrathecal production of Lyme antibodies helps distinguish Lyme disease from other causes of diffuse encephalic disease. Acrodermatitis chronica atrophicans is a late cutaneous change of Lyme borreliosis in which the skin at acral sites becomes atrophic, cigarette paper thin. The condition is rare in the United States but frequent in Europe.

Diagnosis of Lyme borreliosis is clinically based on epidemiologic considerations, consistent symptoms and findings, plus a borderline or positive ELISA test confirmed by Western blot analysis (Table 19–5). Early disease is diagnosed based on exposure, the correct time of the year, and the presence of ECM at a time in which the antibody response has just been mounted. This explains an initial negative ELISA test in over 50% of stage 1 cases. In most of these cases a repeated ELISA 4 to 6 weeks later will be positive.

Immunoglobulin M antibodies reach their peak between the third and sixth week after disease onset and IgG antibodies are highest months or years later. Diagnostic documentation is feasible by borrelia culture of a skin biopsy (4–7 mm punch) obtained at the edge of an EM lesion. Because these cultures require several weeks and are expensive, they are mainly used for research. In disseminated or late disease, IgG antibodies can be demonstrated in over 90% of cases. Titers are particularly high in patients with arthritis. Because of the high false positive rate of ELISA and immunofluorescence assays, Western blotting is now required for confirmation. Demonstration of intrathecal production of Lyme antibodies settles the diagnosis of CNS borreliosis. Unfortunately, different from European cases, this is a rare finding in American cases. *B. burgdorferi* DNA can now be demonstrated in tissue samples, SF, and CSF by the polymerase chain reaction (PCR). This is a cum-

---

TABLE 19–4
CLINICAL MANIFESTATIONS OF LYME BORRELIOSIS

STAGE 1

Erythema migrans (absent in 25% of cases)
Regional lymphadenopathy
Minor constitutional symptoms

STAGE 2

Headache, fever, chills, mild stiff neck, migratory arthralgias, profound malaise,* fatigue*
Secondary annular skin lesions, lymphocytoma (common in Europe, rare in United States)
Meningitis,† encephalitis, facial palsy,† motor and sensory radiculoneuropathy,† mononeuritis multiplex, chorea, myelitis; lymphocytic pleocytosis of about 100/m³; elevated CSF protein
Atrioventricular block, acute myopericarditis, LV dysfunction, cardiomegaly, pancarditis
Migratory arthralgias

STAGE 3

Intermittent oligoarthritis affecting knees (chronic arthritis in some patients)
Encephalopathy, axonal polyneuropathy, leukoencephalitis
Acrodermatitis chronica atrophicans (common in Europe, rare in United States)

*Constant.
†Tend to occur in cluster.

TABLE 19–5

CAVEATS IN LABORATORY DIAGNOSIS OF LYME DISEASE

CULTURE

Only positive on biopsies taken from the advancing edge of EM
Low yield
Expensive

TISSUE STAINS

Artifacts may appear as borrelias

IMMUNOFLUORESCENCE

Too many false positives

ENZYME-LINKED IMMUNOSORBENT ASSAY (ELISA)

Needs interlaboratory standardization
False positives in *T. denticola* peridontal infection, JRA, RA, SLE, infectious mononucleosis, SBE, Rocky Mountain spotted fever, syphilis (Lyme antibodies result in positive treponemal tests but are negative on VDRL)
Negative in 50% of EM cases*
Often positive after cure of the disease
May be negative in late CNS disease

WESTERN BLOTTING

More sensitive and specific than ELISA
Required to sort out borderline and positive ELISA results

T-CELL PROLIFERATIVE ASSAY

Poor reproducibility
Expensive
Specific marker of exposure
May be used in the diagnosis of seronegative CNS disease

POLYMERASE CHAIN REACTION (PCR)

May have false positives due to contamination
Expensive
Important in diagnosis of seronegative CNS and joint disease

*If documentation of Lyme borreliosis is needed, a second sample may be tested 4 to 6 weeks later.

bersome and expensive test that implies DNA extraction from the specimen, PCR amplification, agarose gel electrophoresis, and DNA probe hybridization. PCR studies should be reserved for cases of possible CNS Lyme borreliosis and for research. Proliferative assays are useful in the diagnosis of seronegative CNS Lyme borreliosis as long as they are performed in a reliable laboratory. Pitfalls in the laboratory diagnosis of Lyme borreliosis are listed in Table 19–5.

Diagnosis

Summary of Diagnosis

LYME BORRELIOSIS

- Exposure in an endemic area, early summer, and a typical lesion of ECM are diagnostic of early Lyme disease.
- ELISA demonstration of IgG and IgM antibodies only becomes possible several weeks after the onset of ECM.
- Because of a high rate of false positives, ELISA or immunofluorescence positivity is valid only when confirmed by a positive Western blot assay.
- Proliferative T-cell assays, which are used mainly to diagnose seronegative CNS Lyme disease, have had inconsistent results and remain a research tool.
- PCR demonstration of *B. burgdorferi* DNA, mainly a research tool, may be used clinically in suspected cases of Lyme CNS involvement and in suspected chronic Lyme arthritis.

Natural History

Expected Outcome

Most manifestations of Lyme borreliosis are self-limited in the untreated patient. A small proportion of late arthritis cases become chronic (particularly in patients with the histocompatibility complex allel HLA-DR4) and may result in permanent joint damage. Even in these cases arthritis eventually dies down. The course of untreated Lyme encephalitis is not well characterized.

Treatment

Methods

Prevention measures are listed in Table 19–6. Treatment of early Lyme borreliosis is with doxycycline 100 mg orally bid or amoxicillin 500 mg orally qid for 10 days to 1 month depending on severity of illness and treatment response. Neurologic disease is treated with I.V. ceftriaxone 2 g/day for 2 weeks in early disease and for 4 weeks in late disease. Facial palsy, cardiac abnormalities, and intermittent arthritis respond well to oral regimes for 30 days. Late disease arthritis may be treated orally with doxycycline or amoxicillin for 1 month. Chronic

TABLE 19–6

LYME DISEASE PREVENTION RECOMMENDATIONS (PARTICULARLY IMPORTANT BETWEEN THE MONTHS OF MAY AND SEPTEMBER)

1. Most important is the avoidance of tick vector (avoid tall grass and ground cover).
2. Wear closed shoes; tuck pants under socks or shoes; wear long-sleeved shirt; use light-colored clothes to spot ticks more easily.
3. Inspect skin carefully (including hair) upon returning indoors.
4. Inspect children frequently after they have been outdoors.
5. Check pets as they come indoors.
6. Use insect repellants.
7. Promptly remove ticks with tweezers (infection is unusual with less than 36 hour attachment).
8. Place tick in a jar and bring to your doctor or health department for identification.
9. The issue of antibiotic prophylaxis of tick bites cannot be clearly answered. In areas with a high infection rate in tick nymphs, such as in the Northeast (10%–50%), it is probably better to treat. In areas with a low rate, such as in California (1%–3%), it is not.

arthritis may be treated with ceftriaxone 2g/day for 2 to 4 weeks, but treatment often fails in these cases.

Expected Response

EM lesions resolve within days. Fatigue, headaches, and arthralgias may persist 1 or 2 weeks. Persistence of symptoms for several weeks, or recurrence of symptoms, usually indicates treatment failure. Late Lyme arthritis takes 1 to 3 months to resolve. Interestingly, a substantial number of patients with late arthritis who responded to oral antibiotics subsequently developed neuroborreliosis. Treatment of early disease may prevent Lyme antibody formation, but cellular immunity to Lyme antigens will usually be positive. Some of these patients do progress to seronegative stage 3 disease. Antibiotic treatment of early seropositive disease may result in negativization, but positive titers often persist. Some of these patients go on to develop late disease. Thus, there is evidence that viable *B. burgdorferi* organisms may persist in secluded areas with or without eliciting an antibody response, with a potential to result in seropositive or seronegative late disease.

When to Refer

Early disease should be treated by primary care physicians. Cases of late disease, or when diagnosis is in question, should be referred to a rheumatologist or infectious disease specialist with expertise in Lyme borreliosis.

Key Points

> **LYME BORRELIOSIS**
> - Diagnosis of early Lyme borreliosis is clinical.
> - Early disseminated disease and late disease may be suspected clinically, but a positive ELISA or immunofluorescence test confirmed by Western blot is required for diagnosis.
> - Diagnosis of late Lyme CNS disease and chronic Lyme arthritis requires familiarity with the late manifestations of the disease as well as studies of cellular immunity, intrathecal production of Lyme antibodies, and demonstration of borrelial DNA by PCR.
> - An imprudent interpretation of a positive ELISA or immunofluorescence test has resulted in countless needless treatments for Lyme borreliosis.

Suggested Reading

Centers for Disease Control. Proceedings of the Second National Conference on Serologic Diagnosis of Lyme Disease. Association of State and Territorial Public Health Laboratory Directors. Washington, DC, 1–111, 1994.

Kalish R. Lyme disease. Clin Rheum Dis 19:399–426, 1993.

Magnarelli LA. Current status of laboratory diagnosis for Lyme disease. Am J Med (suppl 4A)98:10S–12S, 1995.

Steere AC, Levin RE, Molloy PJ, et al. Treatment of Lyme arthritis. Arthritis Rheum 37:878–888, 1994.

Syphilis

Treponema pallidum infection may result in several musculoskeletal conditions. Periostitis causes pain and increased radiographic bone density and may lead in disseminated cases to confusion with osteopetrosis. In late disease, the sensory changes of tabes dorsalis may lead to a neuropathic joint, usually in the knee. More common and more relevant from a general medicine standpoint is the polyarthritis that often occurs in secondary syphilis. The present discussion is limited to rheumatologic aspects of secondary syphilis.

Presentation and Progression

Cause

Synovitis in secondary syphilis results from hematogenous synovial seeding.

Presentation

The typical patient with syphilitic synovitis presents with a subacute oligo- or polyarthritis, often with tenosynovitis involving PIPs, MCPs, knee, or ankles. Pain is minimal. Additional manifestations of secondary syphilis, that is, generalized lymphadenopathy, a nonpruritic papulosquamous rash, mucous plaques in mouth, throat, or perigenital area (condyloma lata), indicate the true nature of the condition. Synovial fluid aspirates reveal mildly inflammatory fluids with WBC counts ranging from 4,000 to 30,000 per mm^3 with about 50% of PMN cells. Spirochetes should be looked for by immunofluorescence.

An unusual presentation has been polyarthralgias and the acute onset of bilateral sternoclavicular pain, noted in two patients in Reginato's series. Leukopenia, thrombocytopenia, and low-titer ANA may be present, particularly in HIV-infected patients, suggesting SLE. Finally, there is potential for confusion with Lyme borreliosis. In Lyme, however, the rash and the articular manifestations are completely different and should not suggest secondary syphilis. If this error occurred, a positive treponemal test for syphilis may be found but the VDRL would be negative. Because the sequence of testing in syphilis is (1) VDRL, and (2) a treponemal test, the latter situation should not arise.

Diagnosis

Summary of Diagnosis

> **SYPHILITIC ARTHRITIS**
> - Subacute or chronic nonmigratory oligo- or polyarthritis.
> - Tenosynovitis, osteitis.
> - Concurrent papulosquamous rash.
> - Concurrent oral or perigenital mucous plaques.
> - Moth-eaten, patchy alopecia in some patients.
> - Lymphadenopathy.
> - Moderately inflammatory synovial fluid.
> - Obtain VDRL and a treponemal test.
> - Potential confusion with SLE, particularly in cases with concurrent HIV infection.

Natural History

Expected Outcome

The condition is fully reversible with the treatment of secondary syphilis.

Treatment

Methods

They parallel current treatment of secondary syphilis.

Complications

A Herxheimer reaction may occur following penicillin treatment.

When to Refer

A clinically ambiguous situation would call for rheumatologic consultation. A correct diagnosis by the primary care physician based on the lymphadenopathy, the rash, the orogenital lesions, plus a history of a chancre, would lead to immediate treatment and the rapid cure of the patient, including the synovitis.

Key Points

> **SYPHILITIC SYNOVITIS**
>
> - Syphilitic synovitis should be suspected in all patients with a subacute or chronic oligo- or polyarthritis.
> - A thorough physical examination looking for adenopathy, skin lesions, and orogenital lesions would provide strong diagnostic clues.
> - Confusion with SLE may occur, particularly in cases with concurrent HIV infection.
> - There should be no confusion with Lyme borreliosis.
> - Penicillin treatment rapidly cures syphilitic synovitis.

Suggested Reading

Burgoyne M, Agudelo C, Pisko E. Chronic syphilitic polyarthritis mimicking systemic lupus erythematosus/rheumatoid arthritis as the initial presentation of human immunodeficiency virus infection. J Rheumatol 19:313–315, 1992.

Reginato AJ, Schumacher HR, Jiménez S, et al. Synovitis in secondary syphilis. Clinical, light, and electron microscopic studies. Arthritis Rheum 22:170–176, 1979.

Skillrud DM, Bunch TW. Secondary syphilis mimicking systemic lupus erythematosus. Arthritis Rheum 26:1529–1531, 1983.

CHAPTER 20

Osteoarthritis

Osteoarthritis, a degenerative disease of cartilage with secondary changes in bone, is the most prevalent rheumatic disease worldwide. Radiographic evidence of OA is present in most people by the age of 65 and in 80% by the age of 75 or over. Many joints may be affected, such as the distal interphalangeal joints (DIPs), or just a few in particular, such as the hip and the knee. Because OA is present in most older people, and because most older people complain of joint pain, an unfortunate tendency exists to blame OA for any ache or pain they have. However, pain in a patient with OA may be caused by a number of conditions other than OA. For instance, fibromyalgia has its greatest prevalence in individuals 50 to 75 years old, polymyalgia rheumatica is an old-age disease, and RA and lupus may begin in old age.

Leaving aside systemic conditions and focusing on a patient with a painful, obviously osteoarthritic joint, the following questions should be asked: (1) Are there soft tissue problems contributing to, or explaining, the pain? (2) Does the pain have a remote origin (e.g., spinal disease causing deep pain or radicular pain)? (3) Is a concurrent joint condition causing, or adding to, the symptoms (e.g., a ruptured meniscus, bacterial infection, or crystal-induced synovitis)?

Mechanical, genetic, metabolic/endocrine, and age-related factors play a pathogenetic role in osteoarthritis. Overuse of a joint such as the added load placed on the knee or hip by obesity or a decreased contact surface (increased load per surface unit) from osteonecrosis or bone erosion clearly cause osteoarthritis. Genetic factors include mutations in the collagen type II gene seen in familial osteoarthritis and mutations in the collagen type X gene in some osteochondrodysplasias. Metabolic conditions such as calcium pyrophosphate dihydrate (CPPD) deposition disease and ochronosis and endocrine conditions such as acromegaly result in an altered cartilage that is prone to wear out.

Finally, aging per se may be a contributory factor, since with advancing age articular cartilage becomes increasingly susceptible to fatigue failure. Grossly, osteoarthritic cartilage first swells and then frays, ulcerates, and wears, exposing bare bone. Histologically there is fissuring, chondrocyte proliferation (clones), and proteoglycan depletion (proteoglycans are hydrophilic macromolecules that soak up water, distend the type II collagen network, and give cartilage its turgescence). Turnover studies, however, show an increased synthesis of proteoglycans that is insufficient to keep up with the loss. As a secondary phenomenon bone proliferates at the joint margins presumably to restrict motion, increase stability, and protect the damaged joint. Another secondary phenomenon is synovial inflammation. Lymphocytic infiltrates and synovial proliferation are prominent in the vicinity of the most damaged area of the joint. Radiographically, osteoarthritic joint space narrowing is typically uneven within a given joint, as a result of cartilage loss. Subchondral bone sclerosis and marginal osteophytes sooner or later appear. Well-demarcated subchondral cysts are also characteristic of OA.

Hand Osteoarthritis

The hand is frequently affected by OA (Table 20–1). Sites of predilection for this lesion include the DIP joints (Heberden's nodes), PIP joints (Bouchard's nodes), and first carpometacarpal joint (Figure 20–1). The MCP joints are only affected in patients with chondrocalcinosis, hemochromatosis, and diabetes and in certain epiphysial dysplasias.

Presentation and Progression

Cause

A role of mechanical factors in hand OA is suggested by an increased frequency and severity of lesions in the dominant hand. Indeed, manual workers with various repetitive tasks seem to damage specific hand joints. Thus, cottonmill workers required to use fine pincer grip had more DIP OA than workers involved in power grip. However, there are odd locations of Heberden's nodes (e.g., in the ulnar digits), and in familial osteoarthritis all digits are involved. Interestingly, overweight not only increases the risk of hip and knee OA but of hand OA

TABLE 20–1

THE AMERICAN COLLEGE OF RHEUMATOLOGY CRITERIA FOR THE CLASSIFICATION AND REPORTING OF OSTEOARTHRITIS OF THE HAND

Hand pain, aching, or stiffness and 3 or 4 of the following items:
  Hard tissue enlargement of 2 or more of 10 selected joints*
  Hard tissue enlargement of 2 or more DIP joints
  Fewer than 3 swollen MCP joints
  Deformity of at least 1 of 10 selected joints*

*The 10 selected joints are the second and third distal interphalangeal (DIP), the second and third proximal interphalangeal, and the first carpometacarpal joints of both hands. This classification method yields a sensitivity of 94% and a specificity of 87%. MCP = metacarpophalangeal.

From Altman R, Alarcón G, Applerouth D, et al. The American College of Rheumatology criteria for the classification and reporting of osteoarthritis of the hand. Arthritis Rheum 33:1601–1610, 1990.

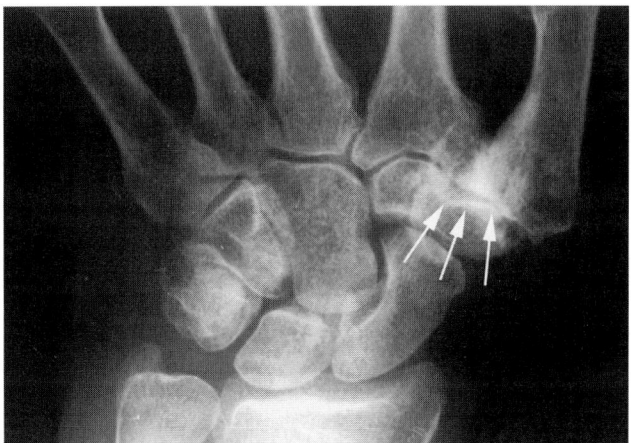

FIGURE 20–1. *Osteoarthritis.* Detail of hand x-rays in a 67-year-old woman with a "square hand" and bulky swelling at the base of the thumb. There is sclerosis of the articulation between the trapezius and the first metacarpal, the trapezius and trapezoid, and the first intermetacarpal joint.

as well, a finding that suggests the existence of systemic factors leading to cartilage breakdown. Heberden's nodes often associate with tibiofemoral osteoarthritis. They may also appear in isolation in hereditary forms of the disease, following trauma, and as a result of soft tissue contracture.

Presentation

The chief symptom in hand osteoarthritis is pain. Involved joints become exquisitely sensitive to an unexpected knock, however subtle. Different from other joints, early DIP (and sometimes PIP) OA features remarkable inflammation. Bony knobs known as Heberden's nodes at the DIPs and Bouchard's nodes at the PIPs as well as flexor deformity subsequently develop. Next most frequently involved is the first carpometacarpal (CMC) joint causing pain at the base of the thumb. Patients with first CMC OA complain of a weak grip, and a joint effusion may be present. Pressure at the joint line in the anatomic snuffbox is exquisitely tender. The typical deformity of first CMC joint OA is the "square hand" in which the osteophytic joint projects out off the radial wrist. De Quervain's tenosynovitis, radiocarpal osteoarthritis, the carpal tunnel syndrome, and distal compression of the superficial branch of the radial nerve (bracelet syndrome) must be distinguished from this condition. There is a useful maneuver to determine that pain originates at the first CMC joint: Hold the patient's thumb and press the metacarpal, while applying to it torque motions, against the trapezius: Bone grinding and pain certify the presence of first CMC osteoarthritis. However, two or more conditions that cause radial wrist pain may coexist.

Less Typical Presentations

Beware of inactive Heberden's nodes that suddenly flare: Late inflammation (as opposed to early inflammation, which is caused by osteoarthritis) should raise the suspicion of superimposed MSU gout, the so-called nodal gout. The same applies to the first MTP, only that in this joint one may be dealing with CPPD pseudogout as well as MSU gout.

Chapter 20 • Osteoarthritis

Diagnosis

Summary of Diagnosis

> **HAND OSTEOARTHRITIS**
> - Hand osteoarthritis includes Heberden's nodes (DIPs), Bouchard's nodes (PIPs), and first CMC OA.
> - Early Heberden's nodes are characteristically inflammatory. Late lesions are bony knobs.
> - Late inflammation of Heberden's nodes suggest gout (nodal gout).
> - Bouchard's nodes cause pain and flexor deformity of the joint, weakening grip.
> - First CMC OA causes the "square hand" deformity and a painful and weak grip.
> - Hand x-rays.
> - CBC, ESR, creatinine, serum uric acid.

Natural History

Expected Outcome

Heberden's nodes, after months of redness and sometimes extreme tenderness, settle down as painless, cold bony knobs. Involvement of several or all digits may be synchronous; in other patients one or two fingers are affected at a time, with some DIPs quieting down as others become inflamed. The dominant hand is the one most affected. Past the initial painful stage, Heberden's nodes pose minimal functional impairment (DIP flexor deformity is not disadvantageous for most people). Severe PIP osteoarthritis, however, not only causes a flexor deformity but significantly limits finger flexion, thus taxing power grip and fine-tuned finger motion. First CMC osteoarthritis causes significant pain, weakens grip, and drastically limits hand function.

Complications

Mucinous pseudocysts (described with ganglia) sometimes complicate DIP osteoarthritis. Another frequent complication, particularly in older women with renal failure, hypertension, or cardiac failure who are chronically receiving diuretic agents, is the previously described nodal gout. Important hand disability may result from PIP and first CMC osteoarthritis. Finally, there may be considerable disfiguration from the condition, particularly in early-expressed familial cases. Although little can be done to prevent deformity, something can be done to correct it in the appropriate patient, as is discussed later.

Treatment

Methods

Patients with hand OA should be given the hand exercises described in the appendix. A paraffin tank (that the patient may purchase if it proves effective in the occupational therapy office) or alternating warm and cold baths are often helpful as well as cost effective in painful OA involving the hand. Acetaminophen 4 g per day is almost as good as NSAIDs for the control of osteoarthritic pain with minimal risk to the patient.

Should acetaminophen not work, low doses of ibuprofen such as 400 mg qid, nabumetone 1 to 1.5 g per day, or a nonacetylated salicylate may be used. The addition of capsaicin may forestall the need for full doses of a NSAID. Full doses of a NSAID are often problematic past the age of 65 because of an increased risk of gastric, renal, cardiovascular (arterial hypertension), and CNS toxicity. Concurrent misoprostol therapy appears to be cost effective in these patients. Corticosteroid injections, which are quite difficult to administer in DIP joints, may be very effective in suppressing inflammation. PIP and first CMC injections are much easier to perform (see the appendix) but still require the skills of a rheumatologist, a hand surgeon, or a general orthopedist.

Expected Response

With the use of analgesics and NSAIDs, painful DIPs joints improve but seldom become fully asymptomatic. Skillfully performed corticosteroid infiltrations (the steroid placed inside rather than about the joint) may at least temporarily eliminate PIP and DIP pain. First CMC joints improve, often dramatically and for several months at a time, following corticosteroid infiltration. Rapid recurrence of pain is an indication for orthopedic referral.

Complications

Complications of therapy are the ones expected in individuals taking NSAIDs (see section on NSAIDs). Abuse of intraarticular corticosteroid infiltrations may result in capsular calcification, joint instability, and destructive arthropathy.

When to Refer

Patients with acute DIP inflammation should be referred to a rheumatologist to evaluate the possibility of superimposed gout. Also, patients with painful DIPs, PIPs, and first CMC joints resistant to NSAIDs should be referred for possible corticosteroid infiltration. There are patients with DIP OA in whom serious joint instability develops. These joints may be fused, and results are excellent. Also, gross Heberden's nodes causing disfiguration may be surgically rimmed and the joint fused, with excellent cosmetic results. Severe PIP OA causes severe dysfunction: a painful and incomplete grip. If MCP function is normal, fusion of the PIP in slight flexion terminates pain and improves hand function. There are several surgical procedures available for the first CMC joint with excellent results. In contrast, prosthetic first CMC and PIP joints have had poor results including rupture of the prosthesis, subluxation, and deformity. Needless to say, referral to a skilled hand surgeon is essential for good results. Rheumatologists work closely with hand surgeons and can provide crucial advice on surgical referral.

Key Points

> **HAND OSTEOARTHRITIS**
> - The course of Heberden's nodes is spontaneous regression of inflammation.
> - Bouchard's nodes often result in flexor deformity of the digit.
> - Bouchard's nodes and first CMC OA may be quite painful and cause hand disability.
> - Treatment of hand OA includes hand exercises, non-opioid analgesics, NSAIDs, and intraarticular corticosteroid infiltrations.
> - Hand surgeon referral should be obtained for patients with painful PIP and first CMC OA unrelieved with conservative therapy, and, if requested by the patient, for the cosmetic correction of Heberden's nodes.

Suggested Reading

Egger P, Cooper C, Hart DJ, et al. Patterns of joint involvement in osteoarthritis of the hand: The Chingford study. J Rheumatol 22:1509–1513, 1995.

Fam AG, Stein J, Rubenstein J. Gouty arthritis in nodal osteoarthritis. J Rheumatol 23:684–689, 1996.

Felson DT. The epidemiology of osteoarthritis: Prevalence and risk factors. In: Kuettner KE, Goldberg VM (eds). Osteoarthritic Disorders. American Academy of Orthopaedic Surgeons, Rosemont, 13–24, 1995.

Kellgren JH, Moore R. Generalised osteoarthritis in Heberden's nodes. BMJ 1:181–187, 1952.

Pelletier J-P, for the Organizing Committee. Osteoarthritis: Challenges for the 21st century. J Rheumatol (suppl 43)22:1–160, 1995.

Osteoarthritis: The Knee

Knee osteoarthritis (Table 20–2) occurs in about 6% of the adult population, and its prevalence increases to 10% in people over the age of 65. Different from inflammatory processes in which there is generalized involvement of the joint, knee OA is inherently uneven, affecting the patellofemoral compartment or the medial or lateral tibiofemoral compartments. Although in advanced disease all compartments exhibit OA changes, damage still predominates in the initially involved compartment.

Presentation and Progression

Cause

Obesity is a major factor in knee OA. There is now good evidence that obesity leads to OA rather than the opposite; that is, inactivity resulting from a painful knee leads to weight gain. Furthermore, weight reduction per se appears to protect against knee osteoarthritis. Other definite causes of knee OA include age, meniscectomy, chondrocalcinosis, prior inflammatory disease such as RA, sports participation with abnormal joints, and occupations such as mining and dockyard work that imply much knee bending and lifting. High-impact, high-intensity competitive sports may also predispose to knee OA. Interestingly, obesity and meniscectomy cause tibiofemoral OA but appear to have little effect on the patellofemoral joint. In other words, the weight-bearing portion of the joint is the one that develops degenerative changes.

Presentation

Knee OA causes mechanical pain, that is, pain made worse by activities and improved by rest. There are, in addition, findings that indicate cartilage wear in a portion of the joint, for example, the patellofemoral joint or the medial or lateral tibiofemoral compartments. Findings in patellofemoral disease include anterior knee pain made worst with stairs (especially walking downstairs due to deceleration), patellofemoral crepitus, exacerbation of pain by sustained (1 minute) passive flexion of the joint, and a positive "shrug sign" (exquisite pain triggered by active upward patellar motion while the bone is being firmly pressed against the femur). In contrast, patients with medial or lateral compartment disease have a genu varum or valgum deformity, respectively; increased knee pain with stressing the diseased compartment; and there is often evidence of anserine bursitis. The latter brings up a critical issue in osteoarthritis management: Is this patient's knee pain due to the osteoarthritic findings (clinical, radiologic) present in the knee? Two sets of confounding problems should be considered: (1) concurrent soft tissue problems, and (2) referred pain from the spine or hip. The main confounding soft tissue condition is anserine bursitis. Other problems include an anteromedial plica syndrome, and prepatellar and infrapatellar bursitis. All of these conditions are dealt with in Chapter 28. Referred neurologic pain should be suspected when passive hip and knee motion is painless. The patient may have a lumbar spine, lumbar plexus, or femoral nerve condition. The patellar reflex may be absent and the reversed Lasègue sign may be positive (see Chapter 26). Osteoarthritic knees often contain an effusion, that is typically cold and minimally inflammatory, that is, less than 3000 cells/mm^3; predominance of mononuclear cells; and unusual presentations.

Diagnosis

Summary of Diagnosis

TABLE 20–2

THE AMERICAN COLLEGE OF RHEUMATOLOGY CRITERIA FOR THE CLASSIFICATION AND REPORTING OF OSTEOARTHRITIS OF THE KNEE

Note: These criteria may be used based on clinical findings and laboratory studies, clinical findings and x-rays, or clinical findings only.

CLINICAL AND LABORATORY

Knee pain plus at least 5 of 9:
  Age > 50 years
  Stiffness < 30 minutes
  Crepitus
  Bony tenderness
  Bony enlargement
  No palpable warmth
  ESR < 40 mm/hour
  RF < 1:40
  SF OA
(92% sensitive, 75% specific)

CLINICAL AND RADIOGRAPHIC

Knee pain plus at least 1 of 3:
  Age > 50 years
  Stiffness < 30 minutes
  Crepitus plus osteophytes
(91% sensitive, 86% specific)

CLINICAL*

Knee pain plus at least 3 of 6:
  Age > 50 years
  Stiffness < 30 minutes
  Crepitus
  Bony tenderness
  Bony enlargement
  No palpable warmth
(95% sensitive, 69% specific)

*Alternative for the clinical category would be 4 of 6, which is 84% sensitive and 89% specific.
ESR = erythrocyte sedimentation rate (Westergren); RF = rheumatoid factor; SF OA = synovial fluid signs of OA (clear, viscous, or white blood cell count < 2000/mm^3).
From Altman R, Asch E, Bloch D, et al. Development of criteria for the classification and reporting of osteoarthritis of the knee. Arthritis Rheum 29:1039–1049, 1986.
© American College of Rheumatology.

KNEE OSTEOARTHRITIS

- Older age of patient.
- Obesity, chondrocalcinosis, previous inflammatory disease, athletic trauma, and previous meniscal surgery are significant predisposing factors.
- Pain increased by activity and relieved by rest.
- Check for joint effusion.
- Check for patellofemoral disease (patellar pain sign, shrug sign).
- Check for angular deformity (varus or valgus).
- Is there evidence for anserine bursitis, prepatellar bursitis, infrapatellar bursitis, or a plica syndrome?
- Is there evidence for referred neurologic pain (spine, plexus, femoral nerve) or hip disease?
- X-rays: standing films and a lateral from each knee for tibiofemoral OA; add axial (patellar) views when patellofemoral OA is a consideration. Joint space narrowing, eburnation of subchondral bone, subchondral cysts, osteophytosis.
- Joint aspiration if fluid present to rule out crystalline disease and to rule out infection in the appropriate setting.

Natural History

Expected Outcome

Knee osteoarthritis may reach a clinical and radiographic plateau or follow a slowly progressive course. Patients move from radiologic to clinical disease, and from mild, to moderate, to severe symptoms in the course of years or decades. Factors that accelerate course in some patients are unknown. Increased symptoms should bring into consideration comorbid joint conditions, in particular crystal-induced disease and fibromyalgia (that has its highest prevalence in old age), soft tissue factors, and radiating pain.

Complications

Osteoarthritic knees may become subacutely or acutely inflamed. Inflammatory episodes in OA may be caused by a superimposed crystal disease such as MSU gout, CPPD pseudogout, or basic calcium crystal-induced inflammation; concurrent inflammatory disease such as RA; or infection. The latter should be suspected in cases that follow a corticosteroid injection and in patients with bacteremia or a possible portal of entry such as skin or urinary infection. Another condition to be considered is a spontaneous (fatigue) tibial or femoral subchondral fracture. Characteristically, these patients have unbearable pain on weight bearing as well as bony tenderness over the femoral condyle or tibial condyle. Knee x-rays may not be initially revealing. Early lesions are best picked up by bone scan or by MRI (Figures 4–3 through 4–5). Baker's cysts are often present (up to 40%) in osteoarthritic knees. Different from RA, however, because OA effusions contain a dearth of inflammatory mediators, a florid pseudothrombophlebitic syndrome only rarely occurs in ruptured OA cysts.

Treatment

Methods

Medical management of knee OA starts with a search for possible aggravating factors such as obesity and excessive recreational activities. Implementation of a sensible weight reduction program is essential, preferably under the guidance of a nutritionist. Certain types of sports such as jogging and racquetball are to be discouraged. Excessive recreational activities are those that cause prolonged pain and/or a joint effusion. It is common sense that an activity which causes postexercise pain for more than 2 hours, or additional symptoms the next day, is excessive and should be reduced to the previously tolerated level. Swimming is an excellent alternative to stay fit. Particular attention should be paid to muscles spanning the joint, such as the quadriceps and the gastrocnemius. Isometric strengthening of the former, and stretching exercises for the latter, are essential (see exercises in the appendix).

The importance of using a cane should be emphasized. A cane is often viewed as a shameful public acknowledgment of a disability. This narrow view neglects the sound biomechanical basis for cane use, the safety it provides, and the elegance with which a cane may be used. Indoors, significant energy conservation can be achieved with the use of a walker.

Associated soft tissue conditions may lead to additional pain, or may even be responsible for the entire pain and should therefore be sought and treated. Anserine bursa corticosteroid infiltrations may be function saving in patients with anserine bursitis. It has long been argued whether OA pain should be treated with nonopioid analgesics or with anti-inflammatory drugs. The tide is now leading away from the latter. Not only do NSAIDs have sometimes prohibitive toxicities in older patients, but there is also evidence that certain NSAIDs such as indomethacin may actually increase the rate of cartilage deterioration. Acetaminophen in 4 g per day doses may be quite effective in pain control. Patients failing to improve should be tried on low-dose NSAIDs, if necessary, in addition to the acetaminophen. Capsaicin may be quite useful in the control of residual symptoms. Prior to stepping up therapy to full-dose NSAIDs, intraarticular corticosteroids should be tried. Techniques of injection and doses are discussed in the appendix. In general, it is recommended that not more than three corticosteroid injections be given per year. Full doses of a NSAID require concurrent gastric protection with misoprostol (see section on analgesics and NSAIDs).

Patients with OA who fail to improve in the face of a well-structured medical and physical therapy program should be offered tidal joint irrigation or arthroscopy. The latter has the advantage of allowing loose bodies removal, sectioning of tight plicae, and smoothing of grossly ulcerated cartilage. Following lavage, patients may experience prolonged relief.

Finally, progressive or unrelieved disease may require surgical correction. Surgical treatment of knee OA includes total joint replacement (replacement arthroplasty) and osteotomies. Generally, patients who are younger than 60 or severely obese are not candidates for a replacement arthroplasty. Also, patients who are candidates for a replacement arthroplasty should realize that heavy exercise will not be allowed postoperatively. They can do golf, biking, and swimming.

On the other hand, unicompartmental disease may be treated with osteotomy at any age. In this procedure a bone wedge is removed laterally from the tibia to correct medial compartment disease (varus malalignment), and medially from the femur to correct lateral compartment disease (valgus malalignment). Arthrodesis (joint fusion) is a salvage procedure that has excellent long-term results but enjoys little popularity among patients, even those who have been left with a painless, steady limb. This should be no surprise because patients, for instance, may be precluded from using an airplane toilet, which does not accommodate an extended leg.

Expected Response

Unless a correctable extraarticular factor is present, full pain relief seldom occurs in OA. On the other hand, a thoughtful treatment strategy often results in satisfactory pain relief and improved function.

Complications

The advanced age of OA patients inherently increases the risks associated with the use of NSAIDs. Septic arthritis is an extremely infrequent complication of intraarticular corticosteroid injection.

When to Refer

Patients with OA who are not relieved with analgesics, low-dose NSAIDs, exercises, and the use of a cane should be referred to a rheumatologist for evaluation. Severe nocturnal pain is an indication of advanced disease and an indication for surgical evaluation.

Guidelines for the Disorder

Recent ACR guidelines for the medical treatment of knee OA are shown in the appendix.

Key Points

> **KNEE OSTEOARTHRITIS**
> - Knee OA may involve preferentially the patellofemoral compartment, the medial compartment, or the lateral compartment of the joint.

- Always search for an extraarticular cause of pain: Finding anserine bursitis, for instance, indicates a reversible component in the patient's condition.
- Exercises, nonopiate analgesics, the addition of low-dose NSAIDs, capsaicin, and the use of a cane represent the first line of treatment in knee OA.
- Full doses of a NSAID require gastric protection with misoprostol.
- Joint lavage or arthroscopy is indicated when physical therapy measures and medications fail to meaningfully relieve symptoms.
- Tibial or femoral osteotomy and total knee arthroplasty are last-resort measures in knee osteoarthritis. Obesity and age younger than 60 preclude total joint replacement.

TABLE 20–3

THE AMERICAN COLLEGE OF RHEUMATOLOGY CRITERIA FOR THE CLASSIFICATION AND REPORTING OF OSTEOARTHRITIS OF THE HIP

Combined clinical (history, physical examination, laboratory) and radiographic classification criteria for osteoarthritis of the hip, traditional format: Hip pain and at least 2 of the following 3 features:

ESR < 20 mm/hour
Radiographic femoral or acetabular osteophytes
Radiographic joint space narrowing (superior, axial, and/or medial)

This classification method yields a sensitivity of 89% and a specificity of 91%.
ESR = erythrocyte sedimentation rate (Westergren).

From Altman R, Alarcón G, Appelrouth D, et al. The American College of Rheumatology criteria for the classification and reporting of osteoarthritis of the hip. Arthritis Rheum 34:505–514, 1991.

Suggested Reading

Cooper C. Occupational activity and the risk of osteoarthritis. J Rheumatol (suppl 43)22:10–12, 1995.

Felson DT. Weight and osteoarthritis. J Rheumatol (suppl 43)22:7–9, 1995.

Felson DT, Zhang Y, Hannan MT, et al. The incidence and natural history of knee osteoarthritis in the elderly. Arthritis Rheum 38:1500–1505, 1995.

Osteoarthritis: The Hip

Presentation and Progression

Cause

Etiologic factors in hip OA (Table 20–3) largely overlap with knee OA. This applies to the effects of overweight; age; inflammatory disease with erosion (for example, RA); and possibly heavy occupational labor such as farming and athletic overuse in high-impact, high-load sports. Additional causes leading to OA that are peculiar to the hip include developmental disorders such as congenital dislocation of the hip, slipped upper femoral epiphysis, and Perthes's disease; and osteonecrosis of the femoral head.

Presentation

The typical patient with hip OA is an otherwise healthy, sometimes obese individual who develops mechanical hip pain, that is, pain related to activity and relieved by rest. Remember that hip (coxofemoral joint) pain projects primarily into the groin and anteromedial thigh and often extends to the greater trochanter region and the gluteal area. Absence of the groin component should raise doubts about hip origin of the pain. Pain is intermittent at first, for example, while getting in and out of a car. Relatives or friends may have identified a minor limp unbeknownst to the patient. Physical findings at this stage may be subtle, particularly a deficit in flexion and some painful limitation in internal rotation and abduction. Later in the course a fixed flexor deformity develops and there is gross restriction of motion, particularly flexion and internal rotation. On gait inspection, patients with hip pain have a shortened stance time on the affected side (antalgic gait). The *Trendelenburg's lurch* describes the shift of the body's center of gravity closer to the affected hip. The *Trendelenburg sign* is the drooping of the pelvis to the opposite side from the affected hip.

Atypical presentations of hip OA include pain in the knee region or near the greater trochanter. Conditions that may cause pain erroneously attributed to hip OA include trochanteric bursitis, iliopsoas bursitis, the snapping hip syndrome, ilioinguinal or genitofemoral neuropathy, meralgia paresthetica and its mimickers, femoral neuropathy, lumbar plexitis, and an L3 or L4 radiculopathy. Clinical differentiation is made primarily by a careful analysis of passive motion. Articular disease hurts in all endpoints of motion (even if some motions are affected more than others). Trochanteric bursitis is tender on the greater trochanter and passive motions are normal; iliopsoas bursitis only hurts on passive flexion and passive internal rotation; in ilioinguinal and genitofemoral neuropathy, hip motion is normal and there is groin hypoesthesia; in meralgia paresthesica pain is anterolateral and there is sharp tenderness 1 cm medial to the anterior superior iliac spine; finally, in femoral neuropathy, lumbar plexitis, and L3 or L4 radiculopathy there is a weakened or absent patellar jerk and the reverse Lasègue, in which hip hyperextension pulls the femoral nerve, is positive.

Diagnosis

Summary of Diagnosis

HIP OSTEOARTHRITIS

- Older age of patient.
- Developmental disorder of the hip joint; obesity; joint erosion (e.g., RA); occupational factors (e.g., farmers).
- Pain triggered by activity and relieved by rest.
- Restricted passive motion (flexion, internal rotation).
- Rule out mimicking conditions: trochanteric and

- iliopsoas bursitis, spinal disease, and various types of neuropathy.
- Hip x-rays: joint space narrowing (superior, medial); osteophytes; degenerative cysts.

Natural History

Expected Outcome

Hip osteoarthritis follows a progressive course. As in the knee, there may be unpredictable exacerbations in pain. Disease progression may lead to severe symptoms and the need for total joint arthroplasty.

Complications

Synovial effusions in hip OA may distend the iliopsoas bursa, compress neurovascular structures at the proximal thigh, and result in quadriceps weakness and diffuse leg edema.

Treatment

Methods

Hip and knee OA are treated rather similarly. Weight reduction should be attempted in obese patients. A properly used cane provides stability and reduces pain. High-impact sports such as jogging and racket sports, which may entice patients with early disease, are to be avoided. Lying prone in bed for 20 minutes once a day stretches the iliopsoas muscles and anterior capsule, discouraging flexor deformity. Gluteal, quadriceps, and hip extensors isometric exercises help maintain stability and further discourage hip flexor contractures. Activities of daily living such as walking, bathing, and toileting may be severely limited. A raised toilet seat, a dressing stick, and wall bars for getting in and out of the tub may significantly improve patient's independence. Aerobic conditioning, preferably by swimming or walking in a pool, should be encouraged. The medication program follows the hierarchy used in knee OA, with the possible exception of capsaicin as an analgesic aid. Unimproved patients, particularly those who are unable to sleep because of pain, should be considered for surgical treatment. Osteotomies (pelvic or intertrochanteric), which are designed to move diseased articular bone away from the contact area, should be considered in younger patients with hip OA resulting from developmental disorders or trauma. Total joint replacements are usually reserved for patients who are 60 years of age or older.

Expected Response

Conservative treatment may significantly improve pain in hip OA and thus result in increased independence and a sense of well-being. Total joint replacement has excellent results in more than 90% of patients.

Complications

Mishaps in the treatment of hip OA have traditionally resulted from the indiscriminate use of NSAIDs, for example, a massive GI bleed, a perforated ulcer. The treatment program just outlined, which largely draws from the ACR Guidelines for Management of Hip Osteoarthritis, is designed to avoid these risks and to incorporate basic occupational and physical therapy measures that contribute to pain control and a patient's independent living.

When to Refer

Patients with hip OA who fail to improve with the program outlined here should be referred to a rheumatologist to determine if further conservative therapy is warranted or if the patient should be referred to an orthopedic surgeon.

Guidelines for the Disorder

The appendix contains recently published American College of Rheumatology guidelines for management of hip osteoarthritis.

Key Points

HIP OSTEOARTHRITIS

- The source of pain in a patient with hip OA must be carefully ascertained; look for extraarticular causes of pain (soft tissue, neurologic).
- Any correctable extraarticular source of pain must be treated.
- The use of a cane significantly reduces the load on the affected hip.
- Any limitation for activities of daily living must be attended to.
- Medications should be given along the hierarchy described under knee OA.
- Surgery is indicated in patients with unrelieved night pain or severe discomfort during daily activities. The usual procedure is a total joint replacement.

Suggested Reading

Brandt KD. Management of osteoarthritis. In: Kelley WN, Harris ED Jr, Ruddy S, et al. (eds) Textbook of Rheumatology, 4th ed. W.B. Saunders, Philadelphia, 1385–1399, 1993.

Hochberg MC, Altman RD, Brandt KD, et al. Guidelines for the medical management of osteoarthritis. I. Osteoarthritis of the hip. Arthritis Rheum 38:1535–1540, 1995.

CHAPTER 21

Infiltrative Conditions

Infiltrative joint conditions include sarcoidosis, amyloidosis, and hemochromatosis. Marked synovial swelling may occur in the the first two conditions. Although diagnosis is usually suggested by extraarticular manifestations, the articular findings are at times characteristic. Features of hemochromatosis have already been alluded to in Chapter 20 concerning hand osteoarthritis and are briefly discussed here.

The arthropathy looks like rheumatoid arthritis but on palpation the swelling is bony; there is minimal synovial proliferation and seldom if ever effusion. Pain on motion is severe, but morning stiffness is minimal. Radiographically, the features of hemochromatotic arthropathy are those of osteoarthritis except location: Prominent findings are present at the second and third metacarpophalangeal joints and the radiocarpal joints, in addition to more standard sites such as the hip and the knee. Approximately 20% of hemochromatosis arthropathy cases also exhibit chondrocalcinosis. Indeed, the wrist and hand arthropathies of chondrocalcinosis and hemochromatosis are identical. Treatment of hemochromatosis has no effect on the arthropathy.

Sarcoidosis

Sarcoidosis is a systemic noncaseating granulomatous disease of unknown origin. Chest manifestations are prominent in most patients. When skin, ocular, musculoskeletal, kidney, or neurologic involvement prevail, connective tissue disease or vasculitis may be erroneously diagnosed.

Presentation and Progression

Cause

Multiple etiologic agents have been considered in sarcoidosis. Current thinking postulates a granulomatous reaction to an unidentified environmental antigen, or a primary dysfunction of the immune system resulting in granulomatous disease. Sarcoid granulomas are comprised of epithelioid cells and multinucleated giant cells surrounded by a rim of helper-inducer lymphocytes. Organ dysfunction occurs chiefly by distortion of normal architecture and therefore depends on granulomatous load. Fever, acute anterior uveitis, erythema nodosum, and painful periarthritis indicate a prominent role of phlogistic mediators. In addition, ectopic 1-alpha-hydroxylation of 25(OH)D by macrophages within sarcoid granulomas causes increased intestinal absorption of calcium, hypercalcemia, and hypercalciuria in some sarcoidosis patients. The critical step is ruling out an infectious or neoplasic origin of the granulomas. A foremost consideration is distinguishing sarcoidosis from tuberculosis. It should also be realized that sarcoid-like granulomas may be found in additional conditions including mycobacterial, fungal, and *T. whippelii* infections; neoplasic disease; connective tissue diseases; foreign body reactions; exposure to environmental agents; and in an obscure febrile disease, granulomatous hepatitis.

Acute sarcoidosis presents with fever, malaise, and a dry cough. Typical chest x-ray findings include bilateral hilar and paratracheal adenopathies. Patients may have painful ankle arthritis and periarthritis, tender red nodules on the anterior surface of legs (erythema nodosum), and acute anterior uveitis. Articular findings may be quite dramatic in these patients to the point of suggesting gout. Facial nerve palsy and parotid enlargement occasionally occur. Subacute or chronic sarcoidosis causes malaise, dyspnea, and cough. Interstitial pulmonary disease with reticulonodular or acinar changes and less frequently scarring disease or pleurisy are characteristic of this form of the disease. Hilar or paratracheal adenopathies may or may not be present. Chronic sarcoidosis features indolent infiltrative lesions rather than phlogistic findings. Chest findings are as in the subacute form of the disease. Typical of chronic sarcoidosis are skin nodules or plaques, bone lesions (intraosseous granulomas have a cystic appearance), synovial thickening, and in some cases brain, heart, peripheral nerves, and kidney infiltration. Musculoskeletal findings in chronic sarcoidosis may be prominent. They include rheumatoid-like arthritis, proliferative tenosynovitis, painful expanding bone lesions in the digits (dactylitis), and myositis that may be polymyositis-like or nodular. Many instances of sarcoidosis are asymptomatic and found on screening chest x-rays.

Diagnosis

Summary of Diagnosis

> **SARCOIDOSIS**
> - Malaise, fever, dry cough, dyspnea.
> - Chest x-rays abnormalities: adenopathies, interstitial changes, scarring, rarely pleural disease.
> - Acute ankle periarthritis in acute sarcoidosis; rheuma-

- toid-like findings, proliferative tenosynovitis, and bone changes such as dactylitis in chronic sarcoidosis.
- Heerford-Waldenström's syndrome: fever, parotid enlargement, facial nerve palsy, anterior uveitis.
- Loefgren's syndrome: erythema nodosum, lower extremity periarthritis, bilateral hilar adenopathies.
- Skin anergy.
- Increased serum levels of angiotensin-converting enzyme in 75% of cases; hypercalcemia and hypercalciuria in some patients.
- Diagnosis can be made clinically in Loefgren's syndrome, but most cases require histologic confirmation preferably by transbronchial biopsy.
- Infectious granulomas, in particular histoplasmosis (yersiniosis in Scandinavian countries), mycobacterial disease, AIDS, and neoplastic disease must be considered in all cases.

Natural History

Expected Outcome

Most of the acute and some of the subacute cases of sarcoidosis resolve spontaneously. Some chronic cases spontaneously arrest leaving sequelae. Overall, chronic progression occurs in approximately 20% of cases. Chronic pulmonary disease rarely leads to pulmonary hypertension. Hypertrophic osteoarthropathy is very uncommon. Cases of myocardiopathy and encephalopathy have a grim outlook.

Treatment

Acute sarcoidosis may be treated with NSAIDs. Leg elevation and warm packs are useful in erythema nodosum. Chest findings in acute sarcoidosis do not require therapy. Subacute and chronic cases should be watched for a few months to determine disease progression. Progressive cases are treated with oral corticosteroids, usually prednisone 1 mg per kilo per day for 4 to 6 weeks followed by a slow taper. Other medications such as hydroxychloroquine or immunosuppressants may be used as steroid-sparing agents, but a beneficial effect has not been conclusively shown. Cyclosporine has been used with reported success in chronic extrapulmonary sarcoidosis involving vital organs.

Resolution of acute sarcoidosis occurs in weeks to a few months. Treatment response in chronic sarcoidosis is slow and difficult to assess. Parameters to follow include clinical findings, serum levels of angiotensin-converting enzyme, serial gallium 67 lung scans, and serial bronchoalveolar lavage.

Complications of treatment are the usual for high-dose, long-term corticosteroids.

When to Refer

Cases of possible sarcoidosis based on the association of lower extremity arthritis and erythema nodosum, chronic arthritis, proliferative synovitis, or bone lesions should be referred to a rheumatologist for diagnostic evaluation and treatment recommendations. Cases with predominant chest findings should be referred to a chest physician.

Key Points

SARCOIDOSIS

- Sarcoidosis is usually diagnosed based on respiratory symptoms and chest x-ray findings.
- In a substantial proportion of cases, articular, bone, or skin findings predominate. Chest x-ray findings suggest the diagnosis.
- Histologic proof (noncaseating granulomas) is required for diagnosis in most cases.
- Infectious and neoplastic conditions must be excluded in all cases based on clinical, pathologic, and microbiologic data.
- An exception is Loefgren's syndrome. This entity is so characteristic (provided that histoplasmosis, coccidioidomicosis, and yersiniosis are excluded by epidemiologic data) that a clinical diagnosis is justified.
- Chronic sarcoidosis arrests spontaneously in approximately half of cases.
- Corticosteroids are the treatment of choice in progressive disease.

Suggested Reading

Canoso JJ. Infiltrative, neoplastic, and endocrine causes of musculoskeletal injuries. In: Kelley WN (ed) Textbook of Internal Medicine, 3rd ed. Lippincott-Raven, Philadelphia, 1182–1186, 1997.

Mañá J, Gómez Vaquero C, Salazar A, Valverde J, Juanola X, Pujol R. Periarticular ankle sarcoidosis: A variant of Löfgren's syndrome. J Rheumatol 23:874–877, 1996.

Schumacher HR Jr. Sarcoidosis. In: McCarty DJ, Koopman WJ (eds) Arthritis and Allied Conditions, 12th ed. Lea & Febiger, Philadelphia, 1449–1455, 1993.

Amyloidosis

Studied under light microscopy, amyloid appears as a homogeneous proteinaceous material that stains pink with Congo red. For many years, such a description made people consider amyloidosis a "boring" disease that some unfortunate people would get as a complication of chronic infection, inflammation, myeloma, heredity, or sometimes for no apparent reason.

This all has changed. A very useful characteristic that allows detection of small quantities of amyloid is a striking apple green birefringence when Congo red–stained sections are inspected under polarized light. Unexpectedly, electron microscopy studies in the early 1960s revealed that amyloid was microfibrillar rather than amorphous. Following this landmark observation, an explosion of new knowledge has taken place in the last three decades in the amyloidosis field. Amyloidosis has been found relevant to such diverse conditions as Alzheimer's disease and hemodialysis-related shoulder pain.

The field is fascinating, but only those forms of amyloidosis that are relevant to arthritis and connective tissue diseases are discussed in this chapter. The following discussion is limited to immunoglobulin light chain (AL type) amyloidosis, hemodialysis-related (AH) amyloidosis caused by beta-2 microglobulin deposition, and the amyloidosis that results from tissue precipitation of the acute-phase reactant serum amyloid A protein

(AA type) in chronic inflammatory conditions. Heredofamilial forms of amyloidosis, the amyloidosis of aging, central nervous system amyloidosis, and amyloidosis confined to a single organ (localized amyloidosis) are not discussed.

Presentation and Progression

Light chain amyloid (AL) occurs in the setting of a monoclonal gammopathy, be it multiple myeloma, Waldenström macroglobulinemia, or monoclonal gammopathies of unknown significance (MGUS). Clinical findings relate to (1) tissue deposition of light chains, and (2) inherent characteristics of the underlying disease. One or more of the following AL-related findings are present in these patients: skin findings including a tendency to bleed upon shaving and waxy papules in face and friction areas, macroglossia, bulky shoulders, cardiomyopathy, peripheral neuropathy, carpal tunnel syndrome, which is usually bilateral, and rheumatoid arthritis–like articular thickening and limitation. The enlarged tongue from amyloidosis is characteristically stiff on two-finger palpation and indented on the edges if the subject is not edentulous (Figure 21–1).

Cardiac involvement features various types of arrhythmia; low-voltage QRS; and thickening of both ventricular walls and septum, hypokinesia, and a characteristic "sparkling appearance" on echocardiography. Findings inherent to the monoclonal gammopathy range from none in cases associated with MGUS to bone pain, anemia, a very high ESR, and Bence-Jones proteinuria when multiple myeloma is present. A well-known clinical scenario in AL amyloidosis is the onset of RA-like arthritis with firm synovial infiltration and bilateral carpal tunnel syndrome in an older individual. Subcutaneous nodules may be present. Characteristically, the ESR is very high, the RF test is negative, and some degree of proteinuria is often present. The condition should be distinguished from late-onset RA and polymyalgia rheumatica.

Hemodialysis-related amyloidosis (AH) presents with bilateral shoulder pain and bilateral carpal tunnel syndrome. Cystic changes in the humeral head are frequent x-ray findings. The cervical spine has been involved in some patients.

Serum protein A (SA) amyloidosis presents with proteinuria from glomerular deposits and hepatosplenomegaly from heavy tissue infiltration in these organs. The condition may present as an asymptomatic proteinuria or a frank nephrotic syndrome. Either finding in a patient with chronic inflammatory or infectious disease should make the physician consider AA amyloidosis. Other causes of proteinuria must of course be ruled out, particularly drug-induced renal damage. Colchicine treatment of familial Mediterranean fever (FMF) has virtually eliminated AA amyloidosis as a late complication of the condition. Previously, approximately 25% of FMF patients developed amyloidosis, which was often fatal.

Diagnosis

Summary of Diagnosis

> **AMYLOIDOSIS**
>
> - Clinical suspicion.
>
> **In All Cases**
> - Tissue biopsy stained with Congo red and inspected under polarized light. Green birefringence is typical of amyloid.
> - Pretreatment with potassium permanganate abolishes the green birefringence of Congo red–stained amyloid in AA and AH amyloid but not in AL amyloid.
> - Least problematic biopsy is by needle aspiration of subcutaneous abdominal fat.
> - Usefulness of abdominal fat biopsy: AL > AA > AH.
>
> **Suspected AL**
> - Serum/urine electrophoresis.
> - Immunoelectrophoresis if an M component appears to be present.
> - Bone marrow biopsy if an M component is confirmed.

Natural History

Amyloidosis is a progressive disease, but some cases have an inherently slow tempo. If the primary condition can be brought under control, or cured, amyloid deposits may experience at least partial regression. Myocardial involvement in AL has a very poor prognosis.

Complications of amyloidosis depend on the type and progression of the disease. Death in AL with myocardiopathy usually occurs from arrhythmia. AH may be a disabling condition but is not lethal. Nephrotic syndrome and renal insufficiency have a dire prognosis in AA.

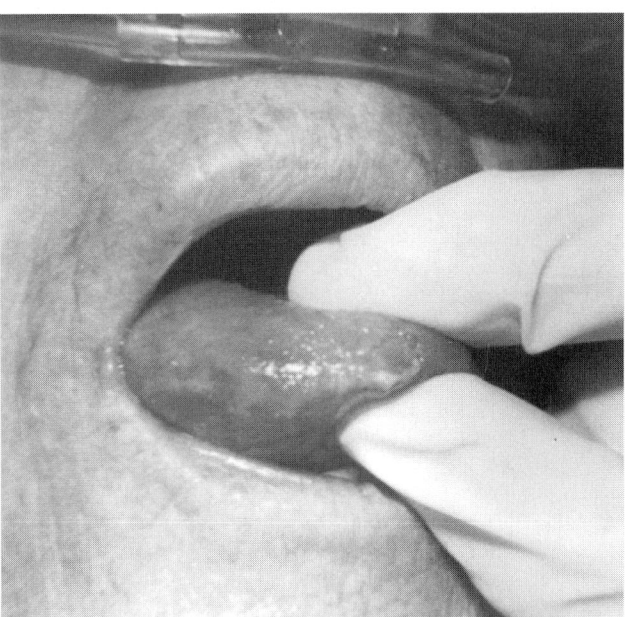

FIGURE 21–1. *Amyloidosis.* Hard, rubbery tongue in a 70-year-old woman admitted with heart failure and bilateral carpal tunnel syndrome. A monoclonal component was identified in her serum. Amyloidosis was diagnosed by fat pad aspiration biopsy.

Treatment

Many treatments have been used in an attempt to halt or reverse amyloidosis. Aggressive treatment of the underlying B-cell condition may help in AL. A commonly used regime includes intermittent courses of melphalan and prednisone. Clinical myocardial disease has a dismal prognosis; some cases have been treated successfully with chemotherapy. Recently, patients with AL amyloidosis have been treated with I.V. melphalan with blood stem-cell rescue, and early results are very encouraging.

Hemodialysis-related amyloidosis may be treated with carpal tunnel decompression surgery and open or arthroscopic debridement of the shoulder such as used in other causes of obstructive subacromial impingement. The condition may be arrested by renal transplantation. The course of AA may be significantly slowed by controlling the underlying inflammatory or infectious disease process. Occasional cases have been cured by radical surgery of chronic osteomyelitis. Colchicine delays or prevents experimental AA. In humans, FMF attacks are prevented by colchicine and as a result AA does not appear. Based on these reasons, low-dose oral colchicine has been used as an adjunct of treatment of AL and AA. Renal transplantation has been used with success in cases of AA with terminal kidney failure.

When to Refer

Amyloidosis is a rare and serious disease that should be handled by specialized physicians. There are several research centers across the country where amyloid patients may be evaluated. If referral to one of these centers is not possible, patients should be followed by a subspecialist with experience in the evaluation and treatment of amyloidosis, usually a rheumatologist, a nephrologist, or a hematologist.

Key Points

> **AMYLOIDOSIS**
>
> - Amyloidosis should be viewed as a miscellany of unrelated conditions that share histopathologic and electron microscopic features.
> - It is more appropriate to consider "amyloidoses" rather than "amyloidosis."
> - Three types of amyloidosis—AL, AH, and AA—are particularly relevant to rheumatic and connective tissue disorders.
> - AL resembles RA, AH results in disabling shoulder disease, and AA often mimics other types of renal involvement in chronic arthritic and infectious conditions.
> - Myocardial involvement in AL and kidney involvement in AA may result in death.
> - Treatment in AL and AA hinges on the successful treatment of the underlying disease.
> - Chronic colchicine administration prevents the development of AA in FMF and may slow down progression in other forms of amyloidosis.

Suggested Reading

Bardin T, Lebail-Darne JL, Zingraff J, et al. Dialysis arthropathy: outcome after renal transplantation. Am J Med 99:243–248, 1995.

Cohen AS. Amyloidosis. In: Isselbacher KJ, Braunwald E, Wilson JD, et al. (eds) Harrison's Principles of Internal Medicine, 13th ed. McGraw-Hill, New York, 1625–1630, 1994.

Dubrey S, Mendes L, Skinner M, Falk R. Resolution of heart failure in patients with AL amyloidosis. Ann Intern Med 125:481–484, 1996.

PART III

BONE DISEASES

CHAPTER 22

Bone Diseases

Bones are made up of cortical bone and trabecular bone. The proportion of each varies among bones as well as within each bone depending on the area. For example, in the shaft of the radius the proportion of cortical to trabecular bone is 96 to 4, and in the distal epiphysis it is 35 to 65. Overall, 80% of the total bone mass is cortical and 20% trabecular.

Cortical bone is made up of haversian units arranged side by side, each comprised of a central vessel and concentric layers, or lamellae, of mineralized collagen. Periosteal cortical bone and endosteal cortical bone differ functionally, the balance in the former being toward apposition and growth, and in the latter toward resorption. Trabecular bone, which is also comprised of layers of mineralized collagen, is arranged along weight-transmission lines.

Both types of bone are affected by an ongoing process of remodeling whose yearly rate is 25% in trabecular bone and 3% in cortical bone. Bone remodeling involves two cell types: osteoclasts, which derive from hematopoietic precursors stimulated by interleukins 6 and 11, and osteoblasts, which derive from mesenchymal cells under the influence of interleukin-1, tumor necrosis factor, parathyroid hormone, and 1,25-dihydroxyvitamin D $[1,25(OH)2D_3]$ or calcitriol. The sequence of remodeling events includes activation of osteoclast precursors, bone resorption by osteoclasts, invasion by pro-osteoblasts that differentiate into osteoblasts, new matrix (osteoid) formation by osteoblasts, and matrix mineralization and maturation into haversian or trabecular lamellae. Osteoblasts contain and release bone-specific alkaline phosphatase; osteoclasts contain tartrate-resistant acid phosphatase. These enzymes have been used as markers of bone synthesis and resorption, respectively.

The bone matrix is comprised of glycoproteins, proteoglycans, and noncollagen proteins of which some are synthetized by osteoblasts and some are absorbed from plasma. Among osteoblast-synthetized matrix proteins is osteocalcin, which is specific for bone and dentin. Serum levels of osteocalcin are a reliable marker of bone formation. The prevailing bone protein (90%), which is also synthetized by osteoblasts, is type I collagen. Because of the abundance of hydroxyproline in collagen, conditions in which bone resorption is grossly increased, such as Paget's disease, characteristically increase the urinary excretion of hydroxyproline. Collagen molecules are stabilized within the matrix by cross links involving pyridinoline (Pyr) and deoxypyridinoline (D-Pyr), which are peculiar to bone. Urinary excretion of Pyr and D-Pyr crosslinks is a sensitive and specific marker of bone resorption. Calcium exists in bone in the form of hydroxyapatite crystals (calcium phosphate) that are tightly packed onto collagen fibers, between them, and in the ground substance. Increased urinary calcium can be used as a marker of bone resorption.

The physiologic control of bone metabolism involves the integrated function of kidneys, intestine, parathyroid glands, and bone. The kidneys regulate the excretion of Ca, P, and Mg, and excrete aluminum and beta-2 microglobulin. In addition, the kidney is a target organ for the action of parathormone (PTH) as well as a degrading site for PTH. PTH decreases urinary Ca excretion, increases Ca absorption from bone (an osteoclast-mediated function), and increases the renal synthesis of calcitriol. Calcitriol enhances the intestinal absorption of Ca, increases the release of Ca from bone, and contributes to the inhibitory control of PTH secretion. Thus, both PTH and calcitriol elevate serum Ca levels. Hypocalcemia increases both PTH and calcitriol levels; in hypercalcemia both levels are decreased.

Methods of Assessment

Conventional radiography is insensitive to early osteoporotic changes, since 20% to 40% of the calcium content must be lost before osteopenia (the radiographic designation of bone loss, regardless of mechanism) becomes discernible. However, spinal x-rays are important in the baseline assessment of patients as well as in following the course of the disease. Also, x-rays may show unexpected pseudofractures, a reliable marker of osteomalacia. Vertebral osteoporotic findings include increased radiolucency, thinning of cortical margins, decreased horizontal trabeculation, increased vertical trabeculation, and accentuated vertebral endplates.

Dual x-rays absorptiometry (DXA) (Table 22–1) is a widely used projectional method for assessing bone mass at the vertebral spine, proximal femur, or whole body. The technique permits one to focus, within a given region, on areas with a different cortical to trabecular bone ratio. A drawback of the method has been that spinal osteophytes falsely increase bone mineral content in standard PA measurements. This source of error has been corrected with lateral spinal measurements. The radiation involved in the procedure is minute. With current scanners the procedure is completed in approximately 2 minutes.

Quantitative computed tomography (QCT) is an older but still widely used method that allows determination of bone mineral content in a tridimensional fashion for each individual vertebra. The technique can be used for both spinal and peripheral bone densitometry. QCT involves more radiation than DXA. Also, precision is slightly less and accuracy error slightly greater than with DXA.

TABLE 22-1
TECHNIQUES FOR MEASURING BONE MINERAL DENSITY

Technique	Precision Error (%)	Accuracy Error (%)	Effective Dose Equivalent (uSv)*
RADIOGRAPHY			
PA lumbar spine			~550
Lateral lumbar spine			~450
SPA	1–2	4–6	< 1
DPA			
Lumbar spine	2–3	2–11	5
Proximal femur	2–5		3
DXA			
PA lumbar spine	1	1–10	1
Lateral lumbar spine			
Decubitus	2–6		3
Supine	1–2		3
Proximal femur	1–2		1
Forearm	~1		< 1
Whole body	1		3
QCT			
SEQCT	2–4	5–15	50
DEQCT	4–6	3–6	100
pQCT	0.5–1	2–8	< 1

*PA chest film, 50 uSv; annual background irradiation, 2400 uSv.
SPA = single photon absorptiometry; DPA = dual-photon absorptiometry; DXA = dual x–ray absorptiometry; QCT = quantitative computed tomography; SEQCT = single-energy QCT; DEQCT = dual-energy QCT; pQCT = peripheral QCT.
Modified from Jergas M, Genant HK. Current methods and recent advances in the diagnosis of osteoporsis. Arthritis Rheum 36:1649–1662, 1993.

Markers of bone formation and resorption do not allow discrimination between trabecular and cortical bone.

Markers of Bone Formation: Serum *alkaline phosphatase* levels are not useful in osteoporosis but are excellent in Paget's disease. Best determination is with monoclonal Ab that recognizes the bone fraction. Serum *osteocalcin* levels are increased where there is increased bone turnover: Paget's, hyperthyroidism, hyperparathyroidism, and acromegaly. They are decreased in hypoparathyroidism, hypothyroidism, and during glucocorticoid treatment. Measurement is by radioimmunoassay.

Markers of Bone Resorption: Plasma *tartrate-resistant acid phosphatase* levels are not specific for osteoclasts. Their usefulness as a marker of bone resorption is unclear. Fasting *urinary calcium* measured on a morning sample and *corrected for creatinin excretion* is useful if increased, but the technique lacks sensitivity. Owing to various factors, including liver metabolism, *urinary hydroxyproline* represents only a fraction of collagen catabolism. Its correlation with Ca kinetics and bone histomorphometry is poor. *Urinary pyridinoline* (Pyr/D-Pyr) is very useful as a marker of bone degradation. In osteoporosis, Pyr/D-pyr correlate with bone turnover as determined by Ca kinetics and histomorphometry.

Bone Turnover at Menopause: With menopause there is a drastic increase in bone turnover with an excess of resorption over formation that peaks 1 to 3 years after cessation of ovarian function and slows down over the ensuing 20 years. Serum osteocalcin and urinary Pyr/D-Pyr are increased and return to premenopausal levels after a few months of estrogen replacement, which prevents the rapid initial postmenopausal bone loss as well as about 50% of osteoporotic fractures. Osteoporotic patients with high bone turnover exhibit greater remineralization upon initiation of antiresorptive therapy than those with a low turnover. As shown in Table 22–2, there are well-defined correlates of BMD. Increased BMD correlates with weight, height, age at menopause, estrogen use, muscle strength, thiazide use, dietary calcium intake, non-insulin-dependent diabetes mellitus, and recent or past activity. Decreased BMD correlates with increasing age, history of fracture in mother, current smoking, and gastric surgery.

Elderly Patients with Hip Fracture: In this population there is increased urinary Pyr/D-Pyr (increased resorption), decreased serum osteocalcin (decreased formation), and increased levels of serum noncarboxylated osteocalcin (carboxylation is vitamin K dependent), suggesting nutritional deficiency.

Suggested Reading

American Society for Bone and Mineral Research. Favus MJ (ed) Primer on the Metabolic Bone Diseases and Disorders of Mineral Metabolism, 2nd ed. Raven Press, New York, 1993.

TABLE 22-2
CORRELATES OF AXIAL AND APPENDICULAR BONE MINERAL DENSITY*

Variable	Lumbar Spine	Femoral Neck	Distal Radius
Age	—	—	—
Weight	+++	+++	+++
Height	++	++	
Fracture in mother	—	—	—
Age at menopause	+	+	++
Estrogen use	+++	+++	+++
Quadriceps strength		++	
Grip strength			+++
Thiazide use	+++	++	+++
Nonthiazide diuretic use	++		
Current smoker			—
Cumulative alcoholic drinks	+		
Dietary calcium intake		++	+
Non-insulin-dependent diabetes mellitus		+++	+++
Osteoarthritis (hip or knee)		++	
Gastric surgery			—
Recent or past activity	+	+	

*Symbols used indicate positive (+) and negative (−) effects on bone mineral density. Adapted from data from Orwoll ES, Bauer DC, Vogt TM, et al. Axial bone mass in older women. Ann Intern Med 1996. 124:187–196, and Burger H, van Daele PLA, Odding E, et al. Association of radiographically evident osteoarthritis with higher bone mineral density and increased bone loss with age: The Rotterdam Study. Arthritis Rheum 39:81–86, 1996

Eriksen EF, Axelrod DW, Melsen F. Bone Histomorphometry. Raven Press, New York, 1994.
Jergas M, Genant HK. Current methods and recent advances in the diagnosis of osteoporosis. Arthrits Rheum 36:1649–1662, 1993.
Manolagas SC, Jilka RL. Bone marrow, cytokines, and bone remodeling. N Engl J Med 332:305–311, 1995.
Orwoll ES, Bauer DC, Vogt TM, et al. Axial bone mass in older women. Ann Intern Med 124:187–196, 1996.

Osteoporosis

In osteoporosis, the most prevalent of bone diseases, a decrease in trabecular bone plus endosteal resorption of cortical bone results in a lower bone mass per unit volume, which weakens bone. Silent for years or decades, late osteoporosis is marked by spontaneous vertebral compression fractures as well as femoral neck and radial (Colles) fractures upon relatively minor trauma. It is a sad situation indeed that in what is a largely preventable condition and also a treatable condition in its early stages, efforts are usually applied too late.

Presentation and Progression

Cause

Osteoporosis has multiple etiologies (Table 22–3). The usual form of the condition, involutional osteoporosis, reflects the normal decline in bone mass that occurs with aging in both sexes. Peak bone mass is reached between 25 and 35 years of age. Mean peak bone mass of healthy young individuals is known as T-score or young z-score. During a lifetime total bone loss amounts to 20% of cortical bone and 30% of trabecular bone in females. The strength of bone and therefore the fracture risk is chiefly determined by the bone mineral density (BMD). The World Health Organization has recommended using the label osteopenia for individuals who have a 1.0–2.5 SD reduction in BMD below normal peak bone mass. Women with bone mass reductions greater than 2.5 SD are labeled osteoporotic. This arbitrary cut-off was chosen because 95% of women who fracture have BMD below this level. Physical inactivity results in a lower BMD. A family history of fractures strongly associates with a low BMD and suggests a strong influence of still unidentified genetic factors. A less frequent but nevertheless important factor of osteoporosis in both sexes is long-term corticosteroid use, even in doses of less than 10 mg of prednisone a day. Other causes include, as examples, thyrotoxicosis, gonadal deficiency, and chronic renal insufficiency.

Osteoporosis per se is a silent condition. Symptoms and physical findings nearly always reflect fractures, and these come late in the disease.

Osteoporotic vertebral fractures have a predilection for the middle and lower dorsal spine and the upper lumbar spine. Excruciating back pain with intercostal and inner arm radiation (T1–T3); purely intercostal radiation (T4–T6); intercostal and abdominal radiation (T7–T11); or subcostal, inguinal, lateral gluteal, and thigh radiation (T12, also known as subcostal nerve); or inguinal and anterior thigh (L1–L2) brought about by coughing or an awkward motion is characteristic of the condition. Paralytic ileus caused by both the pain and the analgesia may be the dominant finding in older patients. In other patients progressive dorsal kyphosis

TABLE 22–3
CAUSES OF OSTEOPOROSIS

GENERALIZED	
Insufficient calcium intake during the first three decades of life	Chronic corticosteroid use
Milk intolerance	Hyperthyroidism
Northern European or Asian ethnicity	Juvenile osteoporosis
Small body frame (weight < 127 lbs)	Plasma cell dyscrasias
Sedentary life	Leukemias
Anorexia nervosa	Lymphomas
Vegetarian diet	Systemic mastocytosis
Cigarette smoking	Heparin induced
Excessive alcohol consumption	Gaucher disease
Late menarche	Scurvy
Nulliparity	Pregnancy or lactation related
Oophorectomy	Hypophosphatemia
Excessive exercise producing functional amenorrhea	Insulin-dependent diabetes mellitus
Hyperprolactinemia	**LOCALIZED**
Hypothalamic amenorrhea	Inflammatory (paraarticular)
Early menopause	Disuse
Postmenopausal	Sympathetic dystrophy
Male hypogonadism	Transient osteoporosis of the hip
Involutional	Migratory osteoporosis

"widow's hump," back pain based on paraspinal muscle spasm, and height loss are the main features of the condition. Finally, the initial manifestation of osteoporosis may be a Colles fracture or a hip or tibial fracture caused by minor trauma. Primary or metastatic tumor as well as osteomalacia must obviously be ruled out in these patients.

Spine radiographs in established osteoporosis show generalized demineralization, increased vertical striae, accentuation of the vertebral endplates, and ballooning of intervertebral discs leading to biconcave vertebrae. Osteoporotic fractures are wedge-shaped due to a decrease in the anterior height.

PATIENT 27 A 58-year-old man was seen for evaluation of back pain and the appearance of a pointy bone in the middle of his back. Three weeks before, while dressing in the morning, he felt as if something had struck him in the middle of his back. When he touched the area, he felt a bony prominence that had not been there before. There was no pain, but he felt unable to hold anything. That night pain began in the low dorsal area and rapidly became unbearable. Pain was steady and agonizing, worse at night, for the ensuing 3 days. From then on pain was worse during the day in relation with his activities. X-rays (Figure 22–1) showed pronounced spinal osteopenia and a wedged fracture of T10. An MRI revealed that the fracture had a displaced posterior fragment that impinged on the anterior cord (Figure 22–1B). No abnormal signal suggested neoplasm or infection. The patient was quite osteoporotic (3.5 SD below the mean bone mass of the young). There was no electrophoretic evidence of myeloma. Because he had lost libido several months before, an endocrinologic evaluation was undertaken. Very high levels of prolactin led to head MRI, which revealed a pituitary microadenoma. Bromocriptine, calcium, and alendronate treatment was begun.

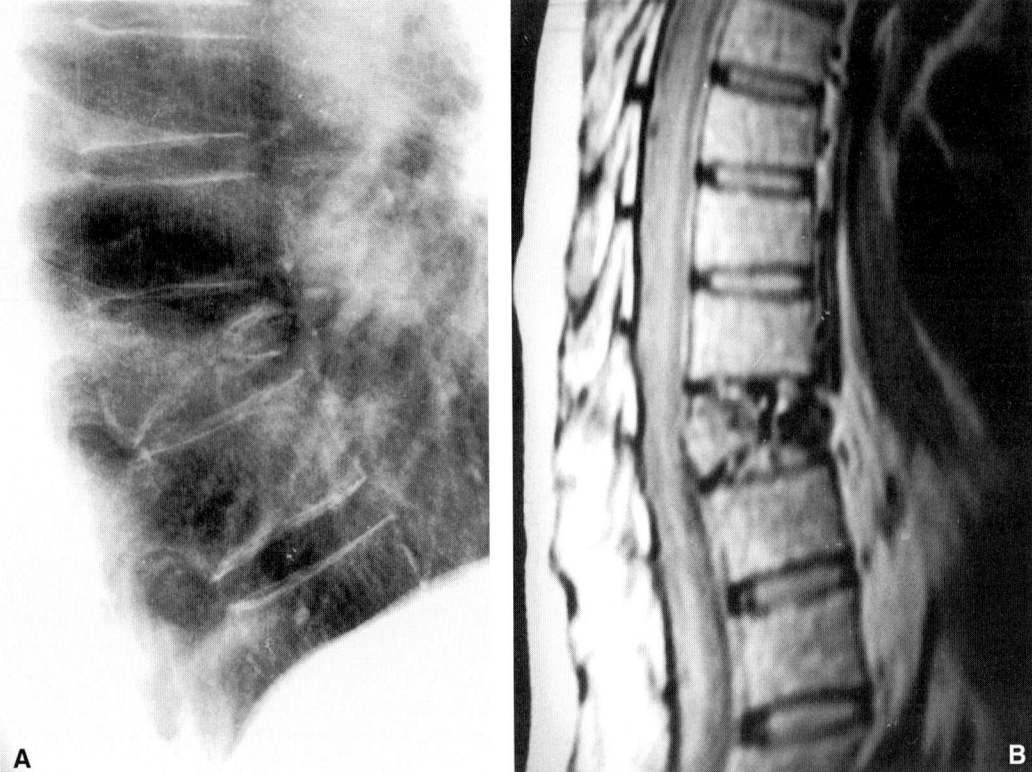

FIGURE 22–1. *Patient 27. Osteopenia, spinal fracture.* A, Dorsal spine films show osteopenia and compression fracture of T10. B, MRI reveals the fracture in great detail, including a large vertebral fragment with posterior displacement that impinges on the cord.

An amazing feature of this case is that the T10 fracture was painless for at least 12 hours after which typical bone pain (continuous, worse at night) set in. But then, this may not be that uncommon, since elderly women often have one or more collapsed vertebrae without having experienced acute, fracture-type back pain. The characteristic x-ray finding in peripheral bones is cortical thinning. This is best estimated at the mid-diaphysis of the second metacarpal in which a normal cortex should be at least one-quarter of the width of the bone.

Laboratory findings in osteoporosis depend on the rate of bone turnover. Some women have an increased bone turnover as shown by hypercalciuria, increased urinary excretion of Pyr/D-Pyr cross-links, and elevated serum levels of osteocalcin. In most patients, however, laboratory tests are normal except for transiently elevated serum alkaline phosphatase levels following a fracture episode. Low serum phosphorus and 25-(OH)D levels should alert the physician to concurrent or mimicking osteomalacia.

Diagnosis

Summary of Diagnosis

> **OSTEOPOROSIS**
> - Risk factors assessment.
> - Spine x-rays in symptomatic patients.
> - Bone densitometry in perimenopausal women.
> - If x-rays show osteopenia or BMD values are > 2.5 BD below the mean peak bone mass, determine:
> - ESR; thyroid tests; serum alkaline phosphatase, Ca, P, and 25(OH)D3; fasting urinary calcium corrected for creatinine excretion; urinary pyridinoline.

Natural History

Expected Outcome

Pain from a vertebral fracture lasts about 1 week, and full resumption of activities can be expected in 4 to 6 weeks. A vertebral fracture portends additional fractures at irregular and unpredictable intervals. As a result, height shortens, dorsal kyphosis appears, lumbar lordosis flattens, and the abdomen becomes protuberant. The prognosis of hip fractures is good in terms of healing, but the overall mortality is high as a result of comorbid conditions. Very significantly, having sustained a first fracture increases the risk for a second fracture at least 2-fold, independently of BMD.

Treatment

Treatment of osteoporosis includes prophylactic measures applicable to each stage of the disease to decrease or overcome continuing bone loss, plus the treatment of fractures and their attendant complications. Prophylactic measures aim at (1) increasing bone mineral density before peak bone mass is reached, (2) reducing the normal decline that follows, (3) preventing the negative consequences of gonadal deficiency, and (4) halting further bone loss (and ideally increasing bone mass) once osteoporosis is radiographically overt or fractures have occurred. As in coronary artery disease, prophylactic measures in osteoporosis make far more sense than the treatment of established disease.

Agents used in osteoporosis are as follows: *Estrogens* effectively prevent the bone loss that follows castration and reduce the rate of postmenopausal fractures by 50%. A commonly used preparation is conjugated estrogens 0.625 mg/day for the first 25 days each month. Because estrogens produce endometrial hyperplasia and increase the risk of uterine cancer, a progestin such as medroxyprogesterone 2.5 to 5 mg/day may be added to the last 12 days of estrogen administration in patients who have an intact uterus. Some authors favor the continuous administration of these agents, which has the advantage of inducing amenorrhea. Unfortunately, although the increased risk of uterine cancer is averted by the progestin, there is an increased risk of breast cancer in postmenopausal women treated with estrogens, with or without the addition of progestin, for more than 5 years. This risk is greatly increased when there is a family history of breast cancer. On the other hand estrogens decrease the risk of ischemic heart disease and possibly colon cancer. It is expected that the net health effect of estrogen use will be elucidated by the currently underway Women's Health Initiative study. Meanwhile, the author favors the early use of estrogens plus progestins when the uterus is intact for the prevention of osteoporosis in patients at an average risk of breast cancer. When used therapeutically, estrogens result in a yearly BMD gain of about 4% in the lumbar spine and 2% in the femoral neck.

Calcium supplementation may help by building up a higher peak bone mass and by decreasing premenopausal bone loss. The effect of calcium supplementation after menopause is less clear but has been shown to be beneficial 5 years or more after menopause.

Calcitonin has analgesic properties, decreases bone resorption, and is particularly helpful in high-turnover osteoporosis. Another indication is the prevention of corticosteroid-induced osteoporosis. Synthetic salmon calcitonin is available in a parenteral and a nasal spray form. Nasal spray administration is more convenient; reduces significantly the bothersome side effects of subcutaneous calcitonin such as flushing, nausea, and vomiting; and decreases the rate of resistance. Rhinitis and other types of mucosal injury occur in about 10% of patients. One spray daily (200 U of synthetic calcium calcitonin) in one nostril, plus calcium 1000 mg per day and vitamin D 400 IU per day supplements, results in a 2% to 3% increase in lumbar spine BMD per year but has a negligible effect on the femoral neck.

Bisphosphonates, carbon-substituted synthetic pyrophosphate analogues, bind tightly to hydroxyapatite crystals, are resistant to endogenous phosphatases, and because they are released during bone resorption they inhibit osteoclast function. Bisphosphonates have been shown to decrease bone resorption and increase spinal mineral density more than at peripheral sites. An impact on disease progression can be expected, as well as a decreased fracture rate. Two bisphosphonates are in use: etidronate and alendronate. Continuous etidronate administration impairs new bone matrix mineralization and induces osteomalacia. Cyclical administration circumvents this effect. Thus, etidronate is administered daily for 2 weeks followed by 11 to 13 weeks of calcium supplementation alone. Alendronate, in contrast, is used continuously at a dose of 10 mg daily. This agent is very potent in inhibiting osteoclast-mediated bone resorption at doses that do not inhibit bone mineralization even when given in daily doses. A recent trial of alendronate versus placebo (both groups receiving calcium supplement) in postmenopausal women showed in the treated group a steady increase in BMD over the 3 years of the trial, and a 48% reduction in the proportion of women with new vertebral fractures. Bisphosphonates may be used in the treatment of postmenopausal osteoporosis and in the prophylaxis of corticosteroid-induced osteoporosis. Used therapeutically, alendronate results in a yearly increase of 4% to 5% in the lumbar spine and 1% in the femoral neck.

Vitamin D metabolites act on the intestine by antagonizing the inhibitory effect of glucocorticoids on calcium absorption and have the potential to prevent steroid-induced osteoporosis. To prevent hypercalcemia, calcium supplementation should only be used by individuals with an insufficient intake. Vitamin D may be absorbed from the diet or synthetized in the skin under adequate sun exposure. Vitamin D (D_3) is a derivative of 7-dehydrocholesterol under ultraviolet radiation with a wavelength between 290 and 315 nm. Vitamin D is transported to the liver where it is metabolized to 25 hydroxyvitamin D [25(OH)D_3]. A second hydroxylation occurs in the kidney to form 1,25 hydroxyvitamin D [1,25(OH)2D_3] or calcitriol, which is the only active metabolite of vitamin D. 1,25(OH)2D_3 or calcitriol is available in 0.25 or 0.5 µg capsules. Calcitriol treatment 0.25 µg twice daily improves calcium balance and decreases fractures. Hypercalcemia rarely develops.

Thiazide diuretics decrease urinary calcium loss, raise serum calcium, suppress parathyroid function, inhibit the synthesis of 1,25(OH)D_3, and decrease intestinal calcium absorption. They are useful in patients with high-turnover osteoporosis and hypercalciuria and may be beneficial in other forms of osteoporosis as well.

Fluoride stimulates osteoblast proliferation and new bone formation and thus has long attracted workers in the osteoporosis field. However, a double-blind study of sodium fluoride published in 1990 showed that although vertebral mineral density was greatly increased in the treated group, the rate of vertebral fractures was not decreased and there was a hint of an increased tendency to hip fractures. In addition, gastric irritation was frequent and patients often developed a painful condition of feet and legs presumably as a result of microfractures. The interest in fluoride was rekindled by a more recent study in which a slow-release sodium fluoride preparation was used in cycles of 25 mg twice a day 12 months on, 2 months off *plus* calcium citrate 400 mg twice a day. Although the study results favored fluoride, conflicting data have continued to appear, and the drug has not been approved by the Food and Drug Administration for the treatment of osteoporsis.

Prophylaxis of Osteoporosis

1. Encouragement to follow a healthy diet beginning in childhood and aimed at achieving a high-peak bone mass by the third or fourth decade of life. Daily calcium intake should be 1500 mg for adolescents, 1000 mg for premenopausal women, and 1500 mg for postmenopausal women. The American diet provides about 300 mg of calcium; a cup of milk, a cup of yogurt, and a thick slice of cheese each provide 250 to 300 mg of calcium.
2. Encouragement to live an active life and remain fit.
3. Cessation of cigarette smoking and excessive alcohol intake.
4. Discouragement of excessive thinness.
5. The early postmenopausal administration of estrogens (testosterone in men with gonadal deficiency) to prevent bone loss (see later). Alendronate may be considered an alternative to estrogen use.
6. Vitamin D supplementation (800 units) in addition to 1500 mg of calcium in elderly people.

Treatment measures once a decreased bone mass has been detected by incidental x-rays, bone densitometry, or, more frequently, the occurrence of fractures, include calcium supplementation, estrogen administration, and bisphosphonates or calcitonin for patients who are unable or unwilling to use estrogens. Women over the age of 75 may not benefit from the use of estrogens or calcitonin and should be treated with calcium supplementation plus vitamin D.

Peripheral osteoporotic fractures are treated, similar to any fracture, with immobilization and analgesia; union is not delayed. In general, long bone fractures should be managed with early surgical stabilization to achieve early weight bearing in lower extremity fractures and rapid restoration of function in upper extremity fractures. Vertebral osteoporotic fractures occur within the vertebral bodies, and the posterior elements are rarely compromised. These fractures are stable and surgical stabilization is seldom required. Patients with symptomatic osteoporotic vertebral fractures should be restricted to bed rest for a few days and given analgesics, generally acetaminophen with codeine. Transcutaneous nerve stimulation (TNS), which has the theoretical advantage that sensorium is not altered and there is a lesser tendency to develop a paralytic ileus, probably only has a placebo effect. A low-profile corset or polypropylene brace may reduce muscle spasms and pain; however, its use is seldom required. Measures to prevent falls in elderly people are essential including the prudent use of sedatives, avoidance of dehydration, use of a cane or walker, and supervision.

When to Refer

Probably all perimenopausal women, but especially those with one or more risk factors for osteoporosis, should be referred for bone densitometry study (preferably by DXA) and have biochemical studies of bone turnover. Consultation with a physician specialized in bone conditions, usually an endocrinologist or a rheumatologist, should be implemented in patients with radiographic osteoporosis and patients with > 2.5 SD bone mass loss as compared with peak bone loss in healthy young individuals.

Key Points

> **OSTEOPOROSIS**
> - Osteoporosis is caused by an imbalance between bone formation and bone resorption resulting in a decreased bone mass.
> - An increased turnover magnifies any tendency to bone loss.
> - Fracture rate roughly doubles per each standard deviation (SD) decline below peak bone mass of healthy young individuals.
> - Measures to increase peak bone mass (sufficient Ca and vitamin D intake, an active life) are important in prophylaxis and should be implemented beginning in childhood.
> - Estrogen replacement prevents the accelerated bone loss that follows menopause.
> - Perimenopausal women, unless already committed to estrogen use, should be studied by bone densitometry and possibly biochemical markers of bone turnover.
> - A bone mass more than 1 SD below normal peak bone mass (T-score), particularly if associated with an increased bone turnover, is an indication for estrogen, bisphosphonate, or calcitonin treatment.
> - Vitamin D deficiency should be suspected in elderly patients who sustained a spontaneous or minimal trauma fracture.

Suggested Reading

Aloia JF, Vaswani A, Yeh JK, et al. Calcium supplementation with and without hormone replacement therapy to prevent postmenopausal bone loss. Ann Intern Med 120:97–103, 1994.

Colditz GA, Hankinson SE, Hunter DJ, et al. The use of estrogens and progestins and the risk of breast cancer in postmenopausal women. N Engl J Med 332:1589–1593, 1995.

Liberman UA, Weiss SR, Broll J, et al. Effect of oral alendronate on bone mineral density and the incidence of fractures in postmenopausal osteoporosis. N Engl J Med 333:1437–1443, 1995.

Lucas TS, Einhorn TA. Osteoporosis: The role of the orthopaedist. J Am Acad Orthop Surg 1:48–56, 1993.

Miller PD, Bonnick SL, Rosen CJ. Consensus of an international panel on the clinical utility of bone mass measurements in the detection of low bone mass in the adult population. Calcif Tissue Int 58:207–214, 1996.

Corticosteroid-Induced Osteoporosis

Presentation and Progression

Corticosteroid treatment has a profound impact on mineral and bone metabolism and is an important cause of osteoporosis. Glucocorticoids directly inhibit pro-osteoblast replication, which results in osteoblast depletion and decreased matrix synthesis. Furthermore, calcium intestinal absorption is decreased, leading to parathormone (PTH) increase and thus increased osteoclastic activity. Trabecular bone is more severely affected than cortical bone. The condition affects patients of all ages. Low-dose corticosteroids (10 mg of prednisone or less) such as used in the treatment of inflammatory bowel disease, polymyalgia rheumatica, or as an adjunct in the treatment of rheumatoid arthritis also cause bone loss. Although individual patients vary in susceptibility, there are well-known risk factors of corticosteroid-induced osteoporosis including cumulative dose, young age, perimenopausal status, old age (in both sexes), presence of inflammatory joint disease, and inactivity.

Symptoms and clinical findings are similar to involutional or estrogen deficiency osteoporosis.

Diagnosis

Summary of Diagnosis

> **CORTICOSTEROID-INDUCED OSTEOPOROSIS**
> - Increased bone loss is unavoidable in prolonged (more than 1 month) corticosteroid treatment.
> - Additional osteoporosis risk factors should be assessed.
> - Baseline bone densitometry and bone turnover markers determination should be obtained when perimenopausal or postmenopausal women are placed on corticosteroids.
> - Early prophylaxis is important in the prevention of fractures.

Natural History

The greatest bone loss (12%–15%) occurs in the initial 12 to 18 months of corticosteroid therapy. Discontinuation of corticosteroids leads to a rebound of osteoblastic activity that only partially corrects the BMD loss. Fractures affecting spine, ribs, and ends of long bones are the main complications of corticosteroid-induced osteoporosis.

Treatment

Methods

Prophylaxis is essential here. It begins with an assessment as to whether corticosteroids are really needed in the clinical situation at hand. If they are, the lowest possible effective dose should be used. Patients should be encouraged to perform weight-bearing exercises, particularly walking. All patients, regardless of steroid dose, should be given a 1000 to 1500 mg calcium supplement plus 400 to 800 units of vitamin D. Patients who are hypercalciuric may benefit from the addition of hydrochlorotiazide 25 mg twice a day. Perimenopausal and postmenopausal women should be offered, unless contraindicated, estrogen/progestin replacement. If estrogens cannot be used, patients receiving high-dose corticosteroids especially (prednisone 30 mg per day or more or equivalent) should be offered a bisphosphonate or calcitonin. Established corticosteroid-induced osteoporosis should be similarly treated with the strong recommendation of using estrogens if possible, a bisphosphonate, or calcitonin. Osteomalacia and multiple myeloma should not be missed in these patients.

Complications

Possible complications of treatment include hypercalcemia, which is more likely to occur when calcium and vitamin D are administered together with hydrochlorotiazide. There is an increased risk of breast cancer in patients taking estrogens, with or without progestin, and therefore these patients should be under close surveillance to identify early lesions should they occur.

When to Refer

Expert advice is suggested for treatment decisions in perimenopausal women and also when overt osteoporosis is diagnosed.

Key Points

> **CORTICOSTEROID-INDUCED OSTEOPOROSIS**
> - The condition occurs with high- or low-dose corticosteroids and relates to total cumulative dose.
> - Pathogenesis includes decreased osteoblast function, decreased calcium absorption, and increased urinary calcium loss.
> - Prophylaxis includes weight-bearing exercises, calcium and vitamin D supplementation, and hydrochlorotiazide in hypercalciuric patients.
> - Estrogens, bisphosphonates, or calcitonin may be used prophylactically in peri- or postmenopausal women as well as for treatment of established osteoporosis.

Suggested Reading

Dequeker J, Westhovens R. Low dose corticosteroids associated osteoporosis in RA and its prophylaxis and treatment: Bones of contention. J Rheumatol 22:1013–1017, 1995.

Laan RFJM, van Riel PLCM, van de Putte LBA, et al. Low-dose prednisone induces rapid reversible axial bone loss in patients with rheumatoid arthritis. Ann Intern Med 119:963–968, 1993.

Sambrook PN, Jones G. Corticosteroid osteoporosis. Br J Rheumatol 34:8–12, 1995.

Osteomalacia and Rickets

Deficient mineralization of bone matrix characterizes both osteomalacia and rickets. Whereas the former occurs in adults, the latter occurs during bone growth, which explains the skeletal deformities of rickets. There is a susceptibility to fractures. Hypophosphatemic myopathy may or may not be apparent. Both osteomalacia and rickets may be caused by vitamin D $[1,25(OH)2D_3]$ deficiency; defects at the vitamin D receptor; plus a miscellany of conditions such as chronic acidosis, renal tubular acidosis, aluminum intoxication, chronic administration of anticonvulsant drugs, renal insufficiency in children, chronic hemodialysis, and certain tumors (tumoral osteomalacia). In turn, vitamin D deficiency may be due to a lack of exposure to solar radiation, nutritional factors, impaired intestinal absorption of vitamin D, or a congenital or acquired failure of liver (25-hydroxylase) or kidney (1-hydroxylase) vitamin D hydroxylation. Vitamin D deficiency decreases serum calcium by decreasing absorption in the gut and mobilization from bone, hypocalcemia results in increased parathormone (PTH) secretion, and increased PTH increases serum calcium and increases phorphorus renal excretion, which causes the hypophosphatemia (Table 22–4).

Presentation and Progression

Cause

Most cases of osteomalacia occur in the elderly population. The typical patient is a feeble nursing home resident who has little direct exposure to sunlight and eats a marginal diet (no milk, no vitamin D supplement). Upon a minor injury the patient suffers a fracture and radiographs reveal osteopenia. In such a patient the usual tendency is to diagnose involutional osteoporosis. However, the astute clinician suspects osteomalacia and requests serum calcium and phosphorus levels. Calcium may be normal or low, but phosphorus is markedly reduced (lowest limit of normal 0.9 mmol/L (2.8 mg/dl) supporting a diagnosis of osteomalacia.

Another setting in which osteomalacia should be suspected goes like this: A 35-year-old man progressively develops diffuse achiness, low back stiffness, and an overwhelming feeling of weakness. Ankylosing spondylitis is considered based on radiographically abnormal sacroiliac joints. The astute clinician has some problems accepting this diagnosis: The achiness is not articular or enthesial (at tendon or ligament attachments); there is proximal muscle weakness; and there is a 3 cm nodule in the left thigh that the patient says has been present for years. Serum alkaline phosphatase is high, and both serum phosphorus and 1,25(OH)2D$_3$ levels are low. A tentative diagnosis of tumoral osteomalacia secondary to a soft tissue hemangiopericytoma is made. Salient clinical findings in rickets are shown in Table 22–5.

TABLE 22–4

BIOCHEMICAL DETERMINATIONS IN OSTEOMALACIA AND RICKETS

SERUM

Low or normal calcium
Low phosphorus
Markedly elevated alkaline phosphatase
Creatinine and phosphorus elevated in renal failure
PTH levels elevated if hypocalcemia is present
25(OH)D low in nutritional, malabsorption, or cholestatic liver disease vitamin D deficiency
1,25(OH)2D normal or high owing to secondary hyperparathyroidism (if enough vitamin D is available)
1,25(OH)2D low in tumoral osteomalacia

TABLE 22–5

CLINICAL MANIFESTATIONS OF RICKETS

Softened calvarium and frontal bossing*
Kyphoscoliosis
Prominent chondrocostal joints (rachitic rosary)
Sternal indentation
Lower ribs indentation (Harrison's groove)
Bowing deformity of long bones

*In younger infants.

Diagnosis

Summary of Diagnosis

OSTEOMALACIA

- X-rays of affected part: fracture (s) involving spine, pelvis, ribs, or hip; osteopenia; pseudofractures (Looser's zones); widened epiphyseal plates in rickets.
- Serum biochemistries: Ca low or normal, P low, alkaline phosphatase high (this is a normal finding after a fracture).
- Serum 25(OH)D$_3$ low, serum 1,25(OH)2D$_3$ normal or high due to secondary hyperparathyroidism if there is enough 25(OH)D$_3$ substrate in nutritional osteomalacia.
- Diffuse achiness, myopathic weakness, serum 1,25(OH)2D$_3$ decreased: Consider tumoral osteomalacia.
- In appropriate situations rule out anticonvulsant use (phenobarbital, phenytoin, carbamazepine), vitamin D–dependent rickets, intestinal malabsorption, renal failure, renal tubular disorders, and hypophosphatasia.

Natural History

Recurrent fractures and end results parallel osteoporosis, although multiple rib fractures are more frequent than in osteoporosis; disability may occur if myopathic weakness is present. The potential exists for confusion with rheumatic disease, particularly fibromyalgia, polymyalgia rheumatica, and ankylosing spondylitis.

Treatment

Methods

Treatment in nutritional osteomalacia consists of the administration of vitamin D$_2$ (ergocalciferol) or D$_3$ (cholecalciferol) 800 to 4000 IU (0.02–0.1 mg) daily for 6 to 12 weeks followed by 200 to 400 IU per day.

Expected Response

Improvement in achiness and strength occurs within a few weeks. Pseudofractures heal within 6 months. In tumoral osteomalacia all biochemical and clinical abnormalities resolve with complete resection of the tumor. Inoperable cases benefit from a combination of calcitriol [1,25(OH)2D$_3$] and phosphorus supplementation.

When to Refer

Both identification and treatment of nutritional osteomalacia in the elderly fall within the scope of primary care physicians. Other forms of osteomalacia should be evaluated by an endocrinologist, gastroenterologist, or nephrologist, depending on the nature of the underlying condition.

Key Points

OSTEOMALACIA AND RICKETS

- Nutritional osteomalacia is frequent in the geriatric group where it tends to be confused with osteoporosis.
- Tumoral osteomalacia is more frequent than previously believed; it should be considered in patients with diffuse achiness, myopathic weakness, and low serum phosphate. It may also explain weakness and disability in some patients with known cancer.
- Multiple additional conditions associate with osteomalacia.
- Treatment of nutritional osteomalacia is with vitamin D supplementation; symptoms and findings, including unhealing fractures, resolve within 6 months of treatment.
- Tumoral osteomalacia reverses with the successful removal of the tumor. If surgery is not possible, patients may be treated with calcitriol [1,25(OH)2D$_3$] and phosphate supplementation.

Suggested Reading

Cai Q, Hodgson SF, Kao PC, et al. Brief report: Inhibition of renal phosphate transport by a tumor product in a patient with oncogenic osteomalacia. N Engl J Med 330:1645–1649, 1994.

Drezner MK. Tumor-associated rickets and osteomalacia. In: Favus MJ (ed) Primer on the Metabolic Bone Diseases and Disorders of Mineral Metabolism. Raven Press, New York, 282–288, 1993.

Osteitis Fibrosa Cystica (OFC): Hyperparathyroidism

Hyperparathyroidism, because it causes OFC, affects muscle function, and leads to connective tissue calcification, often results in rheumatic symptoms which may closely mimic rheumatic disease. Clinicians should be aware of the range of findings in hyperparathyroidism lest diagnosis and an opportunity to achieve a cure be missed.

Presentation and Progression

Cause

Hyperparathyroidism results from autonomous or compensatory (secondary hyperparathyroidism) excess PTH secretion. Primary hyperparathyroidism is due to parathyroid adenomas in 80% and glandular hyperplasia in 15%. About 10% of parathyroid adenomas are ectopic, occurring in the thyroid, the thymus, or elsewhere in the mediastinum. Parathyroid carcinomas are a rare cause of the syndrome (less than 1% of cases). Secondary hyperparathyroidism is a physiologic response to hyperphosphatemia in patients with renal insufficiency and presupposes some degree of PTH resistance. Tertiary hyperparathyroidism designates the emergence of monoclonal parathyroid tissue in the same setting, for example, renal insufficiency, hyperphosphatemia, and relative resistance to PTH.

Increased PTH levels cause increased bone resorption, increased renal synthesis of 1,25(OH)2D$_3$ (which enhances intestinal Ca absorption), and decreased Ca clearance in the kidney, all contributing to hypercalcemia. Calciuria is increased but given the decreased Ca clearance is less than expected for the degree of hypercalcemia. Pathologically, OFC is characterized by a decreased number of trabeculae, increased numbers of giant multinucleated osteoclasts, and marrow fibrosis caused by activation of mesenchymal cells, differentiation into fibroblasts, and collagen production that occupies peritrabecular spaces. Hypercalcemia impinges negatively on muscle function and drives ectopic calcification of connective tissue. CPPD crystal deposition in cartilage results in chondrocalcinosis and prepares the ground for pseudogout.

Presentation

Before discussing OFC and other musculoskeletal concomitants of hyperparathyroidism, it is pertinent to review how the condition comes to be identified. About 50% of primary cases are diagnosed in the asymptomatic stage by the routine use of biochemical profiles. In another 30% to 40% hyperparathyroidism is identified during evaluation for nephrolithiasis or renal insufficiency. Musculoskeletal disease leads to diagnosis in the remaining 5% to 10% of cases. These proportions are reversed in secondary hyperparathyroidism, which is usually diagnosed following musculoskeletal complaints. As discussed in the next chapter, however, renal osteodystrophy (the umbrella term for renal failure–related bone disease) is pathogenetically heterogeneous, and only half of patients have OFC as the basis for their symptoms.

What is the range of musculoskeletal findings in hyperparathyroidism? Most common is silent osteopenia as a result of chronic osteoclast stimulation with predominant loss of cortical bone. Other patients have diffuse bone pain, one step higher in the ladder of osteitis fibrosa cystica. Further bone damage may result in a rheumatoid-like syndrome that may be diagnosed as RA except that laboratory studies are normal and hand x-rays, rather than fusiform soft tissue swelling, periarticular osteopenia, and perhaps early marginal erosions, feature ragged periosteal resorption in the radial side of the middle phalanges and resorption of digital tufts indicative of OFC. Another form of presentation of

OFC is focal bone pain resulting from a "brown tumor," a cystic lesion often expansile and aggressive that is composed primarily of multinucleated osteoclasts. As mentioned, CPPD crystal chondrocalcinosis is frequent in hyperparathyroidism and may be a cause of recurrent pseudogout. Interestingly, despite the scarcity of complaints, up to 40% of patients with primary hyperparathyroidism will have one or another of the radiographic findings of the disease. Along this line, hyperuricemia is said to be present in 40% of hyperparathyroid individuals, making gout frequent in this setting. Finally, in some patients myopathic features of hyperparathyroidism predominate and proximal muscle weakness and atrophy may mistakenly suggest polymyositis.

Diagnosis

Summary of Diagnosis

> **OSTEITIS FIBROSA CYSTICA (OFC): HYPERPARATHYROIDISM**
>
> - Diagnosis may be suspected clinically if the primary or secondary hyperparathyroidism is known, and requires a high degree of clinical acumen if the underlying diagnosis is not known.
> - Features of OFC include osteopenia, fractures, diffuse bone pain, rheumatoid-like symptoms, focal bone pain and tumor (brown tumors), and destructive arthropathy.
> - Chondrocalcinosis (with or without pseudogout) and myopathy are additional musculoskeletal manifestations of hyperparathyroidism. Gout may occur from the commonly associated hyperuricemia.
> - Laboratory diagnosis of hyperparathyroidism is based on (1) demonstration of persistent hypercalcemia, plus (2) an elevated serum PTH concentration by a method that is sensitive, specific, and reliable.
> - Radiographic findings in OFC include osteopenia, subperiosteal bone resorption (phalangeal, distal clavicles, sacroiliac joints), osteosclerosis (mainly in secondary cases), and cystic lesions (brown tumors) that occur in association with subperiosteal resorption.

Natural History

Expected Outcome

Osteitis fibrosa cystica in any of its forms, pseudogout, and hypercalcemic myopathy are progressive as long as the hyperparathyroid state remains unchecked. A particular concern is progression of osteopenia superimposed on the involutional osteoporosis women are subject to.

Treatment

Methods

A detailed discussion of how hyperparathyroidism is treated is beyond the scope of this book. However, some principles are reviewed here.

Although surgical treatment of hyperparathyroidism can be always justified in the absence of contraindications, surveillance is acceptable in individuals who are at least 50 years old and only have a minimal hypercalcemia. Below the age of 50 parathyroid surgery is always indicated. Additional indications for surgery include a marked elevation of serum Ca (more than 1–1.6 mg/dl), a history of life-threatening hypercalcemia, a bone mass more than 2 SD below the young normal mean, calciuria greater than 400 mg per 24 hours, significant renal failure, and urolithiasis.

Expected Response

With surgery, reversal of bone pain and myopathic weakness may be expected. Patients with OFC usually become severely hypocalcemic after surgery, and recurrent attacks of pseudogout, if the patient has chondrocalcinosis (akin to the increased frequency of gout attacks once hypouricemic treatment is started), are to be expected postoperatively.

When to Refer

Patients with suspected OFC should be referred to an endocrinologist for further evaluation and a decision on therapy.

Key Points

> **OSTEITIS FIBROSA CYSTICA (OFC): HYPERPARATHYROIDISM**
>
> - OFC is seen most frequently in patients with renal failure (secondary hyperparathyroidism).
> - Hyperparathyroid osteopenia cannot be distinguished from osteoporosis based solely on bone densitometry. Bone biopsy may be important in this setting.
> - Several rheumatic conditions may be mimicked by osteitis fibrosa including fibromyalgia (diffuse bone pain), RA, and bone tumors. In addition, hyperparathyroidism may lead to chondrocalcinosis and pseudogout and myopathic weakness.
> - Profound hypocalcemia following parathyroidectomy is likely in patients with OFC.

Suggested Reading

Potts JT Jr, et al. Proceedings of the NIH Consensus Development Conference on Diagnosis and Management of Asymptomatic Primary Hyperparathyroidism. J Bone Miner Res (suppl 2)6:S1–S166, 1991.

Renal Osteodystrophy

Renal osteodystrophy is a multifactorial disorder of bone remodeling seen in patients with end-stage renal failure. Renal failure results in hyperphosphatemia, decreased ionized Ca, increased synthesis of PTH, and decreased synthesis of $1,25(OH)2D_3$. Serum levels of PTH are typically high, and serum levels of $1,25(OH)2D_3$ are typically low. The conditions are given for the development of osteitis fibrosa cystica (OFC) and osteomalacia. In addition, aluminum and beta-2 microglobulin accumulate. Aluminum is incorporated into bone and inhibits osteoblast function causing osteomalacia and adynamic renal bone disease, a condition characterized by hypocellular bone surfaces and no remodeling. Beta-2 microglobulin accumulates within bone and in capsulo/ligamentous tissues. All of these factors negatively affect bone structure and strength.

Presentation and Progression

Cause

Factors involved in renal osteodystrophy include (1) bone mineral loss to buffer organic acids generated by the diet (osteopenia); (2) secondary hyperparathyroidism (OFC); (3) $1,25(OH)2D_3$ or calcitriol deficiency (osteomalacia?); (4) accumulation of aluminum from water (osteomalacia and adynamic bone disease); (5) cysts and osteoarthropathy from accumulation of beta-2 microglobulin (beta-2 microglobulin amyloidosis); and (6) other factors, particularly cytokines and growth factors. It has been estimated that at the start of treatment for end-stage renal failure, 50% of patients have OFC, 7% osteomalacia, 13% both osteitis fibrosa and osteomalacia, and 27% adynamic bone disease.

Presentation

OFC may present with fractures and osteopenia. There is a poor correlation between bone mineral density and bone strength in OFC because the accumulated woven bone is much weaker than normal trabecular bone. Patients with renal osteodystrophy often have severe bone pain on weight bearing predominantly in the heels, ankles, legs, hips, and lower back. Bone pain is particularly severe in aluminum-related bone disease. Proximal muscle weakness and non-healing rib and pelvis fractures and pseudofractures (Looser's zones) are common in renal osteodystrophy. Serum $1,25(OH)2D_3$ is characteristically decreased in renal osteodystrophy. Other laboratory studies help in predicting the type of bone lesion present: Elevated alkaline phosphatase and PTH levels are diagnostic of osteitis fibrosa; minimally elevated alkaline phosphatase and normal PTH level suggest adynamic bone disease; and high-serum aluminum indicates aluminum-related bone disease. Ectopic ossification or tumoral calcinosis occurs in renal osteodystrophy when P serum levels raise to 8 to 9 mg/dl and the Ca X P product exceeds 75.

Ectopic calcific masses may be silent or cause acute inflammation. In extreme cases ectopic calcification may result in livedo reticularis, ulcers, and eschars of skin progressing to deep ulcers and confluent patches of necrosis (calciphylaxis). Visceral calcification may also occur, such as in the lung. Children with renal osteodystrophy suffer skeletal growth retardation and bone deformity, particularly slipped femoral epiphyses and flared methaphyses, the same as in rickets. The accumulation of beta-2 microglobulin leads to amyloid deposits in the shoulders (pain and limitation, bone cyst formation), the carpal tunnel (carpal tunnel syndrome), the cervical spine (instability, compression), and elsewhere, resulting in pain and a variety of compressive syndromes. This condition is typically seen in patients on long-term hemodialysis.

Diagnosis

Summary of Diagnosis

RENAL OSTEODYSTROPHY

- Renal osteodystrophy should be suspected in all patients with end-stage renal failure.
- Clinical findings include bone pain, fractures, pseudofractures, bone cysts, tumoral calcinosis, and deformity.
- Radiographic findings include osteopenia; subperiosteal erosions in the radial side of digital phalanges, resorption of distal end of clavicles, and erosive changes in sacroiliac joints; patchy osteosclerosis; "rugger jersey spine"*; pseudofractures (Looser's fractures through osteoid seams); and ectopic calcification.
- Serum P, Ca, alkaline phosphatase, aluminum, $1,25(OH)2D_3$, and parathormone are important in predicting the type of bone lesion present.
- Bone densitometry results are unreliable because they tend to overestimate trabecular bone.
- Bone biopsy remains the gold standard to clarify the prevailing mechanism of renal osteodystrophy.

*Sclerotic bands that resemble the stripes in rugby jerseys.

Natural History

Expected Outcome

The condition is chronic and progressive; however, measures can be taken to slow progression and achieve at least partial remission of findings.

Treatment

Methods

Control of Serum Phosphate: A low-phosphate diet, by generating less endogenous acid, is essential in the treatment of renal osteodystrophy. Lower serum phosphate levels decrease acidosis-induced osteoclastic activation, raise ionized Ca, and decrease PTH secretion. Thus, lowering serum phosphate decreases bone resorption, prevents ectopic calcification, and improves secondary hyperparathyroidism. In addition to dietary restriction, the use of an intestinal phosphate binder such as Ca carbonate or Ca acetate is useful to maintain a normal serum phosphate concentration. Calcium carbonate should be ingested with meals to inhibit maximally phosphate absorption. Daily doses range from 4 to 14 g/day. Hypercalcemia is a definite risk in patients using Ca carbonate.

Control of Serum Ca: Serum Ca concentration should be maintained in the high normal range to suppress PTH secretion. This goal can usually be achieved by adjustments of Ca concentration in the dialysate.

Use of Calcitriol: Calcitriol levels are uniformly low in renal osteodystrophy. Calcitriol administration, 0.25 to 1.5 µg/day, which improves secondary hyperparathyroidism, has been helpful to decrease bone pain, increase muscle strength, and improve posture. Histologic changes of OFC can be reverted with this agent. Patients with high P levels should not be given calcitriol, which increases Ca concentration and thus enhances the risk of ectopic calcification.

Parathyroidectomy: If aluminum-related bone disease has been excluded and OFC has been proven by bone biopsy, parathyroidectomy may be indicated to control (1) persistent hypercalcemia not due to excessive Ca or calcitriol intake, malignancy, or sarcoidosis; (2) intractable pruritus; (3) severe bone pain and recurrent fractures; (4) progressive ectopic calcification; and (5) calciphylaxis.

When to Refer

Patients with renal osteodystrophy should be followed primarily by a nephrologist or jointly by a primary care physician and nephrologist. Specific painful processes may require the expertise of a rheumatologist or endocrinologist interested in bone conditions for diagnosis and treatment recommendations.

Key Points

RENAL OSTEODYSTROPHY

- Renal osteodystrophy comprises the skeletal manifestations of end-stage renal disease.
- Lesions according to frequency: OFC > adynamic renal bone disease > OFC plus osteomalacia > osteomalacia.
- Laboratory studies are useful in predicting type of bone lesion and mechanisms involved.
- X-ray findings are subtle in many cases and require high-quality films for assessment.
- Bone densitometry is unhelpful if normal.
- Bone scan is very useful in the assessment of fractures and pseudofractures.
- Treatment is based on the use of a low P diet, phosphate binders, control of serum Ca (Ca concentration in the dialysate), and calcitriol.
- Parathyroidectomy is reserved for refractory hypercalcemia, intractable pruritus, progressive ectopic calcification, and calciphylaxis.
- Osteitis fibrosa cystica must be proven by biopsy prior to parathyroidectomy.

Suggested Reading

Bargmann JM. Calciphylaxis, calcinosis and calcergy—separate but not equal. J Rheumatol 22:5–7, 1995.

Goodman WG, Coburn JW, et al. Renal osteodystrophy in adults and children. In: Favus MJ (ed) Primer on the Metabolic Bone Diseases and Disorders of Mineral Metabolism, 2nd ed. Raven Press, New York, 304–323, 1993.

Hruska KA, Teittelbaum SL. Renal osteodystrophy. N Engl J Med 333:166–174, 1995.

Paget's Disease of Bone

Paget's disease is a localized disorder characterized by a structurally disorganized, metabolically active bone compromising part of a bone, an entire bone, or several bones (polyostotic Paget's) (Figure 22–2). Mature lamellae and woven bone are randomly interspersed. There is an abundance of large multinucleated osteoclasts eroding bone and an equally expanded population of osteoblasts filling the holes osteo-

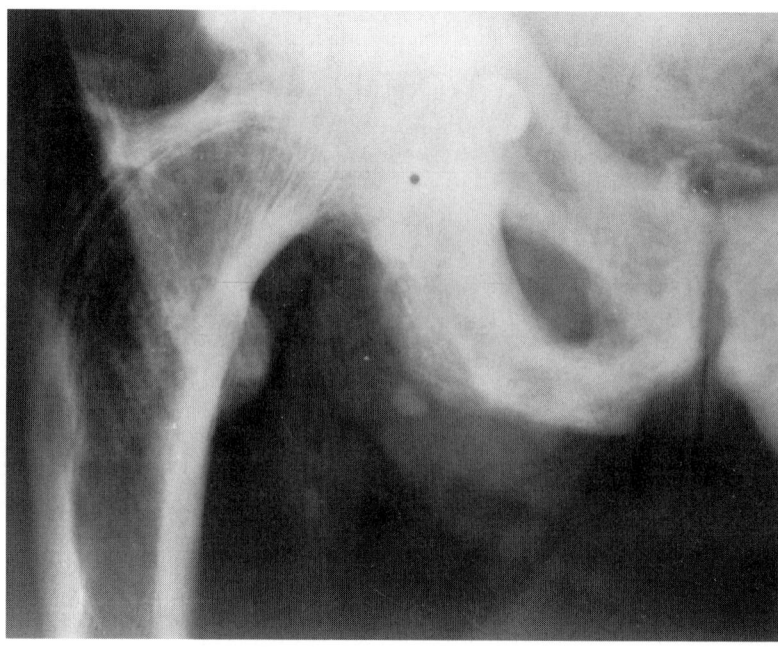

Figure 22–2. *Paget's disease.* There is marked cortical thickening and coarse trabeculation involving femur, iliac bone, and pubis bilaterally.

clasts leave. The cause of Paget's disease is unknown, but evidence suggests that both genetic factors (increased prevalence of the HLA-DQW1 antigen, additional family members affected in 15%–30% of cases) and viral infection (paramyxovirus-like particles within osteoclasts) play a role in the condition.

Presentation and Progression

Paget's disease affects 1% to 2% of the North American population. Most cases are found in the sixth decade of life. Before the age of 40 the condition is definitely rare. Pelvis, femur, spine, skull, and tibia are the most frequently involved bones. Paget's disease is often asymptomatic with the diagnosis being made (1) during evaluation of an increased serum alkaline phosphatase level found on routine examination, or (2) during radiologic evaluation of a fracture or a joint condition that is responsible for the symptoms. Focal pain characterizes symptomatic Paget's disease; pain may be continuous and worse at night or may appear upon weight bearing or during joint motion in lesions that abut on a joint. The involved area often feels warm on palpation, reflecting the increased vasculature of the lesion.

There are several unusual presentations of Paget's disease. Cranial involvement enlarges the head and often causes constricting headaches. The function of cranial nerves may be affected. Bowing of the femur or tibia may be prominent. A lytic lesion may be the dominant abnormality on x-rays, suggesting a neoplasm (Paget's disease always extends to at least one end of the bone). At the other end of the spectrum, a single carpal bone may be involved; these lesions are sclerotic. Finally, angioid streaks may be found in the retina (similar to the lesion seen in pseudoxanthoma elasticum), particularly in polyostotic cases.

Diagnosis

Summary of Diagnosis

> **PAGET'S DISEASE OF BONE**
> - Focal pain, pain on weight bearing, or asymptomatic.
> - Findings on x-rays: an advancing lytic edge ("flamed shaped" or "blade of grass"), sclerosis, trabecular coarsening and disorganization, expanded bone, compromise of at least one end of the bone.
> - Increased serum alkaline phosphatase.
> - Increased urinary excretion of hydroxyproline and pyridinoline.

Natural History

Paget's disease usually remains confined to the initially involved bone(s). Disease extent and disease activity are reflected on laboratory parameters. Serum alkaline phosphatase levels may be increased 10-fold in active polyostotic cases with skull involvement. Lesser elevations are seen in cases without skull involvement and in monostotic disease. Bone resorption is reflected in the urinary excretion of hydroxyproline and pyridinoline. The condition runs a chronic and progressive course in most cases; however, even without treatment some lesions "burn out" clinically, radiologically, and biochemically.

Complications of Paget's disease may be local, compressive, and systemic. Local complications include fractures, damage in a neighboring joint, and neoplastic transformation. Fractures may be incomplete and affect the convex side of bowed bones. This is a frequent cause of enhanced local pain. Complete traumatic or pathologic fractures may complicate pagetic involvement of the proximal femur. Paget's disease is known to cause or aggravate osteoarthritis in a neighboring weight-bearing joint. Finally, neoplasic transformation may occur. Benign osteoclastic masses may grow out of a pagetic lesion. Also, malignant neoplasms complicate approximately 1% of pagetic lesions, particularly when the pelvis, femur, or humerus is involved. Histologic types include osteogenic sarcomas, fibrosarcomas, and chondrosarcomas. Malignant transformation should be suspected when a previously inactive or controlled lesion once again begins to hurt. Compressive complications may result from malignant transformation or, more frequently, because pagetic bone expands. Well-known complications of vertebral enlargement include cord compression and spinal stenosis; cranial involvement may result in hearing loss and cranial nerve palsies; and invagination of the odontoid process through the foramen magnum may rarely cause brain stem compression or hydrocephalus. Systemic complications include hypercalcemia, which may occur when patients with extensive disease are immobilized or if hyperparathyroidism develops, hyperuricemia (of unclear origin), and high-output cardiac failure in polyostotic cases with massive shunting through pagetic bone.

Treatment

Methods

Before considering treating a pagetic lesion, make an effort to determine whether the pain originates in the lesion or in a concurrently involved structure (e.g., a neighboring osteoarthritic hip). Also, tailor treatment to the extent and degree of activity of the lesion (Table 22–6). Determining the source of pain implies a careful assessment of aggravating factors and the results of physical examination. Intrinsic pain is constant and often worse during the night. In this regard, pagetic pain resembles the pain of primary and metastatic bone tumors and osteoid osteoma. Pain that originates in a neighboring joint increases with weight bearing and by bending the joint (e.g., osteoarthritic knee or hip pain in tibial or femoral Paget's, respectively).

Painless lesions serendipitously discovered may or may not require treatment. Lesions in the tibia, femur, spine, and skull (especially when the latter is extensively involved) as well as lesions located near major joints, even if asymptomatic, should be treated to prevent complications. Also, antipagetic treatment should be administered when elective surgery is contemplated to reduce the vascularity of the lesion and decrease the chance of bleeding.

Current treatment of Paget lesions is with calcitonin or a bisphosphonate. Both agents inhibit osteoclast function and thus stabilize and partially reverse the lesions. Two forms of

TABLE 22–6
INDICATIONS FOR DRUG THERAPY IN PAGET'S DISEASE
1. Bone pain
2. Treatment of hearing loss, spinal stenosis with nerve dysfunction, and high-output congestive heart failure
3. Prevention of fractures or skeletal deformity in patients with rapidly progressive osteolytic lesions
4. In preparation for orthopedic surgery

synthetic salmon calcitonin are available: the injectable, which is administered subcutaneously, and the nasal spray. Subcutaneous calcitonin is administered daily, 100 IU or 0.5 cc for 6 months, then decreased to 50–100 U every other day or 3 times a week. The intranasal form is administered 1 spray (200 U) daily is one nostril, on the same schedule as the subcutaneous form.

Bisphosphonates are the other mainstay of Paget's treatment. Most experience has been gathered with etidronate at a daily dose of 5 mg/kg/day (usually 200–400 mg/day) for 6 months followed by 6 months of no treatment. This cycle is repeated for several years. Cyclic treatment is essential to avoid complications. Newer bisphosphonates such as alendronate 40 mg daily for 6 months are not only more potent, but their effect lasts longer and they are less likely to induce osteomalacia and fractures.

Nonspecific treatment in Paget's disease includes the use of walking aids such as a cane, physical therapy, in particular for the strengthening of pelvic and lower extremity muscles, and analgesics or nonsteroidal anti-inflammatory agents for the control of arthritic symptoms.

Orthopedic treatment includes total joint replacement in cases in which intraarticular anesthetics prove articular origin of pain, tibial osteotomy to correct knee pain in patients with pronounced tibial bowing, spinal decompression in pagetic spinal stenosis, and the treatment of accidental or pathologic fractures. Preoperative treatment with bisphosphonates or calcitonin decreases intraoperative bleeding. A reduction of serum alkaline phosphatase to 50% of preoperative values indicates adequate control.

Expected Response

With either agent, symptomatic improvement is seen in a few weeks and biochemical parameters improve after 3 to 6 months of treatment.

Complications

Salmon calcitonin often loses potency with time. Loss of potency may be less with intranasal administration. A frequent side effect of subcutaneous calcitonin is nausea and facial and ear flushing occurring minutes to a few hours after each injection. As mentioned, intranasal administration circumvents this side effect. Symptoms may be lessened by administering the agent at night or by reducing the dose. As mentioned, the main problem with etidronate has been the induction of osteomalacia and fractures by noncyclic administration or with the use of higher than recommended doses.

When to Refer

Patients with Paget's disease should be referred for evaluation to an expert on metabolic bone conditions, usually an endocrinologist or a rheumatologist. Treatment may or may not be recommended. Also, orthopedic imput may be required in some patients. Treatment of Paget's is best done concurrently with an expert.

Key Points

PAGET'S DISEASE OF BONE

- A frequent condition often identified in the fifth decade of life.
- Wide range of extent and severity.
- Clinical activity is determined by assessment of serum alkaline phosphatase and urinary hydroxyproline and pyridinoline.
- Multiple complications may occur at the lesion proper, in a neighboring joint, by neural compression, and systemically.
- Rapid worsening of pain or deformity should be investigated by x-rays plus bone biopsy if suspicion of malignancy arises.
- Treatment should contemplate whether symptoms result from the pagetic lesion, a compressive lesion, or concurrent joint disease.
- Current anti-Paget therapies, calcitonin and bisphosphonates, are helpful in improving symptoms and correcting biochemical parameters of activity.
- Ancillary therapies, including analgesic and anti-inflammatory medications, physical therapy, and orthopedic surgery, should be used as needed and add importantly to the successful treatment of Paget's disease.

Suggested Reading

Kaplan FS, Singer FR. Paget's disease of bone: Pathophysiology, diagnosis, and management. J Am Acad Orthop Surg 3:336–344, 1995.

Osteonecrosis

Osteonecrosis is a generic name that literally implies bone death. It may occur as an idiopathic process affecting an entire bone or part of a bone (these processes, which are best known to radiologists and orthopedic surgeons, are listed in Table 22–7), or it may be acquired as a result of local or systemic processes that have predilection for certain bones. A local acquired osteonecrosis is exemplified by the necrosis of the femoral head that follows a subcapital fracture. The prototype condition of acquired systemic osteonecrosis is corticosteroid-induced aseptic necrosis of bone. Only systemic causes of osteonecrosis are discussed in this chapter.

Presentation and Progression

Cause

There are multiple causes of systemic osteonecrosis and the most common are listed in Table 22–7. Particularly relevant causes are prolonged corticosteroid treatment, alcoholism, and sickle-cell disease. The common denominator in systemic osteonecrosis is interference with bone microcirculation at the epiphyses. Factors held important include blood stasis, hypercoagulability, and damage to endothelial cells. In hypercorticism and alcoholism the main obstructing element appears to be fat globules released into the circulation by a fatty liver. In sickle cell disease deformed erythrocytes get tangled in the capillaries and obstruct microcirculation. In systemic lupus erythematosus (SLE), close to 20% of patients eventually develop osteonecrosis. At a particularly high risk are patients who take 60 mg of prednisone a day or more, have vasculitis, or have Raynaud's phenomenon. An associated antiphospholipid syndrome, with the attendant thrombosis in the microcirculation, may also play a role in SLE-associated osteonecrosis.

Usual Symptoms and Signs

The typical patient in steroid-induced osteonecrosis has systemic lupus erythematosus, asthma, or inflammatory bowel disease and has been taking intermediate to high corticosteroid doses (e.g., prednisone 20 to 60 mg per day) for many months or years. On the other hand, it is believed that osteonecrosis may be induced by any prednisone dose greater than 20 mg per day for 1 month. The initial symptom is gradually mounting hip pain experienced at the groin, anterior thigh, or greater trochanter area. Physical examination may disclose little or no limitation. Initial x-rays are often normal. This should not deter the physician from obtaining additional studies. A bone scan in a very early lesion (stage I) will reveal focal decreased uptake (a cold lesion) in the femoral head. MRIs are falsely negative in these lesions, but soon after (3–4 days) an edema pattern will be identified. Past the initial negative phase and before x-rays show collapse (stage II), the most efficient method of diagnosing osteonecrosis is MRI, which shows a low-intensity band representing the revascularization front beneath the necrotic zone. Asymptomatic contralateral lesions are often found. In due time the radiolucency that may be shown in stage II is followed by sclerosis, collapse (stage III), and secondary osteoarthritis (stage IV). Typically, osteonecrosis-induced osteoarthritis affects first the femoral head and only later the acetabulum. Other frequently affected bones include the femoral condyles, the upper tibia, the humeral head, and the talus.

Osteonecrosis may be difficult to diagnose when the underlying condition features synovitis. Thus, in a patient with rheumatoid arthritis (RA) or SLE, hip pain from osteonecrosis may be attributed to synovitis. The astute clinician will suspect the correct diagnosis based on one or more of the following: (1) new hip synovitis should not be expected in quiescent RA or SLE; (2) isolated hip involvement is unusual in SLE, even in active disease; (3) "ankle arthritis" unresponsive to therapy may in fact represent an osteonecrotic talus that is best shown on MRI; and (4) acute medial or lateral knee pain upon standing or walking with painless passive motion and normal x-rays may in fact indicate tibial or femoral osteonecrosis. Equally difficult may be the identification of evolving osteonecrosis in a patient with sickle-cell disease who is having multiple sickle-cell crises. Sickle-cell disease associates with several bone lesions. Bone ischemia results in excruciatingly painful bone crises. Osteonecrosis tends to develop in patients with repeated bone crises. Osteonecrosis involving the femoral head eventually occurs in 10% to 40% of sickle-cell patients at an average age of 25 years old.

Diagnosis

Summary of Diagnosis

TABLE 22–7

CAUSES OF OSTEONECROSIS

SYSTEMIC

Sickle-cell disease and other hemoglobinopathies	Hyperlipemia Types II or IV
	Obesity
Alcoholism	Chronic liver disease
Hypercortisonism (idiopathic, iatrogenic)	Renal transplantation
	Pancreatitis
Primary and secondary antiphospholipid syndrome and other hypercoagulable states	Gaucher's disease
	Fabry's disease
	Dysbarism (decompression sickness, high altitude exposure)
Systemic lupus erythematosus (glucocorticoids, vasculitis, antiphospholipid antibodies)	Carbon tetrachloride poisoning
	Chemotherapy
Oral contraceptives	Radiation therapy
Pregnancy	Idiopathic

LOCAL

Traumatic

Trauma with disruption of arterial blood supply to bone

Idiopathic

Wrist:	Kienböck's malacia (lunate)
	Preiser's disease (scaphoid)
Elbow:	Osteochondritis dissecans (capitellum)
Spine:	Scheuermann's disease (apophyseal rings of vertebral bodies)
Hip:	Legg-Calvé-Perthes disease (femoral head)
Knee:	Osteochondritis dissecans (medial femoral condyle)
Talus:	Osteochondritis dissecans
Tarsum:	Knoller's disease (navicular)
Metatarsals:	Freiberg's infarction (usually second metatarsal head)

OSTEONECROSIS

- Clinical suspicion (SLE, corticosteroid treatment, alcoholism, sickle-cell disease).
- Joint pain on loading in excess of pain during passive motion.
- Relatively preserved range of motion.
- X-rays may be normal in early stages.
- Bone scans show early focal decreased uptake followed by increased uptake around the lesion.
- MRIs are most efficient in diagnosis past the initial 3 to 4 days of the lesion and before x-rays are positive.

Natural History

Expected Outcome

Once the lesion appears, a progressive course may be expected. In many patients, after the first lesion, further lesions appear in other locations, for example, the contralateral hip, the humeral head, and the talus. The appearance of an additional site of pain in an osteonecrosis patient always has an ominous connotation and should be considered seriously. Additional lesions may appear even if the corticosteroids have been discontinued.

Complications

Osteonecrosis is usually complicated by collapse of necrotic bone at the site of bone repair and sooner or later causes severe degenerative changes in the involved joint. Different from the femoral head and other weight-bearing bones, osteonecrosis in the humeral head may cause little functional limitation.

Treatment

Methods

The bone should be protected from weight bearing. However, only a few lesions are shown to heal with non–weight bearing alone. External electrical stimulation using pulsed electromagnetic fields has been used experimentally alone and as an adjunct to core decompression in early lesions with limited success. Treatment of established osteonecrosis remains surgical. Stages I (cold spot only) and II (positive MRI, no collapse) femoral head lesions are often treated with core decompression biopsy, which proves the diagnosis and is thought to delay or halt progression in some cases. Bone graft is often added to this procedure. However, in a randomized trial of core decompression versus non–weight bearing with crutches in early-stage osteonecrosis, core decompression afforded initial pain relief but failed to prevent collapse of the femoral head. In stage III lesions (radiologic focal collapse), a hemiarthroplasty or total joint replacement is usually required. Hemiarthroplasties work well in symptomatic shoulders. In the hip, some cases with less than 25% involvement of the femoral head may be saved by rotational osteotomy. In most instances, however, total hip replacement is needed. Stage IV lesions with continuous pain and osteoarthritis on both sides of the joint can only be offered total joint replacement. Outcome of total hip replacement in sickle-cell patients has a relatively poor prognosis, with a 30% chance of revision within 4.5 years.

Expected Response

There are no firm data supporting the effectiveness of core decompression surgery or electrical stimulation. The results of joint arthroplasties are excellent.

Complications

Because osteonecrosis often occurs at a relatively early age, long-term complications of the prostheses, such as wearing and loosening, may be expected to occur.

When to Refer

Patients with suspected osteonecrosis should be referred to a rheumatologist or orthopedic surgeon. This is the kind of lesion that should not be missed in its early stages.

Key Points

OSTEONECROSIS
- Should be suspected whenever focal bone pain appears in a patient with known risk factors: for example, SLE, steroid use, alcoholism, or sickle-cell disease.
- Once a lesion is present, its course is progressive and has the potential, if left untreated, to destroy the joint.
- Additional lesions may appear.
- Treatment of early lesions is with core decompression biopsy. The usefulness of this technique has not been fully documented.
- Most advanced lesions eventually need arthroplasty.

Suggested Reading

Acurio MT, Friedman RJ. Hip arthroplasty in patients with sickle-cell haemoglobinopathy. J Bone Joint Surg 74:367–371, 1992.
Conway WF, Totty WG, McEnery KW. CT and MR imaging of the hip. Radiology 198:297–307, 1996.
Jones JP Jr. Concepts of etiology and early pathogenesis of osteonecrosis. Instructional course lectures. Am Acad Orthop Surg 43:499–512, 1994.
Koo K-H, Kim R, Ko G-H, et al. Preventing collapse in early osteonecrosis of the femoral head. J Bone Joint Surg 77B:870–874, 1995.
Petri M. Musculoskeletal complications of systemic lupus erythematosus in the Hopkins lupus cohort: An update. Arthritis Care Res 8:137–145, 1995.

Osteomyelitis

An early diagnosis of osteomyelitis is essential to prevent complications such as epidural abscesses, chronic osteomyelitis, or irreversible damage to a neighboring joint. Unfortunately, clinical findings in osteomyelitis may be difficult to elicit, fever and other markers of infection may be subdued or altogether missing, and imaging abnormalities may take days to weeks to develop depending on the technique used. Primary care physicians should be highly sensitized to osteomyelitis and have the tools to act appropriately and with the right kind of help. Pediatric aspects of osteomyelitis are only mentioned here for general information and to highlight contrasting findings with adult disease.

Presentation and Progression

Cause

Osteomyelitis may be caused by hematogenous infection (the most common form of the condition), by a contiguous focus such as in osteomyelitis secondary to septic arthritis, or by direct innoculation as seen in the ulcerated diabetic foot or following spinal or hip surgery. Hematogenous infection occurs via the systemic circulation in cases that follow skin or respiratory tract infection, or by way of Batson's venous system that connects pelvic organs to the lumbosacral spine. Predisposing conditions include parenteral drug use, alcoholism, HIV infection, or disturbances in the bone microcirculation such as in sickle-cell disease, neuropathic ulcers, sternotomy incisions, spinal surgery or instrumentation, and total joint arthroplasties. The most frequently involved agent in adult hematogenous osteomyelitis is *Staphylococcus aureus,* followed by Enterobacteriaceae, and streptococci. If the patient is black, a sickle-cell preparation should be obtained and if positive, *Salmonella* coverage should be added. *Staphylococcus aureus* causes most instances of osteomyelitis in parenteral drug users. Foot osteomyelitis in diabetics is usually polymicrobial including aerobic cocci, bacilli, and anaerobes. Immunocompromised patients may develop *Candida, Aspergillus, Cryptoccocus,* or *Pneumocystis* osteomyelitis. *M. tuberculosis* and *Brucella* affect the spine more frequently than peripheral bones. Additional pathogens in certain endemic areas include *Histoplasma, Coccidioides,* and *Blastomyces.*

Usual Symptoms and Signs

Pain is the main symptom except in cases that occur in anesthetic areas such as the diabetic foot. Osteomyelitic pain is relentless and made worse at night. Local tenderness may be elicited by direct pressure or percussion. Palpation, to be useful, must be done with anatomic precision. For instance, if the patient has severe pain in the knee region it must be determined whether the tender area is located at the femoral condyle, the tibia, or the joint proper, since the usual differential diagnosis in this location is between osteomyelitis and septic arthritis. When spinal osteomyelitis is suspected, it is useful to have the patient lying prone with a folded pillow supporting the abdomen. In this position the spinous processes spread apart and contracted paraspinal muscles relax. Firm pressure is then applied on each spinous process; reproducible tenderness is consistent with vertebral damage be it osteomyelitis, a fracture, or malignant disease.

In addition to having pain and bone tenderness, most patients are febrile. Fever need not be high or associated with shaking chills. Indeed, the clinician should be aware that low-grade fever is quite common in osteomyelitis and that in some cases there is no fever at all. Similar considerations apply to leukocytosis and neutrophilia, which tend to be present in patients with acute inflammatory symptoms. An elevated ESR is almost the rule, the exception being cases in which the ESR cannot be raised due to shape abnormalities in the erythrocytes, such as in sickle-cell disease, and in conditions associated with low serum fibrinogen levels. C-reactive protein levels may be quite useful in the evaluation and follow-up of these cases. The diagnostic value of the various imaging procedures is shown in Table 22–8.

Various unusual situations may occur. In a denervated foot with a plantar ulcer, if a probe directly hits bone osteomyelitis is likely to be present. Plain x-rays may or may

TABLE 22–8
IMAGING IN OSTEOMYELITIS

Imaging Modality	Time Lag to Positive Findings	Typical Findings	Differential Diagnosis
Conventional radiography	Up to 2 weeks	Parametaphyseal soft tissue swelling (child.); bone lucency at metaphysis surrounded by sclerotic rim (Brodie's abscess, child.); periosteal reaction; subperiostal resorption; cortical erosion; lytic osseous lesions; sequestra.	Posttraumatic and nonspecific (varicose veins) periosteal reaction
Conventional tomography	N.A.	Shows details of bone lesion better and sequestra better than conventional radiography but has been superseded by computed tomography	
Radionuclide scanning	Few days	Positive three-phase uptake (flow, 1–2 minutes; pool, 5–10 minutes; delayed, 2–4 hours postinjection)	Cellulitis: positive uptake in first and second phases alone Arthritis: tracer deposition in both sides of the joint
Computed tomography	Less than 2 weeks	Excellent demonstration of cortical destruction and sequestra. Good to detect adjacent soft tissue extension and abscesses. Increase in intramedullary density an early finding. Intraosseous gas pathognomonic of osteomyelitis	Increased intramedullary density also seen in hemorrhage, stress fracture, or irradiation
Magnetic resonance imaging	Few days	Early demonstration of increased intramedullary water and abscesses. Excellent for demonstration of adjacent arthritis, epidural and paraspinal abscesses. Excellent to distinguish osteomyelitis from cellulitis in the diabetic foot	Trauma and malignancy of bone and soft tissues may cause similar findings

N.A. = Not available.
After Aliabadi P, Nikpoor N. Imaging osteomyelitis. Arthritis Rheum 37:617–622, 1994.

not show osteolysis, but diffuse bone marrow changes on MRI are diagnostic of osteomyelitis. Another difficult situation arises in sickle-cell patients with chronic bone pain from multiple sickle-cell crises and bone infarction.

Osteomyelitis is suggested by fever, malaise, local bone tenderness, leukocytosis, and an increased ESR. Conversely, osteomyelitis may be relatively silent in addition to being afebrile. This is frequent in Brodie's abscess, a pediatric form of osteomyelitis characterized by metaphyseal involvement of a long bone. Tuberculosis as a cause of osteomyelitis in affluent countries continues to be rare even though with the recent surge of drug-resistant tuberculosis in HIV-infected patients a rise is expected. A high index of suspicion is therefore appropriate when evaluating focal bone pain in HIV-infected individuals and also in immigrants from poor regions of the world.

Diagnosis

Summary of Diagnosis

> **OSTEOMYELITIS**
> - Focal bone pain.
> - With or without fever.
> - With or without leucocytosis.
> - ESR usually elevated.
> - A positive probe test in infected pedal ulcers (detection of a rock hard structure at the ulcer base) is proof of osteomyelitis and imaging procedures other than admission x-rays are unnecessary.
> - If plain x-rays are normal, obtain bone scan; if positive, document further by MRI or CT (Table 22–8).
> - Unless blood cultures are positive, a bone biopsy or aspiration should be obtained for culture to arrive at a positive diagnosis and choose an appropriate antibiotic agent.

Natural History

Expected Outcome

Bone infections often extend to the surrounding soft tissues, and abscess migration may occur along fascial planes. Among the soft tissue extensions, epidural abscesses are most feared. Compromise of a neighboring joint is particularly common in children. Untreated osteomyelitis results in necrotic bone in approximately 10 days, although radiographic identification of a sequestrum may be delayed several weeks. Patients with chronic osteomyelitis experience repeated episodes of bone pain, tenderness, pus discharge through a sinus tract, and occasionally low-grade fever. Each episode is accompanied by an increased ESR. Many such episodes, each associated with elevated levels of serum amyloid A (SAA) protein, may result in systemic amyloidosis.

Treatment

Methods

Osteomyelitis treatment requires prolonged administration of an appropriate antibiotic in the same high doses as used in bacterial endocarditis. Initial treatment while blood or bone biopsy cultures results are pending should be guided by the findings of a gram-stained specimen from bone or an abscess plus the most likely agent for that particular host. Intravenous antibiotics should be used at first followed by oral agents for a period of 4 to 6 weeks or more. Epidural abscesses constitute a neurosurgical emergency. Treatment requires laminectomy and drainage of the collection followed by appropriate antibiotics.

Treatment of chronic osteomyelitis requires the removal of all necrotic tissue and sequestra. This is followed by the same treatment course as in acute osteomyelitis. Some patients prefer intermittent antibiotic courses rather than the pain of one or more complicated surgical procedures. In diabetic pedal ulcers, antibiotic choice is based on the results of blood cultures and wound cultures. Osteomyelitis, suggested by a positive probe test, is proven by needle biopsy or open surgical debridement. These patients require a prolonged course of intravenous antibiotics followed by oral antibiotics to a total of 10 weeks, or equivalent.

Expected Response

Successful antibiotic therapy results in slow improvement of pain. Radiographic changes may increase initially and then undergo resolution over several months.

When to Refer

All patients with osteomyelitis should have the benefit of an infectious disease consult. Orthopedic assessment is essential to determine risk to an adjacent joint and to have a plan of action if a sequestrum is present or becomes obvious during treatment. All patients with vertebral osteomyelitis should be assessed by MRI. Presence of epidural abscesses calls for immediate neurosurgical or orthopedic evaluation. A pedal ulcer complicated by osteomyelitis requires the involvement of a vascular surgeon and an infectious disease specialist.

Key Points

> **OSTEOMYELITIS**
> - Osteomyelitis should be suspected whenever focal bone pain develops.
> - Lack of fever and a normal peripheral WBC count are not inconsistent with a diagnosis of osteomyelitis.
> - The ESR is almost always elevated.
> - Routine x-rays may or may not be abnormal. The assessment of possible osteomyelitis justifies the early use of radionuclide bone scanning, and if this is abnormal, an MRI.
> - Successful treatment results in gradual improvement in symptoms followed by ESR normalization and radiologic healing of the lesion.
> - Early consultation with an infectious disease specialist, orthopedic surgeon, and vascular surgeon (in osteomyelitis-complicating pedal ulcers) is essential for optimal treatment results.

Suggested Reading

Aliabadi P, Nikpoor N. Review: Imaging osteomyelitis. Arthritis Rheum 37:617–622, 1994.
Epps CH Jr, Bryant DD III, Coles MJ, et al. Osteomyelitis in patients who have sickle-cell disease: Diagnosis and management. J Bone Joint Surg 73:1281–1294, 1991.
Grayson ML, Gibbons GW, Balogh K, et al. Probing to bone in infected pedal ulcers. A clinical sign of underlying osteomyelitis in diabetic patients. JAMA 273:721–723, 1995.

Hypertrophic Osteoarthropathy (HOA)

Hypertrophic osteoarthropathy is definitely one of the most interesting conditions in rheumatology and one that is likely to yield, on systematic study, key knowledge in rheumatic disease pathogenesis. For the moment, however, HOA remains a useful marker of serious internal disease.

Presentation and Progression

Cause

HOA may be hereditary, but it is more frequently seen with pleuropulmonary, cardiac, and gastrointestinal disease. The many causes of HOA are shown in Table 22–9.

Presentation

The clinical markers of HOA are digital clubbing, periostosis, and noninflammatory synovial effusions, particularly in lower extremity joints. Digital clubbing may be described as a bulbous expansion of distal digital soft tissues and nails. As a result, the angle between the nail and the dorsum of the distal phalanx, as seen from the side, is lost, and compression of the nailbed gives the impression of pressing on a rubber pad.

Periostosis, a term that implies periosteal activation, is characterized by periosteal new bone laid down at the diaphy-

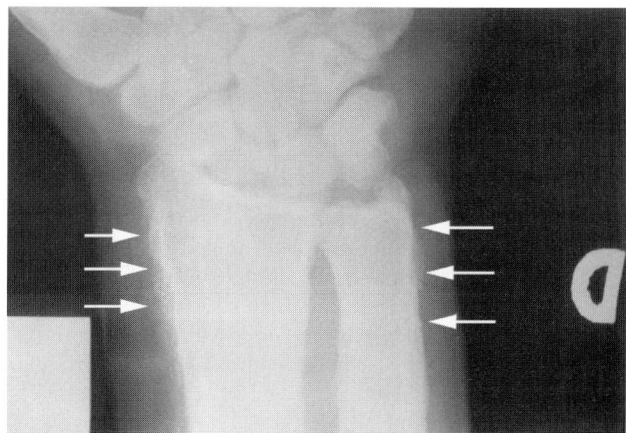

Figure 22-3. *Hypertrophic osteoarthropathy.* Coarse periosteal new bone formation in the distal ulna and radius (arrows) in a patient with cyanotic congenital heart disease. (Courtesy of Dr. Manuel Martínez Lavín, México City.)

ses of appendicular bone (Figure 22–3). HOA may also present cylindrical nonpitting edema in the lower extremities and the skin may be thickened and redundant (pachydermoperiostosis), particularly in the forehead, which gives the patient a leonine appearance. Cutaneous changes are most prominent in hereditary forms of the disease. The condition may be asymptomatic, presenting only with clubbing, or extremely painful due to periostosis as in cases of lung cancer. There are cases of symmetric HOA that resemble RA. There are also unilateral cases, usually in the lower extremities, such as in cases of aneurysms or infected endarteritis of the iliac artery.

Diagnosis

Summary of Diagnosis

> **HYPERTROPHIC OSTEOARTHROPATHY (HOA)**
> - Digital clubbing.
> - Dyaphyseal pain and tenderness from periostosis.
> - Noninflammatory joint effusions.
> - Sometimes cylindrical edema, paresthesias, and redundant and hyperpigmented skin.
> - X-rays of appendicular bones to determine periosteal new bone formation.
> - Bone scan useful for the early diagnosis of periostosis.
> - Obtain chest x-rays looking for lung cancer and other intrathoracic pathology.
> - Consider subacute bacterial endocarditis (SBE).
> - Consider gastrointestinal disease (cirrhosis, inflammatory bowel disease).
> - Consider hereditary forms of HOA.

Natural History

Expected Outcome

Hypertrophic osteoarthropathy persists and slowly gets worse, particularly in terms of bone pain, as long as the

---

TABLE 22–9
CAUSES OF HYPERTROPHIC OSTEOARTHROPATHY

INTRATHORACIC

Lung cancer, primary or metastatic	Mesothelioma
Pulmonary A–V fistulas	Right-to-left cardiac shunts
Lung abscesses	Infective endocarditis
Cystic fibrosis	Esophageal carcinoma
Lung granulomas	Thymoma
Pulmonary fibrosis	Achalasia

INTRAABDOMINAL

Inflammatory bowel disease (Crohn's, UC)	Polyposis
Malabsorptive syndromes	Intestinal malignancies
Laxative abuse	Cirrhosis of the liver
	Hepatocarcinoma

MISCELLANEOUS

Heredofamilial	Thalassemia
Hyperthyroidsm (thyroid acropachy)	Nasopharyngeal and other carcinomas

underlying condition is not arrested and symptomatic treatment is not begun.

Treatment

Methods

Treatment of HOA can be approached in two ways. One is by removing its cause, for example, removal of lung cancer, treatment of SBE, closure of AV shunt, control of inflammatory bowel disease. If any of these can be achieved, slow resolution of HOA will follow, including the bony changes. Symptomatic control is achieved with NSAIDs, in particular indomethacin.

When to Refer

Not all cases of HOA are clear cut. For instance, a patient with IBD with knee effusion and ankle tenderness may have IBD arthritis, crystal-induced synovitis, and HOA among other causes. There are also many reasons why a patient with primary biliary cirrhosis, or SBE, has bone and joint pain. Joint aspiration is very helpful diagnostically. Diagnosis of HOA is strongly supported by viscous, clear, noninflammatory synovial fluid.

Key Points

HYPERTROPHIC OSTEOARTHROPATHY (HOA)

- Hypertrophic osteoarthropathy is a red flag for a variety of serious conditions.
- Synovial fluid examination, long-bone x-rays, and bone scan in early cases are important for diagnosis.
- Once the cause is identified, if a curative treatment exists (e.g., antibiotic treatment of SBE), full remission of HOA will follow.
- Symptomatic treatment is with NSAIDs, particularly indomethacin.

Suggested Reading

Martínez-Lavín M. Hypertrophic osteoarthropathy. In: Klippel JH, Dieppe PA (eds) Rheumatology. Mosby Year Book, 7 40-1-4, 1994.

Pineda C, Fonseca C, Martínez-Lavín M. The spectrum of soft tissue and skeletal abnormalities of hypertrophic osteoarthropathy. J Rheumatol 17:773–778, 1990.

Schumacher HR. Articular manifestations of hypertrophic pulmonary osteoarthropathy. Arthritis Rheum 19:629–635, 1976.

PART IV

MUSCULOSKELETAL CONDITIONS
(Regional Rheumatic Diseases)

Musculoskeletal conditions are among the most poorly taught subjects in medical school. Even in orthopedic and rheumatology training programs they tend to remain on the fringes, which explains the ambiguous terms *medical orthopedics* used by orthopedists and *nonarticular rheumatism* used by rheumatologists. These ailments are extremely common in medical practice, and primary care physicians would do well to learn current principles of diagnosis and treatment. The musculoskeletal conditions discussed here include tendinitis, tenosynovitis, bursitis, fasciitis, enthesopathy, and compression neuropathies. Each of these processes may involve anatomic regions such as the hand, wrist, elbow, shoulder, neck, upper back, lower back, hip, knee, ankle, heel, midfoot, and forefoot. Overuse, repetitive strain, compression, and aging play a major pathogenetic role in many of these syndromes. The biochemical and cellular mechanisms underlying these changes have just started to be unraveled (for an eloquent statement, read Cawston TE, Riley GP, Hazleman BL. Tendon lesions and soft-tissue rheumatism—great outback or great opportunity? Ann Rheum Dis 55:1–3, 1996).

Because such diverse conditions as rheumatoid arthritis, reactive arthritis, gonococcemia, gout, sarcoidosis, and amyloidosis, to name a few, may lead to quite similar syndromes, the astute clinician should not overlook clues to underlying systemic diseases. A detailed analysis is made of the most common syndromes including trigger finger; carpal tunnel syndrome; tennis elbow and its mimickers; shoulder pain in its different varieties; neck pain; mechanical low back pain including disc herniation, facet joint syndrome, and spinal stenosis; meralgia paresthetica; trochanteric bursitis; anserine bursitis; heel pain; hallux valgus; ordinary cramps; and joints that rub, squeak, or snap, among others. Prior to discussing each of the regional conditions a few concepts of clinical anatomy are reviewed. It would be helpful, although by no means necessary, to read these sections with an outline of anatomy at hand.

Suggested Reading

Jenkins DB. Hollinshead's Functional Anatomy of the Limbs and Back, 6th ed. W.B. Saunders, Philadelphia, 1991. (A beautifully illustrated, updated classic. Very useful for the student of regional limb anatomy.)

McKinnon P, Morris J. Oxford Textbook of Functional Anatomy, Vol. 1. Musculoskeletal System. Oxford University Press, New York, 1994. (Clinically oriented; excellent illustrations that make difficult points understandable.)

O'Rahilly RO. Anatomy. A Regional Study of Human Structure, 5th ed. W.B. Saunders, Philadelphia, 1986. (A detailed, well-organized general anatomy textbook; outstanding descriptions of limb, back, and neck anatomy plus relevant thoracic and abdominopelvic anatomy.)

CHAPTER 23

Hand and Wrist Pain

The hand and wrist are frequently involved in regional rheumatic disease. Data from the history and physical examination are usually sufficient for diagnosis. Conditions discussed in this chapter are Dupuytren's contracture, ganglia, trigger finger (digital stenosing tenosynovitis), de Quervain's tenosynovitis, acute digital tenosynovitis, proliferative tenosynovitis, and carpal tunnel syndrome. In the aggregate these conditions account for the bulk of regional disturbances of the hand. Before approaching the specific entities some anatomic and functional aspects of the hand are discussed including the palmar fascia, tendon sheaths, nerves, and superficial landmarks that are germane to the topic.

Looking at my hand fom the palmar side (Figure 23–1) I see the digits and thumb, the palm with the thenar and hypothenar eminences, and the volar wrist. The creases between digits and palm are unrelated to the metacarpophalangeal (MCP) joints except in the thumb in which both structures overlap. Both the MCP and the A_1 pulley of the digital tendon sheaths (Figure 23–2) correspond to the proximal palmar crease in the index finger, the distal palmar crease in the annular and little fingers, and between the two creases in the middle finger. These are important landmarks because the flexor tendon sheath nodules in the trigger finger involve the A_1 pulley, which is also the site of the corticosteroid infiltrations used in this condition.

At the wrist, the flexor retinaculum that binds anteriorly the carpal tunnel extends from the scaphoid tubercle and the crest of the trapezium laterally to the pisiform and the hook of the hamate medially. The proximal edge of the flexor retinaculum corresponds to the distal crease of the wrist. The tendons of the palmaris longus (absent in 10% of persons) and the flexor carpi radialis can be readily identified. As it enters the carpal tunnel the median nerve runs deep to the palmaris longus and medial to the flexor carpi radialis.

Viewed from the radial side with the thumb in extension the anatomic snuffbox stands out. Its anterior border corresponds to the extensor pollicis brevis and abductor pollicis longus tendons, which run enclosed in a common sheath. The posterior border corresponds to the extensor pollicis longus. By deviating the wrist ulnarly, the scaphoid becomes palpable just distal to the radial head. The cleft of the first carpometacarpal joint, in turn, is apparent 1 cm distal to the scaphoid. Important dorsal landmarks include Lister's tubercle at the radial head, and the ulnar styloid. The flexor sheath of the thumb always extends to the wrist (within the carpal tunnel, this sheath is known as the radial bursa). The flexor sheath of the little finger connects in 80% of cases with the ulnar bursa, a synovial expansion that layers the flexor digitorum tendons within the carpal tunnel.

The flexor sheaths of digits 2, 3, and 4 are usually independent and extend just proximal to the A_1 pulley. In approximately 9% of cases, however, one of these sheaths extends more proximally and connects with the ulnar bursa. These anatomic features determine the proximal extension of infection in cases of suppurative flexor tenosynovitis.

Normally, we can bend the thumb toward the base of the little finger (full flexion), and stretch it out radially (full extension), project it vertical to the palm (full abduction), and bring it back to the radial border of the hand (full adduction). The lesser fingers may be flexed to contact with the palm and may be extended fully, perhaps achieving a dorsal extension (hyperextension) of 5 degrees. Opposition movement brings the tip of the thumb in contact with the tip of each of the lesser digits (index, long, ring, and little fingers). Each of the

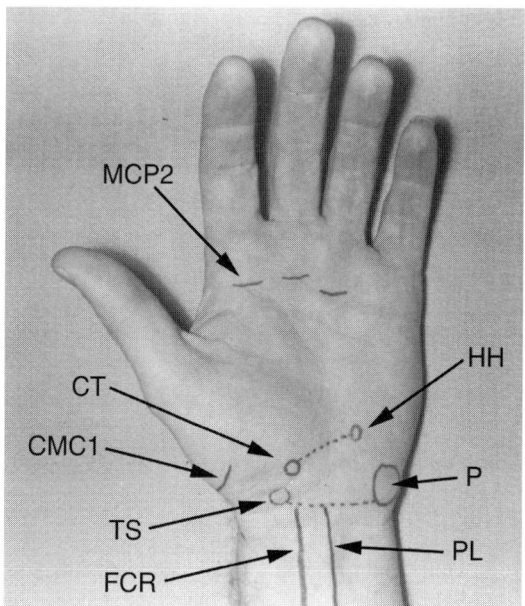

FIGURE 23–1. Hand seen from the palmar side to identify some important landmarks: MCP2 = Second metacarpophalangeal joint. HH = Hook of hamate. P = Pisiform. PL = Palmaris longus tendon. FCR = Flexor carpi radialis tendon. TS = Tubercle of scaphoid. CMC1 = First carpometacarpal joint. CT = Crest of trapezium. HH, P, TS, and CT represent the attachments of the flexor retinaculum that binds anteriorly the carpal tunnel. The median nerve is placed between PL and FCR. Thus, to inject the carpal tunnel, the needle should be entered just ulnar to PL.

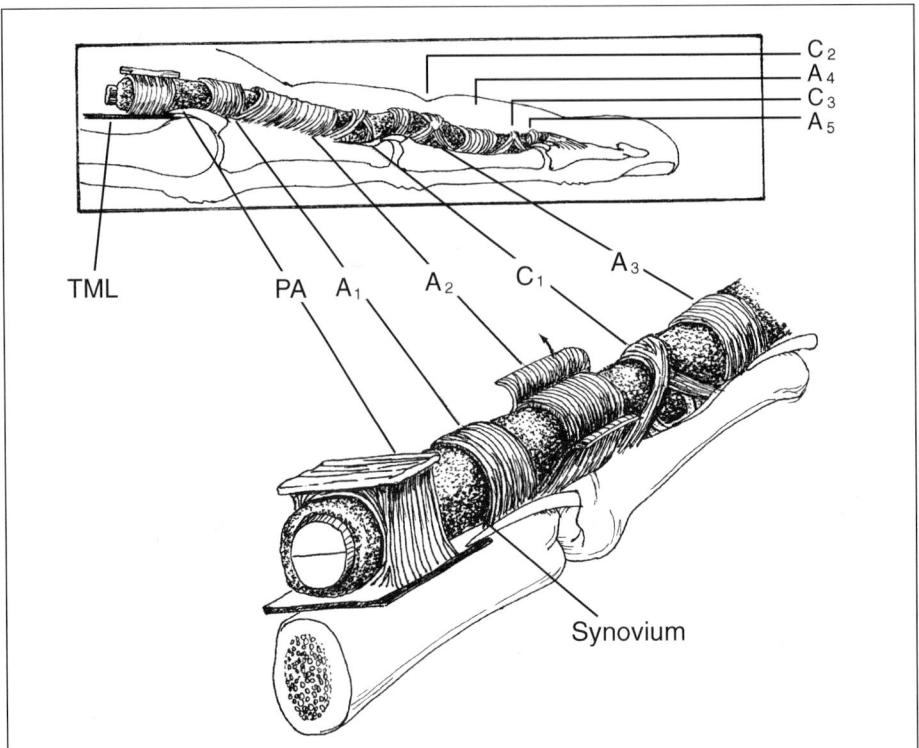

FIGURE 23–2. *The digital flexor tendon sheath.* TML = Transverse metacarpal ligament. PA = Palmar aponeurosis. A_1 to A_5 = Annular pulleys 1 to 5. C_1 to C_3 = Cruciform pulleys 1 to 3. Nodules in trigger finger involve A_1. Rheumatoid tenosynovitis and other chronic inflammatory conditions involve the entire synovium of the sheath. (After Doyle RR. Anatomy of the flexor tendon sheath and pulley system: A current review. J Hand Surg 14A:349–351, 1989.)

lesser digits has two flexor tendons, the superficialis and the profundus, that attach to, and flex, the middle and distal phalanges, respectively. In the thumb a long flexor attaches to the distal phalanx, and a short flexor, a thenar eminence muscle, attaches to the proximal phalanx and radial sesamoid.

The little finger, index, and thumb have two extensor tendons, and the middle and ring fingers have one. Needless to say, extensor digital tendons have no synovial sheaths. Their insertion is through the extensor hood, a roughly triangular fibrous sheath to which extensor tendons and intrinsic muscles (lumbricals and interossei) attach. By virtue of their direction of pull, which is volar to the MCP and dorsal to the proximal interphalangeal (PIP) and distal interphalangeal (DIP) joints, intrinsic muscles flex the MCP and extend the PIP. The palmar fascia, which is the site of involvement in Dupuytren's contracture, is a triangular fibrous membrane that overlies the tendons in the palm. Proximally, its apex merges with the palmaris longus tendon and is anchored to the flexor retinaculum. Distally, the palmar fascia divides into four pretendinous bands, each attaching to the fibrous tendon sheath and to the phalangeal margins. Lateral expansions of these bands constitute the superficial transverse metacarpal ligament, which together with the A_1 and A_2 pulleys prevent tendon bowstringing during finger flexion. Here are some simple maneuvers that help assess tendon integrity:

1. The extensor tendons may be tested passively by the "tenodesis effect." The maneuver consists of watching what happens to the fingers during passive extension and flexion of the wrist. In extension, all digits flex. In flexion, provided that the extensor apparatus is intact, all digits extend. A failure to extend means tendon rupture, which in rheumatoid arthritis patients occurs at the ulna styloid, or attenuation of the extensor apparatus itself.

2. To test the extensor pollicis longus tendon, the patient is asked to place the hand palm down on a flat surface and raise the thumb. Normally, the extensor pollicis longus tendon stands out. If the tendon is ruptured, which in rheumatoid arthritis patients occurs at Lister's tubercle, the tendon fails to show and a hollow is noted instead.

3. If the patient is able to straighten the index and little finger while third and fourth fingers are held flexed under the thumb, the extensor indicis and the extensor digiti minimi (additional individual extensor tendons for these digits) are intact.

4. To test the flexor digitorum profundus tendon, the patient is asked to attempt flexion of the digit while the middle phalanx (the proximal phalanx in the thumb to test the flexor pollicis longus) is held in extension.

5. Swan-neck deformity, which consists of hyperextension of the PIP joint and flexion of the DIP joint, may result from various mechanisms, one of which is abnormal intrinsic muscle tension. Normally, passive flexion of the PIP is the same with the MCP in extension as it is in flexion. If intrinsic muscle tension is present, PIP flexion will be normal with the MCP in flexion, and reduced or impossible with the MCP in extension. The reason for this clinically useful phenomenon is that MCP exten-

sion stretches the shortened intrinsics, leaving no slack to allow passive flexion of the PIP.

Suggested Reading

Canoso JJ. Bursae, tendons and ligaments. Clin Rheum Dis 7:189–221, 1981.

Canoso JJ. Hands, wrists and elbows. In: Cohen AS, Bennett JC (eds) Rheumatology and Immunology, 2nd ed. Grune & Stratton, Orlando, 1–9, 1986.

Dupuytren's Contracture

Presentation and Progression

Cause

Dupuytren's contracture, a condition that affects predominantly middle-aged and older individuals of northern European descent, results from fibrotic thickening and contracture of the palmar fascia. Usually bilateral and unequal, severity of findings is unrelated to handedness. An association with diabetes, local trauma, alcoholism, and the use of antiseizure medication have long been suggested.

Presentation

Dupuytren's contracture develops slowly, and patients are often unaware of its presence in early disease. Nodules and then string formation in the mid-palmar region usually affect the fourth ray, but also the third and fifth follow. Unsightly palmar retraction, finger contractures, and hand disability characterize late Dupuytren's disease. Additional (concurrent or sequential) fibrotic lesions speak of a "Dupuytren's diathesis." These include firm nodules at the extensor surface of PIP joints (knuckle pads), penile fibrosis resulting in a curved erection (Peyronie's disease), and troublesome plantar fascia nodules. An association with trigger finger, carpal tunnel syndrome, lateral epicondylitis, and frozen shoulder has been noted in diabetes mellitus. Unilateral, rapidly progressing Dupuytren's contracture may develop in the aftermath of sympathetic dystrophy.

Finally, a paraneoplastic condition known as Medsger's syndrome features painful palmar swelling followed by retraction (Figure 23–3), joint contractures, and bilateral frozen shoulder. Medsger's syndrome is seen predominantly in patients with cervical or uterine neoplasms, lung cancer, and other malignant conditions but may also arise in patients with benign ovarian teratoma and endometriosis, and during antituberculous therapy. By the time this condition develops, most patients are known to have malignant disease. However, Medsger's syndrome may precede the clinical appearance of the neoplasm for up to 2 years.

Diagnosis

Summary of Diagnosis

> **DUPUYTREN'S CONTRACTURE**
>
> - Diagnosis is based on the identification of nodular or stringlike palmar fibrosis.
> - A "Dupuytren's diathesis" is suggested by the association of "knuckle pads," Peyronie's disease, and plantar fibrotic nodules.
> - Diabetes should be ruled out when two or more of the following overlap: trigger finger, carpal tunnel syndrome, lateral epicondylitis, and frozen shoulder.
> - Atypical, inflammatory cases suggest an underlying neoplasm (Medsger's syndrome).

Natural History

Expected Outcome and Complications

Dupuytren's contracture has an unpredictable course. Early in the disease palmar nodules are prominent and there is no retraction. Mitotically active, hypercellular lesions convey a worst prognosis in terms of recurrence after fasciectomy. An intermediate signal on MRI identifies these lesions. However, since nodules are so readily seen, the expense of the test can hardly be justified. As the lesion evolves nodules are replaced by strings and hand retraction develops. Early in the disease it is not possible to distinguish cases that will not progress, which represent the majority, from those heading to disfiguration and function loss. The latter is heralded by difficulty to place the hand into a pocket; the bent fingers get in the way. Finger contractures, usually involving the third, fourth, and fifth digits, cause a major handicap in manual workers and musicians. Of paramount therapeutic importance is to distinguish finger contractures due to fascial fibrosis from the late results of concurrent stenosing tenosynovitis. Presence of the latter is suggested by antecedent finger triggering. Attenuation of the extensor

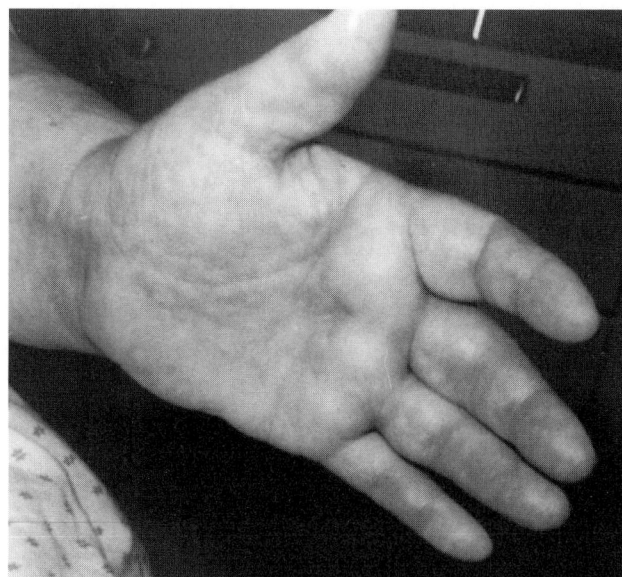

FIGURE 23–3. *Medsger's syndrome.* This woman, aged 62, with a history of cervical cancer treated by surgery and radiotherapy 2 years prior, suddenly developed edema and bluish indurations in the palmar aspect of both hands. Surgical biopsy revealed excess dermal mucopolysaccharides and increased cellularity. Over the course of weeks, widespread palmar fascia induration followed, resembling Dupuytren's contracture but more extensive across the palm. Platelets were in the 700,000/mm³ range. Local recurrence of the malignancy involving the pelvic floor was shown.

tendinous apparatus in long-standing PIP contractures negates a beneficial effect of surgery.

Treatment

Methods

Multiple systemic treatments have been empirically tried. Nonsteroidal anti-inflammatory drugs appear ineffective. Oral colchicine has a theoretical inhibitory effect on collagen synthesis, but an in vivo effect has not been shown. Corticosteroid infiltrations (except in cases in which stenosing tenosynovitis coexists) and DMSO have also been used without proof of effectiveness. Wire traction of the fascia reverts clinical and histologic findings, but contracture promptly recurs as traction is released. Treatment of Dupuytren's contracture remains surgical. Subtotal fasciectomy is reserved for patients with late disease in whom finger limitation develops, and for cosmesis.

Expected Response

Surgical results are highly dependent on the stage of the disease. Recurrences are frequent in patients operated in the nodular stage. On the other hand, long-standing finger contracture, by causing attenuation of the extensor apparatus, may negate the beneficial effect of surgery. Attenuation of the extensor apparatus can be recognized intraoperatively by a negative tenodesis effect (fingers do not extend when the wrist is passively flexed). An extension splint used for 3 weeks after surgery often solves this problem.

Complications

Dupuytren's contracture may cause function loss and disfigurement from both finger contracture and unsightly knuckle pads. Penile deviation from Peyronie's disease is a cause of pain during sexual intercourse. Plantar fibromatosis causes severe plantar pain and poses perplexing treatment problems.

When to Refer

Patients with hand dysfunction and those cosmetically concerned should be evaluated by a hand surgeon. Plantar fibromatosis should be evaluated by an orthopedic surgeon interested in soft tissue tumors (the point here is not to miss sarcoma).

Key Points

DUPUYTREN'S CONTRACTURE

- Its cause is unknown.
- Middle-aged and elderly individuals are affected.
- There is fibrosis of the palmar fascia. Other fibrotic processes are often present.
- Progression is unpredictable.
- Systemic and local therapies (drugs, injections) are ineffective or of unproven value.
- Functional limitation or cosmetic concern should trigger consultation with a hand surgeon.
- Palmar fasciectomy has excellent results.

Suggested Reading

Adams RF, Loynes RD. Prognosis in Dupuytren's contracture. J Hand Surg 17A:312–317, 1992.

Makela EA, Jaroma H, Harju A, et al. Dupuytren's contracture: The long-term results after day surgery. J Hand Surg 16B:272–274, 1991.

Terek RM, Jiranek WA, Goldberg MJ, et al. The expression of platelet-derived growth-factor gene in Dupuytren's contracture. J Bone Joint Surg 77A:1–9, 1995.

Yacoe ME, Bergman AG, Ladd AL, et al. Dupuytren's contracture: MRI imaging findings and correlation between MR signal intensity and cellularity of lesions. AJR 160:813–817, 1993.

Ganglia

Presentation and Progression

Cause

Ganglia are benign cystic lesions with a clear mucinous content. They usually grow in the hand and wrist, occasionally elsewhere in the soft tissues, and rarely within bone (intraosseous ganglia). Ganglia represent the most common tumorous condition in the hand and wrist, followed in frequency by inclusion cysts and nodular pigmented synovitis. Multiple lesions are uncommon, although individual lesions can be shown pathologically to be composed of a larger central cavity surrounded by several smaller cavities with thin or thick septae separating them.

The origin of ganglia is controverted. Some authors consider them to be true cysts in which focal myxoid degeneration of the connective tissues is followed by cavitation. The prevailing opinion, however, is that ganglia represent expanded outpouches of a joint. This view is supported by high-pressure arthrography studies in which contrast material was seen to pass from the joint into the cyst. Because the reverse was not true, the presence of a Bunsen-type valve consisting of a tortuous narrow duct the walls of which collapse under direct cyst pressure has been postulated (Figure 23–4). These findings, plus ganglia that are unrelated to joints or tendon sheaths, suggest that both pathogenetic theories may be true.

Presentation

Most ganglia (60%–70%) occur in the dorsal wrist in relation with the scapholunate and trapezium-trapezoid joints. Next in frequency (18%–20%) are volar wrist ganglia that grow between the tendons of the flexor carpi radialis and brachioradialis. These lesions are quite close to the radial artery. Less common locations include the carpal tunnel, proximal digital flexor tendon sheaths, the vicinity of distal interphalangeal joints (digital mucinous pseudocysts), various sites elsewhere in the connective tissues, and even bone (intraosseus ganglia).

An early symptom is intermittent pain experienced after heavy use of the hand, with or without a lump. Ganglia may also present as a painless, slowly growing mass. A smooth sur-

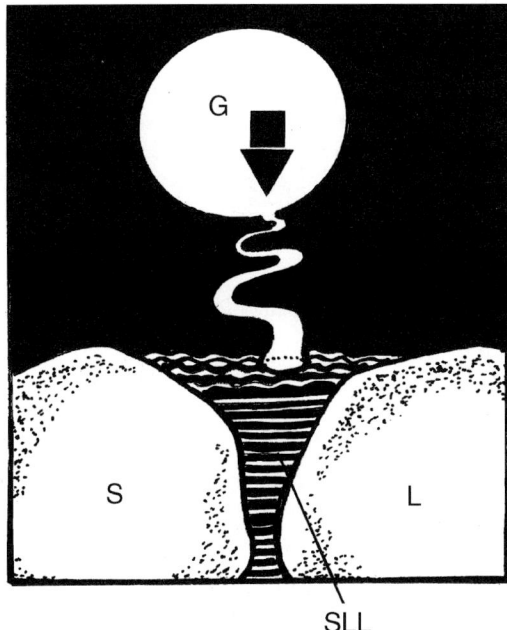

FIGURE 23–4. *Ganglion.* There has been controversy on the origin of ganglia. In certain locations, such as the dorsum of the wrist, ganglia routinely connect with the underlying joint. Here a ganglion (G) is shown that originates at the scaphoid-lunate ligament in the dorsum of the wrist. Its convoluted thin neck becomes compressed when the cyst's pressure increases and opens up when the pressure gradient favors the joint (Bunsen-type valve). S = Scaphoid. L = Lunate. SLL = Scaphoid-lunate ligament. (After Angelides AC, Wallace PF. The dorsal ganglion of the wrist: Its pathogenesis, gross and microscopic anatomy, and surgical treatment. J Hand Surg 1:228–235, 1976.)

face is characteristic. Ganglia become tense and painful during flares and soft and painless as the episode resolves either spontaneously or with the help of a splint. In ganglia, symptoms and findings parallel the use of the hand. This very characteristic makes mandatory ruling out more straightforward synovial outpouches that coincide with synovial effusions and can be easily emptied by pressure. Other tumoral lesions tend to be invariant. Atypical presentations stem from unusual size or location of the lump. Digital mucinous pseudocysts occur in the dorsal distal phalanx in relation with an osteoarthritic distal interphalangeal joint. These lesions are superficial, may be translucent, and commonly associate with a linear nail deformity. Compressive neuropathies, and rarely a compartmental syndrome, may result from ganglia growing at nerve passages or within confined spaces. Examples include carpal tunnel ganglia compressing the median nerve, and ganglia at the scapular notch causing a suprascapular nerve compression neuropathy. Ganglia about the radial wrist must be differentiated from radial artery aneurysms. Although transmitted pulsations may closely resemble aneurysmal pulsations, particularly in ganglia located at an arterial fork, careful palpation may distinguish the two lesions. Ganglia at the popliteal fossa may mimic a Baker's cyst or a popliteal artery aneurysm. Ultrasonography is an effective method to distinguish ganglia from aneurysmal lesions and should be used whenever doubts remain.

Finally, intraosseous ganglia, also known as juxtaarticular bone cysts, are well-defined osteolytic lesions with surrounding sclerosis filled with mucoid material located in the epiphyseal subchondral bone. A communication with the joint is not found in the majority of cases. Common locations include the upper end of femur and tibia, the medial malleolus, and the carpal bones. Intraosseous ganglia may develop by penetration of an extraosseous ganglion into bone, or more frequently, as a primary lesion. These lesions may be silent or may produce pain, particularly after ambulation. Ganglia should also be distinguished from juxtaarticular myxomas. These are benign, multilocular cystic lesions with a myxoid or mucinous content that typically occur around the knee and in the vicinity of the acromioclavicular joint. A joint connection cannot be demonstrated in juxtaarticular myxomas.

Because ganglia are noninflammatory lesions, ESR and other routine tests are normal. X-ray studies show nonspecific focal soft tissue increase. Although ganglia are clearly demonstrated by CT with contrast and MRI, the use of these techniques is unjustified except when a malignant lesion is a consideration. Ultrasound studies are very helpful in the diagnosis of ganglia. Ganglia are typically cystic and unicameral, although they may be septated. Heterogeneous lesions have a high probability of being malignant and should be further investigated by MRI. Aspiration of ganglia yields an extremely viscous, mucinous, crystal clear fluid with a few large vacuolated cells. These findings are pathognomonic of the lesion.

Diagnosis

Summary of Diagnosis

> **GANGLIA**
>
> - Diagnosis is based on the characteristics of the lesion on physical examination: smooth surface, tense, typical location around the wrist are characteristic.
> - Deep ganglia require ultrasound investigation: homogeneous, smooth-walled lesions represent ganglia.
> - MRI is indicated when malignancy is suggested clinically or by heterogeneous findings on ultrasound examination.
> - A clear, highly viscous fluid is characteristic of ganglia.

Natural History

Expected Outcome

Ganglia may resolve without treatment. This is said to occur in about 40% of the lesions. In the author's experience, however, true resolution is far less frequent; what one may be seeing is rather a long asymptomatic period between flares. Small ganglia may represent an intermittent nuisance, becoming symptomatic only after heavy use of the hand. Large ganglia (> 3 cm in diameter) fluctuate in size but seldom go away.

Complications

Large dorsal wrist ganglia are unsightly. They may also compress superficial branches of the radial nerve and cause hand dysesthesia. Volar wrist ganglia under the flexor retinaculum are a well-known cause of the carpal tunnel syndrome. A deeply seated palmar ganglion may compress the deep palmar branch of the ulnar nerve and cause intrinsic muscle atrophy. Ganglia at the suprascapular or spinoglenoid notch may impinge on the suprascapular nerve and result in posterolateral shoulder pain and atrophy of the supra- and infraspinatus muscles (this syndrome may be confused with an advanced rotator cuff impingement lesion). Finally, ganglia at the proximal tibiofibular joint, by growing under the unyielding fascia, may cause an anterior compartment syndrome.

Treatment

Methods

Time-honored treatments include rupture by finger pressure or a sharp blow with a heavy book, cyst puncture with a needle, and the injection of corticosteroids or sclerosing agents. In dorsal wrist ganglia and other accessible lesions, the author uses a large-bore (#18) needle for aspiration (which confirms the diagnosis) followed by the injection of 20 to 40 mg of methylprednisolone acetate or equivalent. Splint immobilization for 2 weeks reduces the likelihood of recurrence. In recurrent lesions, or in cysts growing in potentially troublesome areas such as the carpal tunnel, surgical resection is indicated. The cyst should be removed in toto including its stalk and capsular attachment. Digital mucinous pseudocysts may also be aspirated and infiltrated with corticosteroids. However, in most cases excision with removal of a portion of the joint capsule will be required. Large intraosseous ganglia are treated with curettage and bone grafting.

Expected Response

The success rate of aspiration and corticosteroid injection is approximately 50%. Recurrent ganglia may be reinjected once. Surgical removal cures 85% to 95% of cases.

Complications

One must be sure, prior to aspiration and injection, that the lump represents a true ganglion rather than an arterial aneurysm. Complications of injection are few, mainly skin atrophy and depigmentation. Arterial damage must be quite rare. Complications of surgery, which are infrequent, include a painful scar, infection, the possibility of nerve damage, and postoperative sympathetic dystrophy.

When to Refer

Patients with ganglia larger than 3 cm in diameter and cases with suspected compression neuropathy should be referred to a hand surgeon.

Key Points

GANGLIA
- Benign cystic lesions with a mucoid content that are most frequently found in hand and wrist.
- Disfiguration and compressive neuropathies are important consequences of ganglia.
- Conservative treatment includes aspiration of the jellylike contents and corticosteroid infiltration.
- Success rate of conservative treatment is about 50%.
- Surgical treatment includes removal of the cyst, the feeding duct, and its capsular attachment.
- The success rate of surgical treatment is about 90%.

Suggested Reading

Andrén L, Eiken O. Arthrographic studies of wrist ganglions. J Bone Joint Surg 53A:299–302, 1971.

Angelides AC, Wallace PF. The dorsal ganglion of the wrist: Its pathogenesis, gross and microscopic anatomy, and surgical treatment. J Hand Surg 1:228–235, 1976.

Drapé J-L, Idy-Peretti I, Goettmann S, et al. MR imaging of digital mucoid cysts. Radiology 200:531–536, 1996.

Schajowicz F, Clavel Sainz M, Slullitel JA. Juxtaarticular bone cysts (intra-osseous ganglia). A clinicopathological study of eighty-eight cases. J Bone Joint Surg 61B:107–116, 1979.

Soren A. Pathogenesis, clinic, and treatment of ganglion. Arch Orthop Traumat Surg 99:247–252, 1982.

Young L, Bartell T, Logan SE. Ganglions of the hand and wrist. So Med J 81:751–760, 1988.

Trigger Finger (Digital Stenosing Tenosynovitis)

Presentation and Progression

Cause

The trigger finger, or digital stenosing tenosynovitis, is common in middle-aged and older individuals and also in young children. Females are more frequently affected than males, with a ratio of 2 to 4 to 1. Many tasks predispose to the condition such as wringing clothes, sewing, cutting, and using precision hand tools such as in dentistry. In adults, the obstruction is caused by cartilage metaplasia and fibrosis at the A_1 pulley in the proximal portion of the digital flexor tendon sheath (Figure 23–2) plus minor similar changes in the tendon itself. Pathologic changes are believed to be caused by repetitive high pressures exerted by the tendon on the pulley during finger flexion. A fibrotic diathesis is a contributing factor in diabetes. In children the obstruction is caused by nodular thickening of the tendon rather than the sheath.

Presentation

Patients complain of difficulty and pain upon flexion-extension motions or actual triggering in which a snap is felt and heard when the finger is about two-thirds flexed and extended. In more advanced cases the finger can be actively flexed with a snap, after which it remains locked in flexion. To regain the extended position, which again occurs with a snap, the digit must be helped with the other hand. In late cases the digit remains incarcerated in flexion. One, or less frequently a few fingers, are involved. The association of multiple, bilateral stenosing lesions, carpal tunnel syndrome, tennis elbow, and frozen shoulder should raise the possibility of diabetes.

On examination a tender lump is usually felt volar to the MCP joint and palpation reveals this to be the site of the snap. Superficial landmarks, which correspond to the proximal border of the A_1 pulley, include the MCP flexor crease for the thumb, the proximal palmar crease for the index, the distal palmar crease for the ring and small fingers, and halfway between both creases for the middle finger. The most frequently involved digits in adults (Figure 23–5) are the thumb (one-third to one-half of cases) and the long finger (one-third of cases). The remaining one-third to one-quarter is comprised, in descending order, by the ring, index, and little fingers. Passive flexion, as in all the tenosynovitides, is normal. Multiple stenotic lesions may be idiopathic (50% of cases) or may indicate diabetes (45% of cases), hypothyroidism, ochronosis, multicentric reticulohistiocytosis, and light-chain amyloidosis. In the aggregate, multiple lesions account for 10% to 20% of cases of stenosing tenosynovitis.

In the pediatric population, trigger fingers differ from the adult condition in several ways, for example, the thumbs are most frequently involved with a thumb to lesser digits ratio of 10 to 1, the nodular thickening corresponds to the tendon rather than the sheath, bilateral involvement occurs in at least 25% of cases, and a locked digit is far more frequent than snapping.

Diagnosis

Summary of Diagnosis

> **TRIGGER FINGER**
> **(Digital Stenosing Tenosynovitis)**
>
> - Pain, irregular motion, or snapping at the distal palm caused by motion of one or a few digits.
> - Pediatric cases and late-adult cases often present with a digit incarcerated in flexion.
> - A nodule is usually felt at the A_1 pulley.
> - No evidence of inflammation should be present.
> - Metabolic causes must be ruled out when multiple digits are involved.

Natural History

Expected Outcome

Untreated or treated with only a splint, about 20% of trigger fingers improve. Spontaneous improvement is most likely to occur in patients who consult within the first 2 weeks of symptoms. In the remaining patients the condition persists.

Complications

A trigger finger may cause significant disability in occupations that require fine use of the hand. Untreated adult cases often end up with a permanently flexed digit. Children usually present with the digit locked in flexion.

Treatment

Methods

Trigger finger may be treated with a resting splint, but results are generally poor. Splintage, if used at all, should be reserved for cases of less than 2 weeks' duration. Surgical release of the A_1 pulley, the standard treatment of trigger finger in children, is no longer the treatment of choice in adults because of a high complication rate (complications of surgery are quite few in children), plus the excellent results of corticosteroid

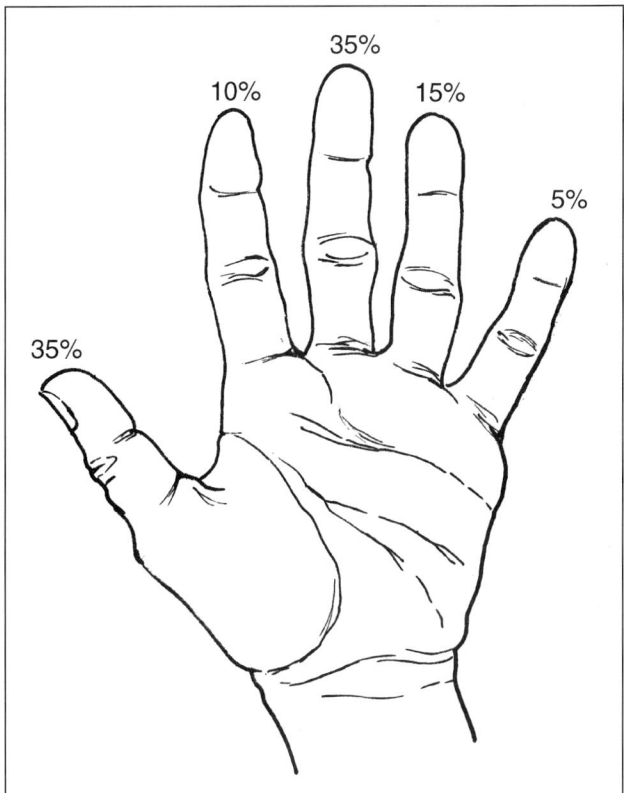

FIGURE 23–5. *Trigger finger.* Frequency of trigger finger according to digit in adults. In children, virtually all cases occur in the thumb.

infiltrations. Techniques of injection, steroid preparations, and doses are shown in the appendix. In idiopathic cases, the success rate of a single infiltration is 50% to 60%. If patients failing to improve are reinjected at 3 week intervals, good results increase to 80% with one reinjection and 90% to 100% with a second reinjection. With a single sham infiltration (local anesthetic alone), the improvement rate is about 20%. In diabetics, particularly in insulin-dependent diabetes, the failure rate of three injections is close to 50%. Surgical release in adults is today reserved for patients who refuse infiltration, patients who present with a permanently locked digit, and failures to improve after an arbitrary maximum of three infiltrations.

Expected Response

Following steroid infiltration, pain relief may be expected in 3 to 5 days and relief of obstruction in a few days to 3 weeks, providing the rationale for the 3 week interval between infiltrations (Table 23–1).

Complications

Surgical release in adults has a 10% complications rate including a failure to improve due to incomplete release of the A_1 pulley; digital nerve injury; sympathetic dystrophy; accidental section of the palmar aponeurosis pulley and the A_2 pulley, which in addition to the intended section of the A_1 pulley results in bowstringing and flexion loss; and infection. If painful scars are also included, the rate of unsuccessful

TABLE 23–1

RESULTS OF CORTICOSTEROID INFILTRATION IN TRIGGER FINGER (STENOSING TENOSYNOVITIS): UNCONTROLLED SERIES

	Patients	Fingers Injected	Fingers Cured (%)
Marks and Gunther, 1989	74	108	86
Faunø et al., 1990	93	104	73*
Newport et al., 1990	251	338	77
Anderson and Kaye, 1991	58	77	88
Panayotopoulos et al., 1992	30	30	89

*Only one injection.
No complications observed in these series.

procedures increases to 30%. Surgical release in diabetics is followed by palmar skin aching and thickening and flexion contracture of the PIP joint in about 20% of cases. Corticosteroid infiltrations, in contrast, offer high effectiveness and a low complication rate. No instances of tendon rupture or infection were reported in extensive series. The only complication of corticosteroid infiltrations the author has seen, which is both unusual and asymptomatic, is focal fat atrophy.

When to Refer

Provided adequate learning (demonstration and some experience under direct supervision by a rheumatologist, hand surgeon, or orthopedist), corticosteroid infiltrations for trigger fingers can and should be administered by primary physicians. Patients with involvement of multiple tendons and cases that fail to improve after one or two infiltrations should be referred for reconsideration of diagnosis and further therapy.

Key Points

TRIGGER FINGER (Digital Stenosing Tenosynovitis)

- Idiopathic cases usually involve one digit.
- Multiple finger involvement should raise the possibility of missed systemic synovitis (RA, psoriatic, etc.), diabetes, hypothyroidism, or some unusual metabolic or infiltrative condition.
- One or more corticosteroid infiltrations succeed in over 90% of idiopathic cases.
- Diabetic stenosing tenosynovitis fails to respond to corticosteroid infiltrations in 50% of insulin-dependent cases and about 25% of non-insulin-dependent cases.

Suggested Reading

Anderson B, Kaye S. Treatment of flexor tenosynovitis of the hand ("trigger finger") with corticosteroids. Arch Intern Med 151:153–156, 1991.
Chammas M, Bousquet P, Renard E, et al. Dupuytren's disease, carpal tunnel syndrome, trigger finger, and diabetes mellitus. J Hand Surg 20A:109–114, 1995.
Griggs SM, Weiss A-PC, Lane LB, et al. Treatment of trigger finger in patients with diabetes mellitus. J Hand Surg 20A:787–789, 1995.
Murphy D, Failla JM, Koniuch MP. Steroid versus placebo injection for trigger finger. J Hand Surg 20A:628–631, 1995.
Sampson SP, Badalamente MA, Hurst LC, et al. Pathobiology of the human A_1 pulley in trigger finger. J Hand Surg 16A:714–721, 1991.

De Quervain's Tenosynovitis

Presentation and Progression

Cause

De Quervain's tenosynovitis, which involves the common tendon sheath of the extensor pollicis brevis (EPB) and abductor pollicis longus (APL), shares determining factors and pathology with the trigger finger (stenosing tenosynovitis). The female/male ratio is 10 to 1. Due to the lifting involved, women with newborn babies are particularly prone to de Quervain's tenosynovitis.

Presentation

Patients complain of pain, usually severe, in the radial aspect of the wrist. Pain radiation up the forearm and down to the thumb is often reported. Patients often drop articles. Certain activities such as wringing clothes or lifting a baby produce excruciating pain.

On examination there is thickening and tenderness at the common sheath of the EPB/APL tendons in the anterior border of the anatomic snuffbox. A pencil-like swelling extends from the radial styloid to the base of the thumb. In about a quarter of cases palpable crepitation occurs with adduction/abduction motions of the thumb (crepitating tenosynovitis).

Ulnar deviation of the wrist acutely increases the pain. This is the basis of Finkelstein's maneuver, which is diagnostic of the condition (Figure 23–6). The maneuver is done as follows: (1) The patient is directed to grasp the fully flexed thumb with the remaining four digits. (2) The wrist is then *very gently* passively deviated to the ulnar side. The appearance of excruciating radial pain allows a diagnosis of de Quervain's tenosynovitis to be made. The condition must be differentiated from local or systemic inflammatory or infiltrative tenosynovitis, compression neuropathy of the superficial branch of the radial nerve (bracelet syndrome), carpal tunnel syndrome, C6 radiculopathy, and osteoarthritis involving the first carpometacarpal joint or the radiocarpal joint (Table 23–2).

Diagnosis

Summary of Diagnosis

DE QUERVAIN'S TENOSYNOVITIS

- Female predominance.
- Pain in the radial wrist.
- A thickened EPB/APL tendon sheath.
- A positive Finkelstein's test.

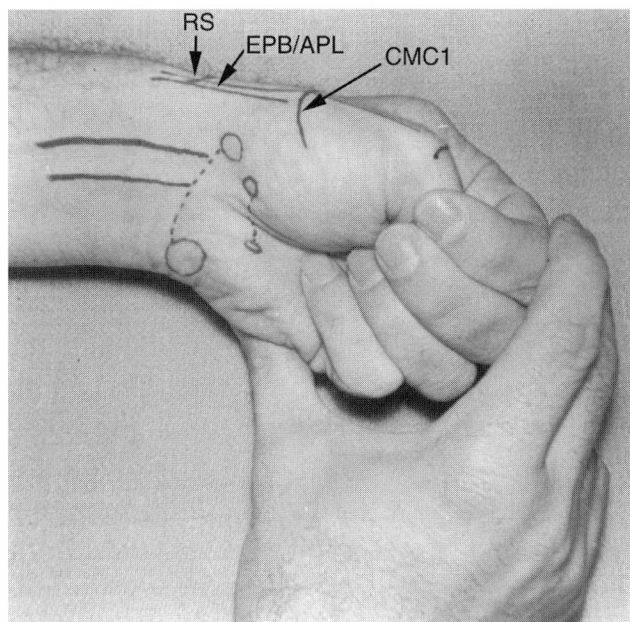

FIGURE 23–6. Finkelstein's test for de Quervain's tenosynovitis. Radial deviation of the wrist stretches the inflamed common sheath of the EPB/APL, causing acute pain. RS = Radial styloid. EPB = Extensor pollicis brevis. APL = Abductor pollicis longus. CMC1 = First carpometacarpal joint.

Natural History

Expected Outcome

Untreated, de Quervain's tenosynovitis causes severe pain and protracted upper extremity disability.

Treatment

Methods

Local corticosteroid infiltrations are highly successful in de Quervain's tenosynovitis (Figure 23–7). Technical aspects of the procedure are discussed in the appendix. The idea is to place the corticosteroid suspension within the involved tendon sheath. In addition, I recommend applying a simple gutter plaster splint in the radial border of distal forearm, wrist, and thumb to be used continuously for 3 days and as a night splint for the following 2 weeks. Relief of symptoms occurs in 60% (single injection) to 90% (up to 3 injections) of cases. Failures of infiltrations may relate to anatomic variations of the sheath such as a loculated sheath and separate sheaths for the EPB and APL (one or more of these variations are present in 34%–75% of individuals). Surgical indications are as in trigger finger.

Expected Response

Pain relief is usually noted within 48 hours of the injection. Patients become asymptomatic in 1 to 2 weeks. A frequent complication is skin depigmentation that may last 1 to 2 years at the site of the infiltration. This is particularly noticeable in individuals with a dark skin. Skin atrophy and echymosis occur predominantly in elderly patients.

When to Refer

Injections for de Quervain's tenosynovitis are technically difficult. Care must be exerted to avoid extravasation with its attendant cutaneous side effects. Referral of de Quervain's tenosynovitis patients to a rheumatologist or an orthopedist is recommended.

Key Points

> **DE QUERVAIN'S TENOSYNOVITIS**
> - Fibrotic stenosis at the APL/EPB tendon sheath.
> - The "bracelet syndrome," carpal tunnel syndrome, radiculopathy, inflammatory and infiltrative tenosynovitides, and carpometacarpal and radiocarpal osteoarthritis must be ruled out.
> - Most cases respond to corticosteroid infiltrations.

TABLE 23–2
DIFFERENTIAL DIAGNOSIS OF RADIAL WRIST PAIN

	Location	Paresthesias	Tinel Sign	Torque Test	Finkelstein Maneuver	X-rays
de Quervain tenosynovitis	Anterior border of anatomic snuffbox	No	Negative	Negative	Positive	Positive (STS)
"Bracelet syndrome," SRN	Outer distal forearm, wrist, hand	Yes	Positive*	Negative	Negative	Negative
Carpal tunnel syndrome	Radial 3 digits	Yes	Positive†	Negative	Negative	Variable‡
First carpometacarpal OA	Base of thumb	No	Negative	Positive	Negative	Positive (OA)
Radiocarpal OA	Radial wrist	No	Negative	Negative	Negative	Positive (OA)

Tinel sign = paresthesias induced by light percussion on nerve trajectory.
Torque test = passive torque motions of thumb metacarpal while applying axial pressure.
SRN = superficial radial nerve.
*Positive at junction of distal one-third and proximal two-thirds of radial forearm.
†Positive in anterior wrist at mid-distance between radial and ulnar borders.
‡It depends on etiology. Dynamic factors and soft tissue pathology do not cause x-rays findings.
STS = soft tissue swelling.
OA = osteoarthritis.

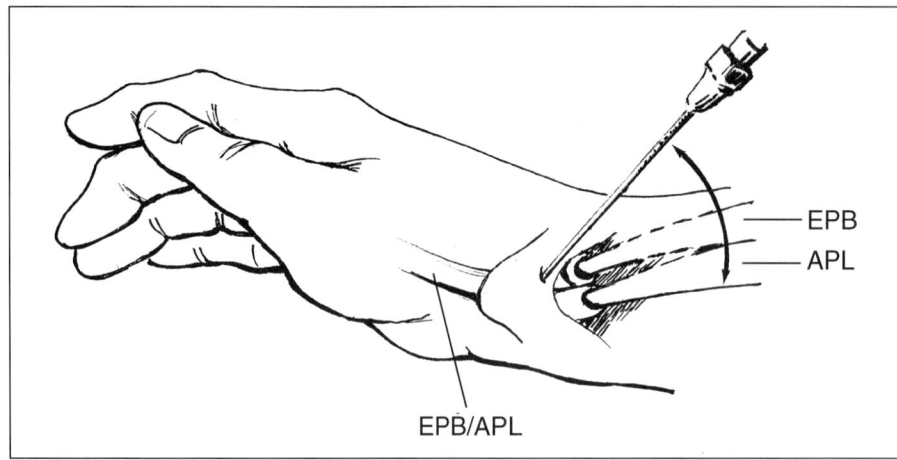

FIGURE 23-7. *Injection treatment of de Quervain's tenosynovitis.* After local xylocaine anesthesia, the needle is inserted aiming at the radial styloid. The steroid preparation is then injected under low pressure. The tendon sheath should be felt to distend throughout its length as distally as the base of the thumb. (See details in appendix.) EPB = Extensor pollicis brevis. APL = Abductor pollicis longus. (After Witt J, Press G, Gelberman RH. Treatment of de Quervain tenosynovitis. J Bone Joint Surg 73A:219–221, 1991.)

Suggested Reading

Anderson BC, Manthey R, Brouns MC. Treatment of de Quervain's tenosynovitis with corticosteroids. Arthritis Rheum 34:793–798, 1991.

Bahm J, Szabo Z, Foucher G. The anatomy of de Quervain's disease. Int Orthop 19:209–211, 1995.

Chen W-S, Eng H-L. Tuberculous tenosynovitis of the wrist mimicking de Quervain's tenosynovitis. J Rheumatol 21:763–765, 1994.

Witt J, Pess G, Gelberman RH. Treatment of de Quervain tenosynovitis. J Bone Joint Surg 73A:219–221, 1991.

Acute Digital Tenosynovitis

Presentation and Progression

Cause

The condition may represent a suppurative infection or a sterile inflammatory reaction triggered by basic calcium crystal deposits. Suppurative cases are caused predominantly by *Staphylococcus aureus* or *Streptococcus pyogenes* and result from direct innoculation.

Particularly worrisome are injuries at the digital creases where the tendon sheaths lie immediately under the skin. *Gonococcus, Meningococcus,* and *T. pallidum* are more likely to produce, by hematogenous seeding, acute tenosynovitis around the wrist. Calcific tenosynovitis occurs in the setting of scleroderma or mixed connective tissue disease. Coexistence with pyogenic infection is common.

Presentation

Acute digital tenosynovitis has an unmistakable presentation. Pain is severe. The involved digit is held in semiflexion. There is volar swelling, erythema, and the digital creases tend to be erased. Dorsal edema is common. Although some passive finger flexion is usually present, passive extension is prevented by excruciating pain. Acute arthritis is excluded by lack of lateral tenderness at the interphalangeal joints. In cellulitis, swelling occurs between creases. Proximal extension of tenosynovitis varies according to the anatomy of the flexor tendon sheaths. Acute tenosynovitis involving the first and fifth rays extends proximally to the wrist. Rarely, a connection between these sheaths results in the so-called horseshoe abscess. In the second to fourth rays proximal extension is limited to the palmar creases. Anatomic variations may result in aberrant clinical findings.

Diagnosis

Summary of Diagnosis

> **ACUTE DIGITAL TENOSYNOVITIS**
> - Finger held in semiflexion.
> - Volar redness, swelling, and tenderness.
> - A preceding puncture wound in septic tenosynovitis; underlying scleroderma or mixed connective tissue disease in calcific tenosynovitis.
> - Proximal extension depends on the digit.
> - X-rays: Amorphous calcium deposits are present in calcific tenosynovitis.

Natural History

Expected Outcome

Untreated suppurative tenosynovitis spreads to the palmar spaces. Secondary interphalangeal joint septic arthritis is a less frequent complication. Tendon sloughing is the unfortunate outcome in neglected cases. Calcific tenosynovitis has a self-limited course; inflammation eventually settles down, and some of the calcium gets reabsorbed.

Treatment

Methods

Suppurative tenosynovitis must be diagnosed early if its dire complications are to be prevented. Hand surgery consultation should be obtained at once. Treatment includes systemic antibiotics and surgical drainage. The latter is accomplished by exposure of the proximal end of the sheath and the insertion of a catheter for lavage and postoperative irrigation. Some surgeons prefer multiple bilateral incisions. Necrotic tendon must be removed, which is accomplished by a zigzag incision along the entire length of the digit.

Calcific tenosynovitis should be looked at critically. Any breakage of the skin should make the case suspect of coexistent suppurative infection. Cases with an intact skin, as long as a hand surgeon concurrently follows the patient and agrees, may be treated with a dorsal splint molded to the digit's curvature and a strong NSAID such as indomethacin 50 mg qid for 2 days followed by dose reduction and discontinuation over 1 week. Alternatively, 40 units of ACTH may be administered I.M., repeating the dose the next day if necessary. Failure to improve should trigger surgical drainage, gram stain, appropriate cultures, and systemic antibiotics pending culture results.

Expected Response

Treated early and appropriately, suppurative synovitis resolves over 1 to 2 weeks. Calcific tendinitis also resolves slowly; the hand should be protected for 1 to 2 weeks.

When to Refer

All patients with acute digital tenosynovitis should be referred to a hand surgeon. Early infectious disease advice is also essential.

Key Points

> **ACUTE DIGITAL TENOSYNOVITIS**
> - The condition may be septic or caused by basic calcium crystals (calcific tendinitis).
> - Any break of the skin in calcific tendinitis should make the case suspicious of coexistent suppurative infection.
> - Early diagnosis and treatment is essential.
> - A hand surgeon should be immediately notified of the case.
> - Suppurative digital tenosynovitis is treated with systemic antibiotics and surgical drainage.
> - Calcific tendinitis is treated with a splint plus NSAID or I.M. ACTH.

Suggested Reading

Abrams RA, Botte MJ. Hand infections: Treatment recommendations for specific types. J Am Acad Orthop Surg 4:219–230, 1996.

Canoso JJ, Barza M. Soft tissue infections. Rheum Dis Clin 19:293–309, 1993.

Proliferative Tenosynovitis

Presentation and Progression

Cause

Subacute or chronic swelling of tendon sheaths has different implications if one is dealing with a single sheath or multiple sheaths. Multiple sheath tenosynovitis usually represents systemic disease, most frequently RA although it may also occur in psoriatic arthritis (pseudorheumatoid type), SLE, and sarcoidosis. Single sheath proliferative tenosynovitis usually represents nodular pigmented tenosynovitis, in which case a single mass is noted (Figure 23–8), indolent infection, or foreign body synovitis. Rare cases occur in sarcoidosis, diffuse pigmented villonodular tenosynovitis (PVNS), and extraarticular synovial chondromatosis. Indolent infection may in turn be caused by mycobacterias (*M. tuberculosis, M. marinum, M. terrae*), fungi (*Exophiala mansonii, Sporotrix schenkii, Phialophora richardsiae*), and even algae (*Prototheca wickerhamii*). Nontenosynovial masses, in particular sarcomas, must be considered in the differential diagnosis lest major errors of diagnosis be made.

PATIENT 28 A 60-year-old man presented with a rapidly enlarging lump in the volar aspect of the left index finger developing during the past 3 weeks (Figure 23–9). The patient felt otherwise well. On examination the mass was fleshy and interfered minimally with finger motion. Rather than a proliferative tenosynovitis it was felt that the patient probably had a soft tissue sarcoma. A chest x-ray showed a large mass in the left lung field (Figure 23–10). Excisional biopsy revealed a monophasic synovial sarcoma. A needle biopsy of the lung mass was obtained, revealing identical tissue.

Presentation

Over weeks or months patients witness the slow growth of an eccentric, elongated, relatively painless lump. Frequent sites

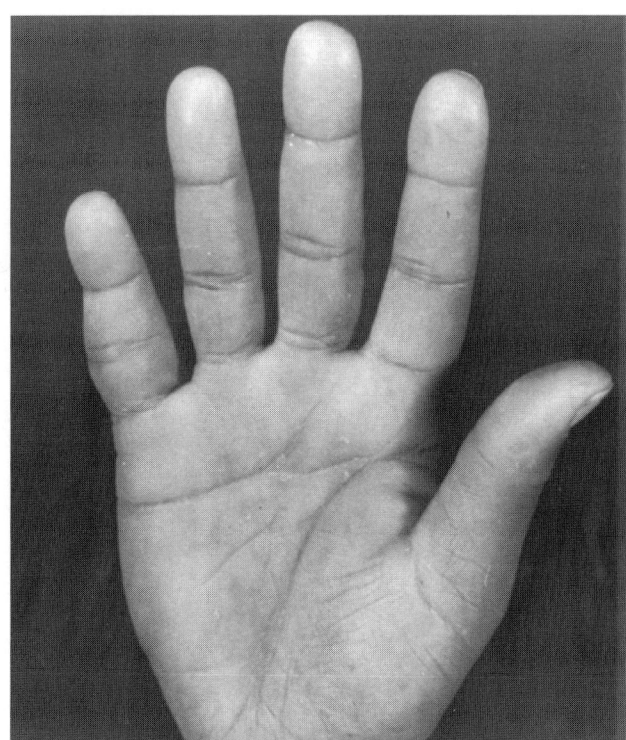

FIGURE 23–8. *Nodular pigmented villonodular tenosynovitis.* A 48-year-old man noted the slow growth of a hard nodule in the palmar aspect of the right little finger. There was no history of puncture wound. The lesion was typical, being composed of multinucleated giant cells, foam cells, hemosiderin, and polyhedric histiocytic cells. Stains and cultures for mycobacterias and fungi were negative.

of involvement include tendon sheaths in the volar aspect of a finger, the wrist, or the ankle. Symptoms of compressive neuropathy may be preeminent, in particular when synovial sheaths within the carpal tunnel syndrome or in the vicinity of the medial malleolus are involved.

Diagnosis

Summary of Diagnosis

> **PROLIFERATIVE TENOSYNOVITIS**
> - With the exception of RA and other systemic synovitides, diagnosis can only be guessed at clinically.
> - The overall yield of x-ray studies is low.
> - Tuberculosis should be considered in immunosuppressed patients, particularly if they have emigrated from endemic areas.
> - Diagnosis in single sheath tenosynovitis requires surgery (tenosynovectomy) with appropriate tissue handling including routine histology, gram, acid-fast, and PAS stain, and bacterial, mycobacterial, and fungal cultures.

Natural History

Expected Outcome

Outcome depends on the etiology of the process. Digital flexor tenosynovitis in RA causes marked functional limitation. Symptoms may be misleading, suggesting articular rather than tenosynovial disease. Tendon ruptures are common in RA. Some forms of single sheath tenosynovitis such as tuberculous tenosynovitis and PVNS may cause significant damage in neighboring bones and joints.

Complications

Complications of proliferative tenosynovitis depend on location and etiology. Systemic and localized proliferative tenosynovitis may cause compressive neuropathies such as carpal tunnel syndrome and tarsal tunnel syndrome. Rupture of the flexor digitorum profundus may be missed on a cursory examination of a rheumatoid hand. Dorsal RA wrist tenosynovitis often causes, over the course of months or years, extensor tendon attenuation and rupture. Rupture of the extensor pollicis longus at Lister's tubercle is another frequent problem in this condition. Tendon, bone, and joint damage may result from tuberculosis and PVNS.

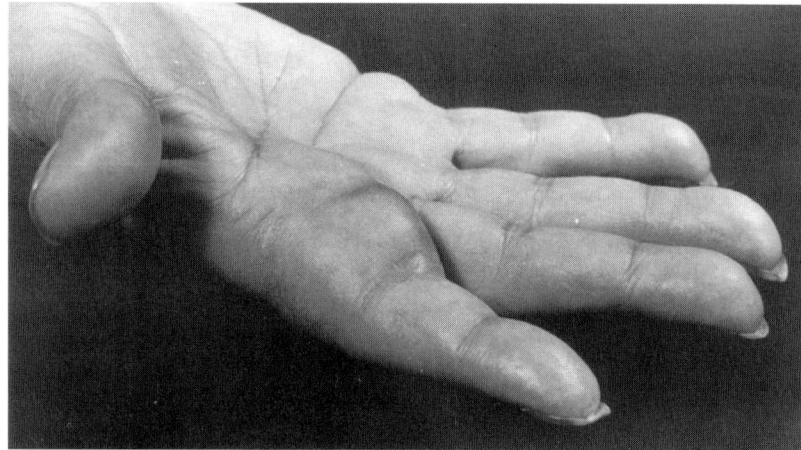

FIGURE 23–9. *Patient 28. Appearance of the index finger. The consistency of the mass was fleshy, suggesting a sarcoma.*

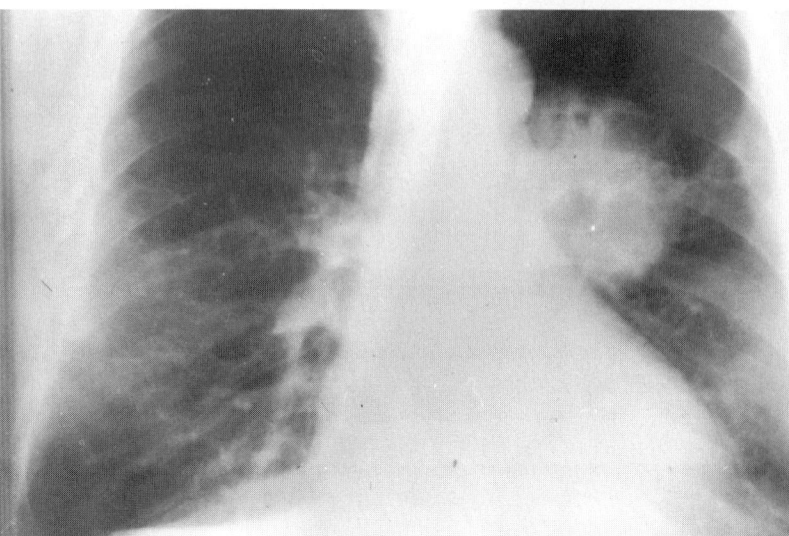

FIGURE 23–10. *Patient 28. A chest x-ray obtained at initial evaluation revealed a huge mass in the left parahilar region. Surgical biopsy of the finger mass and needle biopsy of the lung mass revealed a poorly differentiated synovial sarcoma.*

Treatment

Methods

Treatment in systemic tenosynovitis is aimed at the underlying process. Residual tenosynovitis or particularly severe involvement at one or a few sites benefits from local corticosteroid infiltrations. Directions for tendon sheath injections are given in the appendix. In single sheath tenosynovitis, treatment begins with diagnosis, which in turn requires tenosynovectomy. Once the nature of the process has been unveiled, specific treatment is begun. Tenosynovectomy is curative in nodular PVNS, fibroma of the tendon sheath, and tenosynovial synovial chondromatosis.

When to Refer

All cases of proliferative tenosynovitis deserve rheumatologic evaluation. Orthopedic referral is important in cases of systemic tenosynovitis that pose a threat to tendons (dorsal wrist tenosynovitis) or result in compression neuropathy as well as in single sheath tenosynovitis. Considering the agents involved, infectious proliferative tenosynovitis requires infectious disease consultation.

Key Points

PROLIFERATIVE TENOSYNOVITIS

- It may involve one or multiple tendon sheaths.
- Single sheath tenosynovitis is most often caused by chronic infection.
- Diagnosis in single sheath tenosynovitis requires tenosynovectomy and appropriate histologic and microbiologic studies.
- Complications of proliferative tenosynovitis include tendon rupture, compressive neuropathies, and in some cases, destruction of adjacent bones and joints.
- Treatment depends on the etiology. Corticosteroid infiltrations are quite useful in residual rheumatoid tenosynovitis. Tenosynovectomy is curative in certain localized processes. Antibiotic therapy may be required.

Suggested Reading

Canoso JJ, Barza M. Soft tissue infections. Rheum Dis Clin 19:293–309, 1993.
Puttick MPE, Stein HB, Chan MRT, et al. Soft tissue tuberculosis: A series of 11 cases. J Rheumatol 22:1321–1325, 1995.
Regnard P-J, Barry P, Isselin J. Mycobacterial tenosynovitis of the flexor tendons of the hand. J Hand Surg 21B:351–354, 1996.

Carpal Tunnel Syndrome

Presentation and Progression

Cause

Carpal tunnel syndrome (CTS), or compressive neuropathy of the median nerve at the wrist, is the most common of the compressive neuropathies. The wide range of conditions capable of causing CTS can be explained by anatomic and functional characteristics of the carpal tunnel and the variety of structures traversing this tightly packed passage (Table 23–3).

The carpal tunnel is bound dorsally and laterally by fibro-osseous structures (carpal bones and ligaments) and anteriorly by the flexor retinaculum, a tough fibrous band 2 to 4 mm thick attached laterally to the scaphoid's tubercle and the trapezium and medially to the pisiform and hook of the hamate. The passage contains tendons, tenosynovium, areolar tissue, small vessels, and the median nerve. Superficial landmarks for the median nerve are the palmaris longus and the flexor carpi radialis. The nerve lies beneath the palmaris longus tendon and between this tendon and the flexor carpi radialis. Transverse MRI measurements of the carpal tunnel holding the wrist in neutral position, extension, and flexion reveal smallest cross-sectional areas in both extension and flexion. This is in keeping with intracarpal tunnel pressures, which are known to increase when the wrist is held in either flexion or extension. Similarly, the nocturnal aggravation of symptoms is explained by high pressures recorded in the early morning hours, the highest values being noted at 6 a.m.

Presentation

Patients complain of hand pain and paresthesia. Symptoms are usually bilateral. Pain has an annoying burning or stinging quality and is made worse by activities such as peeling potatoes, wringing clothes, sewing, and repetitive forceful activities of the hand. A general feeling of hand numbness and clumsiness is suggestive of the condition. Night pain and paresthesias are typically relieved by shaking the hand. Sensory symptoms may be limited to the classical median nerve territory, that is, thenar area and palmar aspect of digits 1 through 4, or may affect a more limited or extensive area in the palmar hand. Atrophy of the abductor pollicis brevis, whose belly normally bulges out at the radial border of the hand in full abduction of the thumb (thumb perpendicular to palm), may be noted. Hypoesthesia may be overt, but more frequently two-point discrimination or the use of the

TABLE 23–3

CAUSES OF CARPAL TUNNEL SYNDROME

Idiopathic
Pregnancy
Occupational (repetitive wrist motions)
Diabetes
Myxedema
Acromegaly
Chronic synovitis (RA, polymyalgia rheumatica, psoriatic arthritis, SLE, eosinophilic fasciitis)
Crystal–induced synovitis (gout, pseudogout)*
Median nerve enlargement (leprosy)*
Soft tissue infection*
Hematoma (hemophilia)*
Fractures (especially Colles)*
Amyloidosis (LA, hemodialysis related)
Tumoral calcinosis
Tumors (ganglia, pigmented villonodular synovitis, synovial sarcoma, other)

*Acute carpal tunnel syndrome; may need debridement or drainage. Obtain hand surgery or orthopedic surgery consultation promptly.

Semmes-Weinstein monofilaments is required to elicit the findings.

Classical provocation maneuvers include the *Tinel sign*, in which paresthesias radiate to the middle or index digits following light percussion at the wrist flexor crease; the *Phalen's test*, which is positive if median territory paresthesias occur within a 1 minute flexion of the wrist (the patient is asked to hold the forearms horizontally and allow both hands to drop into complete flexion at the wrist); and the *McMurthry's sign*, in which manual pressure on the nerve at the carpal tunnel reproduces painful symptoms or paresthesia.

Compared with nerve conduction tests as the gold standard, sensory symptoms are highly sensitive (in excess of 90%), but their specificity is below 20%. When symptoms are combined with a positive Tinel test, sensitivity decreases to 62% and specificity increases to 52%. If a positive Phalen's test is also required, sensitivity further declines to 29% and specificity increases to 77%. Electrodiagnostic testing is therefore essential when a definite diagnosis must be established, such as in the preoperative assessment of patients. Unfortunately, the sensitivity of nerve conduction studies is less than 90%. A likely explanation is that nerve conduction studies only test large-diameter fibers; damage to C fibers and sympathetic fibers (which are sensitive to ischemia) is not detected. It is therefore possible that C fibers are those affected in the early painful and dysesthetic forms of the disease.

Less Typical Presentations

Pain from CTS may extend proximally to the arm or shoulder and thus lead to a wrong diagnosis of rotator cuff tendinitis, thoracic outlet syndrome, and cervical radiculopathy. Other cases exhibit unusual symptoms such as diffuse hand pain or symptoms limited to one digit, principally the second or the third. There are also patients, usually in the older age group, in whom muscle atrophy is out of proportion to the subjective complaints. Finally, bona fide CTS may coexist with a higher level of impingement such as median nerve entrapment at the proximal forearm ("pronator syndrome") and cervical radiculopathy. These two-level compressions, which are known by hand surgeons as "double-crush syndromes," are responsible for some failures of carpal tunnel release. Acute CTS deserves special note. The condition is caused by a rapidly expanding lesion within the carpal tunnel and as such is seen in fractures, deep hematomas (hemophiliacs, anticoagulation), necrotizing fasciitis, tumoral calcinosis, crystal-induced inflammation, and sometimes in rheumatoid arthritis (RA) and other inflammatory conditions. In acute cases severe sensory symptoms associate with bulging and tenderness in the volar distal forearm and wrist.

Diagnosis

Summary of Diagnosis (Table 23–4)

CARPAL TUNNEL SYNDROME

- Pain and paresthesias in median nerve territory.
- Nocturnal symptoms.
- Hand numbness and clumsiness.
- Positive provocative tests: Phalen's test, Tinel's sign, or McMurthry's sign.
- EMG and nerve conduction studies if provocative tests are negative and in the preoperative evaluation of patients.
- Assessment, by history and physical examination, of possible underlying etiologies.
- CBC, ESR, TSH, serum protein electrophoresis in the older age group.

Natural History

Expected Outcome

Except in cases associated with pregnancy; the early, activities-related dysesthesic forms of the condition; and cases due to synovitis, acromegaly, or myxedema in which the underlying process can be brought under control, CTS follows a chronic and often progressive course. In late disease, pain, sensory deficit, and weakness of thumb abduction and opposition take a heavy toll on the patient. The rate of progression is by no means established. There are patients with long-standing symptoms in whom minimal or no residual damage can be demonstrated.

Treatment

Methods

A resting splint in the neutral position (which decreases carpal tunnel pressures) is the mainstay of conservative therapy for CTS. As the sole form of therapy, however, splints are only applicable to reversible CTS such as seen in pregnancy, early synovitis for which systemic anti-inflammatory therapy was just begun, and hypothyroidism. Corticosteroid infiltrations, by reducing synovitis, are highly effective in the treatment of CTS in patients with RA, polymyalgia rheumatica, and systemic lupus erythematosus. For less clear reasons,

---

TABLE 23–4

CARPAL TUNNEL SYNDROME: PATIENT EVALUATION

HISTORY

Occupational factors?
Pregnancy?
Diabetes?
Hypothyroidism?
Acromegaly?
Arthritis?

LABORATORY (only if suggested clinically)

TSH
ESR
RF
ANA
Serum protein electrophoresis

albeit transiently, they are also effective in idiopathic and diabetic CTS.

Most cases of idiopathic and diabetic CTS eventually require surgical release. Surgery should be offered without delay to any patient with evidences of ongoing nerve damage such as permanent symptoms, hypoesthesia, weakness of thumb abduction, or early thenar atrophy. To avoid diagnostic errors and disappointments, a positive nerve conduction test should be a prerequisite to surgery (Table 23–5). Finally, decompressive surgery is required in acute CTS except in crystal-induced synovitis, which promptly responds to a splint plus high doses of a NSAID or I.M. ACTH or tiamcinolone acetonide.

Traditional open surgery of CTS has recently been challenged by advocates of endoscopic release. Open surgical release is a well-established procedure. It can be performed in an outpatient setting, is safe, and allows tissue biopsy. Good results can be expected in over 80% of cases with patients returning to work after a median of 4 weeks. Endoscopic carpal tunnel release, a recently developed technique, is equally effective, causes less postoperative pain, and allows an earlier (median 2 weeks) return to work.

Expected Response

Response to splinting and injection is variable. Mild cases and cases due to synovitis usually improve. Patients with idiopathic and diabetic CTS may also improve, but recurrence of symptoms is almost always the rule. With surgical release, complete pain relief 24 hours after surgery portends an excellent outcome. Patients who continue with pain may still have a good outcome, but a third of them do not improve. Maximal resolution of pain and paresthesia occurs within 3 weeks of surgery; grip and pinch strength improve over preoperative levels only after 6 months. Early mobilization after release (no splint or a splint for a maximum of 1 week) is associated with a better outcome (Table 23–6).

Complications

Complications of corticosteroid infiltrations are very rare; the author has only seen an occasional increase in pain, which resolves in 1 to 2 days. Drawbacks of open surgical release include persistent postoperative weakness, a tender scar, pain in the thenar or hypothenar eminences (pillar pain), plus rare instances of sympathetic dystrophy. Problems associated with endoscopic release include nerve and vessel laceration (complications that occur, in experienced hands, in approximately 5% of procedures), incomplete release, scarring and recurrence, greater complexity of the technique, and, surprisingly, higher costs.

When to Refer

Assessment and initial treatment of CTS fall within the realm of primary care medicine. As patients are evaluated an underlying etiology such as RA, diabetes, or hypothyroidism may or may not surface. Idiopathic CTS patients should be injected and provided a splint. Long-term results of conservative therapy are disappointing in this group with less than 20% of patients remaining asymptomatic at 1 year. Referral to a hand surgeon should not be delayed in patients with persistent or recurrent symptoms.

In diabetic patients it is imperative to determine whether one is dealing with CTS or diabetic peripheral neuropathy. Electromyogram and nerve conduction studies should be obtained in these patients, and if CTS is confirmed corticosteroid infiltration may be attempted. Lack of response calls for hand surgery referral. Cases due to RA or other systemic conditions should be treated with a splint and referred to a rheumatologist for evaluation and treatment recommendations. In the older age group, light-chain amyloidosis is a realistic possibility. These patients will have evidence of monoclonal gammopathy in serum and/or urine electrophoresis. Open surgery provides both nerve release and a positive diagnosis when appropriate stains are used.

Key Points

TABLE 23–5

CARPAL TUNNEL SYNDROME WITH NORMAL ELECTRODIAGNOSTIC TESTS

Early or intermittent CTS with C fiber injury only
Compression of the median nerve high in the forearm (flexor digitorum superficialis, pronator teres)
Radiculopathy

TABLE 23–6

RECURRENT OR NONRESOLVING CARPAL TUNNEL SYNDROME AFTER SURGICAL RELEASE

Incomplete section of flexor retinaculum*
Carpal tunnel mass (ganglia, hypertrophic scar, etc.)*
Synovitis
Diabetes
Incomplete diagnosis (double-crush lesions)
Erroneous diagnosis (neuropathy, particularly in diabetes)

*MRI very useful in diagnosis.

CARPAL TUNNEL SYNDROME

- As important as diagnosing CTS is searching for its etiology.
- CTS due to pregnancy, hypothyroidism, and synovitis responds well to a splint plus treatment of the underlying condition.
- Idiopathic and diabetic CTS may transiently respond to conservative therapy, but surgical release is eventually required in most cases.
- A wrist splint in the neutral position is the mainstay of conservative therapy.

- Corticosteroid infiltrations are a helpful adjunct in rheumatoid arthritis and other synovitides.
- Surgical release, whether open or endoscopic, is indicated in failures of conservative therapy, when there is evidence of significant neuropathy, and in acute CTS.
- The chosen procedure should be the one the surgeon is most experienced with.
- Following surgery, resolution of pain and paresthesia occurs within a few weeks; improvement in strength takes several months to 2 years.

Suggested Reading

Brown RA, Gelberman RH, Seiler JG III, et al. Carpal tunnel release. A prospective, randomized assessment of open and endoscopic methods. J Bone Joint Surg 75A:1265–1275, 1993.

Buch-Jaeger N, Foucher G. Correlation of clinical signs with nerve conduction tests in the diagnosis of carpal tunnel syndrome. J Hand Surg 19B:720–724, 1994.

Cook AC, Szabo RM, Birkholz SW, et al. Early mobilization following carpal tunnel release. J Hand Surg 20B:228–230, 1995.

Gelberman RH, Hergenroeder PT, Hargens AR, et al. The carpal tunnel syndrome: A study of carpal canal pressure. J Bone Joint Surg 63A:380–383, 1981.

Katz JN, Fossel KK, Simmons BP, et al. Symptoms, functional status, and neuromuscular impairment following carpal tunnel release. J Hand Surg 20A:549–555, 1995.

Olehnik WK, Manske PR, Szerzinski J. Median nerve compression in the proximal forearm. J Hand Surg 19A:121–126, 1994.

Shinya K, Lanzetta M, Conolly WB. Risk and complications in endoscopic carpal tunnel release. J Hand Surg 20B:222–227, 1995.

Weiss A-PC, Sachar K, Gendreau M. Conservative management of carpal tunnel syndrome: A reexamination of steroid injection and splinting. J Hand Surg 19A:410–415, 1994.

Wintman BI, Winters SC, Gelberman RH, Katz JN. Carpal tunnel release. Correlations with preoperative symptomatology. Clin Orthop 326:135–145, 1996.

CHAPTER 24

Elbow Pain

Elbow conditions are frequently encountered in general medical practices. By far, the most common are the so-called tennis elbow and olecranon bursitis. Elbow involvement is also frequent in RA, CPPD crystal deposition disease, and the spondyloarthropathies. Finally, there are also several tendinitides and nerve compression syndromes that clinicians should be able to identify.

The elbow joint serves as a hinge between forearm and arm and also allows pronation/supination of the forearm. In elbow extension a valgus angulation known as the carrying angle becomes apparent. As the elbow is flexed, this angle changes progressively to a varus angulation so as to bring the hand closer to the mouth. The axis of pronation/supination passes through the radial head, the center of the distal end of the ulna, and the extended little finger. Two radioulnar joints are involved in this motion: the proximal, which is continuous with the elbow joint, and the distal, which is adjacent to, but separate from, the wrist joint. Pronation/supination involves the eccentric axial rotation of the radius around the ulna, which remains stationary in relation to the humerus. To allow flexion and extension of the hinge, the elbow capsule is lax front and back. Tough collateral ligaments reinforce the sides of the joint.

Several adjacent tendon attachments are of clinical importance. Anteriorly, the biceps tendon inserts in the medial side of the radius, thus acting both as a flexor and as a supinator. Beneath the biceps is the brachialis, which by inserting in the ulnar tuberosity acts as a pure flexor. In the medial side, the distal humerus gives insertion to the pronator teres, the wrist flexors, and the flexor digitorum superficialis. Laterally, the distal humerus is the site of insertion for the brachioradialis, wrist and finger extensors, the superficial layer of the supinator, and the anconeus. Posteriorly, the triceps muscle attaches to the proximal olecranon. The radial nerve reaches the forearm anterior to the radial elbow (Figure 24–1). About 1 cm proximal to the joint this nerve divides into a deep and a superficial branch. The deep branch courses in front of the radiohumeral joint before piercing the supinator muscle beneath the arcade of Frohse. This point, which is located 2.3 cm distal to the radiohumeral joint, is the site of tenderness in the compression neuropathy of the posterior interosseous nerve, a leading mimicker of tennis elbow. The ulnar nerve enters the forearm diametrically opposite the radial nerve between the olecranon process and the medial epicondyle under a tough bridging band, the arcuate ligament.

Because the insertions of the arcuate ligament separate from each other approximately 5 mm for each 45 degrees of flexion, elbow flexion reduces the capacity of the cubital tunnel (Figure 24–2). A provocative test for the cubital tunnel syndrome, the elbow flexion test, is based on this encroachment. Posteriorly, the olecranon bursa separates the olecranon process (and the attached triceps tendon) from the underlying skin and contributes significantly to the remarkable motion of

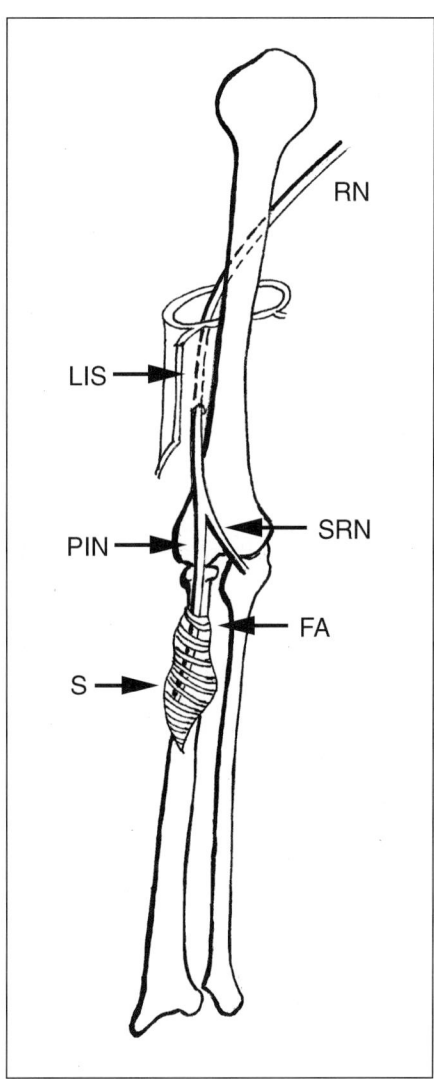

FIGURE 24–1. *Radial nerve anatomy relevant to elbow pathology.* RN = Radial nerve. SRN = Superficial radial nerve (sensory). FA = Frohse's arcade (fibrous border of supinator). S = Supinator. PIN = Posterior interosseous nerve (motor). LIS = Lateral intermuscular septum of upper arm. (After Prasartritha T, et al. A study of the posterior interosseous nerve (PIN) and the radial tunnel in 30 Thai cadavers. J Hand Surg 18A:107–112, 1993.)

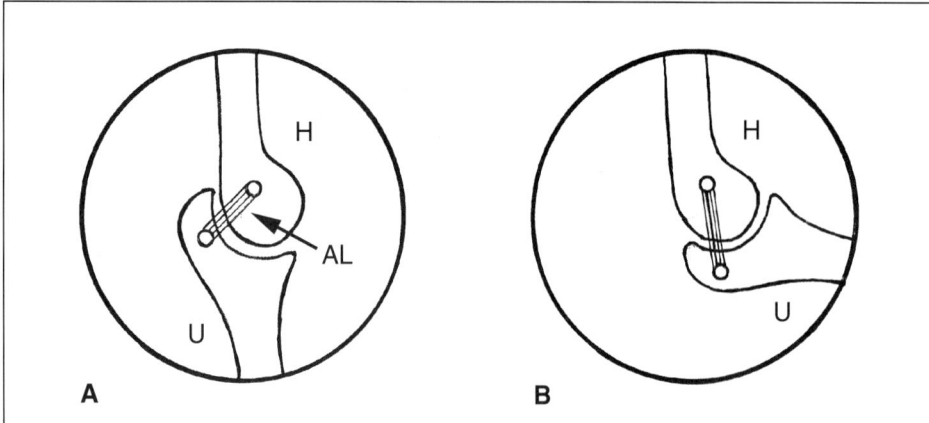

FIGURE 24–2. *The arcuate ligament in the medial elbow.* Because of an eccentric axis of motion, elbow flexion stretches and tightens the arcuate ligament, which compresses the cubital tunnel. H: Humerus, AL: Arcuate ligament, U: Ulna. A, Elbow in extension; B, elbow at 90 degrees flexion. (After Wadsworth TG. The external compression syndrome of the ulnar nerve at the cubital tunnel. Clin Orthop 124:189–204, 1977.)

the skin at the elbow tip. Because of its location, this bursal sac is vulnerable to trauma and infection from skin pathogens. Elbow pain may result from arthritis, ligamentous and muscle attachment tears or inflammation, compressive neuropathy, and bursitis. Pain may also be referred from distant structures, mainly the neck and hand (carpal tunnel syndrome).

Physical examination of the elbow includes flexion/extension (hinge) and pronation/supination. Flexion is limited by the bulk of anterior soft tissues and extension by the locking of the olecranon process in the olecranon fossa. Lateral motions only occur in cases of instability. Pronation and supination are measured with the elbow flexed 90 degrees from radial side up (0 position). In arthritis, effusion, synovial proliferation and inflammation make the elbow adopt a 40 to 50 degree flexion. Swelling is most evident posterolaterally, and in severe cases both flexion and extension as well as pronation and supination are limited and painful. Arthritis, which affects both flexion and extension, should be distinguished from impingement and periarticular soft tissue problems in which findings are asymmetric. In impingements, which may be anterior or posterior, there is painful limitation toward the side of the lesion while the opposite motion is normal. For example, an osteochondroma (a calcified cartilaginous body free-floating in synovial fluid) lodged in the olecranon fossa in the extensor side of the joint will only affect extension. In contrast, in periarticular soft tissue problems such as tendinitis and bursitis, motion opposite to the lesion causes pain from tissue stretching or compression by the skin while passive motion toward the side of the lesion is unimpaired. In addition, the resisted action of an inflamed tendon is painful. Five common conditions are discussed in this chapter: tennis elbow, radial tunnel syndrome and compression neuropathy of the deep branch of the radial nerve, golfer's elbow (medial epicondylitis), cubital tunnel syndrome, and olecranon bursitis.

Tennis Elbow

Presentation and Progression

Cause

Tennis elbow, also known as lateral epicondylitis, is the main cause of lateral elbow pain (Table 24–1). Most cases of the condition occur in non–tennis players. Tennis elbow represents a sports-related or, more frequently, a work-related enthesopathy of the extensor carpi radialis brevis at its insertion in the lateral epicondyle. Operative specimens reveal tendon glycosaminoglycan infiltration, microtears, as well as new bone formation at the attachment site. Both traction injury and ischemia appear to play a role in developing this lesion.

Presentation

Initially there may be an ache in the extensor surface of the forearm. As time elapses symptoms mount and pain becomes localized to the lateral elbow. Grasping an object with the wrist in extension reproduces the pain (the coffee cup sign). There is exquisite tenderness just distal to, or anterior to, the lateral epicondyle. Passive range of elbow motion is normal. Pain is reproduced by resisted dorsiflexion of the wrist and resisted extension of the long finger, which tightens the fascial origin of the extensor carpi radialis brevis. Late in the condition a minimal flexor deformity may develop. This can only be identified if passive elbow extension is checked. Any significant degree of limitation, say a 20 degree lack of extension, cannot be attributed to tennis elbow and should raise the suspicion of arthritis, impingement at the olecranon fossa, or limitation placed by a soft tissue mass somewhere in the posterior aspect of the joint. Tennis elbow symptoms in an active teenager may be an indication of osteonecrosis of the capitulum. Diffuse, deep, aching forearm pain is highly suggestive of the radial tunnel syndrome in which an entrapment neuropathy of the deep branch of the radial nerve (a pure motor branch) presumably occurs. Paresthesias and hypoesthesia in the lateral volar forearm may indicate a compression neuropathy of the musculocutaneous nerve at the elbow if not a C5 or C6 radiculopathy.

TABLE 24–1
CAUSES OF LATERAL ELBOW PAIN
Lateral epicondylitis
Compression neuropathy of the deep branch of the radial nerve
Enthesitis
Radiohumeral arthritis
Fibromyalgia
C5 or C6 radiculopathy

Diagnosis

Summary of Diagnosis

> **TENNIS ELBOW**
>
> - Tennis elbow is diagnosed clinically based on the presence of lateral elbow pain, tenderness just distal to the lateral epicondyle, and pain on resisted wrist dorsiflexion.
> - X-rays should be obtained to rule out calcific tendinitis, exostosis, osteoarthritis at the radiocapitellar joint, and malignancy. A traction spur is present in 20% of cases.
> - Infrared thermography, useful as a research tool, is unnecessary in clinical practice.

Natural History

Expected Outcome

Community cases of tennis elbow tend to be self-limited. As seen in medical practices, however, the condition has a protracted course and may even become intractable.

Complications

Chronic, disabling pain is the only complication.

Treatment

Methods

Most important in treatment is activities modification, not only in terms of how many times the offending task is performed but also how the activity is performed. This is clearly demonstrated in tennis players in whom tennis elbow often represents a red flag that leads to identification of faulty playing patterns. Common errors include inadequate conditioning; a faulty backhand; the use of metal rackets; an incorrect grip size; and heavier, stiffer, and tightly strung rackets. Treatment (Table 24–2) involves the use of a proper technique, a cushioned synthetic grip, and reducing tension on the strings. Counterforce bracing with an upper forearm compression band discourages full muscle action. Pinching and grasping should only be allowed in supination. The exercise program is best instructed and guided by an occupational therapist. Strengthening exercises are prescribed for the entire upper extremity, not just the elbow, emphasizing a graded resistive program for wrist dorsiflexors. General conditioning and cardiovascular fitness should be maintained. A 2 week course of NSAIDs and/or local capsaicin seems reasonable in tennis elbow patients.

Patients who fail to improve after 4 to 6 weeks of conservative therapy may be offered a corticosteroid infiltration. Why this delay in offering a widely used form of treatment? The reasons to be conservative relate to the long-term efficacy and safety of corticosteroid infiltrations. In a recent blinded trial corticosteroid infiltrations were superior to local anesthetic infiltrations at 8 weeks, but outcome at 6 months was similar in both groups. Also, half of corticosteroid infiltrations resulted in severe pain that could last several days. Corticosteroid infiltrations have been found superior to Cyriax-type physiotherapy (deep transverse friction plus manipulation) at 6 weeks, but there were no differences at 1 year with 34% of patients in the steroid group experiencing recurrence.

Finally, in the opinion of leading elbow surgeons, repeated corticosteroid infiltrations may cause chronic pain. Looking back at my own experience, from initially infiltrating most tennis elbows I now seldom use the procedure. Corticosteroid infiltrations should be done with great care (see appendix).

Refractory cases should be referred to an expert elbow surgeon, usually a hand or a shoulder orthopedist. Many operations are available and most have excellent results. A simple procedure involves the lateral release of the common extensor tendon origin under local anesthesia in a day surgery unit. Resection of the involved, disorganized tendon site is preferred by some surgeons. Regardless of technique most patients treated surgically are permanently improved.

TABLE 24–2

TREATMENT OF LATERAL EPICONDYLITIS

Avoid overuse
Hold weights in supination only
Compressive band
NSAID
Isotonic and isometric exercises for the entire extremity
Deep massage and manipulation?
Corticosteroid infiltration?

Expected Response

On conservative treatment (decreased or modified activities, physiotherapy, the use of a forearm compression band, local capsaicin, and an oral NSAID), improvement may be expected in 4 to 6 weeks. With a corticosteroid infiltration, symptoms should abate in 3 to 4 days. Surgical treatment has excellent results, but the procedure should be delayed because many cases will remit on prolonged conservative treatment. The author suggests the following progression of treatment: (1) Conservative treatment for 4 to 6 weeks. (2) Unimproved patients are offered corticosteroid infiltrations (one to three infiltrations given 2 weeks apart). (3) Resistant cases are referred to a surgeon.

Complications

Complications of treatment include the general risks associated with the use of NSAIDs plus the risk of corticosteroid infiltrations in patients so treated, including a 50% chance of transient pain exacerbation.

When to Refer

As hinted earlier, tennis elbow may be wrongly diagnosed. Fibromyalgia features prominent lateral elbow pain, but the presence of symmetric tenderness should prompt a complete review of fibromyalgic points, which settles diagnosis. A prominent mimicker is the radial tunnel syndrome (see next section). An infrequent confounding lesion is the compressive neuropathy of the musculocutaneous nerve at the elbow. This condition is characterized by tenderness just lateral to the biceps tendon at the elbow crease, hypoesthesia in the lateral volar forearm, and increased pain upon full pronation. Amorphous calcium deposits near the lateral epocondyle may cause an acute, self-limited tennis elbow, but symptoms in some patients are protracted. Fluoroquinolone antibiotics are known to cause entheseal pain, the usual site being the Achilles tendon. However, in patients who use the upper extremity heavily, fluoroquinolones may cause an acute lateral epicondylar enthesopathy with typical tennis elbow symptoms. In Panner's disease, also known as little leaguer's elbow, isolated osteoarthritis of the radiocapitellar joint occurs secondary to osteonecrosis of the capitulum. Diagnosis of this condition is radiologic. Chronic pain may rarely indicate bone or soft tissue malignancy. If a mass is palpable the likelihood of neoplasia is high.

PATIENT 29 A 30-year-old man was referred for evaluation of a protracted left tennis elbow. Symptoms had been present for a year and had been progressive despite several corticosteroid infiltrations and formal physical therapy. Unusual features of his condition included severe pain and about 20 degrees of elbow flexor contracture that was attributed to chronicity and lack of use of the extremity. Flexion was full, but extension had a soft tissue endpoint at 20 degrees flexion consistent with impingement-type limitation. Some soft tissue bulging was noted posterolaterally between the olecranon process and the lateral epicondyle. Because a soft tissue mass was strongly suspected, a bilateral CT scan was requested. However, due to cost factors only the left side was examined and findings were considered normal. Given the clinical findings, a CT scan of the right elbow was once again requested, and on comparison with the left side a previously unidentified soft tissue lump was noted at the site of the bulge. The patient had a clear cell sarcoma.

Key Points

TENNIS ELBOW

- Lateral elbow pain that is reproduced by resisted wrist dorsiflexion.
- An enthesopathy caused by a repetitive traction injury.
- The condition is self-limited in mild cases.
- Treatment is empirical. If tendon overuse can be stopped, symptoms cease. Counterforce bracing in the upper forearm discourages full use of the muscles and helps relieve pain. Capsaicin and NSAIDs may afford relief. Corticosteroid infiltrations may be used after failure of conservative therapy.
- Treatment failures may represent diagnostic errors. Have a rheumatologist or orthopedic surgeon review the case.
- Surgery in refractory bona fide cases of refractory tennis elbow has a success rate of near 90%.

Suggested Reading

Coonrad RW. Tendonopathies at the elbow. American Academy of Orthopedic Surgeons Instructional Series 15:25–32, 1991.

Price R, Sinclair H, Heinrich I, et al. Local injection treatment of tennis elbow. Hydrocortisone, triamcinolone and lignocaine compared. Brit J Rheumatol 30:39–44, 1991.

Safran MR. Elbow injuries in athletes. Clin Orthop 310;257–277, 1995.

Verhaar J, Walenkamp G, Kester A, et al. Lateral extensor release for tennis elbow. A prospective long-term follow-up. J Bone Joint Surg 75A:1034–1043, 1993.

Verhaar J, Walenkamp G, van Mameren H, et al. Local corticosteroid injection versus Cyriax-type physiotherapy for tennis elbow. J Bone Joint Surg 77B:128–132, 1995.

Radial Tunnel Syndrome and Compressive Neuropathy of the Deep Branch of the Radial Nerve

Presentation and Progression

Cause

The radial nerve, as it approaches the radiohumeral joint, divides into two branches: the superficial branch that provides sensation to the back of the hand, and the deep branch (that later becomes the posterior interosseous nerve), which is muscular and articular in distribution (Figure 24–1). The deep branch pierces the supinator muscle (actually traverses between the superficial and the deep layers of the muscle) 2.3 cm distal to the joint. The leading edge of the superficial layer of the supinator, which is fibrous in 30%, is known as "arcade of Frohse." There are two forms of compressive neuropathy of the deep branch of the radial nerve. In the most common, known as the radial tunnel syndrome, the nerve is believed to be chronically and intermittently compressed at the arcade of Frohse. This view has been challenged because EMG findings are normal and because nerve conduction across Frohse's arcade is unaffected by sustained supination. An alternative explanation is an overuse tendopathy of the supinator. Similar to tennis elbow, radial tunnel syndrome is particularly prevalent in manual workers such as electricians, machine operators, switchboard operators, and bricklayers who are subject to repetitive pronation and supination or forceful wrist extension.

The second form of the syndrome results from a space-occupying mass compressing the nerve as it enters the supinator. Compressive lesions include rheumatoid synovitis and various tumors including ganglia, fractures, and dislocations of the radial head.

Presentation

Most patients with radial tunnel syndrome are thought initially to have a resistant case of tennis elbow. One or more corticosteroid infiltrations and even a surgical extensor release may have failed. Different from tennis elbow, however, there is deep, diffuse achiness in the dorsal and lateral forearm that is increased by activities but is also present at rest. Pain may be triggered by resisted supination while the wrist is passively kept in dorsiflexion. Finally, rather than at the lateral epicondyle, tenderness occurs anteriorly at Frohse's arcade. To find this landmark the author first marks the cleft between the radial head and the capitulum in the lateral elbow (gentle pronation and supination with the semiflexed elbow facilitates identification of the radial head). The mark is extended anteriorly round the joint. Frohse's arcade is located 2 to 2.5 cm distal to the mark (or 3 cm distal to the flexor crease) between the middle two-thirds and the lateral one-third of the anterior forearm. Interestingly, patients may have both tennis elbow and radial tunnel syndrome and surgical treatment of one of these conditions may relieve both.

Patients with a true compressive neuropathy have shooting paresthesias up and down the course of the radial nerve for days or weeks prior to developing paresis of the extensor digitorum communis and the extensor carpi ulnaris along with poorly localized muscle pain. By this time the patient may be unable to extend the index, long, ring, and little fingers and dorsiflexion of the wrist may be weak and result in dorsoradial deviation. A wrong diagnosis of tendon rupture is frequently made in these patients. Automatic extension of the fingers when the wrist is passively flexed (tenodesis effect) proves that tendons are intact.

Diagnosis

Summary of Diagnosis

RADIAL TUNNEL SYNDROME

- Diagnosis is clinical based on the presence of deep aching pain in the posterolateral muscles of the forearm, tenderness at Frohse's arcade, and pain upon resisted supination of the passively dorsiflexed hand.
- EMGs and nerve conduction studies are normal.

COMPRESSIVE NEUROPATHY OF THE DEEP BRANCH OF THE RADIAL NERVE

- Diagnosis is clinical based on paresis of extension in digits 2 through 5, a positive tenodesis effect, and radial deviation of the wrist in dorsiflexion.
- EMGs show denervation of the paretic muscles.
- MRI gives the highest diagnostic yield in nonrheumatoid cases. Ultrasound may be used as a screening procedure.

Natural History

Expected Outcome

Radial tunnel syndrome is a protracted painful condition that may become chronic. On the other hand, space-occupying lesions result in progressive paresis. The clinical course of this condition is stereotyped: initial involvement of digits 3 through 5, then the index, and then the thumb.

Treatment

Methods

Radial tunnel syndrome is treated like tennis elbow. Corticosteroid infiltrations are not recommended because they are difficult to administer and if misplaced may damage the nerve. Severe symptoms extending beyond 2 months should prompt orthopedic referral for nerve release and removal of any abnormal tissue (Table 24–3). The arm must be pronated and supinated intraoperatively to demonstrate the constricting structure(s). True compressive neuropathies require prompt diagnosis and surgical removal of the space-occupying lesion. If compression results from elbow synovitis, such as in RA, intraarticular corticosteroids should be tried first because they are occasionally successful.

TABLE 24–3

OPERATIVE FINDINGS IN 30 OPERATIONS FOR RADIAL TUNNEL RELEASE*

Compressing Structure†	No.
Tight arcade of Frohse	15
Dense proximal fascial bands	12
Tight superficial component of supinator	10
Compressive vessels	3
None of note	5

*Patients could have more than one compression mechanism.
†Intraoperative pronation and supination help in the identification of the structure at fault.
From Lawrence T, et al. Radial tunnel syndrome. A retrospective review of 30 decompressions of the radial nerve. J Hand Surg 20B: 454–456, 1995.

Expected Response

Conservative treatment of radial tunnel syndrome should lead to progressive improvement within 6 weeks. Surgical release in radial tunnel syndrome has a success rate of approximately 70%. Response to excision of a compressive mass is variable; long-standing compression often causes irreversible paresis.

When to Refer

In the radial tunnel syndrome a failure to improve after 6 weeks of conservative therapy should prompt orthopedic referral for consideration of surgical release. Orthopedic consultation should be promptly obtained, however, in any patient suspected of having nerve compression from an expanding lesion.

Key Points

RADIAL TUNNEL SYNDROME

- Radial tunnel syndrome, a pain syndrome involving the lateral elbow and forearm, is often confused with tennis elbow. Both lesions may coexist.
- Occupational or recreational factors are similar in both conditions.
- Their differentiation is based on the quality and distribution of pain, location of maximal tenderness, and triggering maneuvers.
- Conservative treatment is as in tennis elbow.
- Surgical treatment of chronic cases is often successful.

> **TRUE COMPRESSIVE NEUROPATHY**
>
> - In a true compressive neuropathy of the radial nerve, neurologic findings prevail, namely, neuritic pain and paresis.
> - The space-occupying lesion may be obvious, such as elbow synovitis in RA, or it may be a primary expansive lesion (ganglia, sarcomas, etc.).
> - Prompt orthopedic or surgical oncology consultation should be obtained if a focal lesion is shown.

Suggested Reading

Lawrence T, Mobbs P, Fortems Y, et al. Radial tunnel syndrome. A retrospective review of 30 decompressions of the radial nerve. J Hand Surg 20B:454–459, 1995.

Millender LH, Nalebuff EA, Holdsworth DE. Posterior interosseous-nerve syndrome secondary to rheumatoid arthritis. J Bone Joint Surg 55A:753–757, 1973.

Prasartritha T, Liupolvanish P, Rojanakit A. A study of the posterior interosseous nerve (PIN) and the radial tunnel in 30 Thai cadavers. J Hand Surg 18A:107–112, 1993.

Roles NC, Maudsley RH. Radial tunnel syndrome. Resistant tennis elbow as a nerve entrapment. J Bone Joint Surg 54B:499–508, 1972.

Verhaar JAN, Spaans F. Radial tunnel syndrome. An investigation of compression neuropathy as a possible cause. J Bone Joint Surg 73A:539–544, 1991.

Golfer's Elbow (Medial Epicondylitis)

Presentation and Progression

Cause

Golfer's elbow is the mirror image of tennis elbow. The condition is caused from repetitive traction stress at the medial epicondylar attachment of the pronator teres or flexor carpi radialis muscles. Golfer's elbow often occurs in professional and amateur sports players as well as in manual workers, particularly in bricklayers. Curiously, golfer's elbow is more frequent than tennis elbow in high-performance tennis players whereas tennis elbow tends to occur in inadequately conditioned recreational tennis players 35 to 50 years of age. Golfer's elbow is relatively uncommon, about 5% of the frequency of tennis elbow.

Presentation

Patients complain of medial elbow pain upon manual activities. Pain is increased by resisted wrist flexion and resisted forearm pronation. Ulnar paresthesias from an associated ulnar compressive neuropathy are present in 30% of cases.

Diagnosis

Summary of Diagnosis

> **GOLFER'S ELBOW (Medial Epicondylitis)**
>
> - Golfer's elbow is diagnosed clinically based on a history of medial elbow pain plus the results of resisted wrist flexion and forearm pronation.
> - Differential diagnosis includes calcific tendinitis, bone and soft tissue tumors, ulnar neuropathy, and radiating pain (T1).
> - X-rays findings in golfer's elbow are normal. The study is useful to exclude alternative diagnoses.

Natural History

Expected Outcome

Untreated, golfer's elbow may become chronic. Advanced concurrent ulnar neuropathy may weaken the hand. There are no other complications of the condition.

Treatment

Methods

As in tennis elbow, conservative treatment includes partial rest, local application of capsaicin, a 2 week course of NSAIDs, activities modification, the use of a forearm compression band, exercises for the entire upper extremity, and general conditioning. Resistant cases may be treated by one or two corticosteroid infiltrations given 2 weeks apart.

Expected Response

Patients are expected to improve within 4 to 6 weeks; lack of response is an indication for corticosteroid infiltrations.

Complications

Because the ulnar nerve runs just behind the the medial epicondyle, misplaced injections may damage the nerve. Intra-tendinous injections may result in tendon rupture. The procedure should be left to physicians who are familiar with elbow anatomy.

When to Refer

Patients failing to improve after 4 weeks of conservative therapy should be referred to a rheumatologist or an orthopedic surgeon for possible injection and further treatment recommendations. The threshold for referral should be lower in cases with ulnar neuropathy.

Key Points

> **GOLFER'S ELBOW (Medial Epicondylitis)**
>
> - Elbow pain at the medial epicondyle.
> - Increased symptoms upon resisted wrist flexion and resisted forearm pronation.
> - Association with repetitive manual activities.
> - Treatment includes partial rest, activities modification, a forearm compression band, exercises for the entire extremity, general conditioning, capsaicin, and NSAIDs.

- Corticosteroid infiltrations are reserved for resistant cases.
- Surgical medial release is a last-resort treatment.

Suggested Reading

Coonrad RW. Tendonopathies at the elbow. American Academy of Orthopedic Surgeons Instructional Series 15:25–32, 1991.

Safran MR. Elbow injuries in athletes. Clinical Orthop 310:257–277, 1995.

Cubital Tunnel Syndrome

Presentation and Progression

Cause

Compression of the ulnar nerve at the elbow may result from external pressure, space-occupying lesions, and anatomic variations in the ulnar canal (Figure 24–3). Preventable causes include incorrect positioning on the operating table and lying drunk on the floor with the elbow flexed. Space-occupying lesions include elbow synovitis, ganglia, hematoma, and nerve hypertrophy such as seen in leprosy. More frequently compression results from anatomic variations in the cubital tunnel including (1) an absent retinaculum that allows a free-floating nerve to dislocate and be traumatized; (2) a thick arcuate ligament that is relatively unyielding in flexion; and (3) nerve compression by an atavistic muscle, the anconeus epitroclearis. During elbow flexion the nerve is stretched and the capacity of the cubital tunnel is reduced as the arcuate ligament becomes taut (Figure 24–2) and the medial elbow ligament bulges out.

Presentation

An early complaint is waking up with the elbow flexed and paresthesias in the ulnar part of the hand. Symptoms are promptly relieved by extending the extremity. This may be normal in some individuals. Evolving disease features pain in the ulnar side of the hand and forearm (nerve trunk pain) and permanent dysesthesia in the fourth and fifth digits. Sensory loss, intrinsic muscle weakness, and atrophy indicate late disease.

Several provocative tests may be used for diagnosis. In the flexion test, the subject's elbow is brought to full flexion and kept in this position for 60 seconds. In the pressure test, the examiner's long and index fingers compress the ulnar nerve just proximal to the cubital tunnel, keeping the elbow flexed 20 degrees and with the forearm in supination for 60 seconds. Ulnar paresthesias triggered by either test represent a positive response. In the Tinel sign, paresthesias are elicited by light taps on the nerve. Best results are obtained by applying pressure while the elbow is flexed (sensitivity 0.98, specificity 0.95). Electrodiagnostic studies are expensive, uncomfortable, and add little information in clear-cut cases. They are useful to distinguish double compressions, to rule out diffuse peripheral neuropathy, in cases in which compensation is involved, and for unequivocal demonstration of the condition prior to decompressive surgery.

Diagnosis

Summary of Diagnosis

> **CUBITAL TUNNEL SYNDROME**
> - Diagnosis is clinical based on symptoms, physical findings, and a positive result of provocative tests (flexion, compression, Tinel).
> - Elbow x-rays including a cubital tunnel view should be routinely obtained.
> - Electrodiagnosis is useful in selected cases.

Natural History

Expected Outcome

Patients may have only night symptoms plus a positive provocation test. Other patients go on to suffer permanent,

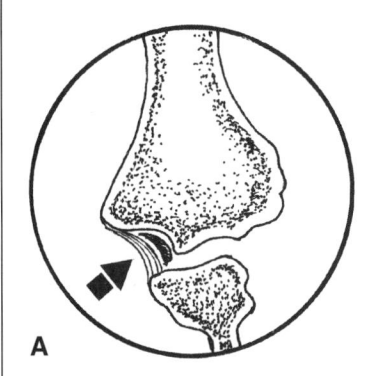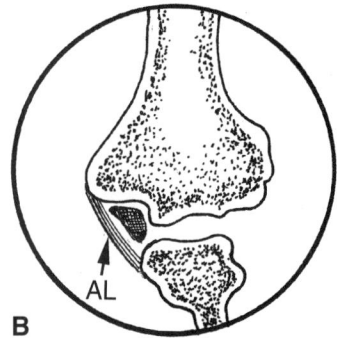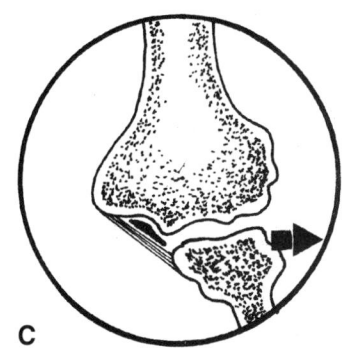

FIGURE 24–3. The external compression syndrome of the cubital tunnel. A, External compression of the ulnar canal such as malpositioning on the operating table. B, Space-occupying lesion (in this case a hypertrophic ulnar nerve). C, Trauma with lateral ulnar shift. AL=Arcuate ligament. (After Wadsworth TG. The external compression syndrome of the ulnar nerve at the cubital tunnel. Clin Orthop 124:189–204, 1977.)

annoying dysesthesia. Permanent symptoms should be considered a red flag because nearly all cases of ulnar palsy progress to intrinsic muscle paralysis. The end result may be a clawed and stiff hand.

Treatment

Methods

NSAIDs and a splint may be tried in early cases, but surgical release will ultimately be required in most patients with permanent symptoms. In the absence of motor involvement the simple incision of the arcuate ligament is often effective to relieve pain and dysesthesia. More advanced cases may be treated by anterior transposition of the ulnar nerve, a larger procedure that carries the risk of nerve ischemia.

When to Refer

Any transition from functional compression (paresthesias in flexion only) to persistent symptoms should trigger orthopedic referral. Timely surgery is highly effective for symptom relief and prevention of irreversible intrinsic paralysis.

Key Points

CUBITAL TUNNEL SYNDROME

- Is a common cause of ulnar neuropathy.
- It should be distinguished from radiculopathy, thoracic outlet compression, and nerve entrapment at the wrist (Guyon's canal).
- A positive provocative test indicates nerve entrapment at the cubital tunnel.
- Persistent symptoms (dysesthesia unrelieved by elbow extension) is an indication for surgery.
- Arcuate ligament section is effective in early neuropathy (sensory symptoms only). Late cases require anterior transposition of the ulnar nerve.

Suggested Reading

Manske PR, Johnston R, Pruitt DL, et al. Ulnar nerve decompression at the cubital tunnel. Clin Orthop 274:231–237, 1992.
Novak CB, Lee GW, Mackinnon SE, et al. Provocative testing for cubital tunnel syndrome. J Hand Surg 19A:817–820, 1994.
O'Driscoll SW, Horii E, Carmichael SW, et al. The cubital tunnel and ulnar neuropathy. J Bone Hand Surg 73B:613–617, 1991.
Wadsworth TG. The external compression syndrome of the ulnar nerve at the cubital tunnel. Clin Orthop 124:189–204, 1977.

Olecranon Bursitis

Presentation and Progression

Cause

The olecranon bursa is a discoid, flattened synovial sac approximately 3 cm in diameter that is interposed between the elbow skin and the underlying olecranon process and adjacent triceps tendon. Owing to its exposure to microtrauma (intermittent compression), plus its immediacy to the skin, the olecranon bursa is prone to traumatic inflammation and infection with skin-derived pathogens. Furthermore, the olecranon bursa, like any synovial structure, may participate in crystal synovitides, rheumatoid arthritis (RA), and connective tissue disorders.

Frequent causes of olecranon bursitis include trauma, bacterial infection, gout, and RA, in decreasing order. Recurrent leaning on the elbow on a hard surface, and rarely a discrete blow, cause the most common form of olecranon bursitis, traumatic bursitis. Second in frequency is septic bursitis in which the usual pathogens are *S. aureus* and *S. pyogenes*. Rare cases are due to anaerobic bacteria, mycobacteria (*M. marinum* and *M. tuberculosis*), and algae such as *Prototheca*. Infection of the olecranon bursa results from direct innoculation. Hematogenous seeding is exceptional even in bacteremias caused by well-known synoviotropic agents such as *N. gonorrhoea* and *H. influenzae*. Conversely, bacteremia is rare in septic bursitis, occurring in less than 5% of cases. Olecranon bursitis occurs in approximately 20% of gout patients. Bursal gout rarely represents the first manifestation of the disease. Tophi may or may not be palpable in the overlying skin. Finally, olecranon bursitis may be prominent in RA and is sometimes seen in SLE and other connective tissue diseases. Rheumatoid olecranon bursitis is a frequent association of gross rheumatoid nodules at the elbow tip.

Presentation

Olecranon bursitis may present as a cold, painless saccular mass at the elbow tip. The lump may have been present for weeks or months causing only a cosmetic concern. These cases are usually traumatic. Rarely are other etiologies involved. Gout, for instance, accounts for less than 10% of cases. Also, there are rare cases of septic bursitis that are quite benign clinically and by bursal fluid analysis; yet gram stain of the sediment is positive and *S. aureus* or *S. epidermidis* grow on culture.

PATIENT 30 A 50-year-old man was transferred to the author's hospital in shock and with a white lung. Three days before he had been seen at a walk-in clinic for evaluation of a swollen, slightly tender olecranon bursa. He was afebrile and felt well. Clear fluid was aspirated and sent for analysis and culture. In the same procedure, because the case appeared to be aseptic, 20 mg of methylprednisolone acetate was injected in the bursa. A day later there was local pain; the patient became febrile, extremely weak, and dyspneic and upon evaluation at a local hospital toxic shock was diagnosed. Retrospectively, the original bursal fluid contained 2000 WBC/mm^3 with 95% polys and gram stain was negative; however, *S. aureus* grew on culture. Upon transfer, the bursa was inflamed and its top was crusted (Figure 24–4). Attempted bursal reaspiration failed due to flocculent debris, and open drainage was undertaken. A picture of his feet, showing the classic desquamation of toxic shock, is shown in Figure 24–5.

This case illustates two points: (1) bursal fluid may look innocent in septic olecranon bursitis, and (2) never inject steroids in a superficial bursa without first having a negative culture

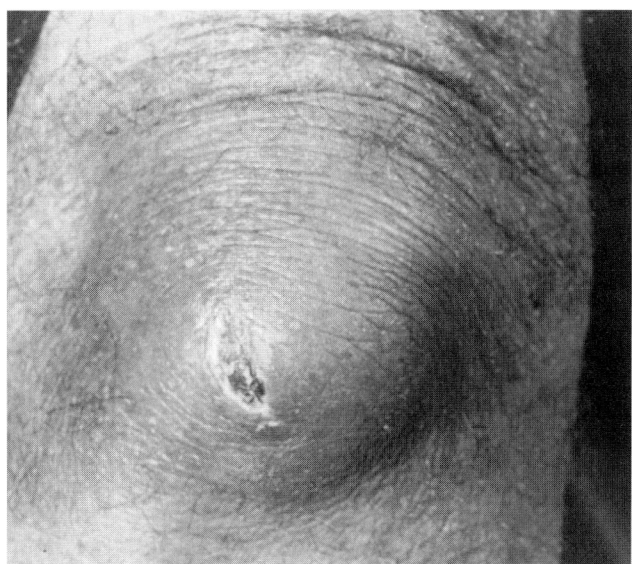

FIGURE 24–4. *Patient 30. Septic olecranon bursitis with toxic shock.* There is swelling, redness, and a small laceration with crusting at the elbow tip suggestive of septic bursitis.

result. Rheumatoid olecranon bursitis may be subacute and moderately inflammatory in concert with exacerbations of arthritis or chronic and cold in grossly nodular disease.

Other cases of bursitis have an acute onset and are clearly inflammatory. There is pain, erythema, local warmth, and the distended sac may be almost buried within a patch of inflamed skin. These cases are (approximately) septic in 70%, gouty in 20%, and traumatic in 10%. Crust, excoriation, or some other evidence of cutaneous injury is present in most cases of septic bursitis (Figure 24–6). Characteristic of the condition is limited and painful elbow flexion due to stretching and compression of the bursal sac. Passive extension, however, if done slowly and gently is both painless and full.

Atypical presentations of olecranon bursitis include upper extremity edema and pseudoarthritis. "Bursitic edema," which results from bursal leakage, extends along the ulnar border of the forearm and sometimes reaches the hand. The swelling may be bland and chronic in leaking rheumatoid bursae or acute and violently inflammatory resembling cellulitis or fasciitis in ruptured septic bursitis. Rarely, extensive inflammatory edema complicates acute cases of gouty and traumatic bursitis.

The pseudoarthritic form is characteristic of septic bursitis. Inflammation is so severe and extensive that acute arthritis is mimicked. It is the difference between severely limited flexion and the full or almost full passive extension that leads the astute clinician to the correct diagnosis.

Diagnosis

Summary of Diagnosis

> **OLECRANON BURSITIS**
>
> - Diagnosis is usually self-evident from the characteristic saccular distension of the bursa.
> - Exceptions to this rule are cases with extensive edema and cases that mimic acute arthritis.
> - In bursitic edema, residual bursal distension at the elbow tip allows a correct diagnosis to be made. In pseudoarthritic cases, normal passive extension suggests bursitis.
> - Etiology may be suggested by clinical findings, but overlapping features result in a high probability of error. Bursal fluid analysis including gross appearance, WBC count and differential, crystal search by polarizing microscopy, and culture is essential for diagnosis.

Natural History

Expected Outcome

Unless the offending cause is removed, in which case the process resolves within 3 months, traumatic effusions tend to persist indefinitely, producing the "chronic hygroma of the elbow." It has been stated that traumatic effusions have a tendency to become infected. In the author's experience this is a very infrequent occurrence except in cases treated with intrabursal corticosteroids. Complications of septic olecranon bursitis are rare. They include (1) rare cases (about 5%) of bacteremia; (2) rupture of very tense bursae causing dramatic inflammatory forearm and hand edema; (3) toxic shock in a few instances of *S. aureus* or streptococcal bursitis; (4) a chronically draining point after unwise aspiration at the bursal apex where the skin lacks recoil; and (5) cortical olecranon osteomyelitis in untreated cases. Acute bursal gout, similar to articular gout, resolves spontaneously in about 10

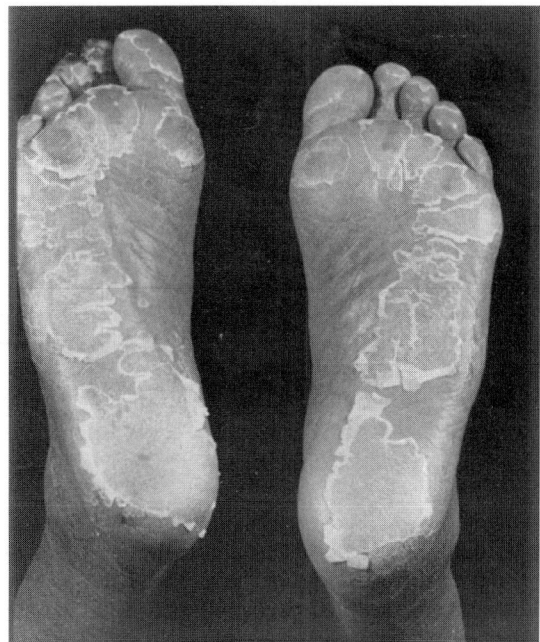

FIGURE 24–5. *Patient 30. Septic shock following staphylococcal olecranon bursitis.* Gross desquamation of plantar surfaces consistent with toxic shock.

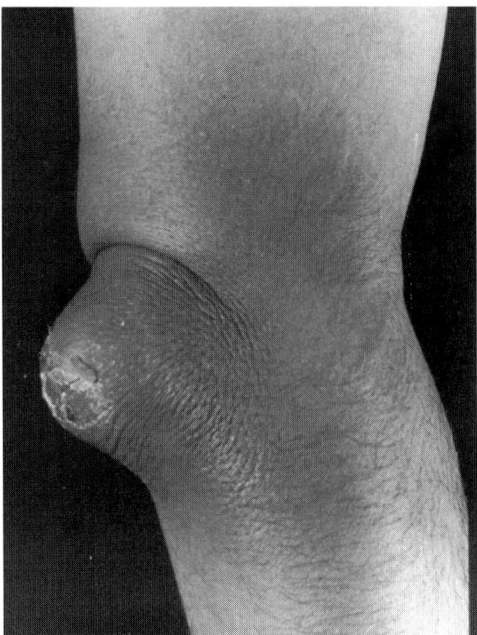

FIGURE 24–6. *Septic olecranon bursitis.* Classic appearance with angry erythema, crusting at tip from antecedent trauma, peribursal edema, and bursal swelling. (From Canoso JJ, Sheckman PR. Septic olecranon bursitis. Report of sixteen cases. J Rheumatol 6:96–102, 1979. By permission.)

days. In contrast, chronically distended bursae containing milky urate effusions are a frequent finding in advanced tophaceous gout. In rheumatoid arthritis, nonnodular bursitis tends to subside as the articular synovitis is brought under control by systemic therapy. Chronically distended sacs containing a milky suspension of cholesterol crystals are characteristic of nodular RA. Aspiration of chronic bursitis, whether gouty or rheumatoid, is followed by prompt reaccumulation of fluid. Multiple aspirations and corticosteroid infiltrations carry a high risk of infection.

Treatment

Methods

Treatment of traumatic bursitis should be based on the removal of its cause: recurrent microtrauma. Thus, patients should be instructed not to lean on the elbow and to avoid activities that in one or another way traumatize the olecranon region. One patient had to carry molded pieces from one room to another, many times each day, through a swinging door that he pushed open with the elbows; another example are drinking people who may lean on a hard counter while holding the head with their hand; and so on. By removing pressure on the elbow, traumatic effusions slowly resolve.

Intrabursal corticosteroids (see technique in appendix) can be used in unimproved patients after 3 months of conservative therapy and in patients who, for one reason or another, want to get rid of the lump as soon as possible. Intrabursal corticosteroids usually terminate the process within 1 week. In a retrospective review of 47 cases of traumatic olecranon bursitis with a negative initial bursal fluid culture result, of which 25 received 20 mg of triamcinolone hexacetonide, the injected bursae improved promptly, usually within a week; the uninjected bursae took several weeks to months to get well. However, 3 of the injected cases developed septic bursitis presumably as a result of the steroid injection, 5 noted skin atrophy at the bursal site, and 7 complained of chronic pain on leaning on the elbow. Minimal complications occurred in the uninjected group. Significantly, outcome at 3 months was similar in the injected and uninjected patients, suggesting that with patience the observed side effects of corticosteroids could have been prevented. However, in a randomized, blind, controlled trial of methylprednisolone acetate 20 mg intrabursally, methylprednisolone plus naproxen 1 g/day, naproxen alone, and placebo, the injected patients (with or without naproxen) improved faster than patients on naproxen or placebo. No instances of infection, pain, or skin atrophy were noted during a follow-up of 6 months. Thus, the less potent methylprednisolone acetate appears to be effective and safer than triamcinolone hexacetonide for the treatment of traumatic bursitis. Because the conservative treatment is physiologic, because each corticosteroid injection at least theoretically carries some risk, and because recurrences may occur if avoidance of trauma is not stressed, the author prefers to use conservative treatment first and offer intrabursal corticosteroids to patients who fail to improve.

Treatment of septic olecranon bursitis should be along guidelines used for soft tissue infections rather than septic arthritis. Surgical drainage or bursectomy has little place in the treatment of olecranon bursitis. Individuals who are otherwise normal should be treated with oral antibiotics such as dicloxacillin 2 g/day to be discontinued 5 days after the first culture negative sample was obtained. Average duration of treatment is 10 days. It has been shown that cases of long duration prior to therapy require more prolonged therapy. Elderly individuals, patients with debilitating conditions, and those on immunosuppressive agents should be hospitalized and treated with parenteral antibiotics such as oxacillin 12 g/day or a cephalosporin, or if the patient is allergic to penicillin, vancomycin for 4 to 7 days followed by oral antibiotics for 7 to 14 days. The bursa should be aspirated daily to assess response. Once sterility of bursal fluid has been achieved, reaspirations should be discontinued. Protracted sterile postinfectious effusions are sometimes observed. Treatment of these effusions is with avoidance of local trauma. Continuing reaspirations should be avoided.

Bursal gout and rheumatoid bursitis should be treated systemically with treatment programs for acute gout and RA, respectively. Chronically distended sacs may improve on long-term allopurinol in gout (since there is a constant association with tophaceous gout) and with disease-modifying treatments in RA. Repeated aspiration and corticosteroid injection are unwise because they are both futile and carry a risk of infection. Bursal resection is unnecessary in both conditions, and in RA is often followed by recurrence of rheumatoid nodules and the formation of a new bursa. Promising results of tetracycline instillation in chronic nodular rheumatoid bursae have recently been reported.

When to Refer

Cases of septic olecranon bursitis that require hospitalization should be followed concurrently with a rheumatologist or infectious disease specialist. Treatment decisions in chronic rheumatoid bursitis should also be made by a rheumatologist.

Key Points

OLECRANON BURSITIS

- Is characterized clinically by a cystic swelling at the elbow tip.
- Etiology of bursitis may be suspected clinically, but aspiration is essential to diagnose bacterial infection and gout.
- Aspiration should be made from the lateral side to avoid chronic leaks and damage to the ulnar nerve.
- Gross appearance of bursal fluid may be deceiving. Hemobursa is nonspecific. Milky fluids may contain urate or cholesterol crystals. "Clear" fluids, although usually traumatic, may also occur in septic bursitis and gout.
- Upon similar disease stimuli subcutaneous bursae respond differently than joints. This includes lower WBC counts, a higher percentage of mononuclear cells, and a poorer mucin clot test.

Suggested Reading

Canoso JJ, Yood RA. Acute gouty bursitis: Report of 15 cases. Ann Rheum Dis 38:326–328, 1979.

Canoso JJ, Yood RA. Reaction of superficial bursae in response to specific disease stimuli. Arthritis Rheum 22:1361–1364, 1979.

Goldin DS, Stangler DA, Canoso JJ. Rheumatoid subcutaneous bursitis. J Rheumatol 8:974–978, 1981.

Ho G Jr, Su EY. Antibiotic therapy of septic bursitis. Its implication in the treatment of septic bursitis. Arthritis Rheum 24:905, 1981.

Smith DL, McAfee JH, Lucas LM, et al. Treatment of nonseptic olecranon bursitis: A controlled, blinded prospective trial. Arch Intern Med 149:2527–2532, 1989.

Weinstein PS, Canoso JJ, Wohlgethan JR. Long-term follow-up of corticosteroid injection for traumatic olecranon bursitis. Ann Rheum Dis 43:44–46, 1984.

Zimmermann B III, Mikolich DJ, Ho G, Jr. Septic bursitis. Sem Arthritis Rheum 24:391–410, 1995.

CHAPTER 25

Shoulder Pain

Shoulder pain is extemely common. At any given time approximately 10% of the adult population will describe current or recent shoulder pain, with a cumulative lifetime frequency that reaches 40%. In two surveys of elderly people over 70 years of age, one performed in institutionalized individuals and the other in the community, the prevalence of shoulder pain was 21%. In the Netherlands, the cumulative incidence of shoulder complaints in general medical practices was 11.2 per 1000 patients per year. Frequent causes of shoulder pain include rotator cuff tendinitis due to subacromial impingement, crystal (basic calcium crystals)-induced inflammation, age-related tendon degeneration, and the frozen shoulder. These and less common conditions of the shoulder are listed in Table 25–1.

To understand shoulder pain a basic knowledge of anatomy is required. The shoulder is a complex joint that includes three diarthrodial joints, the glenohumeral (GH), the acromioclavicular (AC), and the sternoclavicular, and a muscular joint, the scapulothoracic.

Motion is provided by superficial and deep muscles. Superficial muscles include the trapezius, deltoid, latissimus dorsi, teres major, and pectoralis major. These muscles act on the scapula, the clavicle, and the humerus. Deep muscles comprise the rotator cuff muscles: subscapularis, supraspinatus, infraspinatus, and teres minor, plus the long head of the biceps. The humeral insertion of the rotator cuff tendons has the shape of an inverted U: infraspinatus and teres minor in the posterior greater tuberosity, supraspinatus in the superior greater tuberosity, and subscapularis in the lesser tuberosity. Because of this arrangement infraspinatus and teres minor are external rotators, supraspinatus is an abductor, and subscapularis is an internal rotator.

Another relevant muscle in shoulder pathology is the biceps brachii. This muscle, which inserts distally in the proximal radius, has two heads: the short head that inserts in the coracoid process, and the long head whose tendon, after traversing up the bicipital groove, becomes intraarticular and inserts just above the glenoid.

The rotator cuff tendons, which blend with the capsule of the GH joint and interdigitate among themselves forming a common insertion, are in turn separated from the overlying coracoacromial arch and the deltoid by the tenuous subacromial bursa, which acts as a gliding surface. In Codman's view, the subacromial bursa completes to a hemisphere the articulation of the humeral head on the shallow glenoid. In addition to providing humeral motion, rotator cuff muscles are essential in maintaining the internal cohesiveness to the shoulder. Early in arm elevation the deltoid muscle acts nearly vertically on the humerus. Unopposed, the deltoid muscle would ram the humerus under the acromion similar to what happens in patients with a massive rotator cuff tear. Normally, however, the simultaneous contraction of the rotator cuff muscles and long head of the biceps holds the humeral head in place allowing GH motion and preventing self-destruction of the joint. This coordinated action of the rotator cuff muscles (and long head of the biceps) and deltoid, which is essential to shoulder physiology, is known as the shoulder force-couple. The fibrous GH joint capsule attaches medially to the periphery of the glenoid fossa just outside a cartilaginous rim, the labrum glenoidale, and laterally to the anatomic neck of the humerus. A lax inferior capsular recess allows full arm elevation without undue tension.

In the frozen shoulder, fibrosis and capsular retraction absorb this recess and as a result abduction is drastically limited. The GH joint capsule is reinforced anteriorly and inferiorly by the superior, medial, and inferior glenohumeral ligaments, which are important in maintaining joint stability.

Shoulder pain may originate locally (glenohumeral joint, rotator cuff tendon, acromioclavicular and sternoclavicular joints) or at a distant site in the neck, upper extremity, or trunk. Essential in shoulder pain interpretation is an understanding of the segmental innervation of shoulder structures.

Briefly, two possible patterns of shoulder pain exist: C4 pain, which is experienced in the supraclavicular fossa, and C5 pain, which involves the lateral shoulder and upper arm (Figures 25–1 and 25–2). C4 pain may have a local or a

TABLE 25–1

PAIN LOCATION AND CAUSES OF SHOULDER PAIN

SUPERIOR (C4)

Cervical
Acromioclavicular
Sternoclavicular
Diaphragmatic

SUPEROLATERAL (C5)

Rotator cuff tendinitis
Frozen shoulder
Synovitis
Suprascapular nerve entrapment

AXILLARY

Apical tumor
Postoperative
Herpes zoster

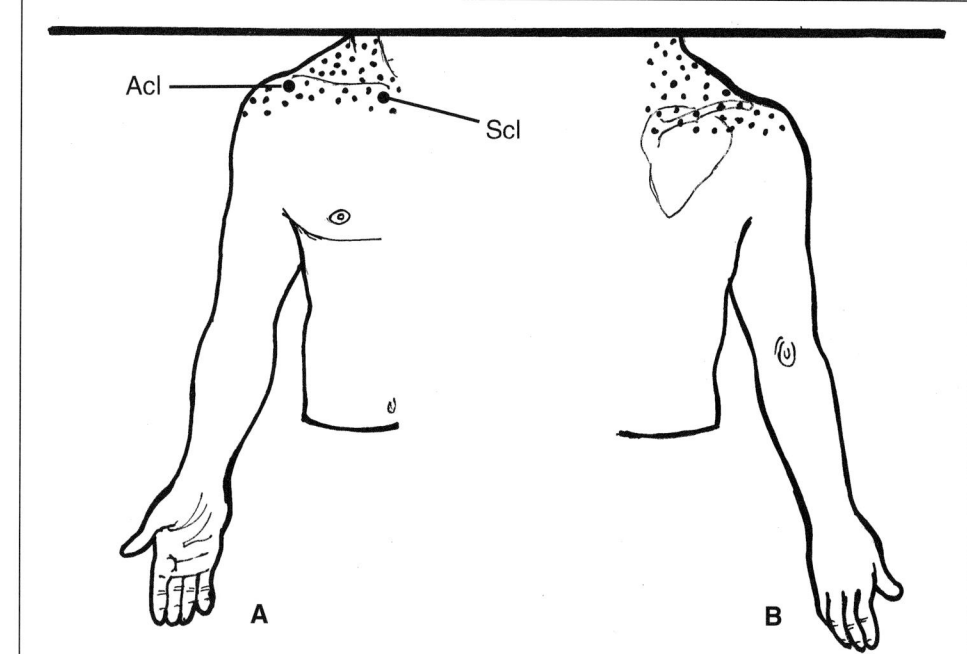

FIGURE 25-1. C4 pain radiation in acromioclavicular and sternoclavicular arthritis. Acl = Acromioclavicular joint. Scl = Sternoclavicular joint. A = Anterior view. B = Posterior view. (After Kellgren JH. In: Scott JT [ed] Copeman's Textbook of the Rheumatic Diseases, 5th ed. Churchill Livingstone, Edinburgh, 62–77, 1978.)

remote origin. Local pain may originate in the acromioclavicular (AC) or stenoclavicular joints, the supraclavicular soft tissues, and the clavicle. Remote causes of C4 pain include thoracic or abdominal processes that impinge on the central, phrenic nerve (C4)–innervated portion of the diaphragm, and neck problems, in particular muscle contracture pain and cervical spondylosis.

The author's system to examine patients complaining of supraclavicular pain is as follows: The patient is first asked to breathe deeply and cough. If pain is not reproduced, a diaphragm-related condition such as basal pleuritis, subphrenic abscess, or splenic infarct can be ruled out.

Neck motion is next explored. Pain may be triggered by homolateral flexion; this pain is dull and persistent in

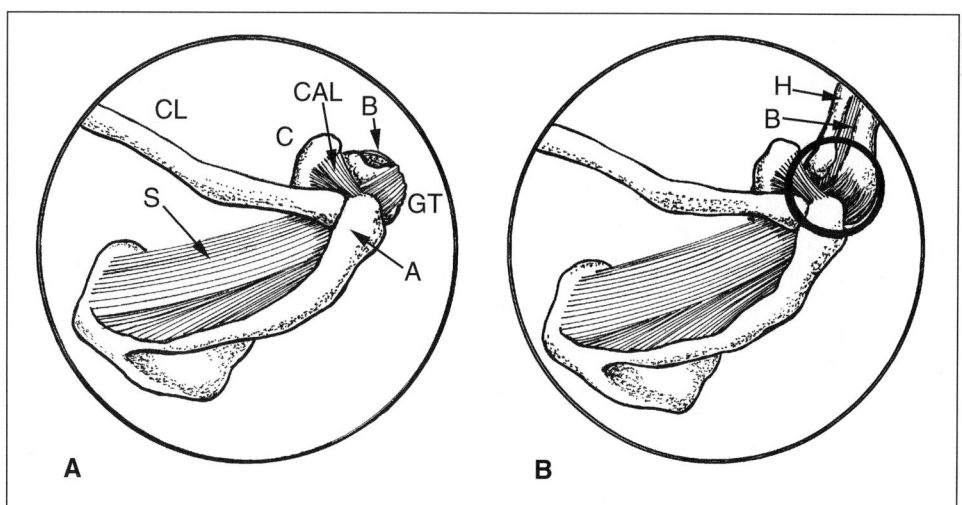

FIGURE 25-2. Anatomy of subacromial impingement. A, As seen from atop, the proximal end of the humerus is partially covered (in its medial half) by the coracoacromial ligament, the anterior acromion, and the acromioclavicular (AC) joint. B, With abduction the greater tuberosity of the humerus squeezes the supraspinatus tendon against the acromion and coracoacromial ligament. Note the close proximity of the biceps tendon, which explains the frequent rupture of the long head of the biceps in chronic impingement. Proliferative conditions of the AC joint, such as osteoarthritis, may also cause impingement. A, Top view of shoulder with arm in dependency. B, Top view of shoulder with arm in flexion and abduction. S = Supraspinatus tendon. CL = Clavicle. C = Coracoid process. CAL = Coracoacromial ligament. B = Biceps tendon within groove (the tendon has been cut). GT = Greater tuberosity of humerus. A = Acromion. H = Humerus.

processes affecting the facet or uncovertebral joints, or sharp and paresthetic when the C4 root is being impinged upon. Pain triggered by contralateral bending, however, is characteristic of muscle contracture pain. If neither coughing or neck motion reproduce the pain, a local cause should be sought. The supraclavicular soft tissues should be carefully palpated seeking a tumor mass, usually a node; then the clavicle; and finally the AC and sternoclavicular joints. In addition to local tenderness, patients with AC arthritis have pain upon full elevation of the arm and when the arm is sharply adducted such as by placing the hand on the opposite shoulder.

C5 pain arises in conditions that affect the glenohumeral (GH) joint, the rotator cuff tendon, and also in the compressive neuropathy of the suprascapular nerve. Distinguishing the two former entities requires an analysis of passive, active, and resisted motion. In GH joint conditions, such as arthritis and the frozen shoulder, motion is restricted in all planes and active and passive motions are equal. In contrast, in tendinous disease, active motion is restricted and passive motion is normal. Furthermore, because inflamed tendons hurt when they are stressed, resisted motions accurately identify the tendon(s) at fault. Resisted motions are tested with the patient's arm at the side of the body and the elbow flexed 90 degrees.

Pain on resisted abduction indicates supraspinatus tendinitis; on internal rotation, subscapularis tendinitis; and on external rotation, infraspinatus and teres minor tendinitis. Suprascapular nerve entrapment is suspected mainly on the basis of antecedent trauma or sports abuse, weakness of abduction and external rotation, tenderness over the suprascapular notch, failure of local anesthetic injections to relieve the symptoms, and positive electrodiagnostic studies.

Suggested Reading

Clark JM, Harryman DT II. Tendons, ligaments, and capsule of the rotator cuff. J Bone Joint Surg 74A:713–725, 1992.
Research Committee, American Shoulder and Elbow Surgeons. A standardized method for the assessment of shoulder function. J Shoulder Elbow Surg 3:347–352, 1994.
van der Windt DAWM, Koes BW, de Jong BA, et al. Shoulder disorders in general practice: Incidence, patient characteristics, and management. Ann Rheum Dis 54:959–964, 1995.
Warner JJP, McMahon PJ. The role of the long head of the biceps brachii in superior stability of the glenohumeral joint. J Bone Joint Surg 77A:366–372, 1995.

Rotator Cuff Tendinitis

Rotator cuff tendinitis may be caused by impingement, calcium crystals–induced inflammation, senile tendon degeneration, shoulder instability, and enthesopathy (inflammation at tendon attachment sites). Common findings in rotator cuff tendinitis include (1) pain in the lateral shoulder and upper arm corresponding to a C5 derivation of the rotator cuff; (2) severe, often catching pain upon certain active movements; (3) normal passive range of motion; and (4) pain- or tear-related weakness in the muscles whose tendons are involved, usually the supraspinatus and the infraspinatus. In the past, acute subacromial or subdeltoid bursitis was a frequent diagnosis. Since most instances of bursal inflammation are secondary to tendon disease or impingement, the condition is not discussed separately.

Impingement

Presentation and Progression

Cause

Impingement of the rotator cuff between the proximal humerus and the coracoacromial arch may occur from anomalies in the coracoacromial arch impinging on the tendon (structural impingement), and from instability due to joint hyperlaxity or weak rotator cuff muscles (functional impingement) (Table 25–2). Coracoacromial arch anomalies may be congenital, such as a hooked acromion, or acquired, such as osteophytes growing into the coracoacromial ligament or at the inferior margins of the AC joint, and calcium deposits in the supraspinatus tendon. As a result of impingement (Figure 25–2), the supraspinatus, the infraspinatus, and the closely related long head of the biceps tendons are subject to recurrent inflammation, accelerated wear, and the prospect of rupture. Impingement-caused tears are usually incomplete in the supraspinatus and infraspinatus, and complete in the long head of the biceps.

Presentation

Structural impingement represents the garden variety of the syndrome. Patients complain of catching pain upon abduction and external rotation movements, superolaterally or anteriorly at the bicipital tendon groove. Pain is triggered or worsened by sustained overhead activities. Night pain precipitated by rolling on the involved shoulder is common in these patients. The typical patient describes having had one or more shoulder infiltrations. Instability-related impingement causes recurrent shoulder pain during and after sports, in particular throwing and overhead sports such as baseball, volleyball, and basketball. In athletes, overuse of the extremity causes attenuation of glenohumeral ligaments. Decreased shoulder stabilization places additional stress on the rotator cuff muscles, resulting in fatigue. Finally, a weakened rotator cuff, overpowered by the deltoid, causes upward displacement of the humeral head, which compresses the supraspinatus tendon against the coracoacromial arch. Findings are similar in structural and functional impingement. Muscle atrophy may be apparent at the supra- or infraspinatus fossae. There is coarse subacromial crepitation on rotations. Focal tenderness may be found around the greater tuberosity or anteriorly at the bicipital tendon groove.

TABLE 25–2 CAUSES OF ROTATOR CUFF IMPINGEMENT	
STRUCTURAL	**FUNCTIONAL**
J–shaped acromion	Rotator cuff weakness
Subacromial spurs	Joint hyperlaxity
AC joint spurs	
Tumoral calcinosis at supraspinatus	

Indeed, most instances of "bicipital tendinitis" are caused by impingement.

Subacromial impingement results in a painful arc of abduction between 70 and 120 degrees keeping the forearms in pronation (palms back) (Figure 25–3). As the arms are being brought down, a painful catch occurs in the midrange. Pain may not occur in supination (palms to front) because in external rotation the greater tuberosity moves away from the coracoacromial arch. Another useful maneuver is to resist external rotation with the patient's arm adducted (elbow pointing forward, arm and forearm in the horizontal plane) and in full internal rotation. Subacromial pain indicates impingement.

As previously mentioned, AC joint osteophytes are an important cause of extrinsic impingement, particularly in elderly individuals. AC joint motion (and therefore pain in AC joint disease) occurs largely past 120 degrees elevation. Thus, in cases of impingement caused by AC joint osteophytes, there is a painful arc of abduction from 70 to 180 degrees; impingement causes pain from 70 to 120 degrees; and AC joint stress from 120 to 180 degrees.

Diagnosis

Summary of Diagnosis

IMPINGEMENT

- History of trauma, sports, and overhead activities.
- Instability maneuvers.
- Impingement maneuvers.
- X-rays.
- MRI if operative treatment is considered.

Natural History

Expected Outcome

Prognosis depends on the patient's age and cause of impingement. High demands placed on the player makes sports-related impingement notoriously difficult to control. In older individuals, associated processes including senile rotator cuff degeneration and cervical spondylosis often preclude a full

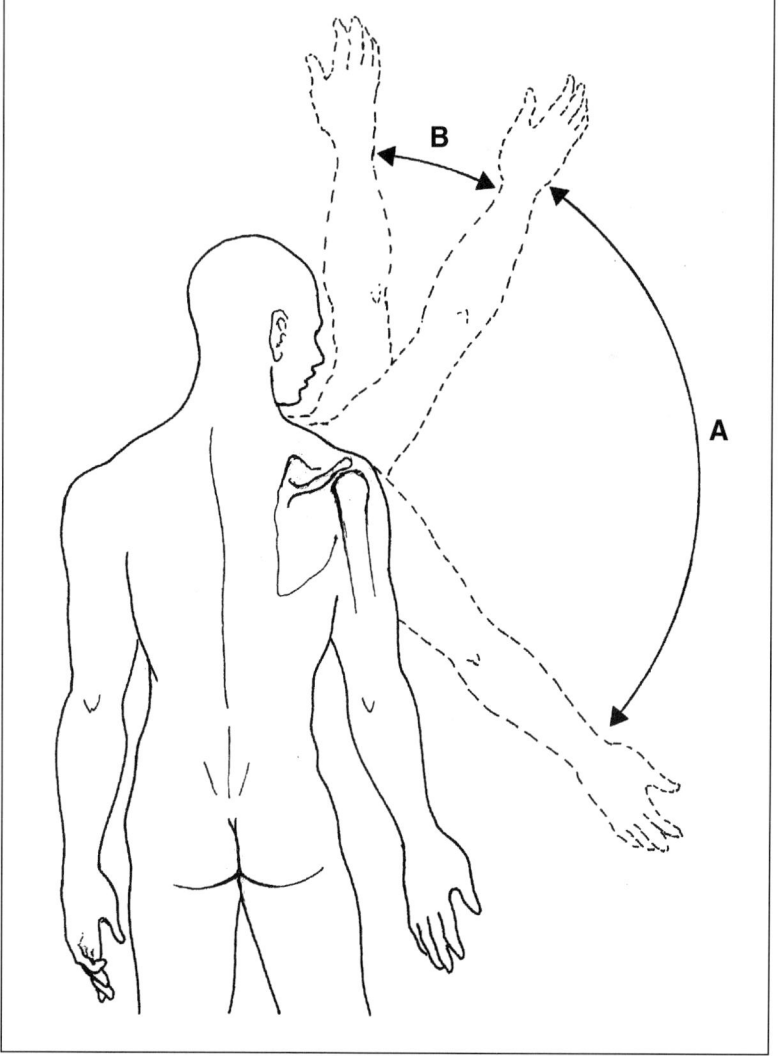

FIGURE 25–3. *The shoulder arc of motion maneuver.* Because the greater tuberosity of the humerus has to clear under the acromion/coracoacromial ligament during abduction, patients with subacromial impingement hurt during arc A. Once the greater tuberosity has cleared, pain ceases in arc B. A similar phenomenon occurs as the arm is brought down: no pain in arc B, pain in arc A, then no pain in full dependency. Because the AC joint has its greatest motion in terminal elevation, patients with AC arthritis hurt in B. Finally, when the AC joint, for example, in osteoarthritis, causes impingement, there will be pain in arc A from impingement, plus in arc B from stress on the diseased joint.

treatment response. In most patients, however, an impingement episode can be controlled without difficulties. A stringent program of home strengthening exercises is essential to prevent recurrences.

Complications

Complications of impingement include the frozen shoulder; rupture of the supraspinatus, infraspinatus, or long head of the biceps tendons; and, in elderly patients with long-standing supraspinatus tears, a feared end-stage lesion known as "recurrent hemorrhagic shoulder of the elderly," "rotator cuff arthropathy," or "Milwaukee shoulder." A *painful, stiff shoulder* complicates immobility. Since motion hurts, to prevent pain ill-advised patients may keep the shoulder still. This causes deconditioning, muscle atrophy and contracture, and further pain. Fibrosis and joint restriction eventually sets in. Spontaneous *tendon rupture* is a frequent complication of impingement lesions. Rupture may be partial (partial thickness tear) or complete (full thickness tear). Spontaneous tears differ in young adult and older individuals. In the younger group tears are partial except when intercurrent trauma, such as a fall onto the outstretched arm, results in a full thickness tear. In older patients, however, complete spontaneous tears are frequent as a result of concurrent senile tendon degeneration.

Clinically, partial tears increase pain and cause only a mild decrease in strength. Full thickness tears behave differently whether they are traumatic or spontaneous. In complete traumatic tears there is an abrupt inability to abduct and any attempts at abduction or external rotation result in excruciating pain. Minimal efforts, such as turning the car key, become impossible. Full thickness spontaneous tears may be asymptomatic or cause pain on motion, weakness of abduction and external rotation, as well as severe nocturnal pain.

Tears may be identified by careful palpation. The patient is examined seated with the arm hanging on the side, elbow flexed 90 degrees. The examiner, standing behind the patient, localizes the greater tuberosity at the proximal end of the humerus. Anterior supraspinatus tears may be felt in external rotation, posterior tears in internal rotation, and infraspinatus tears in hyperextension. Ruptures of the long head of the biceps tendon are usually spontaneous. A hollow area appears in front of the shoulder. Compared with the opposite side, the biceps muscle, held proximally by the short head only, is pulled medially. A local echymosis may follow.

Treatment

Methods

Treatment of impingement depends on its mechanism and stage of the disease. Patients with *functional impingement* are not helped by arthroscopic surgery and are best handled by a sports orthopedist or rheumatologist. It is therefore critical that cases with unstable shoulders be correctly identified. Patients with mild symptoms and stable shoulders are treated with a resting sling for 24 to 36 hours, pendular exercises, and full doses of a NSAID. Recurrent or severe symptoms require that the patient be kept off the offending sport for several weeks. Arthroscopy should be considered in these patients, since possible labral detachments and loose bodies may be successfully treated arthroscopically. Initially, Codman's pendular exercises are used both for analgesia and to maintain range of motion. After 1 to 2 weeks a program of shoulder strengthening exercises is started under physiotherapist supervision, stressing muscle strenghtening for the dynamic control of joint hyperlaxity. Special attention should be paid to the deltoid, the rotator cuff muscles, and the shoulder stabilizer muscles. After several weeks, jointly with the trainer, a decision can often be made about resuming playing. This should be done under modified conditions for several months and with correction of any faulty technique. Full resumption is best delayed for 6 months until tissue healing has been completed.

Corticosteroid infiltrations should be used with great caution in this group, not more than two or three administered 2 months apart (see the infiltration techniques section) with a sterile technique and avoiding intratendinous injections. Successful injections result in some improvement by the next day; full effect is reached at 7 to 10 days.

Structural, subacromial impingement is treated similarly except that the surgical option is open to these patients. A particularly severe or prolonged bout of tendinitis may be shortened by a subacromial corticosteroid infiltration. Infiltrations should be used sparingly, not more than three at 2 to 3 week intervals at a given site.

Expected Response

With the treatment method described patients will be expected to improve or be symptom free and able to return to sedentary or light activities within 1 to 2 weeks. Prognosis in high-performance athletes and in heavy workers is guarded.

Complications

Complications of conservative therapy are rare. In the past, tendon ruptures after shoulder infiltrations for "tendinitis" were thought to be frequent. Although abused or poorly placed injections doubtlessly cause ruptures, current understanding suggests that most instances of tendon rupture are due to the natural progression of the impingement process. With the proper precautions, steroid-induced ruptures must be truly exceptional.

Because surgical treatment of structural impingement has a sound basis as well as excellent results, orthopedic consultation should not be withheld in severely symptomatic patients. As surgery is planned, MRI or CT arthrography are routinely obtained to detect possible tendon rupture. Surgical treatment of structural impingement is based on the partial unroofing of the rotator cuff, which is achieved by partial anterior acromioplasty, resection of the coracoacromial ligament, rimming of osteophytes, possible resection of the AC joint, and resection of a fibrotic subacromial bursa if deemed necessary. The entire procedure can be done by open surgery or arthroscopically.

Pain improvement is dramatic. Compared with open

surgery, arthroscopic unroofing has a shorter rehabilitation period and allows an earlier return to work. There are no differences in cost, however. Small rotator cuff tears can be left alone or treated arthroscopically (they usually involve the articular side of the tendon). Large tears, however, must be repaired if regaining a strong arm is a goal. To restore strength the choices are an open unroofing and tendon repair or an arthroscopic unroofing in conjunction with a small lateral incision for tendon repair. Of the two procedures the best is the one the orthopedic surgeon is most experienced with.

The rehabilitation program is identical in open and arthroscopic surgery. This includes 6 to 8 weeks of passive motion followed by 6 to 8 weeks of active motion. Muscle strengthening is usually begun 3 months after surgery. The expected response after surgical unroofing alone, open, or arthroscopic is major pain improvement in more than 90% of cases. In cases with tendon rupture a successful repair is achieved in approximately 70% of cases. Overall, the results of surgery are highly satisfactory.

Complications of open surgery include the usual anesthetic and infection risks plus dehiscence of the tendon repair. The latter may be documented by echography and corrected with further surgery. Complications of arthroscopy are relatively rare. They include infection, compartmental syndromes from extravasation of the distending fluid, and accidental compressive nerve paralysis. In the aggregate, serious complications occur in less than 1% of patients.

When to Refer

As a general principle, cases of functional impingement in athletes should be referred to a sports orthopedist or an orthopedic surgeon interested in the shoulder. Routine cases of subacromial impingement may be handled by primary care physicians. If an initial corticosteroid infiltration resulted in failure, subsequent infiltrations should be performed by an orthopedist or rheumatologist. Recurrent cases and potentially disabling cases should be referred to an experienced orthopedist for possible surgical decompression.

Key Points

> **IMPINGEMENT**
> - Is a prominent cause of shoulder pain and tendon rupture.
> - Impingement may be structural or functional.
> - Diagnosis is clinical.
> - Keys in diagnosis are a mid-range painful arc of motion and positive impingement maneuvers.
> - Most cases respond to a conservative treatment.
> - Treatment in functional impingement is with muscle strengthening exercises. Arthroscopic inspection may be important in refractory cases to rule out labral tears and other internal derangements of the shoulder.
> - Surgical unroofing is highly successful in refractory cases of structural impingement.

Suggested Reading

Burkhead WZ Jr, Rockwood CA Jr. Treatment of instability of the shoulder with an exercise program. J Bone Joint Surg 74A:890–896, 1992.
Dalton SE. The conservative management of rotator cuff disorders. Br J Rheumatol 33:663–667, 1994.
Fu FH, Harner CD, Klein AH. Shoulder impingement syndrome. A critical review. Clin Orthop 269:162–173, 1991.
Gartsman GM. Arthroscopic treatment of rotator cuff disease. J Shoulder Elbow Surg 4:228–241, 1995.
Hawkins RH, Dunlop R. Nonoperative treatment of rotator cuff tears. Clin Orthop 321:178–188, 1995.
Lyons AR, Tomlinson JE. Clinical diagnosis of tears of the rotator cuff. J Bone Joint Surg 74B:414–415, 1992.
McCarty DJ, Halverson PB, Carrera GF, et al. "Milwaukee shoulder." I. Clinical aspects. Arthritis Rheum 24:464–473, 1981.
Ogilvie-Harris J, Demazière A. Arthroscopic debridement versus open repair for rotator cuff tears. A prospective cohort study. J Bone Joint Surg 75B:416–430, 1993.
Sher JS, Uribe JW, Posada A, et al. Abnormal findings on magnetic resonance images of asymptomatic shoulders. J Bone Joint Surg 77A:10–15, 1995.

Calcific Tendinitis

Cause

Calcium crystal (basic calcium crystals)-induced tendinitis is a condition of young adults. The shoulder location, usually in the supraspinatus or infraspinatus near its attachment, sometimes with spilling into the subacromial bursa, is just one of the many tendon sites the condition may hit. Different from gout, there is no identifiable laboratory marker for the condition. Amorphous calcium deposits appear to build up just preceding the inflammation and often disappear in several months to a few years. They should be distinguished from bone spurs, which are well defined (often with cortical bone), usually asymptomatic, and permanent.

Presentation

Patients with acute calcific tendinitis are in extreme pain and usually arrive at the office holding the arm. Warmth and exquisite tenderness around the greater tuberosity in supraspinatus and infraspinatus tendinitis and in the anterior shoulder in subscapularis tendinitis is characteristic. Muscle inhibition may be complete. The general appearance may be that of an acute infection. The condition is suspected clinically, but diagnosis requires radiologic demonstration.

Diagnosis

Summary of Diagnosis

> **CALCIFIC TENDINITIS**
> - Radiographic demonstration of an amorphous calcium deposit in the vicinity of the rotator cuff tendon.
> - Tangential views may be required.
> - In patients with very acute symptoms, especially if a calcium deposit is not shown, the possibility of a missed posterior shoulder luxation should be considered.
> - Identification of this lesion requires an axillary view.

Natural History

Expected Outcome

Acute calcific tendinitis responds promptly to anti-inflammatory therapy, and prognosis is excellent because the lesion seldom recurs. In some cases, a residual calcific deposit interferes with the free play of the cuff tendon under the coracoacromial arch. Finally, there is a silent phase prior to complete absorption. This phase may last months to years. No complications are expected.

Treatment

Methods

Acute calcific tendinitis is treated with sling immobilization, ice application every 2 hours, plus one of several anti-inflammatory treatments. Full doses of a NSAID such as diclofenac 75 mg bid or naproxen 500 mg tid may be used for 2 to 5 days. Intrabursal (subacromial bursa) corticosteroids, such as methylprednisolone acetate 40 mg, mixed with 2 to 4 mL of 1% lidocaine may also be used. Because of the underlying inflammation these injections tend to be very painful. If the deposit is large enough, aspiration of the calcific material that looks like, and has the consistency of, toothpaste may be attempted, preferably under fluoroscopy or ultrasound guidance with a #16 or #18 needle. Intramuscular ACTH 40 units, such as used in gout, is the author's preferred treatment. If by the next day patients are less than 50% improved, the injection may be repeated. Once pain improves, pendular exercises are begun, to be performed for 2 to 3 minutes at least five times a day.

Expected Response

With the treatments described, marked improvement occurs within 12 to 24 hours, and within 2 to 5 days the episode is over. Pain on active and resisted motion with positive impingement maneuvers may follow. These cases may be improved with a subacromial corticosteroid infiltration. Rarely, persistent impingement may require removal of the calcium deposit or acromioplasty.

Complications

Complications of treatment are rare. ACTH is quite safe. NSAIDs cause GI symptoms frequently, as well as multiple other problems that are reviewed in the NSAID section. However, in the absence of contraindications, a brief NSAID course has little morbidity.

When to Refer

In most instances referral is not required. Patients with residual deposits causing impingement should be evaluated by an orthopedic surgeon.

Key Points

> **CALCIFIC TENDINITIS**
> - Most frequent in young adults.
> - Acute shoulder pain with an inability to move the arm.
> - No history of trauma.
> - An amorphous calcium deposit is seen radiographically in relation with the rotator cuff.
> - Rapid improvement with NSAID, intrabursal corticosteroids, or I.M. ACTH.
> - Impingement by residual deposits may occur.

Suggested Reading

Farin PU, Jaroma H, Soimakallio S. Rotator cuff calcifications: Treatment with US-guided technique. Radiology 195:841–843, 1995.

Rowe CR. Calcific tendinitis. In: Stauffer ES (ed) Instructional Course Lectures, Vol. 34. CV Mosby, St. Louis, 196–198, 1985.

Age-Related Degeneration of the Rotator Cuff

Presentation and Progression

Cause

Age-related rotator cuff tendon degeneration is universal past the age of 50. Changes include fibrovascular proliferation, calcification, fraying, and often tears. Indeed, based on MRI studies in asymptomatic individuals and postmortem studies, up to 70% of elderly individuals have degenerative changes in the rotator cuff, long head of the biceps tendon, and labrum glenoidale. This includes partial tears of the rotator cuff in 26%, and full thickness tears in a surprising 28%. It may not be possible pathologically to distinguish tendon aging from an impingement lesion; indeed, in many cases both lesions coexist. Furthermore, some degree of impingement may result from everyday activities such as holding a book or eating with a fork and knife. Kapandji has commented that any activities implying the use of the hands within the field of stereoscopic vision require some abduction in the scapular plane, a position that may result in supraspinatus impingement.

Presentation

Shoulder pain in elderly individuals is likely to result from overlapping lesions including aging-related rotator cuff tendon degeneration, structural impingement from AC joint osteoarthritic spurs, and concurrent cervical spondylosis with deep pain radiation. Tendon ruptures are frequent in this setting, and within this group some patients with full thickness tears go on to develop the "Milwaukee shoulder."

Diagnosis

Summary of Diagnosis

> **SHOULDER PAIN IN OLD AGE**
> - Usually multifactorial.
> - The predominant lesion is rotator cuff tendon fraying and tears plus subacromial impingement from AC and acromial spurs.
> - A painful stiff shoulder may occur.
> - Cervical spondylosis frequently coexists.

- Unattended, shoulder pain is a frequent cause of disability.
- Accurate diagnosis is essential for successful treatment.

Natural History

Expected Outcome

Senile tendon degeneration symptoms may improve on treatment, but patients seldom return to baseline. Disability for activities of daily living occurs frequently.

Complications

Acute: A common complication in patients with senile tendon degeneration is tendon rupture. This may occur without symptoms and with minimal functional limitation. As previously mentioned, complete ruptures of the supraspinatus or infraspinatus are more common in this age group than in younger people.

Chronic: In some patients, recurrent tendinitis is followed by progressive painful shoulder limitation. Sleep disturbance and disability for daily living activities are frequent complications of rotator cuff disease in the elderly. The Milwaukee shoulder represents the most serious complication of rotator cuff disease. Supraspinatus, infraspinatus, and long head of the biceps tendons are torn. Unopposed, the deltoid muscle pulls the humerus up, and with the constant rubbing of the proximal humerus against the acromion the joint gets destroyed. The shoulder becomes prominent from effusion and tissue proliferation. There is only a bit of excruciatingly painful GH motion. Synovial fluid is often hemorrhagic, and basic calcium crystals may be identified intra- and extracellularly with special stains (Alizarin red) and electron microscopy. Shoulder x-rays reveal bone-on-bone contact between the humeral head and the acromion (normally the supraspinatus tendon accounts for a 1 cm separation) and gross destructive and proliferative changes in the humeral head and glenoid fossa.

Treatment

Methods

The senile shoulder may present as tendinitis, as a painful and restricted shoulder, with sudden weakness following tendon rupture, or the Milwaukee shoulder. An early diagnosis is essential to maintain function. Inadequate diagnosis and suboptimal treatment lead to the poor results that often characterize outcome in the older age group. Even in the best of scenarios, once the condition is accurately diagnosed treatment may be cut short by untoward effects of medications that are so frequent (and often atypical) in this group. Physical therapy should be aimed at the shoulder and also to the general conditioning of the patient. Corticosteroid infiltrations and I.M. ACTH appear to be least problematic in older patients. On the other hand, NSAIDs tend to be poorly tolerated by old people and the risk of mental changes and liver toxicity is significant.

Irreparable tears and even the Milwaukee shoulder may be amenable to surgical treatment. Arthroscopic debridement may partially relieve pain. In the Milwaukee shoulder a hemiarthroplasty procedure may be used. This involves a large humeral head implant that articulates with the glenoid and the acromion. Success in this operation depends on the integrity of the anterior and posterior stabilizers of the shoulder, the subscapularis and the teres minor, respectively.

Suggested Reading

Chard MD, Hazleman R, Hazleman BL, et al. Shoulder disorders in the elderly: A community survey. Arthritis Rheum 34:766–769, 1991.

Kumagai J, Sarkar K, Uhthoff HK. The collagen types in the attachment zone of rotator cuff tendons in the elderly: An immunohistological study. J Rheumatol 21:2096–2100, 1994.

Sher JS, Uribe JW, Posada A, et al. Abnormal findings on magnetic resonance images of asymptomatic shoulders. J Bone Joint Surg 77A:10–15, 1995.

Frozen Shoulder

Presentation and Progression

Cause

The frozen shoulder, also known as adhesive capsulitis, is characterized pathologically by fibrosis (fibroblasts, myofibroblasts, dense collagen) and retraction affecting predominantly the anterior and inferior structures of the GH joint capsule, and expressed clinically by a universal restriction of shoulder motion. A pathogenetic relationship with reflex sympathetic dystrophy (RSD) is suggested by the pain pattern in early cases, regional osteopenia seen in late cases, and the occasional association with RSD in the hand.

Frozen shoulder predominates in women and peaks around age 60. The condition may appear spontaneously or follow minor shoulder trauma, cervical radiculopathy, hemiparesis (occurs in, for example, approximately 25% of patients with hemiplegia due to an aneurysmal bleed), lung cancer, myocardial infarction, or upper extremity cardiac catheterization. Diabetes and thyroid disease may feature an atypical frozen shoulder.

Presentation

The usual patient develops, gradually or abruptly, severe, deep, aching, or boring unilateral shoulder pain that is experienced superolaterally or along the biceps muscle. Pain is particularly severe at night. There may be little initial motion loss, but a rapid loss of passive motion can be witnessed in a matter of days. There are less typical presentations. In bilateral cases diabetes and thyroid disease (both hypo- and hyperthyroidism) should be sought. Diabetic frozen shoulder is seen in poorly controlled disease in association with other fibrotic complications including cheiroarthropathy, trigger finger, and carpal tunnel syndrome. Muscle atrophy may be profound in this setting. Indeed, the author has seen patients who underwent unnecessary muscle biopsy to rule out myositis. A simple evaluation of passive motion would have prevented this error. Occasionally frozen shoulder patients develop a distressingly painful hand swelling. Appropriately, these patients are said to suffer the shoulder-hand syndrome.

Diagnosis

Summary of Diagnosis

> **FROZEN SHOULDER**
> - Fibrotic retraction of the anterior and inferior capsular structures, particularly involving the coracohumeral ligament.
> - Diagnosis is clinical.
> - Shoulder x-rays are normal or show patchy osteopenia (abnormal findings on x-rays or an elevated ESR should put a diagnosis of frozen shoulder in question).
> - Diabetes and thyroid should be investigated, particularly in bilateral cases.

Natural History

Expected Outcome and Complications

Untreated, frozen shoulder evolves in three stages: stage I of nocturnal pain and progressive restriction (lasts weeks to a few months); stage II of restriction and pain with motion (lasts months); and stage III of painless resolving restriction (lasts 1 to 3 years). Examination in late stage I and stage II reveals drastic passive motion loss (only 15 or 20 degrees in each direction) and severe endpoint pain. In stage III restriction slowly resolves, motion is painless, and scapulothoracic motion often provides acceptable function. Within 1 to 3 years from disease onset most patients report having a normal shoulder function albeit with a residual motion loss of 10% to 30% of which they may be unaware.

Interestingly, 10% to 20% of patients develop a contralateral frozen shoulder, usually milder than the first, while the originally involved shoulder is "thawing." Diabetic frozen shoulder has a poor prognosis irrespective of treatment; relentless pain and function loss are probably sustained on a neuropathic basis. Prognosis of thyroid disease–related frozen shoulder has changed. From being poor, particularly in Graves' disease, improved treatment methods result in rapid recovery in most patients.

Treatment

Methods

Many purportedly successful treatment methods of frozen shoulder are in use. They include physical modalities, oral or local corticosteroids, joint distension, nerve blockades, manipulation under anesthesia, and arthroscopic or surgical release, alone or in combination. Most have not been subject to valid study. Furthermore, the few controlled trials have been short term (the longest 8 months), and no treatment has been shown superior to the spontaneously regressive course of the disease. However, low-dose oral corticosteroids for 6 weeks and intraarticular plus subacromial corticosteroid infiltrations were useful for pain relief in the early phase of the process. Thus, treatment of frozen shoulder remains for the most part empiric.

The treatment program used by the author is as follows: Patients seen in stages I and II are offered one to three intraarticular corticosteroid injections, depending on the response, given 15 days apart preferably under fluoroscopic control, or an 8 week course of oral corticosteroids beginning at 20 mg of prednisone a day in one morning dose for 1 week, then reduced by 2.5 mg a week until discontinuation. All patients are instructed on Codman's pendular exercises (see appendix) to be performed for 5 minutes at least five times a day, without weight in the initial 1 to 2 weeks, and then with a 5 lb barbell. In some cases, particularly when sleep is badly disturbed, amitriptyline 25 mg hs or cyclobenzaprine 10 mg hs is added. Acetaminophen up to 4 g/day or a NSAID in full dose may be given in brief courses for the control of residual pain. Patients who are already in stage III should be reassured and given Codman's exercises only.

Diabetic frozen shoulder may be treated with intraarticular corticosteroids (diabetes should be watched, but available evidence suggests that the minimal changes occur after a standard dose) plus Codman's exercises. Amitriptyline in higher doses, perhaps 50 or 75 mg hs, may help in pain control.

Patients who are hyper- or hypothyroid should be treated for the underlying condition and given Codman's exercises and analgesics. Additional treatment may not be required.

Expected Response

On the outlined program patients are expected to make a prompt transition to stage III. Painless restriction of GH motion is well tolerated by most patients. Adherence to Codman's exercises needs to be reinforced on each visit. Whether or not the described treatment program hastens recovery or decreases residual limitation is not known. Only a few patients with idiopathic frozen shoulder fail to improve. As mentioned, prognosis in diabetic frozen shoulder is poor and in thyroid disease is excellent. There is some evidence that refractory cases of frozen shoulder, including the condition in diabetics, may improve with arthroscopic release of anterior and inferior capsular structures.

Complications

There are few. Well-administered intraarticular injections carry a negligible risk of infection. Other local complications are theoretical. Patients who received two or more corticosteroid injections and certainly those treated with oral corticosteroids should be covered with stress doses of corticosteroid for major illnesses and surgical procedures for 2 years. Also, oral corticosteroids will transiently enhance any ongoing osteoporotic process.

When to Refer

Most patients with frozen shoulder can be treated by the primary care physician. Because the condition may cause a great deal of concern, however, early rheumatologic consultation for confirmation of diagnosis and reassurance will be welcomed by the patient. Glenohumeral corticosteroid injections are technically difficult. They should be administered by a rheumatologist, an orthopedic surgeon, or a radiologist.

Key Points

> **FROZEN SHOULDER**
> - Painful restriction of the shoulder joint.
> - Unilateral (a bilateral onset suggests diabetes).
> - Shoulder x-rays are normal or show (late) osteopenia.
> - ESR is normal.
> - Clinical stages: stage I with night pain and progressive restriction; stage II with restriction and pain on motion; stage III of painless resolving restriction.
> - Treatment includes corticosteroids (intraarticular or orally), analgesics, and Codman's exercises.
> - Refractory cases should be evaluated for arthroscopic release.

Suggested Reading

Binder A, Hazleman BL, Parr G, et al. A controlled study of oral prednisolone in frozen shoulder. Brit J Rheumatol 25:288–292, 1986.

Bulgen DY, Binder AI, Hazleman BL, et al. Frozen shoulder: Prospective clinical study with an evaluation of three treatment regimens. Ann Rheum Dis 43:353–360, 1984.

Bunker TD, Anthony PP. The pathology of frozen shoulder. J Bone Joint Surg 77B:677–683, 1995.

Ogilvie-Harris DJ, Biggs DJ, Fitsialos DP, et al. The resistant frozen shoulder. Manipulation versus arthroscopic release. Clin Orthop 319:238–248, 1995.

Shaffer B, Tibone JE, Kerlan RK. Frozen shoulder. A long-term follow-up. J Bone Joint Surg 74A:738–746, 1992.

Suprascapular Nerve Entrapment

Presentation and Progression

Cause

After passing the suprascapular notch, the suprascapular nerve (C5,6) supplies the supraspinatus muscle, the GH joint, the AC joint, and the coracoacromial ligament. It then passes around the lateral scapular spine at the spinoglenoid notch to innervate the infraspinatus muscle. Compression may occur at the suprascapular notch causing weakness of the spinati, or at the spinoglenoid notch affecting the infraspinatus only. Suprascapular nerve entrapment is usually caused by direct trauma or by abuse of sports such as volleyball and baseball that require wide excursions of the scapula. Other cases have been caused by ganglia.

Presentation

Patients present with dull posterior or superolateral shoulder pain. Weakness of abduction and external rotation and tenderness to direct compression of the suprascapular notch are the main findings on examination. Muscle atrophy appears late. To find the suprascapular notch, the scapular spine is bisected and a vertical line is drawn at the midpoint. The notch is located 2 to 3 cm lateral to this intersection, deep in the tissues.

Diagnosis

Summary of Diagnosis

> **SUPRASCAPULAR NERVE ENTRAPMENT**
> - History of direct trauma or heavy sports.
> - Pain in the posterior or lateral shoulder.
> - Weakness of abduction and external rotation.
> - Absence of relief with subacromial xylocaine infiltration.
> - Positive electrodiagnosis: delayed conduction, fibrillation potentials.
> - MRI should be performed to rule out a compressive lesion.

Natural History

Expected Outcome

The condition may regress spontaneously if a reversible factor was involved in causation or may progress causing irreversible atrophy of the supra- and infraspinatus muscles. Unfortunately, cases are often misdiagnosed as subacromial impingement with tendon rupture.

Treatment

Methods

A 1 to 2 month course of physical therapy and observation is indicated in cases in which no compressive lesion is shown on MRI. Patients who fail to improve should have surgical release at the suprascapular notch or at the spinoglenoid notch.

Expected Response

The expected response to surgical release is dramatic pain improvement. Muscle weakness and atrophy recover slowly. About 15% of patients fail to improve.

When to Refer

Patients suspected of having suprascapular nerve entrapment should be evaluated neurologically and referred to an orthopedist who will make a decision regarding surgical release.

Key Points

> **SUPRASCAPULAR NERVE ENTRAPMENT**
> - The entrapment may be at the suprascapular notch or at the spinoglenoid notch.
> - Physical findings resemble those of subacromial impingement with rotator cuff tear.
> - Diagnosis is by exclusion.
> - Delayed conduction and fibrillation potentials in the supra- and infraspinatus muscles are diagnostic.
> - Some cases improve spontaneously.
> - Surgical release is highly effective in pain relief. Muscle recovery may be delayed and incomplete.

Suggested Reading

Vastamäki M, Goranssön H. Suprascapular nerve entrapment. Clin Orthop 297:135–143, 1993.

Acromioclavicular Pain

Presentation and Progression

Cause

Acromioclavicular (AC) pain may be caused by osteoarthritis, osteolysis of the distal end of the clavicle, pseudogout, septic arthritis, the spondyloarthropathies, RA, and juxtaarticular myxomas growing adjacent to the joint. Usual symptoms and signs include pain on top of the shoulder triggered by full arm elevation (terminal portion of the arc of elevation) or adduction, plus swelling noted by palpation at the joint. AC involvement should be actively searched for in any patient complaining of shoulder pain. The author has seen too many patients in whom AC involvement was missed, the pain being attributed to the more frequently involved glenohumeral joint or rotator cuff. Only by purposeful palpation can the process be correctly identified. Osteolysis of the distal end of the clavicle occurs predominantly in weight lifters but may also occur in nonathletic carrying efforts, such as heavy use of a wheelbarrow. Pain has a boring quality and predominates at night.

Diagnosis

Summary of Diagnosis

> **ACROMIOCLAVICULAR PAIN**
> - Suspect by location of pain on top of shoulder.
> - Pain in terminal arc of elevation and with full shoulder adduction.
> - Pain on direct compression of the joint.
> - Acromial view is best to visualize the joint and distal end of clavicle.
> - Aspiration may provide an essential sample for diagnosis (pseudogout, septic arthritis).

Natural History

Expected Outcome

Outcome depends on etiology. AC osteoarthritis produces annoying pain with elevation or adduction motions and has the potential, through inferior spurs, to damage the rotator cuff. Osteolysis of the distal end of the clavicle evolves in three phases: first, pain while bench pressing, then severe pain with night predominance concurrent with joint swelling, followed by remission or progression to AC joint DJD. In pseudogout, acute bouts of pain reflect crystal-induced inflammation. Once the flare quiets down, because CPPD deposition either occurs in damaged joints, or leads to DJD, there is a background of mechanical pain. Septic arthritis of the AC joint may be quite acute, as in cases that complicate indwelling subclavian catheters, but more commonly is subdued and follows a subacute course. Diagnosis may be suspected from subchondral erosions noted on x-rays. Aspiration allows documentation of diagnosis. In the spondyloarthropathies and RA, AC arthritis may follow a protracted course exceeding the duration of peripheral joint flares. Juxtaarticular myxomas, as in the knee, are known to occur in relation with the AC joint meniscus.

Treatment

Methods

In osteoarthritis flares, spondyloarthropathy, and RA, the treatment of choice is an intraarticular corticosteroid injection. The procedure, described in the appendix, is not too difficult. The injection is from the top. Distension of the joint may be noted by placing index and thumb of the nondominant hand at the extremes of the joint. In severe degenerative cases, and also in late cases of osteolysis of the distal end of the clavicle, resection of the distal 1 cm of the clavicle is usually curative. Septic arthritis, because aspirations have little yield and progression to osteomyelitis is frequent as in other tight joints, surgical drainage and debridement is essential.

Expected Response

Outcome is excellent in virtually all forms of AC joint arthritis. One of the reasons for this success is that resection of the distal clavicle is always the choice in late arthritis, regardless of etiology, and the outcome of this procedure is good.

When to Refer

AC joint injections may be given by the primary care physician. Because surgical resection of the distal end of the clavicle is a simple operation with excellent results, orthopedic referral should not be delayed in patients with destructive AC arthritis and severe symptoms.

Key Points

> **ACROMIOCLAVICULAR PAIN**
> - There are multiple causes of AC joint arthritis.
> - AC osteoarthritis can, through inferior spurs, cause subacromial impingement with damage to the rotator cuff.
> - Osteolysis of the distal clavicle affects predominantly weight lifters and can cause secondary AC joint osteoarthritis.
> - Resection of the distal end of the clavicle is successful in most forms of severely damaged AC joint.

Suggested Reading

Cahill BR. Osteolysis of the distal part of the clavicle in male athletes. J Bone Joint Surg 64A:1053–1058, 1982.

Novak PJ, Bach BR Jr, Romeo AA, et al. Surgical resection of the distal clavicle. J Shoulder Elbow Surg 4:35–40, 1995.

Sternoclavicular Pain

Presentation and Progression

Cause

Sternoclavicular pain may result from septic arthritis, spondyloarthropathy, RA, and an obscure osteitis with predilection for the clavicle and other bones in the anterior chest wall seen in association with severe acne and, occasionally, palmoplantar pustulosis. This syndome is known by the acronym SAPHO (S, synovitis; A, acne; P, pustulosis; H, hyperostosis; and O, osteomyelitis). The acne component of SAPHO includes the related skin conditions acne conglobata, acne fulminans, and hidradenitis suppurativa.

Presentation

Patients complain of pain on shoulder motions that imply clavicle motion. Pain may be local or experienced in the supraclavicular fossa and even in the supraspinatus fossa. There is local tenderness. Swelling and redness suggest septic arthritis. Septic arthritis of the sternoclavicular joint, which appears to be more common in intravenous substance abuse and immunosuppressed individuals, is complicated by abscesses in 20% of cases. There is a tendency for these abscesses to grow posteriorly and extend caudally in the anterior mediastinum. In an immunosuppressed patient, there may be minimal superficial inflammation in the face of an extensive mediastinal abscess.

Diagnosis

Summary of Diagnosis

> **STERNOCLAVICULAR PAIN**
> - Local pain.
> - Local tenderness.
> - X-rays (limited yield).
> - CT scan: very useful in the diagnosis of septic arthritis and its complications, abscesses, and osteomyelitis.
> - Aspiration.

Natural History

Expected Outcome

Sternoclavicular arthritis as a complication of spondyloarthropathy or RA usually responds to the systemic treatment of the underlying condition. Intraarticular corticosteroid injections are rapidly effective in relieving symptoms. Medical treatment is usually insufficient in septic sternoclavicular arthritis due to technical difficulties in aspiration and the early presence of osteomyelitis and abscess formation. Surgical treatment is almost always required.

Complications

Complications of septic arthritis include sepsis, osteomyelitis involving the clavicle and sternum, and abscess formation with progression in the anterior mediastinum.

Treatment

Methods

Corticosteroid infiltrations of the sternoclavicular joint, described in the appendix, are technically difficult. Surgical drainage, debridement of osteomyelitic bone, and drainage of abscesses is the treatment of choice in septic arthritis of the sternoclavicular joint.

Expected Response

In the spondyloarthropathies and RA improvement of the sternoclavicular joint may lag behind systemic improvement. These cases may be injected, and improvement is usually rapid, within 1 to 2 days. Improvement of patients operated on for septic arthritis is slow, but this may be due to the precarious general condition of these patients.

Complications

The author has not seen complications of sternoclavicular joint infiltrations or surgical drainage of septic arthritis.

When to Refer

Infiltrations of the sternoclavicular joints are not within the scope of primary care physicians; patients should be referred to a rheumatologist or an orthopedic surgeon. Surgical drainage of septic arthritis often requires the combined efforts of a chest surgeon and an orthopedic surgeon.

Key Points

> **STERNOCLAVICULAR PAIN**
> - Sternoclavicular infiltrations are technically difficult.
> - Sternoclavicular pain in a debilitated individual may be the sole indication of septic arthritis.
> - Septic sternoclavicular arthritis is often complicated by clavicle and sternum osteomyelitis and by abscess formation.
> - CT should be obtained early in patients with suspected sternoclavicular septic arthritis.

Suggested Reading

Kahn MF. Why the SAPHO syndrome? J Rheumatol 22:2017–2019, 1995.
Kahn MF, Chamot AM. SAPHO syndrome. Rheum Dis Clin North Am 18:225–246, 1992.
Olafsson S, Asim Khan M. Musculoskeletal features of acne, hidradenitis suppurativa, and dissecting cellulitis of the scalp. Clin Rheum Dis 18:215–224, 1992.
Wohlgethan JR, Newberg AH, Reed JI. The risk of abscess from sternoclavicular septic arthritis. J Rheum 15:1302–1306, 1988.
Yood RA, Goldenberg DL. Sternoclavicular joint arthritis. Arthritis Rheum 23:232–239, 1980.

Thoracic Outlet Syndrome

The concept of thoracic outlet syndrome is surrounded by an aura of mystery, and rightfully so. Many misdiagnoses of thoracic outlet syndrome have been made in the past in patients who eventually had, for instance, scleroderma. Also, myriad proposed mechanisms of impingement on the neurovascular structures at the root of the upper extremity, plus the diversity of vascular compression–based diagnostic tests, have removed thoracic outlet syndrome from the domain of the uninitiated. Recently, however, new concepts on thoracic outlet syndrome based on pathophysiology rather than dry anatomy have evolved with important implications for diagnosis and therapy.

Presentation and Progression

Cause

Thoracic outlet syndrome occurs far more frequently in females than in males and is a condition of the younger age group. A relative weakness of the muscles that elevate the shoulder and upper arm is often present, and as the shoulder droops the brachial plexus becomes stretched. In addition, because of the sloped clavicle, the costoclavicular space narrows and the axillary artery and vein may become compressed. The actual cause of thoracic outlet syndrome remains elusive in most instances.

There are patients, however, in whom an identifiable neurologic lesion such as brachial plexus palsy or trapezius paralysis is clearly responsible for the syndrome. Very large breasts may drag the clavicle down and result in symptoms. Osseous compression is rare but may result from a cervical rib or a hooked C7 transverse process. On the other hand, presence of a cervical rib is not proof that symptoms are caused by that rib. Variations in the attachment of the scalene muscles on the first rib and congenital fibrous bands are additional, if rare, causes of the syndrome. Glenohumeral joint instability, supraclavicular fossa tumors, and apical lung tumors should be excluded in all patients. Another condition to be excluded is reflex sympathetic dystrophy (RSD) with the caveat that a thoracic outlet syndrome may indeed cause RSD. Symptoms are predominantly neurologic. Patients may present proximal pain involving the trapezius, interscapular region, posterior neck, head, and even chest or may have paresthesia, pain, coldness, cyanosis, weakness, or muscle atrophy in the upper extremity. Involvement of the upper brachial plexus will result in symptoms and signs in the outer upper arm or forearm; lower brachial plexus compromise will affect the ulnar aspect of forearm or hand. Upper and lower findings often coexist. Thoracic outlet symptoms vary with the position of the limb and with the task the patient performs. Nocturnal pain and paresthesias are common.

On examination patients with a thoracic outlet syndrome often have a drooped shoulder on the involved side. A tight brachial plexus may be palpable in the supraclavicular fossa between the anterior and middle scalene muscles, and direct compression or percussion on the plexus causes radiating pain and paresthesia to the upper extremity. Downward shoulder traction in line with the plexus reproduces or increases the symptoms; symptoms cease with upward pulling on the arm. The Adson's and other maneuvers to detect vascular compression should be performed as well (Table 25–3), realizing that pulse extinction has value only when consistent symptoms led to the performance of the test. Sustained (60 second) arm elevation often reproduces the symptoms, and in a significant proportion of patients tests for cubital tunnel syndrome or carpal tunnel syndrome will be positive as well.

Diagnosis

Summary of Diagnosis

Natural History

Thoracic outlet syndrome is a chronic painful condition that untreated results in a high rate of incapacitation. Muscle atrophy occasionally develops as a late complication of the condition.

TABLE 25–3

PROVOCATIVE MANEUVERS TO USE IN PATIENTS WITH SUSPECTED THORACIC OUTLET SYNDROME*

1. Downward traction of the arm for 1 minute.
2. Adson's maneuver: Ask the patient to turn the head to one side, hyperextend the neck, and inhale deeply while checking pulse on that side.
3. Wright's maneuver: Ask the patient to elevate and externally rotate the arm and hold a deep breath. If test is positive with ulnar symptoms, repeat with elbow fully extended to rule out ulnar tunnel syndrome.
4. Shoulder brace position (military brace position).
5. Ask patient to elevate the arms and repeatedly open and close the hands. Maneuver is positive if fatigue and cramps occur within 30 seconds.

*Always do both limbs. Symptoms must be reproduced (a decreased pulse only has no diagnostic value).

THORACIC OUTLET SYNDROME

- Atypical shoulder pain.
- Neurologic or, less frequently, vascular symptoms in the upper extremity.
- A drooped shoulder.
- A positive downward traction maneuver.
- Relief with upward pulling of the arm.
- Examine the supraclavicular fossa for pathology.
- Consider reflex sympathetic dystrophy.
- A positive Adson's or other maneuver for arterial compression (low specificity).
- Obtain cervical spine films (cervical rib and foraminal pathology) and chest x-rays for apical tumors.
- Neurophysiologic tests are almost always normal but are important to detect mimicking or associated conditions (such as a carpal tunnel syndrome).
- A thoracic outlet CT should be obtained preoperatively in cases that are refractory to conservative therapy.

Treatment

Methods

Initial treatment of thoracic outlet syndrome should be conservative and aimed at postural reeducation and periscapular muscle strengthening unless there is motor loss or a significant vascular compromise. Offending positions of the limb and head (head forward position) should be avoided, and an exercise program aimed at correcting posture and stretching shoulder girdle muscles should be prescribed and supervised by an expert physical therapist (see Britt and Novak). Overhead exercises and exercises that involve shoulder bracing are to be avoided. With strict adherence to these measures, partial or complete success is achieved in most patients. Unimproved symptoms after 6 to 8 weeks call for additional therapy. In the past, these patients were referred to surgery. There is now evidence that a strapping device may significantly elevate the shoulder and relieve symptoms in a majority of patients (Nakatsuchi et al.). If this fails to correct symptoms, surgical decompression should be considered. Prior to surgery the anatomy of the region must be carefully determined by CT, and the possible overlapping lesions such as cervical radiculopathy, brachial neuritis, carpal tunnel syndrome, and ulnar neuropathy (particularly the cubital syndrome) should be excluded clinically and by electrodiagnosis. Surgical procedures include resection of the first rib through Roos's approach and scalenectomy; sometimes the two procedures are used in combination. Surgery should be performed by an experienced surgeon. Results are satisfactory provided an accurate diagnosis.

When to Refer

Thoracic outlet syndrome patients may be handled initially by primary care physicians. Instruction on posture and an appropriate exercise program is best achieved with a physical therapy referral. If diagnostic doubts arise, or if patients fail to improve with postural advice and exercises, referral should be made to a physiatrist, neurologist, orthopedic surgeon, or rheumatologist depending on who in the clinician's setting is more familiar with the condition.

Key Points

THORACIC OUTLET SYNDROME

- The condition should be suspected in patients with upper extremity neurologic symptoms or with atypical shoulder, upper back, or neck pain.
- Diagnosis is clinical and is based on symptom reproduction by maneuvers that stretch the brachial plexus.
- A drooped shoulder position accounts for most cases of thoracic outlet syndrome. A head forward position is likely to add to the symptoms. In the remaining cases neuropathic weakness or an anatomic variant (cervical rib, hooked transverse process, fibrous bands) is involved.
- Concurrent compressive neuropathy, most prominently carpal tunnel syndrome, must be excluded.
- Initial treatment includes postural advice and exercises. Improvement with an optimal program approaches 90%. A failure to improve is an indication for supporting bracing. Surgery should be used as a last-resort treatment except in patients with motor loss or ischemia; these patients should be promptly decompressed.

Suggested Reading

Britt LP. Nonoperative treatment of the thoracic outlet syndrome. Clin Orthop 51:45–48, 1967.
Leffert RD. Thoracic outlet syndrome. J Am Acad Orthop Surg 2:317–325, 1994.
Nakatsuchi Y, Saitoh S, Hosaka M, Matsuda S. Conservative treatment of thoracic outlet syndrome using an orthosis. J Hand Surg 20B:34–39, 1995.
Novak CB, Collins ED, Mackinnon SE. Outcome following conservative management of thoracic outlet syndrome. J Hand Surg 20A:542–548, 1995.
Novak CB, Mackinnon SE, Patterson GA. Evaluation of patients with thoracic outlet syndrome. J Hand Surg 18A:292–299, 1993.
Swift TR, Nichols FT. The droopy shoulder syndrome. Neurology 34:212–215, 1984.

Lipomatoses: Shoulder Girdle Lipomatosis, Multiple Symmetric Lipomatosis, and Dercum's Disease

Presentation and Progression

Cause

These are rare conditions. Shoulder girdle lipomatosis is characterized by (so far) left-sided lipomatosis involving the supraclavicular and suprascapular fossae, the deltoid region, and the upper back (dorsal hump) in association with weakness of thoracic girdle muscles from fat infiltration and motor and sensory neuropathy distally in the limb. Symptoms are chronic and clinically resemble thoracic outlet syndrome.

In multiple symmetric lipomatosis, mediastinal lipomatosis and neuropathy often coexist.

Dercum's disease, or "adiposis dolorosa," is a condition of women characterized by the formation of paraarticular lipomatous masses. They are not typical lipomas in that biopsies often reveal giant cell granulomas. The condition should be distinguished from fibromyalgia coexistent with obesity.

Diagnosis

Summary of Diagnosis

LIPOMATOSES

- Fat accumulation in shoulder girdle, regional muscle atrophy, ipsilateral upper extremity neuropathy: shoulder girdle lipomatosis.
- Symmetric lipomatosis, mediastinal fat accumulation, neuropathy: multiple symmetric lipomatosis.
- Tender, discrete lipomas in a paraarticular location: Dercum's disease.

- Electrodiagnosis to diagnose level of neuropathy.
- Thoracic CT in multiple symmetric lipomatosis to detect mediastinal location.

Natural History

Shoulder girdle lipomatosis and multiple symmetric lipomatosis are irreversible. Surgical removal of lipomas offers only temporary help. Dercum's disease causes chronic pain.

Treatment

There is no treatment for shoulder girdle lipomatosis or symmetric lipomatosis. Isolated cases of Dercum's disease have been treated with liposuction with improvement in pain.

When to Refer

Patients with Dercum's disease should be evaluated by a plastic surgeon.

Key Points

LIPOMATOSES

- Both shoulder girdle lipomatosis and symmetric lipomatosis associate with motor and sensory neuropathy.
- Symmetric lipomatosis associates with mediastinal lipomatosis.
- There is no treatment for these conditions.
- Dercum's disease or paraarticular lipomatosis is a cause of chronic pain. It may be difficult to differentiate from fibromyalgia occurring in an obese patient.
- Patients with Dercum's disease should be offered plastic surgery consultation.

Suggested Reading

Dercum FX. Three cases of a hitherto unclassified affliction resembling in its grosser aspects obesity, but associated with special nervous symptoms—adiposis dolorosa. Am J Med Sci 104:521–535, 1892.

Enzi G, Angelini C, Negrin P, et al. Sensory, motor, and autonomic neuropathy in patients with multiple symmetric lipomatosis. Medicine (Baltimore) 64:388–393, 1986.

Anterior Chest Wall Pain: Tietze's Syndrome, Costochondritis, Slipping-Rib Syndrome, Xiphodynia

Presentation and Progression

These conditions, seemingly diverse, have clinical and pathogenic similarities that allow a common discussion. Tietze's syndrome, as described by Alexander Tietze in 1921, is a subacute or chronic painful swelling of the chondrocostal or chondrosternal junction, or the sternoclavicular joint (SCJ). Many conditions may result in this syndrome. A better, more encompassing designation is anterior chest wall pain. Given a patient with anterior chest wall pain, the next step is to identify the structure involved. Determine its location in reference to the sternum (top, side, distal end, manubriosternal junction, the sternum itself) or the costal margin.

1. Pain, tenderness, and swelling just off center at the sternal top indicates SCJ arthritis, osteomyelitis, or osteitis such as seen in the SAPHO. The osteitis component of this syndrome is known in the orthopedic literature as chronic multifocal osteomyelitis.
2. (a) Pain, tenderness, and swelling at the sternal side may indicate chondritis (usually spondyloarthropathy); osteitis (may indicate SAPHO) syndrome; fracture; malignancy; or an abnormally shaped costal cartilage in a patient that really belongs to the category that follows. (b) Pain and tenderness at the sternal side occurs in cardiac ischemia; accessory respiratory muscle overexertion such as in severe cough, asthma, or hyperventilation; fibromyalgia; and occasionally adjacent tumor. Serious mistakes have been made by dismissing chest pain patients just because chest wall tenderness was found. A good history is far more accurate in this setting than the physical examination. Patients with fibromyalgia have symmetric tenderness of which they may be totally unaware, tenderness elsewhere at fibromyalgic points, and a history of chronic pain.
3. Pain and tenderness at the junction between the sternum and the xiphoid best elicited by depressing the xiphoid indicate xiphodynia, an obscure entity that may cause chronic epigastric pain.
4. Pain and swelling at the manubriosternal joint, a fibrocartilaginous joint similar to the pubic symphysis and the joints between the bodies of the vertebrae, occurs almost exclusively in the spondyloarthropathies and in SAPHO syndrome.
5. Pain at the sternum itself may be prominent in acute leukemia and the blastic phase of chronic leukemias, multiple myeloma, and amyloid deposits within the bone in the monoclonal plasma cell dyscrasias.
6. The slipping-rib syndrome is characterized by chronic upper abdominal pain and exquisite tenderness at a specific site in the costal margin. Pain, which may associate with a click, is often caused by movement and certain postures. Relief by local anesthetic infiltration provides further diagnostic assurance.

Diagnosis

Summary of Diagnosis

ANTERIOR CHEST WALL PAIN

- Rule out cardiac ischemia by history and ancillary studies if required.
- Rule out fibromyalgia by history and examination of tender points.
- Consider malignancy, which gives focal or diffuse sternal tenderness.
- Consider spondyloarthropathy.
- Consider SAPHO.
- Consider pectoralis major insertion strain.
- Consider xiphodynia in patients with epigastric pain and tenderness at the xiphoid.

- Consider the slipping-rib syndrome in patients with upper quadrant pain and localized tenderness at the costal margin.
- ESR elevated in spondyloarthropathy, SAPHO, septic arthritis, osteomyelitis, and malignancy.
- X-ray findings in spondyloarthropathy and SAPHO.
- Bone scan useful to locate osteomalacia-related and other fractures and also to locate neoplasic deposits, osteomyelitis, and osteitis.
- CT and MRI best to identify SCJ septic arthritis and sternal, clavicular, or costal osteomyelitis/osteitis.

Natural History

Outcome in anterior chest wall pain syndrome depends on the condition. Most idiopathic cases are self-limited, although it may take months or years for the condition to go away. Fibromyalgic tenderness is chronic, although symptoms have wide variations. Pectoralis muscle strain and cardiac ischemia–related tenderness subside in days to weeks. Chondritis in the spondyloarthropathies and osteitis in SAPHO syndrome cause protracted pain that improves on NSAIDs. Some cases of anterior chest wall pain defy diagnosis and are refractory to therapy.

Treatment

Methods

Mild cases such as in muscle strain are helped by warm packs and acetaminophen. Capsaicin is a plausible alternative. NSAIDs and other agents such as sulfasalazine or methotrexate (if required for the overall condition) help chondritic and SCJ pain in the spondyloarthropathies. Local anesthetic and corticosteroid infiltrations may provide lasting relief and should be tried in protracted nonfibromyalgic chondrocostal pain, xiphodynia, and the slipping-rib syndrome.

Expected Response

Response to treatment is slow, and some cases are refractory to therapy.

When to Refer

Cases of Tietze's syndrome with a normal ESR and no evidence of sacroiliitis or osteitis should be treated by primary care physicians.

Key Points

ANTERIOR CHEST WALL PAIN

- Conditions to keep in mind include cardiac ischemia, excessive respiratory effort, fibromyalgia, spondyloarthropathy, SAPHO syndrome, osteomyelitis, and an underlying chest malignancy.
- Diagnosis requires detailed palpation of the anterior chest wall particularly the SCJs, the manubriosternal joint (a ridge at the level of the second costal cartilages), the costo-chondro-sternal joints, the xiphoid, and the costal margin.
- Most cases are without swelling and are caused by increased accessory respiratory muscle work or fibromyalgia.
- Cases with swelling are either inflammatory (spondyloarthropathy, SAPHO) or due to misshapen costal cartilage.
- An increased ESR speaks of an inflammatory lesion such as chondritis or osteitis, microbial SCJ arthritis, or osteomyelitis.
- Presence of sacroiliitis suggests spondyloarthropathy, SAPHO, and rarely brucellosis.

Suggested Reading

Aeschlimann A, Kahn MF. Tietze's syndrome: A critical review. Clin Exp Rheumatol 8:407–412, 1990.

Carr AJ, Cole WG, Roberton DM, et al. Chronic multifocal osteomyelitis. J Bone Joint Surg 75B:582–591, 1993.

Maugars Y, Berthelot J-M, Ducloux J-M, et al. SAPHO syndrome: A follow-up study of 19 cases with special emphasis on enthesis involvement. J Rheumatol 22:2135–2141, 1995.

Wright JT. Slipping-rib syndrome. Lancet 2:632–634, 1980.

CHAPTER 26

Neck, Dorsal, and Low Back Pain

Neck pain and low back pain are leading reasons why people consult a physician. Low back pain, in addition, is a major cause of work absenteeism and permanent disability. Dorsal pain is infrequent except in older women. Dorsal, cervical, and lumbar pain have a different pathophysiology. The dorsal spine, being more rigid, is more liable to osteoporotic compressive fractures than the cervical and lumbar segments. The cervical spine is the most mobile, followed by the lumbar spine, which by virtue of an almost sagittal orientation of the facet (zygapophyseal) joints has limited lateral motions. Ligamentous and muscle constraints check cervical and lumbar movements and help in shock absorption.

The mechanical advantage of these segments, however, is the very reason for their tendency to wear out, otherwise known as spondylosis. This is particularly true in the lowermost cervical and lumbar segments, C4 to T1 and L3 to S1, respectively. In addition, wearing of the facet joints may lead to forward displacement of the spine above the damaged disc. This process, known as degenerative spondylolisthesis, does not lead to the major displacements seen in spondylolysis-related spondylolisthesis. The clinical spectrum of spondylosis includes, in the cervical spine, asymptomatic limitation, a painful and limited neck, cervical radiculopathy, and cervical myelopathy. In addition, impairment of blood flow may lead to secondary ischemia and vascular myelopathy. In the lumbar spine the clinical spectrum includes asymptomatic limitation, a painful and limited lower back (with or without degenerative spondylolisthesis), and central and lateral lumbar stenosis.

Nucleus pulposus herniation is another major cause of spinal dysfunction. It has long been known that acute loadings on the spine have the potential to burst intervertebral discs. On a normal spine bursts occur through the cartilage plate and bony end plate resulting in nucleus pulposus herniation into the vertebral body (Schmorl nodes). If the annulus fibrosus is damaged, however, the same load, especially if coupled with flexion, squirts some of the nucleus pulposus material out posterolaterally (the medial portion of the canal is protected by the posterior longitudinal segment), impinging on the root. These patients exhibit acute cervical radiculopathy or sciatica due to "disc herniation."

As an individual ages, spondylotic changes are inevitable. On the other hand, not every late middle-aged or older person has neck or lumbar pain. Radiographically advanced spondylosis may be clinically silent, and disabling pain may occur in an individual with nearly normal x-rays. If an MRI is requested and multilevel disc bulging is shown, has the pain been explained? Since any healthy middle-aged person stands a 50% chance of having disc bulgings, plus disc protrusion, disruption of the annulus fibrosus, and facet joint osteoarthritis, the answer is probably not.

What, then, should the clinician do? The same as with any other problem: Obtain a detailed history, examine the patient, generate a hypothesis, and only then, if necessary, request radiologic or other studies. If this path is followed the great majority of patients (those with acute low back pain) will not require additional studies. A small group of patients will remain, however, perhaps 5% to 10% depending on the clinical setting, in whom malignancy, spondylolisthesis, spinal stenosis, spondyloarthropathy, or other pathologic processes will be suspected. In these patients, x-rays and other imaging procedures will not only be indicated, but also cost effective. Similar considerations apply to neck pain.

Neck pain only follows in frequence lumbosacral pain. Its staggering prevalence in the adult and elderly population reflects multiple factors, in particular cervical spondylosis. Pain may originate locally in bone, joints, ligaments, muscles, vessels, and intra- and extraspinal neural structures, or in a distant structure in the head or trunk. Only frequent conditions are discussed in this chapter. For an in-depth discussion of neck pain, refer to Bland's recent comprehensive source.

Acute Nonspecific Neck Pain

Presentation and Progression

Cause

Acute nonspecific neck pain, the most common type of neck pain, predominates in, but is not confined to, young women. Repetitive overuse or a sustained awkward posture at work, unprepared-for movements, mounting stress at home or at the workplace, and impending examinations or marriage are examples of factors involved in causation.

Presentation

Pain is experienced in the posterior or lateral neck. There is often pain radiation to the periscapular region or upper arm, and secondary muscle contracture is common. Frequently involved muscles include the upper trapezius and the suboccipital. The scalenes, the rhomboid, and the levator scapulae are occasionally involved. Onset of symptoms is usually abrupt but may be gradual. In some patients, particularly those with the occupational repetitive stress syndrome, vague distal pain may occur first, followed by neck pain that gradually takes over. Physical examination reveals localized muscle tenderness. An area of muscle contracture may be felt. Trigger points (tender points that upon pressure produce pain in the entire symptomatic area) may be found within the affected muscle. Range of neck motion is typically normal, although motion away from the contracted muscle may result in pain and restriction.

There are several subsets of muscular neck pain. In the *repetitive stress syndrome,* pain is unilateral and tends to involve the lateral neck, the periscapular region, and the proximal upper extremity. If a trigger point is present and compression results in pain in the entire symptomatic area, a diagnosis of *myofascial pain* can be made. In the author's opinion this condition has been overemphasized; further examination of the patient often discloses fibromyalgia. Indeed, overlaps between the repetitive stress syndrome, temporomandibular joint (TMJ) pain, and fibromyalgia are frequent enough to suggest these entities are interrelated.

Muscular pain may also occur as an *add-on to structural conditions* such as cervical spondylosis, disseminated idiopathic skeletal hyperostosis (DISH), rheumatoid arthritis, and ankylosing spondylitis. Limitation of passive neck motion indicates an underlying structural condition. It is important, in assessing patients with cervical muscle contracture pain, not to overlook *fibromyalgia*. In fibromyalgia similar point tenderness is found contralaterally as well as elsewhere in symmetric points.

Diagnosis

Summary of Diagnosis

ACUTE NONSPECIFIC NECK PAIN

- Recurrent lateralized neck pain based on soft tissue factors in patients with normal cervical spine.
- Causative factors include protracted and repetitive physical and psychologic stress.
- If a trigger point is found, myofascial pain may be diagnosed.
- Comorbid structural conditions of the cervical spine are frequent, particularly in the older age group.

Natural History

Generally the condition is self-limited. This is particularly true in patients with short duration of symptoms, that is, 1 to 2 weeks. Symptoms from repetitive stress syndrome and myofascial pain tend to be protracted. Muscular neck pain superimposed on a structural condition of the cervical spine is notoriously recurrent.

Treatment

Methods

Treatment of acute nonspecific neck pain is empiric. Patients may be treated with heat application and gentle stretching of a contractured muscle. A simple technique involves the use of a warm shower. In the shower, the patient aims the water jet on the painful area. After 2 to 3 minutes the head is gently dropped to the opposite side. The analgesic and distracting effect of the water jet allows painless stretching of the contractured muscle. A similar effect may be obtained with warm packs or a heating pad prior to, and during, muscle stretching. The heat-stretch maneuver should be repeated twice daily during the painful period. Full-dose NSAIDs, in severe cases with the addition of acetaminophen, are a helpful adjunct. A soft neck collar may be used during the day as a reminder to avoid offending motions. Massage and local infiltrations with xylocaine may afford additional relief, in particular when a trigger point is present. Patients with myofascial pain and evidences of TMJ dysfunction are said to benefit from the use of a nocturnal palatal brace. Cyclobenzaprine 10 to 20 mg 2 hours before bedtime may be used to induce sleep and favor muscle relaxation. Whether or not these measures shorten the spell is not known. They do provide predictable pain relief while the condition resolves. In patients confronting protracted and unavoidable stress, amitriptyline 25 or 50 mg hs may decrease pain and lessen recurrences.

Expected Response

Improvement in acute nonspecific neck pain is slow, and some residual soreness may linger for 1 to 2 weeks.

When to Refer

Treatment of acute nonspecific neck pain is by the primary care physician. Symptoms that persist or reoccur over several weeks in a specific area, particularly if additional symptoms are present such as a burning quality or paresthesias, indicate neurology referral.

Key Points

ACUTE NONSPECIFIC NECK PAIN

- Predominates in young women under stress.
- Muscle contracture appears to be involved in most cases.
- In the repetitive stress syndrome there is vague distal pain and subsequent involvement of the periscapular region and lateral neck.
- A trigger point may be found. It is imperative in these patients to rule out fibromyalgia. If this is not present, a myofascial syndrome may be diagnosed.
- Treatment includes analgesics, heat application, and stretching of the involved muscle(s).
- Recurrences are common, usually triggered by stress.

Suggested Reading

Sheon RP. Soft tissue cervical spine syndromes. In: Bland JH (ed) Disorders of the Cervical Spine, 2nd ed. W.B. Saunders, Philadelphia, 365–372, 1994.

Whiplash Injury

Presentation and Progression

Cause

Whiplash injuries are caused by an indirect force, usually a low-velocity automobile rear-end collision (Table 26–1). According to the Quebec Task Force, "Whiplash is an acceleration-deceleration mechanism of energy transfer to the neck. It may result from rearend or side-impact motor vehicle collisions, but can also occur during diving or other mishaps. The impact may result in bony or soft-tissue injuries (whiplash injury), which in turn may lead to a variety of clinical manifestations." The victim's neck is said to be subject to a sudden flexion/hyperextension movement, hence the term *whiplash*. However, the prevailing force on the cervical spine is axial and results from the torso sliding up the seat back. Whiplash injuries may result in muscle and ligamentous tears, spinal instability (most often at the C5–6 level), and disc protrusions with radicular compression. In as many as 50% of patients complaining of chronic neck pain after a whiplash injury, pain originates in the cervical facet (zygapophyseal) joints.

Presentation

Immediately following the accident, or sometimes after a day or two, patients experience neck stiffness and occipital or generalized headaches. Pain may be excruciating in some patients. Radicular pain radiation is present in about 10% of cases.

Less Typical Presentations

Memory loss, tinnitus, deafness, masticatory muscle and temporomandibular joint pain, dysphagia, hoarseness, and pupillary asymmetry from sympathetic fibers damage may all occur in whiplash injury patients. The Quebec Task Force has proposed a clinical classification of whiplash-associated disorders, as shown in Table 26–2.

Diagnosis

Summary of Diagnosis

> **WHIPLASH INJURY**
> - Detailed description of circumstances of the accident and symptoms.
> - Neck motion and tenderness.
> - Motor, sensory, and reflex examination.
> - Patients with grade I whiplash (alert, not obtunded by alcohol or drugs) do not require radiographic evaluation. Patients with grade II and III whiplash need radiographic evaluation including AP, lateral, and open mouth films.
> - Additional studies are indicated when the initial radiographic evaluation is equivocal.

Natural History

Expected Outcome

By the sixth week about half of the patients are asymptomatic and have resumed all previous activities. The remaining half will complain of neck pain, radicular pain, as well as less well-defined symptoms in upper extremities including nondermatomal and nonmyotomal paresthesias, and weakness or heaviness in the arms. At 6 months about one-third of patients will still be symptomatic.

Complications

Common complications of whiplash injury include anxiety, hyperirritability, poor sleep, facial paresthesias, dizziness, and

---

TABLE 26–1

INTERVENTIONS DESIGNED TO DECREASE THE RISK OF COLLISION AND THEREFORE WHIPLASH INJURY*

1. Interventions designed to reduce driving while intoxicated (automatic license suspension, enforcement of minimum age for purchase and consumption of alcohol, and legal accountability of merchants who sell alcoholic beverages to intoxicated people).
2. Measures designed to reduce the risk for teenagers (increasing the legal age for license, graduated access to unaccompanied driving, and curfew).
3. Limiting access to driving for individuals on certain medications or with certain medical conditions.
4. Vehicle-related interventions such as improvement in tires, antilock brakes, improved visibility and lighting, and speed control devices.
5. Interventions related to the road environment such as widening, improving surfaces, increasing visibility of the road environment, reducing highway speed limits, not allowing right turns on red lights, and the elimination of hazardous areas or death traps.

*No studies of these measures have so far addressed whiplash injuries, but they are all deemed important by the author.
Adapted from the Scientific Monograph of the Quebec Task Force on Whiplash-Associated Disorders. Spine 208S:1S–58S, 1995.

TABLE 26–2

PROPOSED CLINICAL CLASSIFICATION OF WHIPLASH-ASSOCIATED DISORDERS

Grade	Clinical Presentation
0	No complaint about the neck No physical sign(s)
I	Neck complaint of pain, stiffness, or tenderness only No physical sign(s)
II	Neck complaint and musculoskeletal sign(s)*
III	Neck complaint and neurologic sign(s)†
IV	Neck complaint and fracture or dislocation

*Musculoskeletal signs include decreased range of motion and point tenderness.
†Neurologic signs include decreased or absent deep tendon reflexes, weakness, and sensory deficits.
Symptoms and disorders that can be manifest in all grades include deafness, dizziness, tinnitus, headache, memory loss, dysphagia, and temporomandibular joint pain.
From the Scientific Monograph of the Quebec Task Force on Whiplash-Associated Disorders. Spine 20 8S:1S–58S, 1995.

vertigo. In one study radicular pain usually involving the C6 through C8 roots occurred in 30% of patients and cervical spine instability in about 20%. There are instances of laryngeal, pharyngeal, or sympathetic dysfunction. Protracted symptoms tend to correlate with severity of the injury, older age, and presence of cervical spondylosis. Litigation issues frequently emerge and may cloud interpretation of symptoms.

Treatment

Methods

Reassure patients that whiplash-associated symptoms are almost always self-limited and encourage them to return early to full activities. Initial treatment of whiplash injury includes analgesics for no longer than 1 week, heat application, and, as tolerated, gentle stretching exercises. Neck collars should not be used. At most, patients may be provided a soft neck collar to be used for the first 72 hours only. Mobilization and manipulation only offer transient relief. The prolonged use of rest (4 days or longer), inactivity, and neck collars probably prolong disability. Patients with severe neck pain unimproved by 2 weeks, as well as patients with radicular pain, should have flexion/extension radiographs (to rule out instability) and MRI. Even though the facet joint is the source of pain in at least 50% of cases, intraarticular corticosteroid injections have been ineffective in relieving pain. The rare patients with cervical instability or large disc protrusions may require surgical treatment. Patients with chronic symptoms are best managed by a multidisciplinary team.

Key Points

WHIPLASH INJURY

- Frequent complication of motor vehicle accidents, in particular rear-end collision.
- Mechanism of injury is complex and not well understood; resulting damage includes muscle and ligamentous tears, spinal instability, disc protrusion, and subtle injury to neck organs and sympathetic chain.
- The source of pain is a damaged facet (zygapophyseal) joint in at least 50% of cases.
- Symptoms persist more than 6 weeks in 50% of cases and more than 6 months in 30%.
- Cases with protracted, severe localized neck pain or radicular symptoms should be studied with flexion/extension radiographs and MRI, seeking a surgically correctable lesion.

Suggested Reading

Barnsley L, Lord SM, Wallis BJ, et al. Lack of effect of intraarticular corticosteroids for chronic pain in the cervical zygapophyseal joints. N Engl J Med 330:1047–1050, 1994.
Carette S. Whiplash injury and chronic neck pain [Editorial]. N Engl J Med 330:1083–1084, 1994.
Jonsson H, Cesarini K, Sahlstedt B, et al. Findings and outcome in whiplash-type neck distortions. Spine 19:2733–2743, 1994.
Lord SM, Barnsley L, Wallis BJ, Bogduk N. Chronic cervical zygapophysial joint pain after whiplash. Spine 21:1737–1745, 1996.
Spitzer WO, Skovron ML, Salmi LR, et al. Scientific monograph of the Quebec Task Force on Whiplash-Associated Disorders. Spine 20 8S:1S–58S, 1995.

Cervical Spondylosis

Presentation and Progression

Cause

Cervical spondylosis, the wearing of the cervical spine, involves predominantly the segments C4 to T1. The process originates in the intervertebral discs and secondarily damages diarthrodial joints. Early in the process the jellylike nucleous pulposus loses its avidity for water and shrinks. As a result the annulus fibrosus, unsupported from within, narrows, bulges to the sides, and cracks under the weight of the head. Motions are made irregular, and the segment becomes vulnerable to ligamentous and posterior joints strain. As the distance between vertebral bodies decreases, the stress on facet and uncovertebral joints increases, leading to cartilage wear and osteophytic growths. In the most advanced stages, articular and ring epiphysis osteophytes, disc protrusion or prolapse, and ligamenta flava hypertrophy threaten emerging nerve roots and the cord.

Asymptomatic cases with only limited neck motion are quite frequent. The typical patient with symptomatic cervical spondylosis is a middle-aged or older individual with episodic neck pain and a restricted neck on examination. Pain is experienced posteriorly or laterally in the neck with possible extension to the scapular area, the shoulder, or the upper limb.

Pain radiation in cervical spondylosis may be of the deep pain type or dermatomic. Deep pain radiation from the C6, the C7, and the less frequently involved C5 segments is experienced as a dull pain in the forearm, the radial hand, and the lateral shoulder and upper arm, respectively. Radicular pain occurs when facet joint spurs or disk prolapse impinge on the foramina. Compression of the cervical roots results in pain, numbness and paresthesias, muscle weakness, and reflex changes. The C6 and C7 roots are most frequently involved. C6 radiculopathy is characterized by sensory changes in index and thumb, weakness of elbow flexion, and a decreased biceps reflex. In the C7 radiculopathy there are sensory symptoms in the middle finger, weakness of elbow extension, and a decreased triceps reflex. The C5 and C8 roots are seldom involved. C5 radiculopathy is characterized by sensory changes in the radial border of the extremity short of the thumb. In the C8 radiculopathy the ulnar border of the hand and little finger are involved and the intrinsic muscles of the hand may be weak.

On examination, back and lateral neck bendings are painful and restricted. Prolonged compression of the head in lateral flexion or extension may reproduce the radicular symptoms. Concurrent shoulder limitation is frequent in patients with radiculopathy. Another important association is with the carpal tunnel syndrome (CTS) in the so-called double-crush syndrome. Compressive myelopathy should be suspected in older patients who complain of aching pain in anterior thighs, buttocks, or subcostal area, vertigo, instability, urinary or fecal incontinence, and a tendency to fall. Findings on examination include a combination of upper and lower motor signs in the upper extremities and lower extremities spasticity.

Diagnosis

Summary of Diagnosis

> **CERVICAL SPONDYLOSIS**
>
> - Diagnosis is based on clinical and radiographic data.
> - Middle-aged to older individuals.
> - Neck pain and limitation without evidences of inflammatory disease.
> - Cervical radiculopathy and myelopathy may be present.
> - Cervical spine films (AP, lateral, and oblique views) reveal disc narrowing, osteophytes, and possibly encroachment on neural foramina.
> - Nerve conduction studies and EMG may identify additional impinging lesions such as a coincidental CTS.
> - CT and MRI provide definitive data about the condition.

Natural History

The clinical course of cervical spondylosis is unpredictable, and the correlation between clinical findings and results of imaging studies is poor. Progression is typically slow, giving the illusion that nothing has changed. In cervical myelopathy, vertigo and sensory difficulties in the lower extremities often result in falls.

Treatment

Treatment of cervical spondylosis depends on the clinical findings. Because episodes of neck pain tend to resolve spontaneously in 5 to 10 days, a conservative attitude is warranted in most patients. Uncomplicated neck pain may be treated with acetaminophen, NSAIDs, or a combination of both. Heat applications using warm packs or an electric pad and partial neck immobilization with a soft or semirigid collar are helpful adjuncts for pain control. Cervical traction is reserved for patients with deep pain radiation or radicular pain. Traction should begin at a physical therapy department. Typically, a 7 to 10 lb traction is initially applied. Once the optimal traction has been determined, home traction can be implemented. Surgical decompression is reserved for patients with cervical myelopathy. There are important prophylactic measures that cervical spondylosis patients may benefit from. Attention should be paid to the pillow patients use, the customary position in bed (an elevated arm under the pillow, the prone position), as well as possible awkward neck positions in recreation or at work. The use of a cervical pillow and adopting the fetal position while in bed are beneficial for symptomatic cervical spondylosis. Patients should also be instructed on neck flexibility exercises (see appendix).

When to Refer

Patients with severe root compression symptoms and those with suspected myelopathy should be referred for neurologic or neurosurgical evaluation. Progressive neurologic deficit warrants referral for possible decompressive surgery.

Key Points

> **CERVICAL SPONDYLOSIS**
>
> - Degenerative process of the cervical spine secondary to intervertebral disc failure.
> - Present in 40% above the age of 50; virtually universal above 70.
> - Correlation between clinical findings and imaging abnormalities is poor.
> - Main complications include radiculopathy (C6,7) and myelopathy.
> - Treatment should be temporizing and conservative unless progressive neurologic damage is documented.

Suggested Reading

Bland JH. Disorders of the Cervical Spine, 2nd ed. W.B. Saunders, Philadelphia, 1994.

Buckwalter JA. Spine update: Aging and degeneration of the human intervertebral disc. Spine 20:1307–1314, 1995.

Farbman AA. Neck sprain. Associated factors. JAMA 223:1010–1015, 1973.

Helms CA. Fundamentals of Skeletal Radiology, 2nd ed. W.B. Saunders, Philadelphia, 1995.

McNab I. Cervical spondylosis. Clin Orthop 109:69–77, 1975.

Rothman RH, Marvel JP. The acute cervical disc. Clin Orthop 59–68, 1975.

Dorsal Pain

Dorsal pain has many possible mechanisms. Similar to neck and low back pain, its cause may be in the dorsal spine and its contents, a distant structure, or the posterior chest wall, in particular the paraspinal muscles.

Presentation and Progression

Cause

A common cause of dorsal pain, particularly in elderly women, is a vertebral fracture. Most vertebral fractures are due to osteoporosis. Osteomyelitis (in particular due to *M. tuberculosis*) or septic discitis may involve dorsal vertebrae. Other causes include primary or metastatic malignancy, and trauma. Pain may also occur from root irritation such as in compression of any type (foraminal impingement, neuroma, etc.), and in herpes zoster in which there is reactivation of varicella-zoster virus at the ganglion and along the nerve. Visceral pain radiating to the dorsal region may mean aortic aneurysm, myocardial infarction, pericarditis, esophageal spasm, hiatal hernias, and pancreatic processes including pancreatitis and cancer of the pancreas. Muscle spasm in the paraspinal muscle, or in the trapezium, is a very common pain source. Patients with fibromyalgia may also complain of dorsal pain.

Presentation

Patients may complain of an acutely localized pain at one or more dorsal levels. In muscle contracture-type pain there is not only pain and tenderness medial to the scapula, but radiation may be wide with involvement of neck, shoulder, and upper arm. A trigger point may be located within this area. Indeed, this is the area in which in the author's experience most cases of myofascial pain syndrome occur. Fibromyalgic pain often involves this area. In the spondyloarthropathies, it is common to have pain and tenderness at one or more interspinous ligaments, particularly in the upper dorsal spine. Bone pain is suggested by being persistent, most prominent at night, and markedly aggravated by mechanical factors such as slight flexion or extension motion.

Diagnosis

Summary of Diagnosis

DORSAL PAIN

- Diagnosis is clinical in most cases.
- Muscular pain may feature a bundle of contracted muscle which, when compressed, results in pain radiation to the entire symptomatic area (trigger point).
- In fibromyalgia, there are symmetric tender areas in the dorsal region and elsewhere.
- In the spondyloarthropathies, sharply localized interspinous tenderness may be elicited.
- In bone pain (fracture, malignancy, osteomyelitis) pain is present day and night, there is nocturnal predominance of pain, and marked spinous processes tenderness is present at the involved segment(s).
- If radicular pain is present, consider herpes zoster in addition to bone processes and foraminal impingements. The typical herpetic skin lesion may appear days, sometimes weeks, after radicular pain sets in.
- Always ask yourself if pain could represent radiation from a visceral organ.
- X-rays are not indicated in muscular types of pain or in interspinous pain due to spondyloarthropathy. They are definitely indicated when a bone source is considered.
- If malignancy is considered, a technetium bone scan is useful to identify silent remote bone lesions.
- MRI is superior to CT in defining bone lesions.

Natural History

Outcome depends on the lesion. Muscular contracture pain subsides in 1 to 3 days. Cases with radicular pain radiation, and any case in which a bone source is considered, should be assessed very carefully because compressive complications may be devastating at this level (remember that the spinal cord ends at L1).

Treatment

The same considerations apply as in treatment of neck and low back pain.

When to Refer

Patient referral should be prompt in cases with radicular pain as well as when a bone source is suspected. Neural compression in malignancy, infection, and displaced fractures can be catastrophic.

Key Points

DORSAL PAIN

- Most cases of dorsal pain are due to muscle contracture, fibromyalgia, or bone lesions.
- The most common bone lesion is an osteoporotic fracture.
- Radicular pain radiation and bone-type pain are red flags of potentially catastrophic conditions.
- Neurosurgical or orthopedic referral should be made promptly.

Suggested Reading

Borenstein DG, Wiesel SW, Boden SD. Low Back Pain. Medical Diagnosis and Comprehensive Management, 2nd ed. W.B. Saunders, Philadelphia, 1995.

Low Back Pain

Presentation and Progression

Cause

Low back pain is one of the most common conditions that afflict humankind, the second cause of work absenteeism, and a major cause of disability. The prevalence of back pain in the adult population is shown in Table 26–3. Pain may arise in any of the many structures the lumbar region comprises: muscles, ligaments, bones, joints, and nerves. Each of these structures may be subject to strain, rupture, inflammation, infection, and tumor, not to mention conditions without a known anatomic substrate such as fibromyalgia and myofascial pain. To complicate matters further, low back pain may originate in a more or less distant structure such as the aorta, pancreas, kidney, prostate, and uterus. Faced with this maze, what should a clinician do when confronted with a patient with low back pain?

Presentation

Although many of us would not find it appealing, a probabilistic approach has been proposed that works well.

1. Rule out, on clinical grounds, an expanding abdominal aneurysm, malignant disease, spinal infection, cauda equina compression, a spinal fracture, and referred abdominal or pelvic pain. Complicated abdominal aneurysms occur in late middle-aged or older individuals. Although symptoms are usually anterior, back symptoms predominate in some patients. Tearing left lumbar pain with possible extension to lower extremities, a tender epigastric mass, and/or circulatory collapse indicate a complicated abdominal aneurysm. Such patients should be immediately brought to the attention of a vascular surgeon.

2. Consider the possibility of infection, neoplastic disease, and chronic inflammation. Infection, in particular subacute bacterial endocarditis, should be suspected in patients

who have continuous back pain and fever, with or without shaking chills. A history of intravenous drug use, recent infection in the biliary or urinary tract, a heart murmur, and localized spinal tenderness further support a diagnosis of spinal osteomyelitis. Blood cultures and spine x-rays should be obtained, followed by a bone scan if the x-rays are negative. Typical early radiographic findings include vertebral endplate decalcification and erosion, followed by disc narrowing. Unfortunately, plain x-rays may be negative in the first 2 weeks. A bone scan, showing focal uptake, will afford unequivocal evidence of an ongoing process in these cases. CT, and particularly MRI, detect early vertebral involvement as well as any possible paraspinal or epidural extension. Malignant disease, usually metastatic but sometimes primary, as well as benign tumoral conditions such as osteoid osteoma, cause continuous pain that is characteristically worst at night. There is spinal tenderness at one or more vertebrae. Patients with malignant disease may be anemic or have evidence of a primary tumor. Spine x-rays, followed by a bone scan, will outline most benign and malignant tumors with the possible exception of multiple myeloma. In metastatic disease and multiple myeloma, MRI is superior to CT with contrast in revealing extent of involvement as well as impending neural compression. Spondyloarthropathy, such as in ankylosing spondylitis and the axial arthritis of inflammatory bowel disease and reactive arthritis, characteristically occurs in young men (Table 26–4). Protracted morning stiffness lasting hours is characteristic, and night pain may be severe. Sacroiliac joint inflammation results in buttock and posterior thigh pain. The manubriosternal and sternoclavicular joints may be tender. Sacroiliac and spinal x-rays are normal in early disease. In this situation a positive HLA-B27 determination adds diagnostic certainty. CT and MRI are equally excellent to detect early sacroiliitis. Because of its lower cost CT is the imaging procedure of choice in patients with suspected spondyloarthropathy and a negative HLA-B27.

3. Cauda equina compression may be caused by a massive central disk herniation; extradural bleed, tumor, or infection; and trauma. Patients complain of lumbosacral pain and bilateral lower extremity weakness. Leg weakness, a bilateral straight leg raising sign, perineal anesthesia (saddle anesthesia), decreased anal tone, and in some instances fecal and urine incontinence afford unequivocal evidence of the syndrome. These patients should be immediately seen by an orthopedist or a neurosurgeon for further investigation and treatment.

TABLE 26–3

PREVALENCE OF LOW BACK PAIN AND SCIATICA IN THE ADULT POPULATION

Characteristic	Prevalence (%)
Any low back pain	60–80
Ever had low back pain persisting at least 2 weeks	14
Back pain with features of sciatica lasting at least 2 weeks	1.6
Lumbar spine surgery	1–2

Adapted from Deyo RA, Loeser JD, and Bigos SJ. Herniated lumbar intervertebral disk. Ann Intern Med 112:598–603, 1990.

TABLE 26–4

INFLAMMATORY VERSUS MECHANICAL LOW BACK PAIN

	Inflammatory	Mechanical
Onset	Gradual	Abrupt
Duration	> 3 months	Brief
Morning stiffness	Lasts hours	Lasts minutes
Effect of activity	Diminishes pain	Increases pain
Pain at night	Present	Absent

Calin A, Porta J, Fries JF, Schurman DJ. Clinical history as a screening test for ankylosing spondylitis. JAMA 237:2613–2614, 1977.

4. Spinal fracture should be suspected when an older, osteoporotic patient develops focal pain following a minor lift or an unprepared-for movement, and in younger individuals with back pain following major trauma, such as a fall from a height or a motor vehicle accident.

5. Referred low back pain is also to be ruled out clinically in patients presenting back pain. In general, there are evidences of the retroperitoneal, intraabdominal, or intrapelvic condition causing the pain (see section on referred back pain).

If no clinical evidence favors a complicated aneurysm, cauda equina compression, infection, malignant disease, spondyloarthropathy, or referred pain, the recommendation is to treat symptomatically, as outlined in low back strain, without ancillary studies and wait 4 weeks. The overwhelming majority of patients will do well during this period.

6. Patients treated conservatively who fail to improve or get worse deserve further investigation. This diagnostic tree may be modified by circumstances surrounding each case; some patients will require earlier action; in others the conservative approach will extend well beyond the arbitrary 4 week limit.

Diagnosis

Summary of Diagnosis

LOW BACK PAIN

- A careful history and physical examination, based initially on the exclusion of potentially catastrophic conditions, allows an empirical diagnosis of low back strain in most cases.
- Conditions to be excluded include an expanding abdominal aneurysm; the cauda equina syndrome; referred pain from an abdominal, retroperitoneal, or pelvic source; osteomyelitis; malignant disease; and spondyloarthropathy.
- Based on clinical indications, one or more of an array of tests and imaging procedures are necessary in a minority of patients with persisting or worsening pain.
- Persistence of symptoms beyond 4 weeks justifies a thorough reevaluation.

Natural History

Expected Outcome

The outcome depends entirely on the process; in the usual type, known as low back strain, symptoms typically go away within 1 to 2 weeks; lack of improvement with or without additional findings is enough reason to suspect inflammatory or structural disease, such as spondylolisthesis, and proceed accordingly.

Treatment

Methods

Initial treatment of low back pain is described under low back strain.

Expected Response

As mentioned, in the great majority of patients without initial evidence of serious low back pain, symptoms subside within 2 weeks.

Complications

A clear diagnostic and treatment strategy should minimize the risk of serious complications of conditions featuring low back pain.

When to Refer

The mere suspicion of a leaking abdominal aneurysm should trigger vascular surgery consultation, and cauda equina syndrome calls for a back surgeon or neurosurgeon. Patients suspected of having spinal osteomyelitis should be evaluated in conjunction with an orthopedist and an infectious disease specialist, and if metastatic disease is at issue both an orthopedist and an oncologist should be called in. When spondyloarthropathy is suspected, children and females who might be pregnant should have an HLA-B27. Otherwise, a tilted pelvic radiograph to visualize the sacroiliac joints is a very efficient study in patients with long-standing symptoms. Early rheumatology consultation is highly desirable in these patients.

Key Points

> **LOW BACK PAIN**
> - Initial evaluation is aimed at excluding potentially catastrophic conditions, referred visceral pain, osteomyelitis, malignant disease, and spondyloarthropathy.
> - Most cases run a benign, self-limited course within 2 weeks.
> - Patients who continue symptomatic 4 weeks after initial evaluation should be further investigated to rule out inflammatory disease, structural disease of the spine, and neoplasia.

Suggested Reading

Aliabadi P, Nikpoor N. Review: Imaging osteomyelitis. Arthritis Rheum 37:617–622, 1994.
Borenstein DG, Wiesel SW, Boden SD. Low Back Pain. Medical Diagnosis and Comprehensive Management, 2nd. ed. W.B. Saunders, Philadelphia, 1995.
Frymoyer JW. Back pain and sciatica. N Engl J Med 318:291–300, 1988.
Hall H. Examination of the patient with low back pain. Bull Rheum Dis 33:1–8, 1983.
Jensen MC, Brant-Zawadzki MN, Obuchowski N, et al. Magnetic resonance of the spine in people without back pain. N Engl J Med 331:69–73, 1994.

Referred Low Back Pain

Presentation and Progression

Cause

Retroperitoneal, intraabdominal, and pelvic disease may feature prominent back symptoms that can fool the naive and sometimes the expert. One such cause, a complicated *abdominal aneurysm*, has been mentioned. Pancreatic pain from *pancreatitis or pancreatic carcinoma* is felt primarily in the epigatrium and radiates back to the dorsolumbar junction. Patients with pancreatic cancer may seek relief by leaning forward in the sitting position.

Retroperitoneal tumors, particularly lymphomas, *hematomas*, and *retroperitoneal fibrosis*, may also cause lumbar pain. Retroperitoneal tumors and hematomas, by infiltration or compression of the lumbar plexus, cause uni- or bilateral anterior thigh pain corresponding to the L2 through L4 segments. The patellar reflex (L3, 4) is diminished or absent in these patients, and profound quadriceps muscle atrophy soon sets in. Hyperextension of the thigh, by pulling from the femoral nerve (L2, 3, 4), increases or reproduces the pain. The maneuver is done with the patient lying prone and the knee flexed 90 degrees. Elevation of the thigh from the examining table triggers anterior thigh pain. A patient with relentless anterior thigh pain, malaise, and an increased ESR should be suspected of having a retroperitoneal malignancy. An abdominal CT (not a spinal CT) with attention to the retroperitoneal space should be obtained early in the evaluation of these patients. Retroperitoneal fibrosis is an uncommon lesion in which a mass of fibrous tissue grows in the retroperitoneum compressing ureters and major veins. Patients may present with hydronephrosis, pyelonephritis or renal insufficiency, or uni- or bilateral leg edema. Distressing lumbar pain is a common complaint.

Patients with suspected retroperitoneal fibrosis should be evaluated by a urologist and an oncologist, since retroperitoneal lymphoma needs to be excluded. An abdominal CT helps determine location of the mass. Diagnosis, however, requires surgical exploration and biopsy. Histologic differentiation between retroperitoneal fibrosis and lymphoma may at times prove difficult. A similar fibrotic process may involve the mediastinum compressing the superior vena cava. An association between both retroperitoneal and mediastinal fibrosis and connective tissue diseases such as SLE, Sjögren's, and scleroderma is suggested by multiple reported cases. The antimigraine drug methysergide, now little used, is a known cause of retroperitoneal and mediastinal fibrosis. Most cases of the condition, however, are idiopathic.

Lumbar pain with costovertebral angle percussion tenderness is a classic finding in *pyelonephritis* and *renal* and *perinephric abscesses*. Psoas extension of a perinephric abscess may result in severe groin or leg pain. Patients are febrile, and the urine shows pyuria. Flank pain extending to the iliac fossa and testicle and marked restlessness characterize the passage of a *ureteral stone*. Gross or microscopic hematuria is usually present in these patients. Sacral pain may have a genitourinary origin. Infiltrating *prostate carcinoma* produces relentless suprapubic and sacral pain. Another cause of sacral pain is infiltrating *uterine carcinoma*. Crampy sacral pain extending to the thighs and synchronous with menses may occur in normal women and in patients with *endometriosis*. Pain at the tailbone or *coccygodynia* can be very distressing to the point that patients cannot sit. Fortunately, the process, which is of unknown cause, is often self-limited.

Diagnosis

Summary of Diagnosis

> **REFERRED LOW BACK PAIN**
> - Mounting and tearing or colicky-type pain.
> - Concurrent abdominal or pelvic pain.
> - Bowel, urinary, or gynecologic abnormalities.
> - Ancillary studies tailored to symptoms: urinalysis, occult blood in stools, serum amylase and lipase; ultrasonography, abdominal/retroperitoneal CT scan, colonoscopy, and retrograde ureter pyelography.

Natural History

These are ailments in which delay in action should be avoided; early diagnosis is essential for effective treatment.

Treatment

Treatment varies according to the condition. Protracted cases of coccygodynia may be treated with a corticosteroid infiltration. This can best be administered by an anesthesiologist. Surgical removal of the coccyx is usually successful in the rare patients with refractory pain.

When to Refer

Virtually all patients with referred back pain will require consultation.

Key Points

> **REFERRED LOW BACK PAIN**
> - Cases should be rapidly identified; even in straightforward instances, exclusion by history and physical examination of a complicated abdominal aneurysm and the cauda equina syndrome is necessary.

> - Joint care with a vascular surgeon, gastroenterologist, abdominal surgeon, urologist, or gynecologist is usually required.

Suggested Reading

Borenstein DG, Wiesel SW, Boden SD. Low Back Pain. Medical Diagnosis and Comprehensive Management, 2nd. ed. W.B. Saunders, Philadelphia, 1995.

Deyo RA, Diehl AK. Cancer as a cause of back pain: Frequency, clinical presentation, and diagnostic strategies. J Gen Intern Med 3:320–328, 1988.

Acute Nonspecific Low Back Pain (Back Strain, Lumbago)

Presentation and Progression

Cause

Most cases of acute low back pain belong to this category, which explains the high success rate of the conservative approach to low back pain. Acute low back pain is pathogenetically heterogeneous, and the actual mechanism involved in a given patient can only be speculated on. Muscle contracture probably explains most cases with rapidly resolving symptoms. Jamming of facet joints has been postulated based on anatomic considerations and represents one of the tenets of chiropractic medicine. Ligamentous strain and microtears may play a role in some patients. Kissing of spinous processes due to lumbar hyperlordosis with possible adventitious bursae formation has been considered a cause of recurrent low back pain (Baastrup's disease). Important additional mechanical factors include grossly unequal leg length (difference greater than 2 cm), spondylolisthesis, spondylosis, and disk extrusion. The latter two explain recurrent lumbalgia that merges with root irritation symptoms. A serious underlying condition should always be ruled out clinically (Table 26–5).

Presentation

The typical patient has been in excellent general health until pain develops. Onset of pain is abrupt following unprepared-for movement, unusual effort, prolonged sitting in an awkward position, or a sustained poor posture at work. Similar episodes may have occurred in the past. Pain may be unilateral or may be experienced across the low lumbar area. Radiation to buttock and the posterior thigh is common.

Back examination reveals contractured paraspinal muscles. An area of tenderness may be present between the posterior iliac crest and L4 or L5. The complex anatomy of the area does not allow precise determination of the structure at fault. However, a variable contribution of muscle contracture and ligamentous strain may be inferred from the physical findings. Lumbar spine motion is limited, in particular forward and contralateral flexion as the involved muscles or ligaments are stretched. Hyperextension is painful in muscle contracture and painless in ligamentous strain (damaged ligaments only hurt when they are pulled). However, hyperextension pain may also be caused, for instance, by kissing spinous processes and facet joint osteoarthritis. Leg length

TABLE 26–5

RED FLAGS TO BE CONSIDERED IN INITIAL EVALUATION OF PATIENTS WITH ACUTE LOW BACK PAIN

RED FLAGS FOR MALIGNANCY

Age over 50
A history of malignancy
Unexplained weight loss
Pain increased by rest

RED FLAGS FOR INFECTION

Skin or urinary tract infection
Intravenous drug use
Immunosuppression
Pain increased by rest

RED FLAGS FOR CAUDA EQUINA COMPRESSION

Bladder dysfunction (urinary retention or flow incontinence)
Saddle anesthesia (anus, perineum, genitals)
Loss of anal sphincter tone
Major limb motor weakness

RED FLAGS FOR SPINAL FRACTURE

Preceding trauma relative to age (older, osteoporotic patients may fracture the spine upon a minor fall or a lift effort; in younger patients, spinal fracture requires major trauma such as a fall from a height or a motor vehicle accident)

Modified from Bigos SJ, et al. Acute Low Back Problems in Adults. Clinical Practice Guideline No. 14. AHCPR Publication No. 95–0642. Agency for Health Care Policy and Research, Public Health Service, Rockville, MD, December 1994.

---

may be unequal. Lower extremities have normal strength and the straight leg raising test is either negative or only reveals hamstring muscle contracture.

To be useful the test must be correctly performed. All movements (leg elevation, flexion of individual joints) must be done passively (the physician must provide the force). With the patient lying supine on the examining table the painless side and then the painful side are tested. The leg should be gently raised from the heel asking the patient to keep the knee straight and the muscles relaxed. Patients with L5 or S1 root irritation will experience shooting pain and paresthesias down to the foot between 30 and 70 degrees of elevation (a lesser elevation will not stretch the sciatic nerve enough to reproduce the symptoms). The knee is then gently bent to relax the nerve until root irritation ceases. Finally, with the thigh still raised and the knee semiflexed, the foot is brought to slight dorsiflexion. Reproduction of symptoms is confirmatory of root irritation.

A true positive straight leg raising test should be distinguished from hamstring muscle contracture pain that is a routine finding in patients with low back strain and other mechanical spine problems. Hamstring muscle contracture pain has characteristic findings on the straight leg raising test. As the leg is elevated, posterior thigh pain rather than radicular pain develops. Onset of pain coincides with involuntary contraction of hamstring muscles. From that point, a slight flexion of the knee, by relaxing the hamstring muscles, makes the pain go away. Following this the foot is dorsiflexed.

Absence of pain further excludes radicular irritation. Patients with presumed muscle strain type of backache do not require laboratory studies or x-rays.

Diagnosis

Summary of Diagnosis

BACK STRAIN

- Acute onset following unusual or unprepared-for activity
- Absence of red flags of a serious underlying condition.
- Short duration of symptoms.
- Increasing pain with certain activities and sustained postures.
- Muscle contracture.
- Occasional presence of a trigger point.
- Hyperlordosis and unequal leg length should be sought.
- X-rays are not indicated in these patients.

Natural History

Typically, back strain symptoms subside spontaneously in 2 to 3 weeks. Persistence of pain beyond 3 weeks should raise the possibility of spondylolisthesis, spondyloarthropathy, malignancy, and spinal infection. Overall, only 5% of acute low back pain patients have not had functional recovery at 6 months, although residual symptoms are present in about 30% of patients.

Treatment

Treatment of low back strain includes reassurance, analgesic or anti-inflammatory medications for 7 to 10 days, and transient activities modification. The various modalities of treatment have been admirably reviewed by Katz and Katz. Patients should be told the expected duration of symptoms. Bed rest treatment in acute nonspecific low back pain is no longer justified. In a randomized trial, bed rest for 2 days was as effective as a 7 day rest and resulted in 45% less days of missed work. The results of this work have been further extended by a Finnish study in which three treatment modalities were compared, bed rest for 2 days, back-mobilizing exercises (back extension and lateral bending movements), and continuing routine activities as actively as tolerated. Interestingly, the latter approach led to a faster recovery than the former two treatments. A full dose of a NSAID, such as ibuprofen 3600 mg per day or naproxen 1500 mg per day, reduced after 2 to 3 days may be very helpful in the acute phase of the syndrome. Acetaminophen 4000 mg per day may be added for further analgesia. Muscle relaxants may be required. Low back strain has a tendency to recur. Unequal leg length should be corrected with a shoe insert. Adherence to postural recommendations and exercises is essential in long-term management.

Expected response is pain relief within 2 to 3 weeks. Other than possible recurrence and the attendant work loss there are no complications of back strain per se.

When to Refer

In a recent comparative study of acute low back pain treated by primary care physicians, chiropractors, and orthopedic surgeons, outcome was similar in the three groups but the lowest cost of treatment corresponded to primary care physicians. This study confirms a long-held belief that acute low back pain should be treated by primary care physicians. Since low back pain is such a black box, however, referral should occur any time a primary care physician has a diagnostic or treatment doubt. Also, patients failing to improve over 4 weeks deserve further scrutiny.

Key Points

> **BACK STRAIN**
> - Self-limited, mechanically determined low back pain.
> - The structure at fault cannot be determined from the symptoms.
> - Course is spontaneously regressive with duration of symptoms less than 3 weeks.
> - Laboratory studies and x-rays are not indicated.
> - Treatment is with analgesics, muscle relaxants if required clinically, and local heat. Bed rest should be discouraged.
> - The condition tends to recur; all patients should be instructed on back protection (see the appendix).
> - Persistence of pain beyond 4 weeks dictates the need for further investigation.

Suggested Reading

Bigos SJ, et al. Acute Low Back Problems in Adults. Clinical Practice Guideline No. 14. AHCPR Publication No. 95-0642. Agency for Health Care Policy and Research, Rockville, MD, December 1994.

Carey TS, Garrett J, Jackman A, et al. The outcomes and costs of care for acute back pain among patients seen by primary care practitioners, chiropractors, and orthopedic surgeons. N Engl J Med 333:913–917, 1995.

Katz JN, Katz NP. Lumbar spine disease. In: Weisman MH, Weinblatt ME (eds) Treatment of the Rheumatic Diseases. W.B. Saunders, Philadelphia, 1995.

Malmivaara A, Häkkinen U, Aro T, et al. The treatment of acute low back pain. Bed rest, exercises, or ordinary activity? N Engl J Med 332:351–355, 1995.

Sciatica

Presentation and Progression

Cause

Sciatica, or dermatomic-type pain involving the L5 or S1 roots, which are the main components of the sciatic nerve, is a common condition. Sciatica may occur from a variety of intra- and extraspinal causes. Intraspinal compressions, which are the most frequent, usually result from a herniated nucleus pulposus impinging on a root. Not all potentially compressive lesions cause sciatica or low back pain, however, as attested by the many positive MRIs observed in presumably healthy individuals. Patients who develop nucleus pulposus herniation appear to have a defective annulus fibrosus (posterolateral fissures or diverticula) that favors herniation. Following a low resistance path, nucleus pulposus hernias emerge posterolaterally, lateral to the posterior longitudinal ligament that shields the central portion of the spinal canal. Interestingly, nucleus pulposus herniation exhibits some familial aggregation. The natural history of disc herniation appears to be spontaneous regression by neovascularization and macrophage infiltration in the epidural space. Other etiologies include congenital or acquired spinal stenosis with decreased diameters of the spinal canal; narrowing of the lateral recesses (lateral spinal stenosis) caused by osteophytes, extruded disc material, degenerative synovial cysts, or neurofibromas; anomalous lumbar nerve roots; epidural abscesses; and carcinomatosis.

Because in the lumbar spine nerve roots exit the spinal canal just proximal to the corresponding disc, L4–L5 disc herniations impinge on the L5 root as it travels to the L5–S1 foramen, and L5–S1 disc herniations impinge on the S1 root on its way to the S1–S2 foramen. Symptoms depend on location of herniation as well as the diameters of the spinal canal. The cauda equina syndrome, with compression of multiple lower roots, may be caused by large central hernias, malignancy, infection, dural cysts such as in meningocele and ankylosing spondylitis, intraspinal lipomatosis in primary or iatrogenic Cushing's syndrome, and other lesions.

Usual Symptoms and Signs

Sciatica due to nucleus pulposus herniation is a condition of young individuals in their third or fourth decades of life. Predisposing factors include obesity, occupations that involve prolonged sitting, and smoking. Onset of symptoms may be abrupt or gradual, and there is usually a history of recurrent, nonradiating lumbar pain. Sometimes, as lower extremity pain develops, lumbar pain abates. Sciatica consists of lancinating shooting pains from back to foot extending along the L5 or the S1 dermatomes in 90% of cases. L4 root involvement occurs in less than 10% of cases. Coughing or sneezing increase the pain. Gait, if at all possible, is antalgic keeping the painful limb semiflexed and applying on it the least possible weight. Paraspinal muscles are contractured in the involved side, and upon forward flexion the trunk deviates to one side (list). In the overwhelming majority of patients, symptoms are unilateral.

Root irritation should be distinguished from hamstring muscle contracture pain by the straight leg raising maneuver as described under low back strain. L5 sciatica causes pain and paresthesias in the anterior leg and the dorsal/medial foot. Weakness of great toe dorsiflexion may be present. Reflexes are unaffected. There is an area of hypoesthesia in the great toe and the web space between the first and second toes. In S1 sciatica calf and lateral foot are involved. There is weakness of plantar flexion and the Achilles reflex is either decreased or absent. There is decreased sensation in the posterior calf and the lateral foot. In the uncommon L4 sciatica, sensory changes occur in the medial leg. Because the quadriceps muscle receives inervation from L2 and L3 as well, weakness of knee extension may be difficult to prove. The patellar reflex is often absent in these patients. The possibility that physical findings may be residual from a previous attack should be kept in mind in assessing patients with sciatica.

Less Typical Presentations

Sciatica with a negative straight leg raising test often indicates extraspinal impingement, such as may be caused by a tight piriformis muscle. This muscle, which overlies the sciatic nerve, attaches medially in the anterior sacrum and laterally in the posterior greater trochanter. The piriformis muscle is an external rotator of the extended hip and a hip abductor when the hip is flexed.

To elicit pain in the *piriformis muscle syndrome,* with patient lying prone on the examining table (hip extension) and the knee flexed 90 degrees (leg straight up), the examiner gently brings the leg outward, which results in passive internal rotation of the hip. Reproduction of symptoms with this maneuver, which stretches the piriformis, suggests impingement on the sciatic nerve by a tight piriformis muscle. A thick wallet kept in the back pocket is another cause of extraspinal sciatica. Another lesion that may result in L5 or S1 symptoms with equivocal lumbar symptoms and sometimes a negative straight leg raising test is *herpes zoster*. Pain and paresthesias may precede the typical rash for weeks. Bilateral sciatica suggests compression of the cauda equina. The *cauda equina syndrome* is characterized by bilateral sciatica, saddle anesthesia (perineal and perianal anesthesia that spares the scrotum), and sphincter incontinence.

Diagnosis

Summary of Diagnosis

> **SCIATICA**
> - Acute pain and paresthesias extending along L5, S1, or rarely L4.
> - Preceding recurrent lumbar pain.
> - Reflex changes in L4 (knee jerk) and S1 (ankle jerk) lesions. There are no reflex changes in L5 sciatica.
> - Bilateral sciatica suggests a central hernia or other extensive compressive lesion.
> - A negative straight leg raising test suggests extraspinal compression or neuropathy.
> - Watch for the emergence of cutaneous herpes zoster.
> - Plain radiographs are indicated in patients with neurologic findings to assess spondylolisthesis, fracture, neoplasia, or infection.

Natural History

Sciatica due to nucleus pulposus herniation usually follows a regressive course. Recovery may be complete, or there may be residual reflex loss with or without calf weakness and atrophy. Neurologic sequelae of sciatica are usually mild. Work loss associated with sciatica is considerable, however; 8% of patients may be out of work at 1 year and nearly half will have some work restriction.

Treatment

Methods

Treatment of newly developed sciatica is along the lines of acute back strain. Patients should be reassured about the generally favorable outlook of the condition. Deyo has stressed that early treatment of sciatica should be at home to decrease the chances of dependent behavior and also because traction, the usual justification for admission, does not appear to afford real benefit. Because pain in sciatica tends to be severe and associated muscle spasm is the rule, nonsteroidal anti-inflammatory agents should be supplemented by a time-limited course of codeine (unless there is a reason to withhold opiates) and muscle relaxants such as cyclobenzaprine or carisoprodol.

Bed rest is essential in the early treatment of sciatica. The recommendation should be to spend 1 to 3 days in bed on a firm mattress preferably in the supine position with the hips and knees slightly semiflexed. This can be achieved by placing a pillow under the knees between mattress and sheet, plus pillows on the sides as reminders. In this position muscle contracture is relieved and intradiscal pressures are decreased. The semiflexed position relaxes the sciatic nerve and the iliopsoas muscles. In addition, by flattening the lumbar lordosis the spinous processes separate, and stress on the facet joints is decreased. Rising from bed to use a bedside commode or the bathroom should be done carefully. First, the patient should be changed to the lateral fetal position by rolling en bloc to the side, prior to rising with help.

After 2 or 3 days, as pain and muscle spasm subside, gradual ambulation is encouraged. Return to work is usually allowed 3 or 4 days later. Activities modification should be maintained until symptoms go away. In particular, patients should be discouraged from sitting for prolonged periods. A useful tip is to interrupt desk work every 45 minutes to take a brief walk. Patients should also be instructed on the use of a proper chair (straight), to use a pillow under the small of the back while driving, and to do lifting by holding the object close to the body and using the strength of the legs. Back exercises are then started beginning with abdominal strengthening exercises followed by general strengthening and flexibility exercises (see appendix). Improvement tends to be slow and bed rest may be required for 1 week. Long-term instructions include weight loss, cessation of smoking, and regular exercise.

All patients with sciatica should be watched critically, particularly those without previous back symptoms as well as patients older than 50. Relentless pain and extension of neurologic findings make alternative diagnoses such as neoplasia and infection more likely. Finally, persistence of neurologic findings past 4 weeks of conservative therapy should trigger neurologic or rheumatologic consultation. Imaging studies may be required at this stage.

Expected Response

On conservative treatment approximately 40% of patients are free of symptoms at 1 month and 60% at 1 year. To foster recovery and to avoid deconditioning and muscle atrophy, patients with continuing symptoms should be placed on a spinal rehabilitation program with exercises that emphasize extension (McKenzie's exercises).

Epidural corticosteroid injections administered by an anesthesiologist or a back surgeon are often quite effective in reducing pain; the improvement may last several weeks to a few months and merge with the spontaneous healing of the condition. There is still controversy regarding the value of epidural corticosteroids in the treatment of sciatica, and clinicians should be fully aware of possible risks associated with the procedure.

Surgery, usually open lumbar discectomy, is formally indicated in patients with cauda equina syndrome and may be required in sciatica patients who fail to improve after 6 weeks of conservative therapy, have neurologic deficit, and disk herniation is shown at the corresponding level, usually by CT or MRI. Depression and ongoing litigation affect prognosis negatively but should not be a deterrent for surgery if the preceding criteria are met. The reason to use conservative treatment in most sciatica patients is that although short-term surgical results are superior to conservative treatment, including relief of sciatica at 1 year in 75% of cases and relief of back pain in 70%, follow-up at 10 years shows no difference between surgical and nonsurgical patients. There is, in addition, a small but real possibility of developing surgical complications such as dural sac tears requiring repair (2%–5%), wound infection (2.9%), thromboembolism (1.7%), permanent nerve root injury (very rare), and death (0.2%).

An alternative to open discectomy is *microdiscectomy* in which there is minimal trauma to the soft tissues and stability of the lumbar spine is not compromised. Although formal comparison with open discectomy has not been made, there are reasons to believe that microdiscectomy is successful in a higher proportion of patients, has a lower rate of complications, and patients return to work earlier. The technique is highly dependent on the surgeon's skill, however, and is not generally available. *Chemonucleolysis* is now seldom used in the United States because it is less effective than spinal surgery, anaphylaxis may be induced (0.4%–0.7%), and rare patients develop severe neurologic damage due to intrathecal application of the enzyme including subarachnoid hemorrhage and paraplegia.

When to Refer

Bilateral sciatica should prompt neurosurgical or orthopedic referral because of the possibility of a large central hernia causing a cauda equina syndrome. In the same category are patients with rapidly progressive neurologic deficit. Finally, patients with continuing neurologic deficit after 4 to 6 weeks of conservative therapy should also be referred.

Key Points

SCIATICA

- May have multiple spinal and extraspinal causes.
- Bilateral sciatica and rapidly progressive neurologic deficit call for immediate orthopedic or neurosurgical consultation.
- Most cases of unilateral, single-root sciatica in young individuals are caused by an extruded disc and in older individuals by degenerative changes leading to lumbar stenosis.
- In many instances extruded discs are eventually absorbed in the epidural space.
- Treatment is as in back sprain but improvement is slower.
- In cases due to disc extrusion surgical treatment is better than conservative treatment in the short term, but long-term results may be equal.

Suggested Reading

Bogduk NM. Spine update. Epidural steroids. Spine 20:845–848, 1995.
Deyo RA, Loeser JD, Bigos SJ. Herniated lumbar intervertebral disk. Ann Intern Med 112:598–603, 1990.
Frymoyer JH. Back pain and sciatica. N Engl J Med 318:291–300, 1988.
Katz JN, Katz NP. Lumbar spine disease. In: Weisman MH, Weinblat ME (eds) Treatment of the Rheumatic Diseases. W.B. Saunders, Philadelphia, 1–15, 1995.
Komori H, Shinomiya K, Nakai O, et al. The natural history of herniated nucleus pulposus with radiculopathy. Spine 21:225–229, 1996.
McKenzie EA. Prophylaxis in recurrent low back pain. NZ Med J 89:22–23, 1979.
Postacchini F. Results of surgery compared with conservative management for lumbar disc herniations. Spine 21:1383–1387, 1996.

Spinal Stenosis

The spinal canal comprises a central portion or central canal, which contains the dural sac, and a lateral portion, the root canal, which extends through the foramen and contains the root. Spinal stenosis refers to compression of nerve roots by narrowing of the bony and/or ligamentous boundaries of the central vertebral canal (central spinal stenosis) or its lateral portion (lateral spinal stenosis).

Presentation and Progression

Cause

Spinal stenosis is most often the result of concentric osteophytic and ligamentous encroachment on the dural sac (central spinal stenosis), or osteophytic or disc material impinging on the lateral recesses and foramina (lateral spinal stenosis). The process may be viewed as a result of lumbar disc degeneration leading to secondary osteoarthritic changes of the facet joints; redundancy of ligaments, particularly the ligamenta flava; and osteophytic rims. Where degenerative spondylolysthesis occurs, resulting vertebral displacement further exacerbates root compression. Contributing factors include a congenital or developmental narrow spinal canal (Figure 26–1), disc protrusion, excessive extradural fat such as seen in Cushing's syndrome (primary and iatrogenic) and rarely in obesity, dural and synovial cysts, or any other structure intruding within the spinal canal (Table 26–6). The classic symptom in spinal stenosis is neurogenic claudication (see later). Based on clinical observations and experimental studies, neurogenic claudication indicates two or more levels of compression (Figure 26–2): Two levels of central stenosis cause bilateral neurogenic claudication; one level of central stenosis plus one of lateral stenosis cause unilateral neurogenic claudication.

Presentation

Spinal stenosis typically affects elderly individuals except in age-independent processes such as extradural fat deposition (glucocorticoid or obesity induced). Neurogenic claudication consists of leg, gluteal, or lumbar pain triggered by ambulation and relieved by sitting but not by resting in the erect

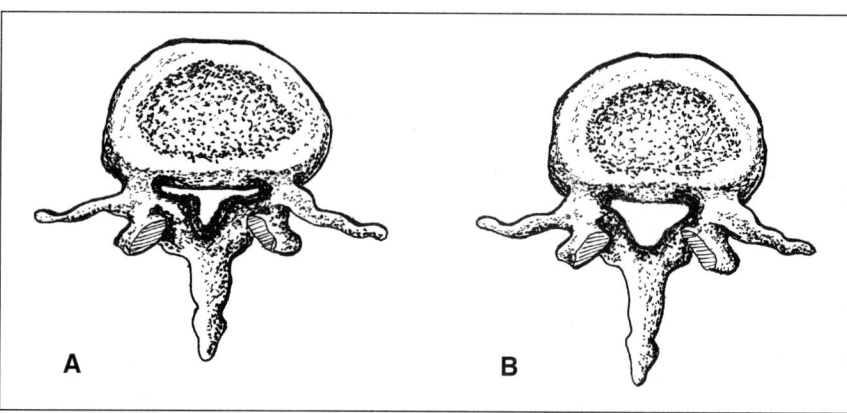

FIGURE 26–1. *Spinal stenosis.* A, A trefoil spinal canal, with reduced diameters, is a frequent predisposing factor of spinal stenosis. Trefoil changes are present through development and become magnified from facet joint hypertrophy, ligamentum flavum hypertrophy, or other impingement mechanism(s). B, A normal spinal canal.

position. Numbness and tingling may be prominent in some patients. The process may be unilateral or bilateral. Characteristics of spinal stenosis are difficulty standing straight and improvement by flexing the lumbar spine. There is an absence of pain while sitting. Patients with advanced disease report lower extremity pain triggered just by standing straight, automatically stoop forward, and avoid lying flat in bed. Patients may have difficulty with activities that require lumbar extension such as walking downstairs, although walking upstairs and bicycling may pose no problem at all. Balance disturbance is prevalent in spinal stenosis.

On physical examination a prominent finding is limitation of lumbar extension. A wide gait and an abnormal Romberg test are often present. Symptoms are characteristically triggered within 30 seconds of lumbar extension. Muscle weakness and reflex loss in the lower extremities may be noted at rest or immediately after bringing up the symptoms by walking. Pulses are usually present, although given the advanced age of the patients they may be absent as a result of atheromatous disease or medial calcification. Interestingly, patients may have both neurogenic and vascular claudication, or the vascular insufficiency may become overt as the neurogenic claudication is surgically relieved. It is estimated that 30% of patients with spinal stenosis have concurrent peripheral vascular disease.

Diagnosis

Summary of Diagnosis

> **SPINAL STENOSIS**
> - Severe lower extremity pain.
> - Neurogenic claudication.
> - Absence of pain when seated.
> - Thigh pain induced within 30 seconds by lumbar extension.
> - Presence of pedal pulses: If absent, check for trophic changes and assess flow by Doppler.
> - Wide-based gait.
> - Romberg sign.
> - Lumbar spine films (spondylosis; primary reduction of lumbar canal diameters; normal in certain cases).
> - MRI or CT of the lumbar spine show the process well. Myelography may also be used.

Natural History

Based on limited data in nonsurgical patients, the course of spinal stenosis is progressive in two-thirds of cases, usually at a very slow pace. The remaining one-third of patients report stable symptoms or some improvement in gait. Late progressive cases may result in an inability to perform activities of daily living, particularly in elderly patients who live alone. Repeated falls occur commonly, with the attendant risk of fractures. Sphincter incontinence and flaccid paraparesis may ultimately occur.

Treatment

Initial cases may be handled conservatively with acetaminophen, lumbar corsets, and back exercises that discour-

---

TABLE 26–6

CAUSES OF SPINAL STENOSIS

CONGENITAL–DEVELOPMENTAL STENOSIS
1. Idiopathic
2. Achondroplasia
3. Hypophosphatemic vitamin D–resistant rickets
4. Morquio's syndrome
5. Conjoined origin of lumbosacral nerve roots
6. Other congenital disorders

ACQUIRED STENOSIS
1. Degenerative (discogenic, spondylolisthesis)
2. Postoperative (laminectomy, fusion, chemonucleolysis, etc.)
3. Posttraumatic
4. Endocrine–metabolic (Cushing, acromegaly, renal osteodystrophy, etc.)
5. Miscellaneous (Paget's disease of bone, ankylosing spondylitis, diffuse idiopathic skeletal hyperostosis, fluorosis, etc.)

COMBINED
1. Developmental plus acquired
2. Cervical plus lumbar (tandem)

Modified from Moreland WW, López-Méndez A, Alarcón GS. Spinal stenosis: A comprehensive review of the literature. Sem Arthritis Rheum 127:127–149, 1989.

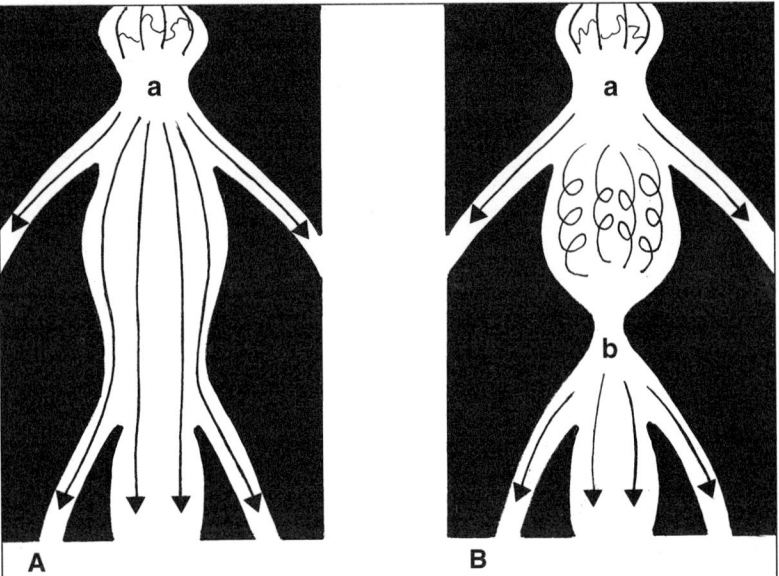

FIGURE 26–2. *Pathophysiology of neurogenic claudication in spinal stenosis.* Single-level central stenosis (A, a) does not cause neurogenic claudication. Two or more levels of central stenosis (B, a plus b) do cause neurogenic claudication, presumably from blood pooling at the entrapped segment. A single level of central stenosis plus a level of lateral recess stenosis cause unilateral neurogenic claudication. (After Porter RW. Central spinal stenosis. Acta Orthop Scand (suppl 251) 64:64–66, 1993.)

age extension of the lumbar spine. This is mainly achieved by strengthening the anterior abdominal musculature. Epidural corticosteroid infiltrations may transiently improve radicular symptoms. They may be used intermittently as the sole form of therapy in patients with significant comorbidity and in those who refuse therapy.

Surgical treatment is indicated in cases with sphincter dysfunction or symptoms that threaten independent living. Preoperative MRI or CT is essential to outline the compressive lesion(s). Surgery involves multilevel laminectomy plus medial facetectomy so that satisfactory release of the compressed dural sac and root(s) is achieved. Fusion is often added in patients with degenerative spondylolysthesis, but its role is controversial; there is substantial morbidity associated with fusion and hospital charges are significantly greater than in patients treated with laminectomy alone. As expected, single-level laminectomy often fails to remove the symptoms.

Expected Response

In Katz's experience, at 7 to 10 years follow-up, 23% of patients had undergone reoperation and 33% continued to experience severe symptoms. However, fully 75% of patients were satisfied with the results of surgery. Worst results are achieved in patients whose main preoperative complaint is low back pain and in patients with significant comorbidity including osteoarthritis, RA, cardiac disease, and chronic bronchopulmonary disease. Patients treated with epidural corticosteroid infiltrations usually have long periods of remission (several months), but symptoms eventually recur.

When to Refer

Patients with suspected spinal stenosis should have the benefit of consultation with a back surgeon. The patient may or may not be offered surgery. Patients who cannot have or refuse surgery should be referred to a pain clinic for possible epidural injection of corticosteroids.

Key Points

> **SPINAL STENOSIS**
> - Spinal stenosis is usually degenerative and therefore affects elderly individuals.
> - Hence there is a high frequency of comorbid conditions.
> - Most cases are slowly progressive.
> - Surgical decompression succeeds in about 75% of patients with degenerative stenosis.
> - Barring severe comorbidity, patients with spinal stenosis should be referred for surgical evaluation.
> - Nonsurgical patients should be offered epidural corticosteroid infiltrations.

Suggested Reading

Katz JN, Dalgas M, Stucki G, et al. Degenerative spinal stenosis. Diagnostic value of the history and physical examination. Arthritis Rheum 38:1236–1241, 1995.

Katz JN, Lipson SJ, Chang LC, et al. Seven to 10 years outcome of decompressive surgery for degenerative lumbar spinal stenosis. Spine 21:92–98, 1996.

Johnson K-E, Rosén I, Udén A. The natural course of lumbar spinal stenosis. Clin Orthop 279:82–86, 1992.

Moreland LW, López-Méndez A, Alarcón GS. Spinal stenosis: A comprehensive review of the literature. Sem Arthritis Rheum 127:127–149, 1989.

Postacchini F. Management of lumbar spinal stenosis. J Bone Joint Surg 78B:154–164, 1996.

Chronic Low Back Pain

Presentation and Progression

An individual presenting low back pain of known or unknown cause that persists, on a seemingly adequate treatment, more than 6 months is said to have chronic low back pain. Underlying conditions include such diverse ailments as sciatica, work-related trauma, spondylolisthesis, spinal stenosis, or one or more surgical procedures for these or other conditions with a sequela of arachnoiditis or epidural scarring.

Patients describe aching lumbar pain, often with radiation to buttocks, and sometimes sciatica, usually triggered by bending or twisting, present day and night. There may be dermatomal or nondermatomal paresthesias. Most patients have been given a back brace. Narcotic dependency is frequently associated. On examination the back is moved reluctantly and with severe pain. Atrophy of paraspinal muscles speaks of disuse atrophy. Lumbar motions are done reluctantly, are very painful, and are often associated with incoordinated muscle contractions. Lower extremities may show a positive straight leg raising test, but more often there is marked, bilateral hamstring muscle contracture. One or more reflexes may be lost. The general appearance is one of physical deconditioning.

Diagnosis

Summary of Diagnosis

> **CHRONIC LOW BACK PAIN**
> - Pain of more than 6 months' duration.
> - Obtain thorough history and perform detailed examination including assessment of depression and fibromyalgia.
> - Review occupational factors.
> - Review available imaging studies.
> - A gadolinium-enhanced MRI provides essential information, particularly in postoperative cases.

Natural History

Expected Outcome

Chronic low back pain patients often receive compensation income or are in the midst of litigation. Narcotic use is frequent. In addition, depression is often present. Treatment of the latter offers a ray of hope. The trend in these patients, however, is to remain unchanged.

Treatment

Methods

Depression and fibromyalgia should be appropriately treated. Any significant leg length discrepancy should be corrected. NSAIDs, often in combination with amitriptyline, cyclobenzaprine, or doxepin, often afford some baseline pain relief. A stable dose of codeine is often useful in chronic low back pain. Periodic epidural blocks with corticosteroid infiltration may afford remarkable relief and improve function. Although facet joints are an important source of pain in many chronic low back pain patients, corticosteroid injection of the facet joints lacked measurable benefit beyond a placebo effect. Likewise, in a randomized trial of traction for nonspecific low back pain in which half of the patients in both the traction group and the sham traction group had had pain for more than 6 months, no demonstrable benefit from traction was shown.

Chronic low back pain patients benefit from attending a back school or a chronic pain clinic. The back school, a concept introduced by neurosurgeons in Sweden, consists of classroom lectures and small-group discussions in which patients are instructed on the anatomic, biomechanical, and epidemiologic aspects of back pain. A pivotal concept in back schools is that patients should take responsibility for the management of their spinal problems. By teaching body mechanics and stressing good body habits, subsequent episodes may be preventable. In chronic pain clinics or units, emphasis is placed on the multidisciplinary treatment of chronic pain as an entity, regardless of its cause. Most patients in chronic pain clinics, however, have chronic low back pain. Most patients arrive at pain facilities unemployed and using large doses of opiates, benzodiazepines, or barbiturates. Treatment includes psychologic support therapies, drug treatments, physiotherapy, nerve blocks, and other modalities used by anesthesiologists. Many patients treated in pain facilities improve and are able to return to some form of gainful employment. In those who fail to improve despite their best wishes and efforts a cord stimulator should be offered, first with an external and then with an implanted device.

When to Refer

Patients with chronic low back pain should be referred to a rheumatologist or back surgeon for reevaluation. Attendance at a back school may be useful. Long-term care of chronic low back pain patients is best done concurrently with a pain unit.

Key Points

> **CHRONIC LOW BACK PAIN**
> - Reassess diagnosis.
> - Identify treatable components, in particular depression, fibromyalgia, and gross leg length discrepancy.
> - If available, offer attendance at a back school.
> - Resilient cases, provided that the patient has a genuine desire to improve, should be referred to a pain service.

Suggested Reading

Beurskens AJ, de Vet HC, Koke AJ, et al. Efficacy of traction for non-specific low back pain: A randomised clinical trial. Lancet 346:1596–1600, 1995.

Bogduk N. Spine update: Epidural steroids. Spine 20:845–848, 1995.

Borenstein DG, Wiesel SW, Boden SD. Pain clinics. Low Back Pain. Medical Diagnosis and Comprehensive Management, 2nd ed. W.B. Saunders, Philadelphia, 676–680, 1995.

Carette S, Marcoux S, Truchon R, et al. A controlled trial of corticosteroid injections into facet joints for chronic low back pain. N Engl J Med 325:1002–1007, 1991.

Katz JN, Katz NP. Lumbar spine disease. In: Weisman MH, Weinblatt ME (eds) Treatment of the Rheumatic Diseases. W.B. Saunders, Philadelphia, 11–13, 1995.

Schwarzer AC, Wang S-C, Bogduk N, et al. Prevalence and clinical features of lumbar zygapophyseal joint pain: A study in an Australian population with chronic low back pain. Ann Rheum Dis 54:100–106, 1995.

CHAPTER 27

Hip Pain

Lay individuals, when asked where the hip is, usually point somewhere between the anterior/superior iliac spine and the greater trochanter. It should therefore be no surprise when patients with pain in the greater trochanter region complain of "hip pain." The potential for confusion is further increased by pain radiation to the knee, anterior thigh, or buttock in conditions affecting the coxofemoral joint. It is therefore important that a patient's words not be taken at face value. If patients report having hip pain, the next question should be, show me where it hurts. If they point to the side (Table 27–1), chances are that the condition will be trochanteric bursitis; to the buttock, radiating lumbar pain or sacroiliac joint pain; to the anterolateral thigh, meralgia paresthetica; and to the groin and anterior thigh, or groin and buttock, or groin and knee, a coxofemoral joint condition, iliopsoas tendinitis (usually calcific), or iliopsoas bursitis.

Trochanteric Bursitis

No one knows with certainty whether the bursa itself is involved in the usual form of this syndrome. True, there are documented cases of trochanteric bursitis due to tuberculosis, pyogenic infection, crystal deposits (CPPD, basic calcium crystals), and occasional cases of trauma. But these rare cases are not the subject of this discussion. At any rate, pain is experienced at the bursal site and no attempt is made to debunk the condition, indeed a very frequent one in clinical practice.

Presentation and Progression

Trochanteric bursitis occurs in situations of repetitive strain on the gluteus medius and minimus muscles. These muscles attach to the lateral and anterior greater trochanter, respectively. There are bursae between the gluteus maximus and the underlying greater trochanter and between the gluteus medius and minimus. Stress may result from a faulty gait such as in leg length discrepancy (a contralateral short leg); in painful conditions of the foot, knee, and hip; and in asymmetries caused by nerve paralysis and scoliosis. In addition, many cases of trochanteric bursitis occur in association with spine disorders, particularly lumbar spondylosis and dorsal kyphosis.

Patients typically complain of lateral hip pain (Figure 27–1) present on walking and also while lying in bed on the affected side. On examination, flexion, extension, and rotations of the hip are full and painless except when the syndrome is caused by coxofemoral joint disease. Resisted hip abduction reproduces the pain in some cases. The typical finding is point tenderness usually at the posterior corner of the greater trochanter. This is easily identified while the patient is lying on the opposite side.

First, palpate the femur from distal to proximal. Where the bone ends, that is the greater trochanter. Now gently walk the digits back, exerting some pressure. Exquisite tenderness will be elicited at the posterior corner of the greater trochanter. The examination is not complete if the musculoskeletal system has not been explored in general including fibromyalgic tender points, back, hips, knees, ankles, feet, and leg length.

Unusually, the trochanteric bursa may be felt distended and painful. These cases are rare but may occur as a result of infection (see earlier) or trauma. It is of utmost importance to remember that the proximal lower extremity is a site of predilection for soft tissue sarcomas.

Diagnosis

Summary of Diagnosis

> **TROCHANTERIC BURSITIS**
> - Pain in the lateral hip region.
> - Absence of paresthesia.
> - Absence of a palpable mass (if present, consider true bursitis and sarcoma).

TABLE 27–1
DIFFERENTIAL DIAGNOSIS OF LATERAL HIP PAIN

Adiposa dolorosa	Prominent panniculus; tender to pinching
Fibromyalgia	Tenderness contralaterally and elsewhere in fibromyalgic points
Hip disease, including stress fracture* and osteonecrosis*	Pain is with all directions of motion; passive limitation usually present
Trochanteric bursitis	Greater trochanter tenderness usually at the posterior corner
Strain of abductor muscles	Tenderness proximal to trochanter; resisted abduction painful
Spinal disease	Pain triggered by motion, usually hyperextension
Compressive neuropathy of subcostal or iliohypogastric nerve	Burning quality; suspect subcostal in pronounced scoliosis; iliohypogastric if there is reproduction with digital nerve compression†
Herpes zoster	The typical rash may be delayed days to 2 weeks

*Hip limitation may be initially minimal or nil.
†Tenderness at the superior margin of iliac crest 10 cm posterior to the anterior superior iliac spine.

- Tenderness at greater trochanter.
- Pain on leaning on the affected side.
- Unusually, pain on resisted hip abduction.
- X-rays are indicated if there are reasons to suspect acute calcific tendinitis or a structural problem of the coxofemoral joint.

Natural History

Trochanteric bursitis is a secondary syndrome rather than a discrete condition and its course parallels its cause; thus, symptoms will persist in uncorrected knee osteoarthritis, plantar wart, and leg length discrepancy, to name some of its causes.

Treatment

Methods

Treatment of trochanteric bursitis includes local measures for symptom relief, and treatment of the condition resulting in gluteus medius and minimus strain to prevent recurrences. Local treatment is by corticosteroid infiltration. Technical aspects of the procedure are described in the appendix. In all patients the cause leading to the process must be sought. This includes examination of the back for scoliosis; pelvis level and lower extremity measurements to detect leg length discrepancy; hip, knee, ankle, and subtalar joint examination for dysfunction; and examination of the plantar surface for nodules, warts, and so on.

Expected Response

Improvement, lasting weeks to months, can be confidently expected after corticosteroid infiltration. As with any corticosteroid infiltration, days must elapse until a definite response is seen. The initial response to the xylocaine infiltration usually forecasts the response to the steroids. Concurrently, measures should be taken to treat, if possible, the underlying process: for example, a shoe lift for a significantly shorter leg, quadriceps strengthening exercises for knee pain, or foot surgery for a painful bunion. With one or two injections 2 weeks apart, over 75% of patients become asymptomatic and most of the remaining patients improve. Approximately 25% of cases recur. Recurrence of symptoms suggests that an underlying condition has been overlooked.

When to Refer

Assessment and initial injection treatment fall well into the domain of primary care physicians. However, if the underlying process cannot be determined, or if after presumed correction the process recurs, consultation with a rheumatologist or an orthopedic surgeon is in order.

Key Points

TROCHANTERIC BURSITIS

- Several mimicking conditions must be excluded, in particular lumbosacral spine conditions and compressive neuropathies (iliohypogastric nerve, subcostal nerve).
- Seek an underlying musculoskeletal disturbance involving the spine, pelvis, or lower extremities.
- Injection treatment is highly effective in the short term, but long-term improvement requires correction or palliation of the underlying problem.

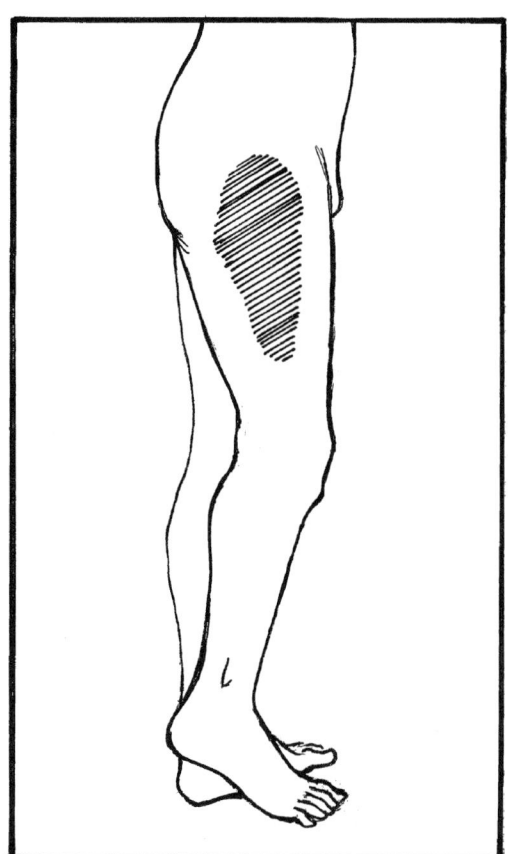

FIGURE 27–1. *Typical location of pain in trochanteric bursitis syndrome.* This is also a frequent pain radiation site for a lumbar spine lesion, various nerve compression syndromes, and hip disease, particularly in osteonecrosis of the femoral head (see text).

Suggested Reading

Collée G, Dijkmans BAC, Vandenbroucke JP, et al. Greater trochanteric pain syndrome (trochanteric bursitis) in low back pain. Scand J Rheumatol 20:262–266, 1991.

Krout RM, Anderson TP. Trochanteric bursitis: Management. Arch Phys Med Rehab 40:8–14, 1959.

Little H. Trochanteric bursitis: A common cause of pelvic girdle pain. Can Med Assoc J 120:456–458, 1979.

Rasmussen K-JE, Fano N. Trochanteric bursitis. Treatment by corticosteroid injection. Scand J Rheumatol 14:417–420, 1985.

Rehm-Graves S, Weinstein AJ, Calabrese LH, et al. Tuberculosis of the greater trochanteric bursa. Arthritis Rheum 26:77–81, 1983.

Traycoff RB. "Pseudothrocanteric bursitis": The differential diagnosis of lateral hip pain. J Rheumatol 18:1810–1812, 1991.

Meralgia Paresthetica

Presentation and Progression

Cause

Meralgia paresthetica (Gr. *meros* = thigh, *algos* = pain) represents a compression neuropathy of the lateral femoral cutaneous nerve (L2 predominantly), a purely sensory nerve. Compression may occur at the nerve's exit from the pelvis behind the inguinal ligament just medial to the anterior superior iliac spine or elsewhere in its spinal, foraminal, retroperitoneal, abdominal, pelvic, or thigh course. Causes include a gravid uterus, massive obesity (particularly with recent weight gain), ascites, local trauma such as laparoscopic herniorrhaphy, a tight belt, and a thick wallet. In many cases the process is unexplained. Diabetes should be ruled out when no cause is found. Multiple sclerosis has eventually surfaced in some of these patients.

The condition is usually unilateral. Patients complain of numbness, tingling, and burning pain over the anterolateral aspect of one thigh. Symptoms may be mild and only surface upon a comprehensive systems review. Findings include decreased pain or touch perception within the symptomatic area and in some patients local tenderness medial to the anterior superior iliac spine. A true Tinel sign with reproduction of sensory symptoms is rare.

Diagnosis

Summary of Diagnosis

> **MERALGIA PARESTHETICA**
> - Paresthesias in anterolateral thigh.
> - Point tenderness medial to anterior superior iliac spine.
> - Hypoesthesia within the paresthetic area.
> - Consider clinically spinal, retroperitoneal, abdominal, and pelvic disease, as well as other causes of neuropathy.

Natural History

Meralgia paresthetica has a protracted course: several months to years. There are no major complications from the condition.

Treatment

Treatment of meralgia paresthetica should be aimed at removing its cause such as weight reduction in obese patients. Local infiltration with xylocaine, followed by a long-acting corticosteroid, may be tried. The site of injection is 1 cm medial to the anterior superior iliac spine. Some authors recommend injecting the deep fascia 4 cm distal to this point. Neurolysis and neurectomy may be tried in refractory cases. Results of surgery are unpredictable.

When to Refer

Patients should be referred to a neurologist or orthopedic surgeon if symptoms are annoying and treatment is required. Also, referral should be implemented when there is reason to suspect that the cause of compression is pelvic, abdominal, retroperitoneal, or intraspinal.

Key Points

> **MERALGIA PARESTHETICA**
> - Symptoms are usually mild.
> - The condition resolves spontaneously in more than half of patients.
> - Metabolic neuropathy; pelvic, abdominal, or retroperitoneal compression; and spinal disease may masquerade for meralgia paresthetica.
> - Treatment includes removal of compression (weight reduction), local infiltration, and in rare cases decompressive surgery.

Suggested Reading

Deal CL, Canoso JJ. Meralgia paresthetica in patients with a big abdomen [Letter]. Ann Intern Med 96:787–788, 1982.

Ecker AD, Woltman HW. Meralgia paresthetica. A report of one hundred and fifty cases. JAMA 110:1650–1652, 1938.

Kitchen C, Simpson J. Meralgia paresthetica. A review of 67 patients. Acta Neurol Scand 48:547–555, 1972.

Iliopsoas Bursitis

The iliopsoas bursa, the largest bursa in humans, separates the anterior aspect of the coxofemoral joint from the iliopsoas muscle. In children and young adults, hip joint and bursa are not connected. However, by the third decade of life, rents appear in the joint capsule that allow communication between both cavities in 15% to 20% of normal individuals.

Presentation and Progression

Cause

Inflammation of the iliopsoas bursa may be primary as a result of trauma but more frequently occurs when a connection with the joint exists in a patient with hip joint pathology. Under these circumstances the bursa may become distended and may participate in the pathologic process affecting the joint. Thus, distension of the iliopsoas bursa may be expected to occur in patients with coxofemoral osteoarthritis, RA, PVNS, synovial chondromatosis, septic infection, TB, and so on.

Patients with primary, irritative iliopsoas bursitis present groin pain that sometimes radiates to buttock or anterior thigh. In these cases, which resemble coxofemoral arthritis, there are no symptoms with passive rotations, but passive flexion triggers groin pain (Table 27–2).

More common, however, is the distension of the iliopsoas bursa in patients with hip disease. These patients will have findings of coxofemoral arthritis, in particular pain and restriction of motion in all hip motions, and, in addition, the mass effects of the distended bursa.

Distensions, if small, may be asymptomatic. Larger disten-

TABLE 27–2

ILIOPSOAS BURSITIS: DIFFERENTIATION FROM ILIOPSOAS TENDINITIS AND HIP DISEASE

	Pain Triggered by:	
	Passive Motion	Resisted Motion
Bursitis	Flexion, internal rotation	0
Tendinitis	0	Flexion, external rotation
Hip	All motions	0

After Fortin L, Bélanger R. Bursitis of the iliopsoas: Four cases with pain as the only clinical indicator. J Rheumatol 22:1971–1973, 1995.

sions may compress vascular and neural structures in the femoral triangle, or the bursa may progress proximally and cause compression in pelvic organs. Thus, iliopsoas bursitis may cause leg edema by venous and lymphatic compression, ischemia by femoral artery compression, and quadriceps weakness and sensory findings in the anterior thigh from compression of the femoral nerve. Proximally migrating bursae may compress the bladder and other pelvic structures.

Diagnosis

Summary of Diagnosis

ILIOPSOAS BURSITIS

Irritative
- Pain in groin, buttock, anterior thigh.
- No pain on rotations or resisted flexion and external rotation.
- Reproduction of pain with passive flexion.

Effusive
- Asymptomatic.
- Edema, ischemia, femoral nerve paralysis, or pelvic organ compression in an individual with coxofemoral joint disease.
- Documentation by ECHO, CT, or MRI that shows cystic collection in front of coxofemoral joint.

Natural History

Expected Outcome

In irritative bursitis symptoms may resolve with relative rest and anti-inflammatories, but a corticosteroid infiltration may be required if symptoms are protracted.

Complications of iliopsoas bursa distensions have already been mentioned: leg edema, ischemic lower extremity symptoms, femoral nerve paralysis, and intrapelvic migration with organ compression, usually the bladder.

Treatment

Methods

Irritative iliopsoas bursitis triggered by trauma or unaccustomed activities usually improves with partial rest, nonsteroidal anti-inflammatories, and avoidance of the initial cause. Refractory cases may be treated with corticosteroid infiltration. This should be administered under fluoroscopic control by an orthopedic surgeon or radiologist. Results of this procedure are excellent. Effusive iliopsoas bursitis is treated by treating the hip joint condition that causes distension of the bursa. Treatment, depending on the condition, may include systemic medications and surgery. Special note should be made of septic arthritis with purulent distension of the bursa. Since septic arthritis of the hip is often drained posteriorly, a bursal abscess may be missed. It is therefore important, prior to surgery, to assess the presence of iliopsoas bursitis by an appropriate imaging procedure.

When to Refer

Patients with irritative iliopsoas bursitis should be treated initially by primary care physicians. They should be particularly careful not to miss hip joint disease. A failure to improve requires consultation with a rheumatologist or an orthopedic surgeon and if injection treatment is deemed necessary, the procedure should be performed by someone proficient with hip aspirations under fluoroscopic control, usually a radiologist or an orthopedic surgeon. Patients with compressive bursitis should be evaluated by a rheumatologist and an orthopedic surgeon. The main task in these patients is to establish the etiology of the underlying hip disease.

Key Points

ILIOPSOAS BURSITIS

- The condition may present with pain resembling hip joint disease.
- These cases, which are due to trauma, respond to rest plus anti-inflammatory medications or to a corticosteroid infiltration.
- In most cases, however, symptoms reveal vascular or neurologic compression in the proximal thigh or compression of pelvic organs by a distended bursa.
- The bursal cyst may be documented by ECHO, CT, or MRI.
- Treatment of iliopsoas bursal distension is the treatment of the hip joint disease that causes the bursal cyst.

Suggested Reading

Fortin L, Bélanger R. Bursitis of the iliopsoas: Four cases with pain as the only clinical indicator. J Rheumatol 22:1971–1973, 1995.

Letorneau L, Dessureault M, Carette S. Rheumatoid iliopsoas bursitis presenting as unilateral femoral nerve palsy. J Rheumatol 18:462–463, 1991.

Meaney JF, Cassar-Pullicino VN, Etherington R, et al. Ilio-psoas bursa enlargement. Clin Radiol 45:161–168, 1992.

Toohey AK, LaSalle TL, Martínez S, et al. Iliopsoas bursitis: Clinical features, radiographic findings, and disease associations. Sem Arthritis Rheum 20:41–47, 1990.

Underwood PL, McLeod RA, Ginsburg WW. The varied clinical manifestations of iliopsoas bursitis. J Rheumatol 15:1683–1685, 1988.

CHAPTER 28

Knee Pain

The Knee

The knee is the largest joint in the economy. Knee motion is only apparently simple. In addition to flexion and extension, there is gliding, rolling, and a complex internal rotation of the femur in reference to the tibia as full extension is approached. In this position the femoral condyles are "screwed home," implying that all of the ligaments of the knee are tight. The knee joint involves three well-defined compartments: the patellofemoral, the medial tibiofemoral, and the lateral tibiofemoral. The patella is in close contact with the femoral condyles only in flexion. Because there is often a valgus angulation, particularly in women, the lateral femoral condyle must be steeper than the medial to prevent lateral patellar subluxation in full flexion. An abnormally flat lateral condyle is often present in individuals who habitually sublux the patella. The patella, a sesamoid bone, is at the apex of the extensor apparatus of the knee. Its proximal portion gives insertion to the quadriceps tendon, and its lower pole is firmly anchored to the tibial tuberosity by the patellar ligament. The prepatellar and the pretendinous bursae are subcutaneous synovial sacs placed anterior to the patella and the patellar tendon, respectively. The convex medial and lateral femoral condyles articulate with the flat tibial tuberosities with the help of two spacers, the medial and the lateral menisci. The menisci, in addition to being a potential source of trouble, are essential in providing the minimal congruence present in the medial and lateral tibiofemoral joints. Understandably, meniscal removal leads to premature compartmental osteoarthritis. Toward their free edge, menisci are avascular and arregenerative. Peripherally, however, ample vascularity received from their capsular attachment assures a tendency to heal. The anterior and the posterior cruciate ligaments, which are placed between the medial and lateral tibiofemoral compartments, check the anterior and the posterior sliding of the tibia on the femur, respectively. Damage to these ligaments, which often accompanies meniscal tears, results in an unstable knee. The knee synovium, which forms a single cavity for the three compartments, has a complex arrangement. In addition to enclosing the articulating surfaces, there are medial and lateral parapatellar expansions, plus a suprapatellar expansion (suprapatellar pouch) that extends proximally 4–6 cm beneath the quadriceps tendon. Given this arrangement, synovial effusions bulge medial, lateral, and proximal to the patella in the form of an inverted U. Knee stability is provided by the extensor apparatus, intraarticular structures such as the menisci and cruciate ligaments, and lateral ligaments that are essential in assuring lateral stability to the joint. The lateral (fibular) collateral ligament is a cordlike structure that extends from the lateral femoral epicondyle to the apex of the fibula. The medial collateral ligament is fanlike and extends from the medial femoral epicondyle to the anteromedial tibia and the medial meniscus. A small bursa is normally placed between this ligament and the joint line.

Important landmarks in the knee region include, *anteriorly* and from proximal to distal, the distal bellies of the vastus lateralis and vastus medialis (the latter is essential to complete knee extension and is the first muscle to waste upon knee immobilization), both poles of the patella, the patellar ligament, and the tibial tuberosity. Fibrous bands from the vastus lateralis attach to the outer edge of the patella, the lateral patellar retinaculum. *Laterally* (knee semiflexed), and from front to back, landmarks in the knee region include the convex rim of the anterior condylar surface; the lateral surface of the femoral condyle with the lateral epicondyle (insertion of the fibular collateral ligament); and the articular cleft, which ends as the femoral condyle meets the tibia under the collateral ligament. The iliotibial tract, which sends fibers to the lateral patellar retinaculum and attaches at Gerdy's tubercle in the anterolateral tibial condyle, is best identified upon flexion-extension movements. In extension, the anterior edge of the iliotibial band covers the lateral epicondyle while in flexion, as the edge moves posteriorly, the lateral epicondyle becomes uncovered. Posterolaterally, the biceps femoris tendon stands out, tenting the skin, as it attaches to the head of the fibula. *Medially,* the articular cleft between the tibial and femoral condyles leads to the medial meniscus. About 5 cm distal to this point the pes anserinus (sartorius, gracilis, and semimembranosus tendons) attaches to the upper medial tibia. This is the site of pain in anserine bursitis. *Posteriorly,* in extension, bulging popliteal fat should not be confused with a Baker's cyst. Proximally, the rhomboid popliteal space is bound by the biceps femoris laterally and the semimembranosus and semitendinosus medially. Distally, the space is bound by the lateral and the medial heads of the gastrocnemius. The popliteal artery pulse is felt at the center of the popliteal space. The tibial nerve, which continues the sciatic nerve, lies lateral to the popliteal artery. Baker's cysts, which occur by distension of a bursa placed between the medial gastrocnemius and the semimembranosus, bulge in the medial one-third of the popliteal space. In contrast, popliteal artery aneurysms bulge at the midline of the popliteal space. Table 28–1 lists common knee conditions according to location.

Iliotibial Tract Syndrome

The iliotibial tract is a thick condensation of the fascia lata that extends from the iliac bone to the upper tibia. There are proximal contributions to the tract from the gluteus maximus posteriorly and from the tensor fascia lata anteriorly.

TABLE 28-1
KNEE PAIN

ANTERIOR

Prepatellar or pretendinous bursitis	Tight lateral retinaculum
Quadriceps tendon tendinitis	Patellar tendon tendinitis
Chondromalacia patella	Osgood-Schlatter disease
Patellofemoral osteoarthritis	Infrapatellar bursitis
Plica medio patellaris	Hoffa's body inflammation

MEDIAL

Anserine bursitis	Medial (tibial) collateral tendon bursitis (no-name, no-fame bursa)
Medial meniscus tears	Semimembranosus bursitis

LATERAL

Iliotibial tract syndrome	Lateral meniscus tears and cysts
Bicipital tendon tendinitis	Popliteal tendon bursitis (posterolateral)

POSTERIOR (pain and/or mass)

Baker's cysts	Mucoid degeneration of popliteal artery wall
Thrombophlebitis	Ganglia
Popliteal artery aneurysms	Sarcomas

Distal insertions include the lateral patellar retinaculum and the anterior surface of the lateral tibial condyle at Gerdy's tubercle. The tract's function is complex; it acts to maintain the knee in the extended position and stabilizes the knee when weight is brought to bear on the semiflexed knee.

Presentation and Progression

In athletes, particularly in long-distance runners, constant flexion/extension movements cause excessive friction between the iliotibial tract and the femoral condyle and result in pain and localized tenderness in the lateral knee 2 cm proximal to the joint line. Pain is increased by standing with the knee 30 degrees flexed. Maneuvers to assess the iliotibial tract may reveal excessive tension. One such maneuver is the Ober test in which the patient lies on the examining table on the unaffected side. Standing behind the patient, the examiner abducts and extends the affected thigh with the knee flexed 90 degrees. Then, he or she gently drops the knee while still holding the foot. If the iliotibial band is normal, the thigh drops. If the iliotibial band is contractured, the thigh remains in abduction.

Diagnosis

Summary of Diagnosis

> **ILIOTIBIAL TRACT SYNDROME**
>
> - Pain in the lateral knee with tenderness 2 cm proximal to articular line.
> - Rarely, lateral trochanteric pain.
> - The Ober's maneuver may be positive in patients with a tight iliotibial tract.
> - X-rays or other imaging studies are unnecessary.

Natural History

Iliotibial tract syndrome is usually sports related. Improvement is expected with activity modification or infiltration.

Treatment

Methods

Treatment of the iliotibial tract syndrome consists of temporarily halting or decreasing the offending activity, applying local heat, and a NSAID for 1 to 2 weeks. If rapid improvement is desired, particularly in the competitive athlete, a corticosteroid infiltration may be administered. Ancillary treatment includes stretching the iliotibial tract and strengthening the abductor muscles.

Expected Response

Treated conservatively (without infiltration), the process is expected to subside in 2 to 3 weeks. With a corticosteroid infiltration, improvement is rapid, usually within 1 week.

When to Refer

Because lateral knee pain may be due to other lesions such as a lateral meniscal rupture, which has the potential to induce secondary osteoarthritis, and popliteal tenosynovitis, patients with presumed iliotibial tract syndrome failing to improve with a 3 week course of conservative therapy should have the benefit of orthopedic consultation to corroborate diagnosis and for possible corticosteroid infiltration.

Key Points

> **ILIOTIBIAL TRACT SYNDROME**
>
> - The condition causes lateral knee pain.
> - Most cases are due to excessive running.
> - A tight iliotibial tract may be shown in some of the patients.
> - Conditions to be excluded include bicipital tendinitis, a lateral meniscus tear, a lateral meniscal cyst, and popliteus tenosynovitis.
> - Patients usually improve with activity modification, local heat, a NSAID, and physical therapy to lengthen a shortened iliotibial tract.
> - Recalcitrant cases should be referred to an orthopedic surgeon to rule out alternative diagnoses and for a corticosteroid infiltration if diagnosis is confirmed.

Suggested Reading

James SL. Running injuries to the knee. J Am Acad Orthop Surg 3:309–318, 1995.

Kaplan EB. The iliotibial tract. Clinical and morphologic significance. J Bone Joint Surg 40A:817–832, 1958.

Orchard JW, Fricker PA, Abud AT, Mason BR. Biomechanics of iliotibial band friction syndrome in runners. Am J Sports Med 24:375–379, 1996.

Renne JW. The iliotibial band friction syndrome. J Bone Joint Surg 57A:1110–1111, 1975.

Prepatellar Bursitis

The subcutaneous prepatellar bursa is superficially placed in the anterior knee. In most instances, the bursa partially overlies the patella and the patellar tendon. Some patients exhibit two discrete bursae, one prepatellar and the other pretendinous.

Presentation and Progression

The condition occurs predominantly in individuals who recurrently traumatize the prepatellar region. This includes occupations such as carpet installers, roofers, and miners. The condition is also common in wrestlers as well as in individuals who repeatedly kneel, for example, to pray. Patients complain of pain, swelling, and tenderness in the anterior knee. Traumatic bursitis causes fairly large, relative painless effusions. In acute cases, bacterial infection and gout are the predominant etiology. Bursal gout may be the first manifestation of the disease; it may occur recurrently or, rarely, affect simultaneously both sides. Alcoholism is frequently encountered in patients with gouty and septic bursitis, and diabetes is an important predisposing factor in septic bursitis (approximately 60% of patients). Inflammatory changes may extend diffusely around the anterior knee as to simulate acute knee arthritis. An important differential point is that individuals with acute prepatellar bursitis keep the knee in full extension or tolerate without pain the extended position.

Concurrent knee joint effusions may occur in two circumstances. One is gout in which acute bursitis and acute arthritis occasionally coexist, resulting in combined physical findings of acute bursitis and acute arthritis. More frequently, especially in cases of septic prepatellar bursitis, a sympathetic knee effusion develops. These effusions are characteristically noninflammatory. The question often arises as to whether or not these effusions should be aspirated. In the author's opinion, if passive knee extension is free and painless in a conscious patient, a diagnosis of sympathetic effusion can legitimately be made. Knee aspiration in these patients is not only unnecessary but carries the risk of infecting the joint. In rheumatoid arthritis, in which olecranon bursitis is common, prepatellar bursitis is rare and occurs almost exclusively in patients with prepatellar rheumatoid nodules, which are rare to begin with.

Diagnosis

Summary of Diagnosis

> **PREPATELLAR BURSITIS**
> - Prepatellar or pretendinous swelling.
> - Fluctuation.
> - Redness and marked tenderness suggest infection or gout.
> - X-rays are unnecessary.
> - Aspirate to diagnose bacterial infection, gout, or trauma by the characteristics of the fluid.

Natural History

Traumatic prepatellar bursitis, diagnosed by a history of recurrent trauma, compatible physical findings, and negative bursal fluid culture and crystal search, spontaneously improves by avoiding kneeling. Gouty bursitis improves spontaneously over the course of several days to weeks; the course of the condition is dramatically shortened by appropriate gout therapy. Septic bursitis, even with optimal treatment, has a very slow resolution. Complications may occur in septic bursitis but are rare.

Treatment

Traumatic Bursitis

Treatment includes initial diagnostic aspiration to exclude other etiologies, and a careful assessment of occupational and other factors that could be determining recurrent local trauma. Unavoidable trauma may be prevented with the use of knee pads. Spontaneous regression of the process occurs over several weeks or a few months. If a speedier recovery is requested, local injection of corticosteroids may be attempted (see appendix). Only the less active steroid preparations should be used, such as methylprednisolone acetate 20 mg, to avoid skin atrophy. Because septic prepatellar bursitis (similar to septic olecranon bursitis) may occur with unimpressive clinical and bursal fluid findings, the procedure should be delayed until a negative fluid culture result is on record. Inadvertent corticosteroid injection in a case of septic bursitis may result in sudden deterioration of the process.

Gouty Bursitis

Treatment is as discussed for gout. Avoidance of local trauma must be emphasized.

Septic Bursitis

Septic prepatellar bursitis should be considered a more serious process than its olecranon bursa counterpart. Hospitalization for a period of 3 to 5 days is justified in most cases to immobilize the knee, administer parenteral antibiotics, and ascertain that the process is being brought under control. Knee immobilization is best achieved with a posterior plaster splint. Since 85% of cases are due to *S. aureus* and the remaining cases are mostly streptococcal, initial treatment with intravenous oxacillin 8 to 12 g/day or a first-generation cephalosporin is most adequate. Bursal drainage may be done by repeated puncture, but in the author's experience is better achieved with a pigtail catheter introduced under ECHO or CT control, or surgically.

In most cases marked improvement occurs in 48 to 72 hours. By the fourth day parenteral antibiotics may be discontinued and oral antibiotics started, usually dicloxacillin 2 g per day. About 30% of patients show persistent sterile effusions that may persist for up to 3 months. For their treatment patients should be encouraged to avoid local trauma.

Complications of septic prepatellar bursitis are rare. They include bacteremia in less than 5% of cases, an anterior compartmental syndrome, fistulization, and cortical patellar osteomyelitis, all of them extremely rare.

When to Refer

Aspiration of the prepatellar bursa is easy when a large effusion is present (as in most cases of traumatic bursitis) but may be very difficult in acute septic or gouty bursitis. In these cases extensive soft tissue inflammation tends to hide bursal effusion. The help of a rheumatologist may be instrumental in securing diagnosis of these patients. Traumatic and gouty prepatellar bursitis fall into the domain of primary care medicine. Similarly, once diagnosed, septic prepatellar bursitis may be treated by the primary care physician with the help of a radiologist to introduce the catheter or an orthopedic surgeon for bursal drainage.

Key Points

PREPATELLAR BURSITIS

- Is often the result of recurrent local trauma.
- Traumatic bursitis tends to be subacute or chronic; septic and gouty bursitis tends to be acute or subacute.
- Diabetes and alcoholism are frequent associations of septic bursitis.
- Acute arthritis may be mimicked. However, in prepatellar bursitis, knee extension is minimally or not at all impaired.
- Septic prepatellar bursitis is a more serious and difficult to treat condition than its olecranon bursa counterpart. It usually requires hospitalization, catheter or surgical drainage, and parenteral antibiotics.

Suggested Reading

Canoso JJ. Bursal membrane and fluid. In: Cohen AS (ed) Laboratory Diagnosis in the Rheumatic Diseases, 3rd ed. Grune & Stratton, Orlando, 79–81, 1986.
Canoso JJ, Barza M. Soft tissue infections. Clin Rheum Dis 19:293–309, 1993.
Ho G Jr, Tice AD, Kaplan SR. Septic bursitis in the prepatellar and olecranon bursae. An analysis of 25 cases. Ann Intern Med 88:21–27, 1978.
Strickland RW, Raskin RJ, Welton RC. Sympathetic synovial effusions associated with septic arthritis and bursitis. Arthritis Rheum 28:941–943, 1985.
Wilson-McDonald J. Management and outcome of infective prepatellar bursitis. Postgrad Med J 63:851–853, 1987.

Anterior Knee Pain

Cause

In addition to prepatellar bursitis, which is an obvious diagnosis on examination, several conditions should be considered in patients with anterior knee pain. A first point in the analysis is to determine whether the patient complains of patellar or parapatellar pain, or if pain location is in the region of the patellar tendon. Patellar pain is sharply localized to the patella and may or may not have medial extension. A common complaint in these patients is difficulty walking downstairs; each down step implies deceleration, which acutely loads the patellofemoral joint. Coarse patellofemoral crepitation is often present on flexion/extension movements, particularly in older patients. In young individuals, usually women, crepitus may be fine or absent.

A patellar origin of the pain may be further documented by one of two maneuvers. In the first, known as the "shrug sign," the patient is asked to relax the knee. Once relaxed (the expectation of pain may preclude examination of the contralateral knee), the patella is gently displaced distally where it is firmly held between the examiner's thumb and index fingers. Finally, while applying some downward pressure, the patient is asked to contract the quadriceps. Acute pain experienced while the patella tracks proximally on the femoral condyles confirms patellofemoral pain.

The second maneuver, known as the sustained knee flexion test, consists in keeping the patient's knee acutely flexed for 1 minute (Figure 28–1). Mounting anterior pain indicates patellar pathology.

Patellar pain in young individuals is usually from a self-limited condition, *chondromalacia patella*. Diffuse anterior knee pain may also be caused by *excessive lateral pressure* by the lateral retinaculum, the fibers of the vastus lateralis that attach in the patella.

Excessive retinacular tightness can be identified with the following maneuver: The examiner stabilizes the medial border of the patella with fingers of both hands while the thumbs are used to pull up the lateral patella, as if raising it out of the trochlea, examining the degree of mobility present. If the lateral patellar border cannot be brought to the horizontal plane, there is excessive retinacular tightness.

Patellar instability is a further cause of anterior knee pain. Maltracking is suggested by the "J sign," which indicates lateral placement or lateral displacement of the patella at termination of extension. With the knee positioned at 30 degrees flexion, lateral displacement when pressure is applied on the medial patella is unequivocal evidence of patellar instability.

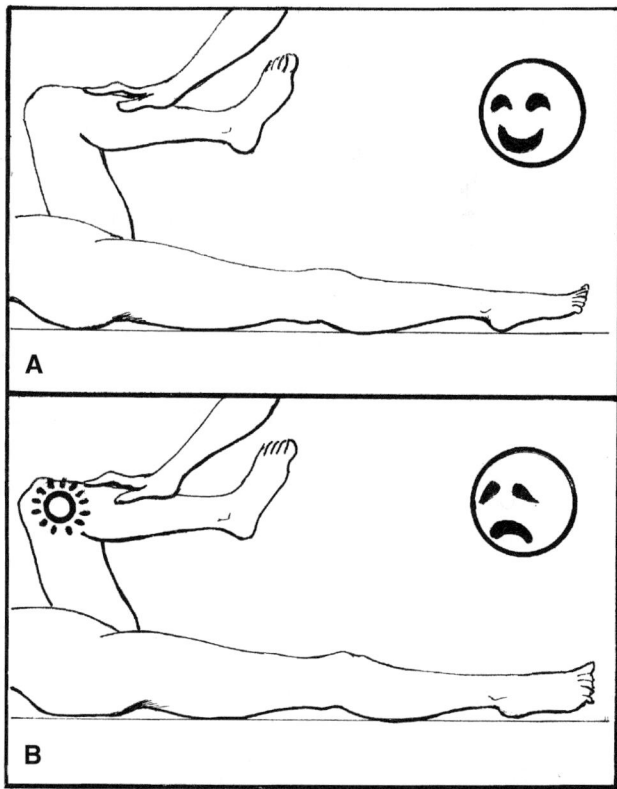

FIGURE 28–1. *The sustained flexion test.* The knee is brought passively to maximal flexion. After 15 to 30 seconds the knee becomes increasingly painful. *A,* Normal individual. *B,* Individual with chondromalacia patella, showing pain. (After Arnoldi K. Patellar pain syndromes [chondromalacia patellae]. Acta Orthop Scand Suppl 261, 65:46–55, 1994.)

In older individuals, however, patellar pain is an indication of *patellofemoral osteoarthritis*, which is a progressive condition. Flexion of the knee while the examiner places posteriorly directed pressure on the patella yields important information about the location of the patellofemoral joint damage: Distal articular lesions will be more manifest in early flexion; proximal articular lesions will cause pain farther into flexion. Exercise-related medial parapatellar pain that may involve the entire medial femoral condyle or generalize, with a click noted upon flexion/extension movements, may be caused by a thickened medial parapatellar plica, a vestigial synovial fold that due to overuse or other factors develops inflammation and fibrosis. This syndrome is known as *plica syndrome*. Pain extension to the medial knee should raise the possibility of a secondary *anserine bursitis*, a process that often develops in patients with patellofemoral disease.

In patients complaining of pain in the patellar tendon region, several conditions must be considered. One is patellar tendon tendinitis. This may occur acutely near its tibial insertion in *acute calcific tendinitis* and also from athletic overuse, "jumper's knee." In the latter, pain occurs at the distal pole of the patella, or at the patellar attachment of the quadriceps tendon. Subacute or chronic cases of distal, insertional patellar tendon tendinitis *or enthesitis* may indicate spondyloarthropathy, particularly in younger males. The latter may be difficult to differentiate from *Osgood-Schlatter disease*, a self-limited traction apophysitis at the tibial tubercle (patellar tendon insertion) seen in athletically active adolescents.

Additional conditions to consider in patients with patellar tendon region pain include infrapatellar bursitis and inflammation of Hoffa's fat body. The infrapatellar bursa is a deep bursa interposed between the patellar tendon and the tibia. Etiologies of the rare *infrapatellar bursitis* include trauma (housemaid's knee), spondyloarthropathy (deep bursal inflammation is common in enthesopathy), gout, and bacterial infection. Hoffa's fat body is placed proximally to the infrapatellar bursa, filling the anterior joint space, so to speak. *Inflammation of Hoffa's body* is usually the result of chronic trauma and as such frequently accompanies patellofemoral osteoarthritis. Careful palpation and consideration of history and associated findings allows distinction between these syndromes. The lateral structures of the knee should also be examined in detail, including the iliotibial tract (vide supra). A final maneuver in patients with anterior knee pain is, with the patient prone, the passive flexion of both knees. Normally, symmetric flexion is possible and heels can be brought to, or near, the buttock. An inability to flex may be due to excessive tightness of the quadriceps extensor mechanism.

Diagnosis

Summary of Diagnosis

ANTERIOR KNEE PAIN

Patellar
- Patellar pain maneuvers.
- Search for associated anserine bursitis.
- Knee x-rays in older individuals (to stage knee osteoarthritis in the three compartments).

Infrapatellar
- Palpate tendon, tibial tubercle, Hoffa's body, infrapatellar bursa.
- Lateral x-rays (amorphous calcifications, tibial tubercle fragmentation in Osgood-Schlatter disease, erosion).
- Axial view of the patella with the Merchant view or the Laurin view to determine the presence of patellar subluxation or tilt.
- Bursal aspiration and HLA-B27 determination may be appropriate in some cases.

Natural History

Outcome of patellar pain depends on its cause. Chondromalacia patella is usually self-limited, although in patients with severe valgus angulation or joint hyperlaxity it may be a long-term, recurrent problem due to lateral patellar subluxation in flexion. Patellofemoral osteoarthritis is likely to give chronic and progressive discomfort. Osgood-Schlatter disease is self-limited with activities modification. A hypertrophic medial plica, patellar tendon enthesopathy, infrapatellar bursitis, and traumatic inflammation of Hoffa's fat body will cause long-term, recurrent symptoms if untreated.

Treatment

Methods

In treating patients with anterior knee pain, consider nonspecific measures, treatment aimed at the condition itself, and treatment of the possible associated anserine bursitis. Because the quadriceps muscle is the major stabilizer of the anterior knee complex, and because any painful knee process will rapidly lead to its atrophy, all patients with anterior knee pain should be prescribed isometric quadriceps exercises to prevent function loss, or to regain function.

Isometric quadriceps exercises are performed with the patient lying in bed and the lower extremities extended. Both sides should be exercised, one side at a time. Since patients may have lost the ability to initiate quadriceps contraction, the unaffected side should be exercised first and then the patient should try to match the contractions achieved in the normal side. This may be difficult at first, and patients may need significant coaching. To initiate the exercise the patient should concentrate on the anterior thigh muscles and contract them as hard as possible, keeping the muscles contracted for 10 seconds (to a count of 10). This is repeated, with 10 second rest pauses in between, six times on each side. This exercise should be done twice daily, most conveniently before getting up in the morning and after retiring at night. Additionally, patients with evidence of a contractured knee extensor apparatus should be instructed on quadriceps stretching (see appendix).

Patients with anserine bursitis should be treated with local corticosteroids (see appendix).

Additional specific treatments depend on the condition. Chondromalacia patella patients should be prescribed a NSAID agent, for a total of 6 weeks. Patients with patellofemoral osteoarthritis may be treated with acetaminofen, NSAIDs, or both if symptoms are severe. Capsaicin may be a useful adjunct. A treatment course of 2 to 3 months should be tried first. Patients with plica syndrome are candidates for arthroscopy; section of the plica may afford lasting relief. Similarly, patients with patellar tilt due to a tight lateral retinaculum may benefit from an arthroscopic lateral release. Patellar tendon enthesopathy responds well to the systemic treatment of spondyloarthropathy. Osgood-Schlatter disease is treated with reduced activities, quadriceps strengthening, and quadriceps elongation. Surgery is rarely needed. Infrapatellar bursitis is treated according to etiology. In all cases kneeling should be discouraged. When occupational factors are involved, the use of a knee pad is a realistic alternative.

When to Refer

Patients with patellar tendon enthesopathy should be referred to a rheumatologist for advice and concurrent care. In the remaining conditions failure to respond within a month, with the possible exception of patellofemoral osteoarthritis in which 2 to 3 months may be required, should trigger orthopedic referral.

Key Points

ANTERIOR KNEE PAIN

- Determine whether pain is patellofemoral, parapatellar, or infrapatellar.
- Determine if secondary anserine bursitis is present.
- Chondromalacia patella, plica syndrome, lateral retinacular tightness, infrapatellar bursitis, patellar tendon enthesopathy, and Osgood-Schlatter disease have a good prognosis.
- Patellofemoral osteoarthritis is a progressive condition.
- The presence of secondary anserine bursitis provides a treatable pain source.
- Isometric quadriceps exercises and quadriceps stretchings if needed are an essential component of treatment.
- Rheumatology input should be sought in enthesopathy.
- Orthopedic consultation should be sought in all other cases if there is a failure to respond to initial treatment.

Suggested Reading

Arnoldi K. Patellar pain syndromes (chondromalacia patellae). Acta Orthop Scand (suppl 261) 65:46–55, 1994.
Boven F, De Boeck M, Potvliege R. Synovial plicae of the knee on computed tomography. Radiology 147:805–809, 1983.
Dandy DJ. Chronic patellofemoral instability. J Bone Joint Surg 78B:328–335, 1996.
Fulkerson JP. Patellofemoral pain disorders: Evaluation and management. J Am Acad Orthop Surg 2:124–132, 1994.
James SL. Running injuries to the knee. J Am Acad Orthop Surg 3:309–318, 1995.

Anserine Bursitis

There are two closely related bursae at the tibial insertion of the conjoined pes anserinus tendons (sartorius, gracilis, and semitendinosus tendons): the bursa anserina proper and, just proximal to this bursa, the subsartorial bursa. For the purpose of this discussion both structures are jointly designated bursa anserina. The bursa anserina must be distinguished from two other bursae present in the medial knee: a bursa beneath the medial collateral ligament and a bursa saddled on the semimembranosus tendon near its insertion.

Presentation and Progression

Anserine bursitis denotes inflammation of the bursa anserina. As in other bursae this should imply swelling of the sac due to effusion and proliferation. This is true only in a minority of cases of anserine bursitis, however. In the usual form of the condition no swelling is noted and the diagnosis rests on the finding of focal tenderness at the bursal site, which is located on the upper inner tibia 5 cm distal to the medial articular line of the knee. The usual lack of swelling places a question mark on the actual pathology of the process, which in the author's opinion is more likely to represent chronic strain of the pes anserine tendon, or sometimes panniculitis, rather than true bursitis.

The typical patient with anserine bursitis is a middle-aged or older woman who complains of knee pain upon walking stairs, particularly upstairs, and limited morning stiffness (< 30 min) in the affected knee. Asked about pain location, patients typically point to the medial upper tibia. A history of previous knee problems may or may not be present. On examination most patients have evidences of patellofemoral osteoarthritis, mainly coarse crepitus on flexion/extension movements. Obesity and valgus angulation of the knee are often present. In younger patients with anserine bursitis, obesity or valgus deformity may represent the only associated finding. On palpation, there is a point of exquisite tenderness in the medial upper tibia at the insertion of the pes anserinus. Diagnostic accuracy may futher be increased by having the patient semiflex the knee and palpating, from proximal to distal, the medial tendinous edge of the thigh until the tibia is met. If this site hurts, diagnosis is confirmed.

Rarely is anserine bursitis a true bursitis featuring cystic swelling of the bursal sac. These cases are exceptional, however.

Diagnosis

Summary of Diagnosis

ANSERINE BURSITIS

- Diagnosis is clinical based on focal tenderness 5 cm distal to the medial articular line of the knee.
- Local swelling may represent a distended anserine bursa, but other lesions affecting soft tissues or bone must be ruled out.
- X-rays should be obtained if indicated for the primary condition affecting the knee.
- X-rays and other imaging procedures, in particular ultrasound and possibly MRI, should be obtained when upper medial tibial swelling is present.

Natural History

Anserine bursitis is always secondary. At times, pain from bursitis overshadows the symptoms of the primary condition; more often it adds pain to an already painful condition.

Since the primary knee condition is usually chronic, anserine bursitis tends to be a persistent problem. Very rarely there is entrapment of the saphenous nerve shown by pain and paresthesias in the medial tibial region with a positive Tinel at the bursal site, from the condition per se.

Treatment

Finding anserine bursitis in a patient with knee pain is usually good news; an element of reversibility has been found in a patient whose underlying process (osteoarthritis, pronounced genu valgum, obesity, etc.) may or may not be amenable to successful treatment.

Once anserine bursitis has been diagnosed, treatment of the underlying condition should be reviewed, in particular adherence to isometric quadriceps exercises and weight reduction. Patients should be offered, in addition, a corticosteroid infiltration at the bursal site. Guidelines for this procedure are given in the appendix. The procedure, if well performed, is almost regularly effective in symptom relief. It is often surprising that patients with advanced knee osteoarthritis, in whom pain was attributed to the damaged joint, suddenly become symptom free after this soft tissue treatment. The rare patient with true cystic swelling of the anserine bursa may be treated with a corticosteroid infiltration (following aspiration of the fluid for analysis) and if this fails, by resection of the bursal sac.

Expected Response

Symptoms of anserine bursitis are immediately relieved after the corticosteroid infiltration as an effect of the local anesthesia. Recurrence of pain may be predicted 1 to 2 hours later until the corticosteroid acts, which usually occurs by the next day. Pain relief, even when the underlying knee condition has not been corrected, persists for several weeks to months. The procedure may be repeated three or four times 2 to 3 months apart. Because the injection is in the soft tissue away from the joint, concerns with multiple corticosteroid joint injections do not apply. There is minimal or no risk of tendon rupture. As complications of the procedure, the author has only seen occasional instances of skin atrophy and ecchymosis.

When to Refer

Anserine bursitis should be treated by primary care physicians once the technique of infiltration has been learned from a rheumatologist or an orthopedic surgeon. Patients who fail to improve and those in whom recurrence of pain leads to an inordinate number of procedures (more than three or four) should be referred to an orthopedic surgeon for reevaluation of the underlying knee condition.

Key Points

> **ANSERINE BURSITIS**
> - A frequent cause of medial knee pain in patients with structural knee problems.
> - Processes that need to be ruled out include medial meniscal tears and bursitis of the medial collateral ligament; painful lipomatosis; fibromyalgia; and when swelling is present, soft tissue tumors and bone tumors affecting the upper medial tibia.
> - Diagnosing anserine bursitis means identifying a treatable process.
> - Corticosteroid infiltration is highly effective in this condition and often renders a painful osteoarthritic knee painless.

Suggested Reading

Brookler MI, Mongan ES. Anserina bursitis. A treatable cause of knee pain in patients with degenerative arthritis. Cal Med 119:8–10, 1973.

Hall F, Joffe N. CT imaging of the anserine bursa. AJR 150:1107–1108, 1988.

Hemler DE, Ward WK, Karstetter KW, et al. Saphenous nerve entrapment caused by pes anserine bursitis mimicking stress fracture of the tibia. Arch Phys Med Rehab 72:336–337, 1991.

Larsson L-G, Baum J. The syndrome of anserina bursitis: An overlooked diagnosis. Arthritis Rheum 28:1062–1065, 1985.

Moschcowitz E. Bursitis of sartorius bursa: An undescribed malady simulating chronic arthritis. JAMA 109:1362, 1937.

Other Bursitides in the Medial Knee

Two bursae in the medial knee (Figure 28–2) may cause symptoms in some patients: the tibial collateral ligament bursa, which is located between the anterior portion of the medial collateral ligament and the joint (also known as the no-name, no-fame bursa), and a closely related bursa saddled around the semimembranosus tendon near its insertion.

Presentation and Progression

Patients present with pain and tenderness in the medial knee following trauma or overexercise. Tenderness may be more pronounced in flexion, which partially uncovers the medial collateral ligament bursa and allows in some cases palpation of a small distended sac. In rare instances the sac may block full knee extension, resembling clinically a medial meniscal tear. Involvement of the semimembranous bursa is more likely to result in swelling at the posterior edge of the medial femoral malleolus.

Diagnosis

Summary of Diagnosis

> **OTHER BURSITIDES IN THE MEDIAL KNEE**
> - Pain after overexercise or trauma.
> - Tenderness (rarely swelling) exposed by knee flexion: collateral ligament bursitis.
> - Swelling, sometimes tenderness around semimembranosus: semimembranous bursitis.
> - MRI distinguishes bursitis from a medial meniscal tear. Both lesions may be present. MRI is important in the prearthroscopic evaluation of these patients.

Natural History

Bursitis develops as a result of trauma or overactivity; its course is spontaneously regressive; a corticosteroid infiltration may foster recovery.

- Treatment of bursitis includes rest, ice, and an anti-inflammatory agent; rapid regression follows a corticosteroid infiltration.

Suggested Reading

Hennigan SP, Schneck CD, Mesgarzadeh M. The semimembranosus-tibial collateral ligament bursa. J Bone Joint Surg 76A:1322–1327, 1994.

Lee JK, Yao L. Tibial collateral ligament bursa: MR imaging. Radiology 178:855–857, 1991.

Stuttle FL. The no-name and no-fame bursa. Clin Orthop 15:197–199, 1959.

Meniscal Tears

A meniscal tear should be suspected in patients with medial or lateral knee pain, particularly in young individuals without clinical evidences of osteoarthritis. This is not to say that patients with compartmental OA do not have meniscal tears; on the contrary, the meniscus may not be just torn in these patients but also ground up.

Presentation and Progression

Meniscal tears in young individuals occur predominantly as a result of sports injury. A typical presentation is acute locking of the knee after a decelerating situation, such as landing on the affected knee, followed by a quick pivot in the opposite direction. Under these circumstances the anterior cruciate ligament is often torn, in association with a meniscal tear. Such a knee characteristically tends to give way in pivoting situations (trick knee), and to lock due to displacement of the loose meniscal portion. Patients with an anterior cruciate ligament tear (Figure 28–3) have a positive Lachman test (positive anterior drawer sign at 25 degrees flexion) as well as symptoms and signs of meniscal entrapment. Signs of a torn meniscus include pain, locking, popping, and joint swelling. A torn anterior cruciate ligament results in the knee's giving way during pivoting motions.

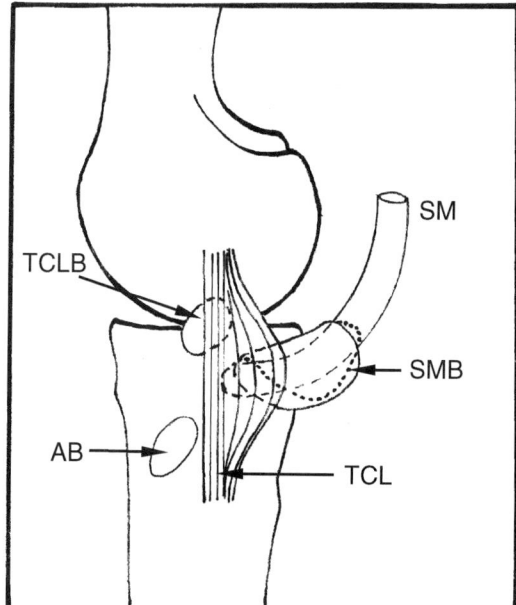

FIGURE 28–2. *Bursae in the medial aspect of the knee.* SM = Semimembranosus tendon. SMB = The semimembranosus tendon bursa, saddled over the distal-most portion of the tendon. TCL = Tibial collateral ligament. AB = Anserine bursa. TCLB = Tibial collateral ligament bursa (also known as no-name, no-fame bursa).

Treatment

Rest for 2 to 3 days, activities modification, cold compresses, and an anti-inflammatory should be prescribed initially. Response to treatment usually occurs within 1 to 3 weeks. Resilient cases, or if the patient needs an early return to work, are indications for a corticosteroid infiltration, which usually relieves symptoms within a few days. Complications of this procedure are exceedingly rare.

When to Refer

Because the differential diagnosis is with a medial meniscal tear, which would have a different treatment, any diagnostic uncertainty should trigger orthopedic consultation. Also, given the anatomic complexity of the medial knee, corticosteroid infiltrations should be done by an orthopedic surgeon or a rheumatologist.

Key Points

OTHER BURSITIDES IN THE MEDIAL KNEE

- Bursitis of the medial collateral ligament bursa is a common condition; bursitis of the semimembranosus bursa is rare.
- Both result in medial knee pain.
- A medial meniscal tear is the main differential diagnosis.
- Bursitis of the medial collateral ligament may block extension, further suggesting a meniscal tear.
- MRI clearly distinguishes these lesions.

Diagnosis

Summary of Diagnosis

MENISCAL TEARS

- History of trauma.
- Pain and possible catching or locking by moving and stressing the damaged compartment.
- A positive Lachman test indicates associated anterior cruciate ligament tear.
- If an effusion is present, aspirate: Hemarthrosis suggests concurrent cruciate ligament tear.
- MRI and arthroscopy, depending on which is available, are diagnostic of meniscal and ligamentous tear.

Natural History

Expected Outcome

The prognosis of untreated ligamentous and meniscal tear is generally poor, as the knee becomes weak, unreliable, and secondary osteoarthritis eventually develops.

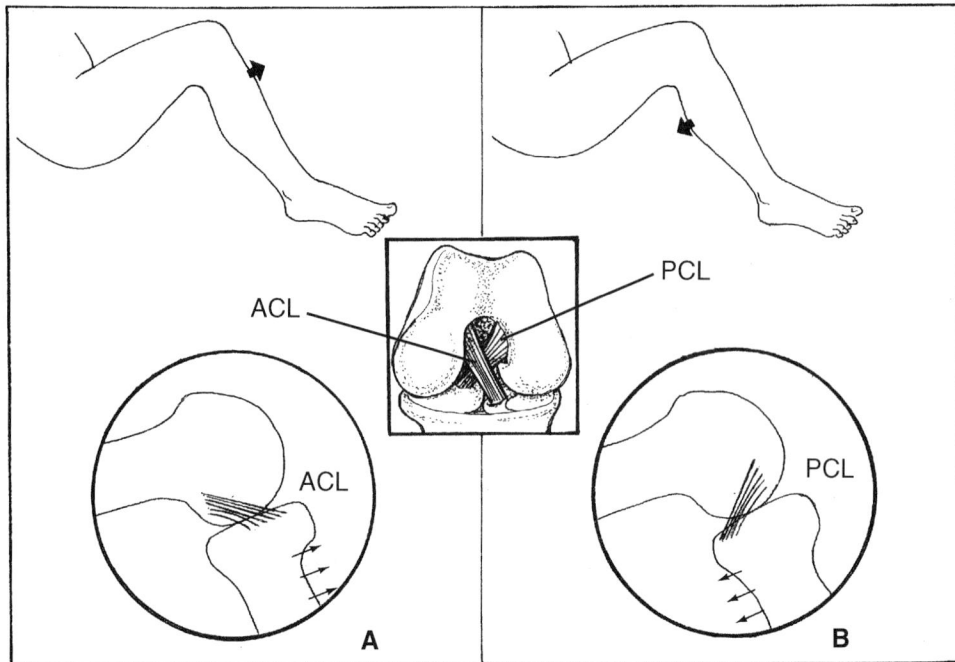

FIGURE 28–3. Anatomy of cruciate ligaments and explanation of the "drawer test." With the knee in semiflexion, the anterior cruciate ligament prevents the tibia from sliding forward ("drawer movement") when the upper leg is pulled forward by the examiner. The opposite happens with the posterior cruciate ligament. A, Anatomy of anterior cruciate ligament. B, Anatomy of posterior cruciate ligament. ACL = Anterior cruciate ligament. PCL = Posterior cruciate ligament.

Treatment

Methods

A general principle is that the meniscus should be saved, totally or partially, whenever possible. Young athletic patients with a meniscal injury, with or without an anterior cruciate ligament tear, should be treated surgically. Lateral meniscal tears involving the vascularized area may be sutured because healing can be expected. More central tears should be treated by removing the loose avascular piece of cartilage. The cruciate ligament itself may be repaired in the same procedure, which may be performed arthroscopically or by open surgery. In osteoarthritis-related meniscal tears, removal of the damaged piece of cartilage may significantly relieve pain.

When to Refer

Patients with a swollen knee after trauma, and also those presenting with pain and evidences of either meniscal tear or anterior cruciate ligament tear, should be referred to an orthopedist for evaluation and treatment.

Key Points

> **MENISCAL TEARS**
>
> - Meniscae are important in joint congruency and an even distribution of loads.
> - Meniscal tears may occur in isolation, in association with an anterior cruciate ligament tear, and in OA of the knee.
> - Findings in meniscal tears include pain, locking, popping, and swelling, with a clear effusion.
> - Anterior cruciate ligament tears result in hemarthrosis and an unstable knee that gives way during pivoting motions.
> - Tears are best diagnosed by MRI.
> - The meniscus should be saved if at all possible; this includes suturing a peripheral tear and removing the loose fragment in central tears involving the avascular zone.
> - Postoperative physical therapy, including continuous passive motion and resistive exercises, is essential to minimize muscle atrophy and for muscle recovery.
> - Hinged protective braces are important in the conservative and postoperative treatment of ligamentous injuries.

Suggested Reading

Shelbourne KD, Patel DV. Management of combined injuries of the anterior cruciate ligaments and medial collateral ligaments. J Bone Joint Surg 77A:800–806, 1995.

Zarins B, Adams M. Knee injuries in sports. N Engl J Med 318:950–961, 1988.

Baker's Cyst

Baker's cysts are well-known synovial cysts that occur in the popliteal fossa. However, not all synovial cysts in the posterior knee represent Baker's cysts. Baker's cysts occur by distension of the gastrocnemius/semimembranosus (G/S) bursa, a synovial sac that separates the semimembranosus tendon from the medial head of the gastrocnemius behind the medial femoral condyle. Although the joint capsule separates the G/S bursa from the knee in the first decade of life, a transverse capsular slit later develops that allows communication between both cavities in 50% of normal individuals by the age of 50. Rarely, other bursae as well as synovial herniations may give rise to popliteal synovial cysts.

TABLE 28–2
A PAINFUL, SWOLLEN CALF: CLUES THAT SUGGEST PSEUDOTHROMBOPHLEBITIS

A history of knee ailment
Knee swelling preceding calf swelling
Presence of a knee effusion
Knee pain preceding calf symptoms, and evidence of structural knee disease
Tenderness at cleft between semimembranosus tendon and medial head of gastrocnemius

Presentation and Progression

Baker's cysts in adults occur by distension of a communicating G/S bursa (Figure 28–4). Thus, a knee condition that causes the effusion must be present in these patients and should be considered a prerequisite to developing a Baker's cyst. Understandably, most adult Baker's cysts occur in individuals with osteoarthritis, ruptured menisci, RA, spondyloarthropathy, crystal synovitides, and infectious processes.

Baker's cysts result in a wide spectrum of symptoms and findings. Many are subclinical and asymptomatic. Symptomatic cysts may cause tension or pain in the popliteal fossa, a visible lump, or complications resulting from mass effect or leakage. Typically, Baker's cysts become hard in extension and soft in knee flexion (Foucher's sign). This characteristic distinguishes Baker's cysts from other popliteal masses (such as popliteal artery aneurysm and tumors) that remain unchanged with knee flexion.

Many Baker's cysts are first identified when complications occur. Thus, unilateral distal leg edema in a rheumatoid patient is often caused by a large cyst interfering with venous and lymphatic return. Neighboring nerves such as the popliteal or its branches may be compressed. Finally, Baker's cysts may rupture, causing pain, swelling, and inflammation in the distal leg; the Homan's sign is positive. This condition, which may resemble thrombophlebitis to perfection, is known as pseudothrombophlebitis (Table 28–2). To make matters more problematic, a ruptured popliteal cyst may be complicated by thrombophlebitis. The condition should be suspected in patients with acute calf symptoms with antecedent knee problems. Rarely, excessive compartmental pressure due to mass effect or leakage may result in a posterior compartmental syndrome.

Baker's cysts in children deserve a special note. As mentioned, during the first decade of life a connection between the knee joint and the G/S bursa has not yet been established. Thus, Baker's cysts in children are usually primary, that is, bursal distension due to repeated irritation or trauma. Interestingly, a high prevalence of Baker's cysts has been recently shown by echography in children with juvenile RA and other forms of arthritis. It is not known whether these cysts occur as a result of early acquired connections, synovial herniation, or synovitis involving an independent G/S bursa.

Diagnosis

Summary of Diagnosis

BAKER'S CYSTS
- Mass in medial one-third of popliteal fossa that softens in flexion (Foucher's sign).
- Antecedent or concurrent joint findings (synovitis, osteoarthritis).

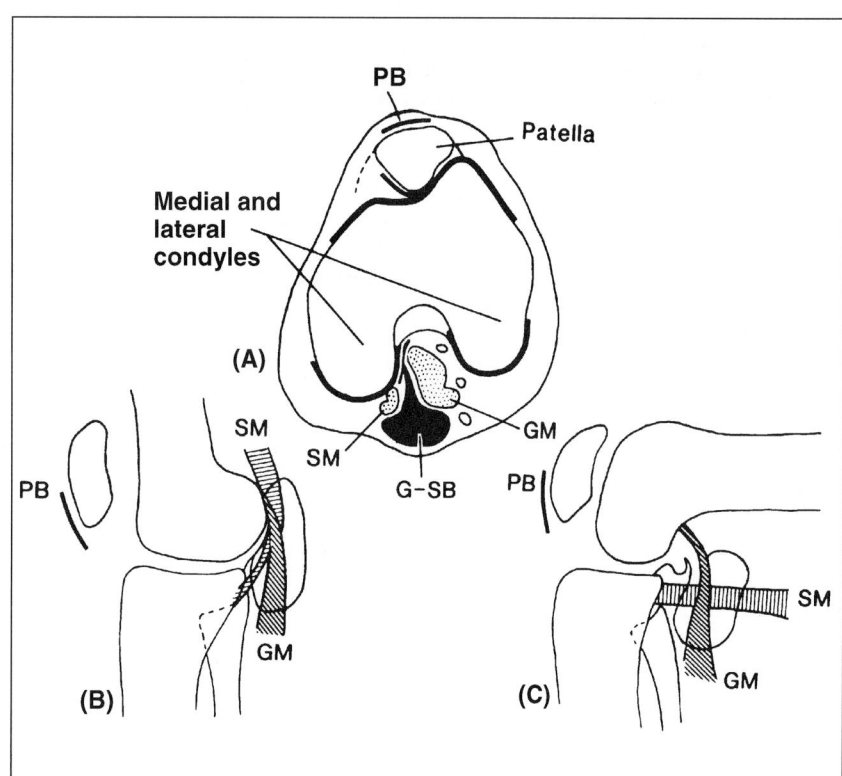

FIGURE 28–4. Pathophysiology of the Baker's cyst. *A*, A slightly distended communicating gastrocnemius/semimembranosus bursa has three portions: A foot that communicates with the joint (a connection between the knee and the bursa exists in 50% of adult knees), a body that is wedged between the gastrocnemius and the semimembranosus muscles, and a superficial expansion under the deep fascia. *B*, In knee extension the gap between the bursa and the knee seals off, the gastrocnemius and the semimembranosus come close together, compressing the bursal sac, and pressure in the superficial expansion increases. *C*, In knee flexion the communication with the bursa is reestablished, the gastrocnemius and the semimembranosus muscles separate from each other, and as a result the cyst's pressure decreases. Baker's cysts, different from other cystic and solid popliteal fossa lesions, typically soften during knee flexion. This feature of Baker's cysts is known as Foucher's sign. (From Canoso JJ. Bursae, tendons and ligaments. Rheum Dis Clin 7:189–221, 1981. After Wilson PD, Eyre-Brook AL, Francis JD. A clinical and anatomical study of the semimembranosus bursa in relation to popliteal cyst. J Bone Joint Surg 20:963–984, 1938; and Lindgren PG. Gastrocnemius-semimembranosus bursa and its relation with the knee joint. III. Pressure measurements in joint and bursa. Acta Radiol (Diagn) 19:377–388, 1978; by permission.)

- X-rays useful in evaluation of the joint; usually do not show the cyst.
- Echography: best to demonstrate intact cysts and for the initial sorting out of other popliteal lesions.
- CT scan and MRI only used for assessment of the underlying joint disease.
- Noninvasive venous studies and sometimes venography are essential to rule out thrombophlebitis. A positive diagnosis of ruptured cyst may be possible by echography, but arthrography is required in some instances.

Natural History

Baker's cysts tend to fluctuate in parallel with the primary joint condition. However, in RA and in rare lesions such as PVNS, inspissated material may result in a persistent popliteal of calf mass. Acute complications, as mentioned, include pseudothrombophlebitis and rarely a posterior compartmental syndrome. Chronic complications include dependent edema, secondary venous insufficiency, and nerve paralysis.

Treatment

Treatment of Baker's cyst should be aimed, if possible, at the articular condition that is responsible for excessive synovial fluid formation. This can be done, for instance, in RA or spondyloarthropathy with an intraarticular corticosteroid injection, in gout or pseudogout with ACTH or a NSAID, and in septic arthritis with repeated joint aspirations or other drainage plus systemic antibiotics. When cysts are very tense and rupture is feared, the knee should be transiently immobilized (with a posterior plaster cast) in semiflexion, since in this position intracyst pressures decrease. Patients with an acutely swollen distal extremity in whom a ruptured Baker's cyst is suspected should be carefully evaluated because anticoagulation in the face of a ruptured cyst may result in a massive popliteal or calf hematoma.

If thrombophlebitis (and articular infection) can be excluded and a ruptured Baker's cyst is shown, intraarticular corticosteroids plus plaster immobilization for 2 to 3 days are quite effective in providing relief. Surgical procedures aimed at the cyst, such as excision, are rarely needed today. However, in the rare patient, excision of a massive symptomatic cyst (with closure of the capsular slit) is still indicated. Baker's cysts in children are treated conservatively (with avoidance of the activity that caused the traumatic effusion), and spontaneous recovery over weeks to months can be expected. Subclinical cysts found by echo obviously do not require treatment above and beyond the rheumatologic treatment of the underlying condition.

When to Refer

The mere presence of a relatively asymptomatic Baker's cyst in a patient with knee osteoarthritis, for instance, is not in itself an indication for referral. Patients with suspected pseudothrombophlebitis are best handled jointly with a rheumatologist. Baker's cysts in RA (except the chronically distended cyst already alluded to) should be taken as an indication of ongoing synovitis and a reason for referral to the rheumatologist who concurrently is following the patient.

Key Points

BAKER'S CYSTS

- Baker's cysts are a frequent cause of popliteal discomfort in patients with knee conditions; they fluctuate with the knee condition, and their basic treatment is the treatment of the knee condition.
- Other tumoral conditions including sarcomas and popliteal artery aneurysms should be considered and excluded based on clinical findings and echography.
- Pseudothrombophlebitis from a ruptured Baker's cyst and thrombophlebitis may be clinically identical. Furthermore, they occasionally coexist.
- Inadvertent anticoagulation in a ruptured cyst may cause serious calf hematoma.
- Symptomatic Baker's cysts in children are usually the result of irritation or trauma, are not associated with a knee condition, and tend to regress spontaneously.
- Baker's cysts occur frequently in children with arthritis; only a minority is symptomatic and therapy aimed at the cyst is not required.

Suggested Reading

Canoso JJ, Goldsmith M, Gerzof SG, et al. Foucher's sign of the Baker's cyst. Ann Rheum Dis 46:228–232, 1987.
Janzen DL, Peterfy CG, Forbes JR, et al. Cystic lesions around the knee joint: MR imaging findings. AJR 163:155–161, 1994.
Katz RS, Zizic TM, Arnold WP, et al. The pseudothrombophlebitic syndrome. Medicine 56:151–164, 1977.
Lindgren PG, Willén R. Gastrocnemius semimembranosus bursa and its relation to the knee joint. I. Anatomy and histology. Acta Radiol (Diagn.) 18:497–512, 1977.
Szer IS, Klein-Gitelman M, DeNardo BA, et al. Ultrasonography in the study of prevalence and clinical evolution of popliteal cysts in children with knee effusions. J Rheumatol 19:458–462, 1992.

CHAPTER 29

Foot Pain

The foot is admirably designed to perform its functions: supporting the weight of the body and propelling and decelerating the body while at the same time being capable of adapting to an uneven terrain as necessary. These functions are subserved by the shock-absorbing property of the plantar fat pad, the elasticity of concave osteotendinous arches supplemented by the plantar fascia, which acts as a windlass, strong ligaments, and the musculotendinous units that both spring up the arches and provide static and translational motion to the foot. If foot anatomy receives little attention during medical training, foot function and pathology are even less well known except by orthopedists, physiatrists, rheumatologists, and podiatrists who are traditionally referred patients with foot complaints. Some aspects of foot anatomy and function that are relevant to our discussion of regional pain syndromes are reviewed next.

As we stand erect, the line of gravity of our bodies passes in front of the second sacral vertebra, behind the hips, and anterior to the knees and ankles. Weight is distributed unevenly in the foot concentrating, on each side, 6/12 in the calcaneal tuberosity, 2/12 in the first metatarsal, and 1/12 in each of the lateral metatarsals. During ambulation, from heel lift to toe off, progressive dorsiflexion of the big toe puts the tibial thrust at the MTP joint. This makes the first MTP joint vulnerable to degenerative changes (as in hallux rigidus) and gout. Overweight and a poorly developed (or depleted) plantar fat pad (Figure 29–1) reduces the pain-free weight bearing of the heel pad or the pads supporting the MTP joints and may result in annoying calcaneal or forefoot pain.

An accurate explanation of how the various foot joints move individually and in concert is beyond the scope of this book. However, some simplifications can be made relevant to physical examination that are useful in interpreting foot pain.

Ankle flexion and extension occur at the *ankle joint* (the tibiofibular mortise over the talus). When inflamed, it hurts all around the ankle, and both passive flexion and extension of the joint produce pain. Inversion (movement of the calcaneus medially) and eversion (movement of the calcaneus laterally) occur at the *subtalar joint,* which is formed by the articulation of the talus on the calcaneus. Patients with subtalar arthritis hurt predominantly on the sides, and passive lateral motions of the calcaneus are painful.

Because both joints hurt in roughly the same general area and inflammation may be diffuse, not infrequently patients with acute subtalar arthritis are wrongly tapped in the ankle, which is the best known of the two joints. Because no fluid is obtained, the erroneous diagnoses of cellulitis or a "dry" inflamed joint are made. The entry to these joints is indeed quite different; the ankle is tapped from the front and the subtalar joint from the lateral side (see appendix). The lesson

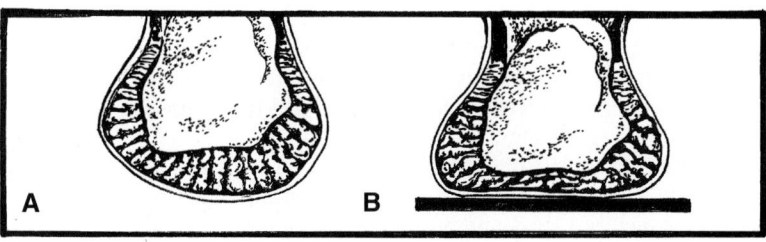
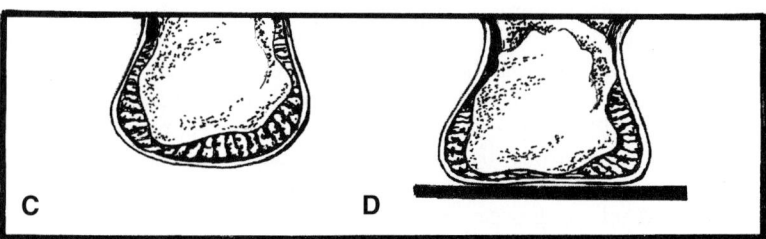

FIGURE 29–1. *Atrophy of calcaneal plantar fat pad. A and B show what happens when a normal individual applies the foot on the ground. Connective tissue septa resist the lateral displacement of the fat pad, maintaining the cushion. In individuals with fat atrophy, C and D, the plantar pad is flabby and weight bearing brings the calcaneus in virtual contact with the ground.*

should be that in any patient with acute "ankle" arthritis, a "dry tap" should be enough of a reason to consider the possibility of subtalar involvement and to act accordingly. If the examiner holds the hindfoot still with one hand, immobilizing the subtalar, and with the other rotates the forefoot in pronation (big toe plantarly) and supination (outer foot plantarly), these motions occur predominantly at the *transverse tarsal joint,* also known as Chopart's joint. This is a biarticular joint comprised dorso-medially by the talonavicular joint and plantar-laterally by the calcaneo-cuboid joint. When one of these joints is inflamed, pain involves the midfoot, dorsally or laterally depending on the joint, and passive torque motions applied to the forefoot cause pain.

Pain originating in the *MTP joints,* particularly the first, has a more obvious origin. If one of these joints is inflamed, and in conditions affecting neighboring soft tissue or bone, gentle squeezing of the entire forefoot will result in pain. The pain source can next be identified by pressing each MTP joint individually, the soft tissues between them, and adjacent bone. Palpation of the lesser MTP joints, which are frequently involved in early RA, requires practice because plantarly the MTPs are far more proximal than the apparent origin of the toes. A similar problem arises in hand examination when the novice attempts to identify the MCP joints on the palmar side. The MTP joints should first be identified on the dorsal side by gently moving the toes. The thumb is then placed in a corresponding plantar site. Tenderness is then elicited by pressing each joint between the thumb, placed plantarly, and the index or long finger on the dorsal aspect of the joint.

Forefoot pain may result from a variety of lesions. Conditions involving the first MTP joint include the hallux valgus deformity, hallux rigidus, gout, and the spondyloarthropathies. An inflamed bunion bursa, whether gouty or as a complication of hallux valgus, causes swelling, redness, and tenderness on the medial aspect of the first MTP joint; the joint itself is not tender on palpation. Synovitis affecting the lesser MTP joints is often a manifestation of RA. In stress fractures involving the lesser metatarsals, the tender area is proximal to the MTP joints. In Morton's neuroma the typical finding is plantar soft tissue tenderness between the third and fourth metatarsal heads, or less frequently between the second and third. Finally, burning plantar forefoot pain may indicate tarsal tunnel syndrome or peripheral neuropathy. The former should be suspected when abnormal findings are present in the medial retromalleolar region, and the diagnosis is further suggested by a positive Tinel sign.

In addition to articular conditions, pain and inflammation in the ankle region may result from tendinitis, tenosynovitis, ligamentous tears, and bursitis. *Medial ankle pain* and swelling with tenderness just distal and posterior to the malleolus suggests posterior tibialis tenosynovitis. If resisted inversion of the foot reproduces the pain and tenderness is present at the navicular tuberosity (the main insertion of the posterior tibialis tendon), a diagnosis of posterior tibialis tenosynovitis is inescapable.

Lateral ankle pain may be caused by collateral ligament damage, tenosynovitis of the peroneal tendons (which run posteriorly and laterally to the lateral malleolus), the painful os peroneum syndrome (os peroneum is a sesamoid in the peroneus longus tendon), or from a stress fracture in the distal fibula. Ankle sprains cause tenderness over the anterior talofibular ligament, and pain is exacerbated by passive inversion of the foot (which stretches the damaged ligament). In peroneal tenosynovitis there is tenderness over the retromalleolar area and pain is elicited by resisted eversion of the foot. In the painful os peroneum syndrome (which may be due to fracture of the os peroneum, attrition or partial rupture of the peroneus longus at the os peroneum, or a giant tubercle on the lateral calcaneus that traps the peroneus longus tendon and the os peroneus), tenderness is distal to the fibula and there is pain on resisted plantar flexion of the first ray. Stress fractures in the distal fibula are seen in obese older women with valgus deformity of the heel as well as in female rheumatoid patients on long-term corticosteroids. Pain is elicited by applying pressure on the fibula just proximal to the malleolus.

Anterior ankle pain and inflammation with unimpaired ankle, subtalar, and mid-tarsal joint examination often indicates tenosynovitis affecting the anterior tibialis or extensor digitorum longus tendons. This condition occurs frequently in RA as well as in individuals who are breaking in tight-fitting boots. True posterior ankle pain is rare; patients with this complaint, when asked about precise location of the pain, usually point to the posterior calcaneal region.

Posterior calcaneal pain occurs in bursitis affecting a superficial bursa between the Achilles tendon and the overlying skin, the retrocalcaneal bursa between the Achilles tendon and the calcaneus, the Achilles tendon proper, or a prominent posterior/superior calcaneal angle (Haglund deformity) impinging from underneath on the Achilles tendon.

Plantar calcaneal pain occurs in individuals with an atrophic calcaneal fat pad, traumatic and inflammatory conditions affecting the insertion of the plantar fascia in the medial calcaneal tuberosity, certain neuropathies affecting branches of the posterior tibial nerve, and stress fractures involving the os calcis. Some of these conditions are discussed here; further details of foot involvement in RA, the spondyloarthopathies, and microcrystalline diseases can be found in the corresponding chapters.

Ankle Sprain

Ankle sprain is the most common athletic injury. It is estimated that in the United States 27,000 ankle ligament injuries occur each day. Orthopedists take care of ankle injuries, but primary care physicians may be on site or may be the first to evaluate the patient. The main issue is to determine whether a fracture is present.

Presentation and Progression

Cause

Ankle ligamentous injuries usually result from forced inversion leading to partial or complete tear of one or more of the three lateral collateral ligaments, beginning with the anterior talofibular ligament that is tight in plantar flexion. Eversion injuries rarely result in rupture of the strong medial deltoid collateral ligament. Approximately 15% of ankle sprains are associated with avulsion fractures. Additional damage may occur, such as tears of the talocalcaneal interosseous ligament. Predisposing factors for ankle sprains include joint laxity, muscle weakness, previous ankle sprains, and developmental abnormalities of the subtalar joint.

Presentation

Patients with ankle or midfoot pain following blunt ankle injuries may or may not be able to bear weight. Immediate (within 1 hour) inability to bear weight that persists to the time of examination and tenderness on palpation at specific bone areas are strong indicators of a fracture and form the basis of the Ottawa Ankle Rules for obtaining x-rays in individuals who sustained an ankle sprain (Figure 29–2). Sprain pain is initially severe, swelling develops within a few hours, and weight bearing may be difficult. In grade 1 sprains there is a partial tear usually involving the anterior talofibular ligament; in grade 2 sprains there is a complete rupture of the anterior talofibular ligament; and in grade 3 tears there is rupture of at least the anterior talofibular and the calcaneofibular ligaments.

Diagnosis

Summary of Diagnosis

> **ANKLE SPRAIN**
> - Inversion or eversion ankle injury.
> - Pain.
> - Swelling developing within a few hours.
> - Difficulty bearing weight.
> - Inability to bear weight and bone tenderness suggest fracture and dictate the need of confirmatory x-rays (see Ottawa Ankle Rules).

Natural History

Expected Outcome

Complications. Unfortunately, chronic discomfort that limits activities occurs in 20% to 40% of patients with ankle sprain, usually as a result of a faulty diagnosis and therapy. Patients complain of diffuse, vague anterolateral ankle pain, a feeling of instability, and sometimes locking or crepitation. Local edema may be present. Secondary changes such as a shortened Achilles tendon often result. In such a patient, x-rays may be normal or abnormal. Cases with normal x-rays should have stress radiography, which is useful to detect instability. Patients with a stable ankle should have bone scan or MRI. Disuse atrophy leading to soft tissue contracture and overt sympathetic dystrophy often play a role in maintaining symptoms. The myriad explanations of a persistently painful ankle after sprain are listed in Table 29–1.

Treatment

Methods

Patients with ankle sprain should be treated with ice packs during the initial 48 hours plus elevation of the ankle in a compression bandage for several days. Crutches are used for ambulation. Ankle range of motion exercises (plantar flexion and dorsiflexion) should be started early, and as pain subsides, strengthening of peroneal muscles should be started.

Expected Response

Most patients should be off crutches and fully ambulatory within 1 week. Grade 3 sprains have been variously treated with surgical repair, functional bracing and early rehabilita-

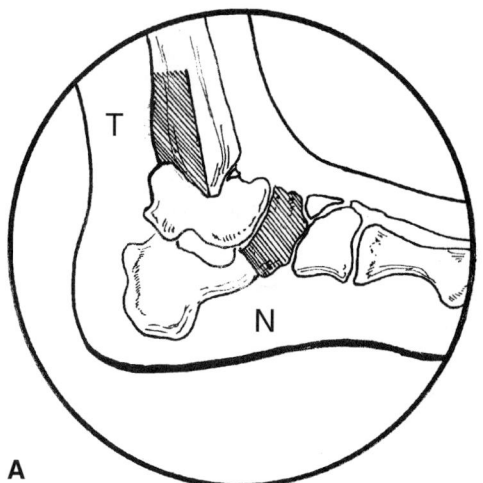
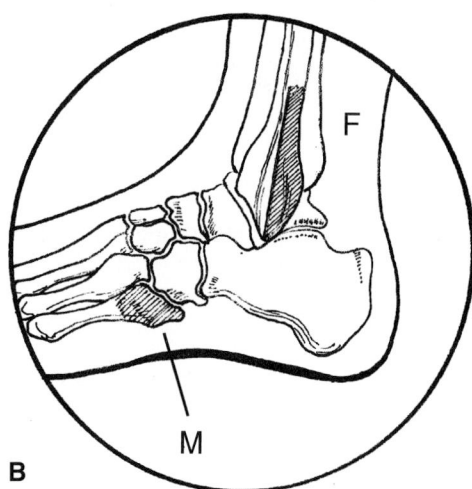

FIGURE 29–2. *The Ottawa Ankle Rules. A,* Medial view of ankle. *B,* Lateral view of ankle. An ankle radiographic series is required only if there is any pain in the malleolar zone and any of these findings: (1) bone tenderness at the posterior edge of distal 6 cm of fibula or tip of lateral malleolus, *or* (2) bone tenderness at the posterior edge of distal 6 cm of tibia or tip of medial malleolus, *or* (3) inability to bear weight both immediately and in emergency department A foot radiographic series is required only if there is any pain in mid-foot zone and any of these findings: (1) bone tenderness at base of fifth metatarsal, *or* (2) bone tenderness at navicular, *or* (3) inability to bear weight both immediately and in emergency department. T = Posterior edge of distal 6 cm of tibia and tip of medial malleolus. N = Navicular. F = Posterior edge of distal 6 cm of fibula and tip of lateral malleolus. M = Base of fifth metatarsal. (After Stiell IG, McKnight RD, Greenberg GH, et al. Implementation of the Ottawa Ankle Rules. JAMA 271:827–832, 1994.)

TABLE 29-1
CAUSES OF PERSISTENT PAIN AFTER ANKLE SPRAIN

Incomplete rehabilitation, most often after grade 3 ligamentous injury
Intraarticular injuries
Chronic instability, mechanical or functional*
Subtalar (talocalcaneal or talonavicular) sprain
Distal tibiofibular syndesmosis pain†
Impingement problems (osteophytes in the anterior rim of tibia or hyalinized tissue between talus and fibula)
Sinus tarsi syndrome‡
Chronic tendon disorders (usually peroneal subluxations or dislocation)
Stress fractures
Nerve injuries
Reflex sympathetic dystrophy
Tumors, incidental
In children, undetected traumatic epiphyseal injuries

*Functional instability is characterized by frequent or recurrent giving way and difficulty in walking on uneven ground.
†Diagnosed by the squeeze test in which compression of the fibula against the tibia in the mid-portion of the calf causes syndesmosis pain.
‡Lateral pain on walking increased by firm pressure on lateral opening of sinus tarsi.
After Renström AFH. Persistently painful sprained ankle. J Am Acad Orthop 2:270–280, 1994.

tion, and immobilization with a lower leg cast for 2 weeks. Best results are obtained with a functional treatment that includes brief ankle protection by brace, bandage, or tape and early mobilization and weight bearing. Rehabilitation in grade 3 sprains is laborious including peroneal and intrinsic muscle strengthening and proprioceptive training with an ankle tilt board. Full patient cooperation is a must. Inadequate rehabilitation explains many cases of protracted post-sprain ankle disability.

When to Refer

All patients with an ankle sprain should have the benefit of orthopedic evaluation.

Guidelines for the Disorder

See the Ottawa Ankle Rules for obtaining ankle or foot x-rays (Figure 29–2).

Suggested Reading

Renström AFH. Persistently painful sprained ankle. J Am Acad Orthop Surg 2:270–280, 1994.
Stiell IG, McKnight RD, Greenberg GH, et al. Implementation of the Ottawa Ankle Rules. JAMA 271:827–832, 1994.

Posterior Calcaneal Pain

Presentation and Progression

Cause

Posterior calcaneal pain (Table 29–2) is a relatively frequent complaint, particularly in young individuals. Pain may be caused by superficial bursitis due to irritation of the heel against the stiffness of a new shoe. Diagnosis of this condition is usually obvious by inspecting the swollen area and the shoe. Chronic heel pain may also result from a prominent posterior superior calcaneal angle (Haglund's deformity) that impinges on the Achilles tendon, creates a pressure area, and causes secondary enlargement of the deep and superficial bursae. The offending bony bump is classically seen just lateral to the Achilles tendon prior to its insertion. Achilles tendinitis from untrained running or as a result of repetitive sports-related impact loading features pain and tenderness 2 to 6 cm proximal to the insertion. In some late cases a tender nodular enlargement develops (probably as a result of interstitial rupture), which often portends gross tendon rupture. With the latter the patient may hear or feel a pop with minimal discomfort. Immediate weakness of push-off is noted followed by pain and swelling. Plantar flexion of the foot will still be possible due to the action of the posterior tibialis, the toe flexors, and the peroneal tendons, but the patient will be unable to perform a single heel rise, and the Thomas test is positive (squeezing the calf does not cause passive plantar flexion).

The spondyloarthropathies are a frequent cause of distal Achilles tendinitis and indeed the back of the heel is the classic site in which enthesopathy develops. Retrocalcaneal bursitis, periostitis, and plantar fasciitis are frequent associations of this condition. Achilles tendinitis and spontaneous rupture may occur in individuals treated with fluoroquinolone antibiotics. Other tendons may also be affected such as the rotator cuff or the common extensor tendon at

TABLE 29-2
FOOT PAIN: COMMON CAUSES

POSTERIOR CALCANEAL PAIN

Superficial bursitis
Achilles tendinitis
Retrocalcaneal bursitis
Haglund's deformity*

PLANTAR CALCANEAL PAIN

Central tenderness
    Fat pad atrophy (primary, secondary to steroid infiltrations)
    Obesity
Medial tenderness
    Compression neuropathy (calcaneal branches, nerve to abductor digiti quinti)
Medial-central tenderness (at medial calcaneal tubercle)
    Plantar fasciitis
    Avulsion fractures
    Fascial microtears
Lateral compression tenderness
    Calcaneal stress fractures
    Calcaneal cysts

PLANTAR FOREFOOT PAIN

Morton's neuroma
Stress fracture
Metatarsophalangeal joint arthritis
Tarsal tunnel syndrome

*A bony bump in posterolateral heel due to a prominent calcaneal posterior superior angle.

the lateral epicondyle. Tendon overuse, the chronic use of glucocorticoids, and renal failure may be predisposing factors for this condition. Finally, nodular involvement of the Achilles tendon and local pain may occur in hypercholesterolemia, gout, and RA.

Diagnosis

Summary of Diagnosis

> **POSTERIOR CALCANEAL PAIN**
> - New shoes, excessive exercise, familial hypercholesterolemia, inflammatory-type back pain, gout, RA?
> - Was a snap felt?
> - Which structure is involved (Achilles tendon, superficial bursa, calcaneus, retrocalcaneal bursa, periosteum)?
> - If Achilles tendon, which portion is involved?
> - Are nodules present?
> - Laboratory studies aimed at proving the likely cause.
> - Lateral x-rays in plantar flexion.
> - MRI when interstitial tendon rupture is suspected.

Natural History

Expected Outcome

Outcome of posterior heel pain depends on the etiology and whether the cause may be removed. Pain caused by superficial bursitis and unaccustomed running has a good prognosis. Calcaneal enthesopathy is usually responsive to the appropriate treatment of spondyloarthropathy. Achilles tendon tophi and xanthomas tend to resolve with the appropriate treatment of gout and hypercholesterolemia. A gross Haglund's deformity may be an indication for surgical treatment. In RA, Achilles tendon nodules tend to persist irrespective of treatment. Spontaneous rupture of the Achilles tendon may occur in late (nodular) overuse tendinitis particularly following corticosteroid infiltrations, in fluoroquinolone-induced tendopathy, the long-term use of oral glucocorticoids, chronic renal insufficiency, and hyperparathyroidism.

Treatment

Methods

Patients with Haglund's deformity or shoe-related superficial bursitis usually benefit from a change in shoe style. A severe Haglund's deformity, however, may require surgical resection of the bump. Resting the tendon with a non-weight-bearing cast for 1 to 2 weeks and NSAIDs, followed by tendon stretching within limits of comfort and a night splint at 90 degrees flexion, are usually effective in early sports-related noninsertional tendinitis. In severe or refractory forms of this condition, surgical treatment is indicated. The procedure involves debriding of the inflamed peritenon and, if fusiform or nodular thickening is noted, longitudinal incisions to visualize areas of necrosis, which should be removed to stimulate healing.

Complete ruptures of the Achilles tendon may be treated by closed and open methods. Closed methods lead to a final tendon strength of 30% and have a rate of rerupture of about 18%. In contrast, open methods result in near-normal strength, and recurrences occur in only 2%. The risks of surgery include pulmonary thromboembolism, infection, suture granulomas, sural nerve injury, stiffness, and skin problems. Patients with spondyloarthropathy and Achilles tendon enthesopathy, which is often associated with plantar fascia enthesopathy, benefit from NSAIDs, appropriate shoes (a heel lift may provide additional help), and stretching exercises. A single intrabursal corticosteroid infiltration may be quite useful in refractory, disabling cases in which the retrocalcaneal bursa is grossly inflamed. This procedure should be done by a rheumatologist who should also review the basic treatment of the underlying condition. Retrocalcaneal bursa injections are technically difficult and, if abused, potentially damaging to the tendon, which may rupture. A single infiltration should be used, and appropriate precautions should be taken to maximize chances of success. This includes the use of a non-weight-bearing cast for 1 to 2 weeks. The treatment of fluoroquinolone-induced tendopathy is empirical and based on removing the offending agent, relative rest, and gentle stretching of the tendon within limits of comfort.

When to Refer

Patients with a severe Haglund's deformity and those who fail to improve with the conservative treatment of sports-related noninsertional tendinitis should be referred to a foot orthopedist. Patients with spondyloarthropathy and calcaneal enthesopathy should be referred to a rheumatologist to supervise the overall treatment of the underlying condition as well as for advice on local measures aimed at the posterior heel pain. Patients with tophaceous gout and those with Achilles tendon rheumatoid nodules should also be evaluated by a rheumatologist.

Key Points

> **POSTERIOR CALCANEAL PAIN**
> - It may be caused by superficial bursitis, Haglund's deformity, sports-related trauma, spondyloarthropathy, and a variety of additional causes.
> - Diagnosis is based on a detailed history and physical examination.
> - In cases of Achilles tendinitis, etiologies associated with a high probability of rupture should be identified.
> - A tender nodule in noninsertional tendinitis indicates interstitial rupture and portends gross tendon rupture.
> - MRI is useful to confirm interstitial rupture.
> - Surgical tendon release and reinforcement is indicated in cases of impending rupture.

Suggested Reading

Canoso JJ, Wohlgethan JR, Newberg AH, et al. Aspiration of the retrocalcaneal bursa. Ann Rheum Dis 43:308–312, 1984.

Clain MR, Baxter DE. Achilles tendinitis. Foot Ankle 13:482–487, 1992.
Jones DC. Tendon disorders of the foot and ankle. J Am Acad Orthop Surg 1:87–94, 1993.
Pavlov H, Heneghan MA, Hersch A, et al. The Haglund syndrome: Initial and differential diagnosis. Radiology 144:83–88, 1982.
Ribard P, Audisio K, Kahn MF, et al. Seven Achilles tendon tendinitis including 3 complicated by rupture during fluoroquinolone therapy. J Rheumatol 19:1479–1481, 1992.

Plantar Heel Pain

Presentation and Progression

In the public, and also among a fair number of physicians, the mere mention of plantar heel pain (PHP) automatically elicits a diagnosis of a "heel spur." Indeed, heel spurs are no more frequent in symptomatic than in asymptomatic individuals. Furthermore, scarring following surgical removal of a spur may result in additional pain.

An important association of PHP is with obesity. In obese individuals the heel pad is compressed by the added load, shock absorption is decreased, and pressure pain results. An analogous situation may occur as a result of a constitutionally thin fat pad and in patients with plantar fat pad atrophy from repeated corticosteroid infiltrations. Fat pad disorders typically result in a tender central heel.

In runners, and also after unaccustomed hikes, fatigue tears of the plantar fascia and avulsion fractures may cause pain at the medial calcaneal tuberosity. The same area is involved in patients with spondyloarthropathy and plantar fascia enthesitis. Insertional plantar fascia pain is typically increased by passive dorsiflexion of the big toe and is located centromedially at the medial calcaneal tuberosity. Annoying heel pain may be caused by an entrapment neuropathy of the calcaneal branches of the posterior tibial nerve or the first branch of the lateral plantar nerve. Since encroachment occurs between the abductor hallucis fascia and the quadratus plantae muscle, maximal tenderness is in the medial border of the heel. Finally, PHP may indicate a stress fracture or the unusual occurrence of an expanding bone lesion such as a calcaneal cyst.

Diagnosis

Summary of Diagnosis

> **PLANTAR HEEL PAIN**
> - Running history, recent weight gain, inflammatory-type low back pain.
> - Location of tenderness (central, at medial calcaneal tubercle, at medial border of heel).
> - Increase in pain by great toe dorsiflexion (plantar fascia enthesopathy).
> - Lateral x-rays of heel to rule out an inflammatory-type spur and a calcaneal lesion.

Natural History

Plantar heel pain, if not addressed, tends to follow a chronic course. Chronic inflammation at the plantar fascia in the spondyloarthropathies may lead to postinflammatory spurs (which are fluffy and associated with erosion). Overweight, bilaterality of symptoms, and long duration of symptoms (more than 6 months) prior to treatment are associated with a poorer outcome.

Treatment

Methods

Conservative treatment of PHP, regardless of etiology, includes a period of rest, the use of a heel cup that cups the soft tissues, increasing the height of the plantar fat pad, Achilles tendon stretching exercises, and possibly the use of a night splint that keeps the ankle joint in neutral. With these measures over 80% of patients become asymptomatic after an average period of 6 months. Patients with spondyloarthropathy and PHP based on enthesopathy, and in general patients with short duration of symptoms are more likely to benefit from NSAIDs. Training errors and using the wrong shoe are important causes of heel pain in long-distance runners and should be sought and corrected. Refractory, disabling cases of calcaneal enthesopathy should be referred to a rheumatologist for a possible corticosteroid infiltration. Other causes of PHP are less likely to improve with corticosteroid infiltrations. Plantar fascia infiltrations are technically difficult and if abused may result in fat atrophy and increased pain. A short leg walking cast may be tried for 6 weeks as an alternative to plantar infiltration. A surgical approach should be considered in patients who fail to improve after a 6 month trial of conservative therapy. Surgical procedures include surgical release of the first branch of the lateral plantar nerve and plantar fasciotomy, often in association with nerve release. Satisfactory results are obtained in approximately 80% of cases.

Key Points

> **PLANTAR HEEL PAIN**
> - It may be caused by fat pad disorders, entrapment neuropathy, enthesopathy (traumatic, spondyloarthropathy related), and heel bone lesions.
> - Physical examination is useful in the initial classification of patients.
> - Running-related pain is usually caused by deficiencies in training and the use of the wrong shoe.
> - Conservative treatment of PHP including rest, a heel cup, and Achilles tendon stretching is successful in approximately 80% of patients.
> - Corticosteroid infiltrations are only indicated in patients with spondyloarthropathy with refractory plantar fascia enthesopathy. The procedure is technically difficult and should be performed by an expert.
> - A short leg walking cast may be tried instead.
> - Surgical procedures should be considered in patients who fail to improve after 6 months of conservative treatment. Usual procedures include nerve release and plantar fasciotomy.

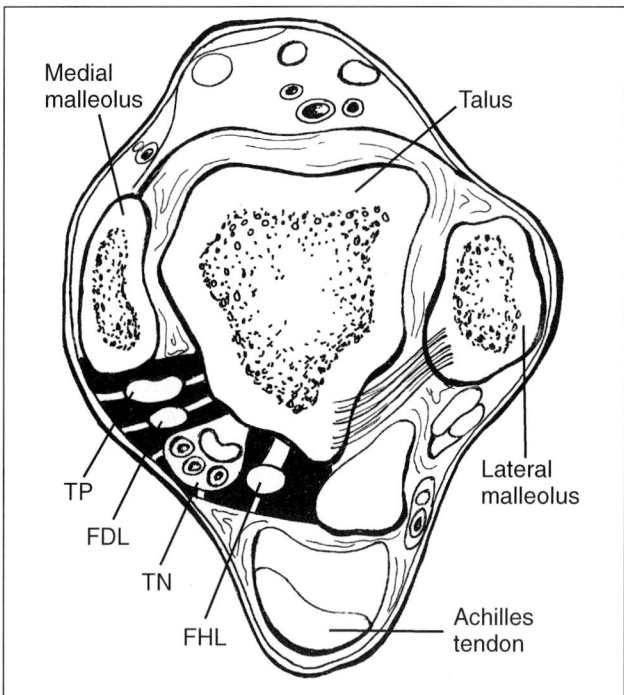

FIGURE 29–3. Anatomy of tarsal tunnel syndrome. Transverse view of ankle. FHL = Flexor hallucis longus tendon. TN = Tibial nerve (single contour), posterior tibial artery, veins. FDL = Flexor digitorum longus. TP = Tibialis posterior tendon. Tendons and neurovascular elements are included into individual fibrous septa that connect periosteum with the deep fascia.

Suggested Reading

Baxter DE, Pfeffer GB. Treatment of chronic heel pain by surgical release of the first branch of the lateral plantar nerve. Clin Orthop 279:229–236, 1992.

Prichasuk S. The heel pad in plantar heel pain. J Bone Joint Surg 76B:140–142, 1994.

Schepsis AA, Leach RE, Gorzyca J. Plantar fasciitis. Etiology, treatment, surgical results, and review of the literature. Clin Orthop 266:185–196, 1991.

Tisdel CL. Chronic plantar heel pain: Treatment with a short leg walking cast. Foot Ankle 17:41–42, 1996.

Wolgin M, Cook C, Graham C, Mauldin D. Conservative treatment of plantar heel pain: Long-term follow-up. Foot Ankle 15:97–102, 1994.

Tarsal Tunnel Syndrome

The tarsal tunnel syndrome results from compression of the posterior tibial nerve at the tarsal tunnel, a fibro-osseous passage located posterior and inferior to the medial malleolus. The floor of the tunnel is comprised of the posterior and inferior medial malleolus, the deltoid ligament, the talus, and the calcaneus. Its roof is the flexor retinaculum, a fibrous band that spans the medial malleolus and the calcaneus. Fibrous subdivisions contain, from medial to lateral, the tibialis posterior tendon, the flexor digitorum longus tendon, the posterior tibial neurovascular bundle, and the flexor hallucis longus tendon (Figure 29–3). Within the tunnel, or just distal to it, the posterior tibial nerve divides into the calcaneal nerves and the lateral and medial plantar nerves.

Presentation and Progression

Cause

The multiple causes of tarsal tunnel syndrome are listed in Table 29–3. The condition is usually unilateral. Patients complain of burning pain and paresthesia, particularly in the plantar forefoot, although a broader area including the heel may be involved. Proximal radiation to the medial leg or calf may occur. Symptoms are at first intermittent and then permanent and are usually aggravated by activity and improve with rest. In some patients, however, burning pain and paresthesia may intensify at night and relief may be sought by getting out of bed or by hanging the limb over the side of the bed. A characteristic finding on examination is a positive Tinel sign posterior to the medial malleolus or somewhat more distally, depending on the site of compression. Decreased sensation and intrinsic muscle weakness are uncommon. In addition, there may be local findings indicative of the etiology. Thus, patients may have a pronounced valgus heel deformity (often in association with a benign hypermobility syndrome) or a lump that may indicate tenosynovitis, ganglion, or exostosis related to tarsal bone coalition. Edema and diffuse tenderness from superimposed sympathetic dystrophy may obscure the diagnosis of tarsal tunnel syndrome.

Diagnosis

Summary of Diagnosis

> **TARSAL TUNNEL SYNDROME**
> - Plantar burning pain and paresthesias.
> - A positive Tinel test behind or just distal to the medial malleolus.
> - A valgus heel or a lump (soft tissue, bone) in the medial retromalleolar area may be present.
> - Decreased sensory conduction velocity or increased distal latencies to abductor hallucis (medial plantar nerve) or abductor digiti minimi (lateral plantar nerve).

Natural History

The natural history of tarsal tunnel syndrome depends on its cause. Plantar numbness and weakness and atrophy of intrinsic foot muscles are the unfortunate end result in

TABLE 29–3
CAUSES OF THE TARSAL TUNNEL SYNDROME
Idiopathic
Tenosynovitis
Varices
Valgus heel
Ganglia
Exostosis related to tarsal coalition
Trauma (fractures, direct trauma to nerve, adhesions)
Melorheostosis
Soft tissue and bone tumors
Variant muscle bellies

untreated cases. Tarsal tunnel syndrome is occasionally complicated by sympathetic dystrophy.

Treatment

Methods

Anti-inflammatory medications and a corticosteroid infiltration may be useful in tarsal tunnel syndrome resulting from chronic tenosynovitis, usually rheumatoid or psoriatic. An orthosis may help cases secondary to a pronounced valgus deformity. Persistent symptoms, however, are an indication for tarsal tunnel release. A preoperative MRI may provide essential information regarding possible compressive lesions. Surgical release of the posterior tibial nerve and its branches affords complete relief in 75% to 90% of patients.

When to Refer

Patients suspected of having tarsal tunnel syndrome should be referred to a foot orthopedist or physiatrist; there is little primary care physicians can do for these patients.

Key Points

> **TARSAL TUNNEL SYNDROME**
>
> - Diagnosis depends on an awareness of the process and the elimination of mimicking conditions: sympathetic dystrophy, L5 or S1 radiculopathy, peripheral neuropathy, and erythromelalgia.
> - The triad of burning plantar pain, positive Tinel, and increased latencies on electrodiagnosis is diagnostic.
> - Conservative treatment of tarsal tunnel syndrome has little value.
> - Surgical release is effective in 75% to 90% of patients.

Suggested Reading

Francis H, March L, Terenty T, et al. Benign joint hypermobility with neuropathy: Documentation and mechanism of tarsal tunnel syndrome. J Rheumatol 14:577–581, 1987.

Goodgold J, Kopell HP, Spielholz NI. The tarsal tunnel syndrome. Objective criteria. N Engl J Med 273:742–745, 1965.

Kaplan PE, Kernahan WT Jr. Tarsal tunnel syndrome. An electrodiagnostic and surgical correlation. J Bone Joint Surg 63A:96–99, 1981.

Takakura Y, Kitada C, Sugimoto K, et al. Tarsal tunnel syndrome. Causes and results of operative treatment. J Bone Joint Surg 73B:125–128, 1991.

Hallux Valgus

Hallux valgus, the familiar pointy first MTP joint with fibular deviation of the first toe, is a frequent source of pain and cosmetic concern. Although adequate footware affords predictable pain relief, many patients understandably object to wearing a big box shoe. The discussion that follows addresses predominantly the surgical option. Based on the history, an informed examination, and appropriate x-rays, the primary care physician should be able to provide helpful advice to hallux valgus patients.

Presentation and Progression

Inadequate footware and hyperlax joints are major contributing factors in the development of hallux valgus. Although largely confined to middle-aged and older women, younger cases of hallux valgus, even in the pediatric group, occasionally occur. Complaints vary; they include local pain, recurrent calluses, an unsightly foot, or difficulty finding appropriate shoes.

Examination should begin with the patient in the standing position. There is a prominent first MTP joint as well as a valgus angle formed by the first metatarsal (deviated medially) and the first toe (deviated fibularly). The degree of deformity ranges from minimal to severe including gross subluxation and overlap of the first and second toes. Prior to testing MTP flexion and extension, an attempt should be made to reduce the hallux valgus manually. This is critical because unrecognized limited motion in the reduced position is likely to persist after surgery. Also, instability of the first metatarsal cuneiform (MC) joint, which is assessed by holding the second metatarsal still and moving the first metatarsal in all directions, should be assessed. Gross MC instability is an indication for MC fusion. Contracture of the Achilles tendon should be recognized. The plantar skin should be inspected for calluses. Finally, particular attention should be paid to pulses, reflexes, and sensation. The examination is completed with weight-bearing x-rays.

Important measurements in planning surgery include *joint congruency* (absence of MTP subluxation), presence or absence of *osteoarthritis, hallux valgus angle* (the intersection of lines bisecting the proximal phalanx and the first metatarsal), and the *intermetatarsal angle,* which is formed by the intersection of the lines that bisect the first and second metatarsals. The choice of surgical procedure is largely influenced by the corrected first MTP flexion and extension, stability of the first MC joint, joint congruency and structural integrity of the first MTP joint, and valgus and intermetatarsal angles.

Diagnosis

Summary of Diagnosis

> **HALLUX VALGUS**
>
> - Inspect feet in the standing position.
> - Look for callosities.
> - Search for joint hyperlaxity and Achilles tendon contracture.
> - Check pulses, reflexes, and sensation.
> - Obtain weight-bearing x-rays.
> - Determine intermetatarsal and hallux valgus angles, and whether first MTP osteoarthritis is present.

Natural History

The course of hallux valgus is inherently progressive. Problems with shoe fit, forefoot pain, and concern with personal appearance tend to increase. A bunion bursa at the apex of the deformity may become inflamed due to trauma, gout, or secondary infection. Rarely, pressure ulcerations develop at this site.

Treatment

All patients with hallux valgus should be offered the conservative option that consists of an appropriate shoe to accommodate the deformity. Extrawide, soft shoes with insole padding relieve pain and prevent pressure point complications. However, because of their bulky box, the best shoes for these patients are a cause of further embarrassment. Thus, most patients with moderate or severe hallux valgus prefer the surgical option. After an initial evaluation by the primary care physician, taking into account the parameters already described, referral should be made to an orthopedic surgeon with broad experience in foot surgery. Surgical procedures range from soft tissue reconstruction and the Keller procedure (resection of base of proximal phalanx plus removal of the medial eminence), applicable to mild disease, to proximal metatarsal osteotomy or first MC joint fusion in advanced cases. Patients should be warned that complete satisfaction with the procedure is achieved in about 75%. Complications of hallux valgus surgery depend on the procedure. They include incomplete correction, excessive correction (hallux varus), recurrence of deformity, infection, nonunion, and avascular necrosis (1% to 2%) when osteotomy is used.

When to Refer

Hallux valgus patients who would like to explore the possibility of corrective surgery should be referred to a skilled foot orthopedist. Patients with vascular insufficiency or peripheral neuropathy should be discouraged from seeking surgery.

Key Points

> **HALLUX VALGUS**
> - Hallux valgus is the most common condition of the first MTP joint.
> - All patients with hallux valgus may be treated conservatively with an extrawide, soft shoe with insole padding.
> - Many patients opt for a surgical correction of the deformity.
> - Patients with vascular insufficiency or peripheral neuropathy should not be operated on.
> - The choice of the surgical procedure depends on the degree and nature of the deformity.
> - Good surgical results are achieved in approximately 75% of cases.

Suggested Reading

Mann RA. Disorders of the first metatarsophalangeal joint. J Am Acad Orthop Surg 3:34–43, 1995.

Hallux Rigidus

Patients with hallux rigidus, the second most common condition affecting the first MTP joint, have reduced motion and as a result have pain on ambulation.

Presentation and Progression

Hallux rigidus affects predominantly young men. The joint changes are those of osteoarthritis, with a predominance of dorsal and lateral osteophytes. The young age of onset in many patients suggests that osteochondritis or epiphyseal dysplasia may be a conditioning factor. Typically, patients experience pain on ambulation. Examination reveals a bulky joint with a deficit of dorsiflexion (Figure 29–4A and B). Periodic flares of the condition superficially resemble acute gout (and many patients with hallux rigidus are taking allopurinol for an erroneous diagnosis of recurrent gout). Radiographic studies reveal a narrowed joint and periarticular osteophytes on the sides and dorsum of the joint.

Diagnosis

Summary of Diagnosis

> **HALLUX RIGIDUS**
> - Recurrent or chronic first MTP pain.
> - Bulky joint; reduced dorsiflexion.
> - Lateral and AP x-rays.

Natural History

As expected in a degenerative joint process affecting a weight-bearing and cyclically loaded joint, the course of hallux rigidus is progressive. In addition to severe pain and limitation of ambulation, hallux rigidus often results in compression neuropathy of the dorsal cutaneous nerve.

Treatment

Hallux rigidus may be effectively treated with wide, extra-depth shoes with a rocker-bottom sole to compensate for the loss of dorsiflexion. Surgery is often successful in this lesion. A simple procedure known as cheilectomy (joint debridement) includes synovectomy, removal of osteophytes, and removal of part of the dorsal metatarsal head, allowing 60 to 70 degrees of intraoperative dorsiflexion. Maximal improvement occurs by 3 to 4 months. Expected benefits include about 25 degrees dorsiflexion and absence of dorsal impingement pain. Patients who fail to improve may be offered joint fusion or a Moberg procedure, which consists of a closing-wedge dorsal osteotomy of the proximal phalanx.

When to Refer

Patients with hallux rigidus should be informed about the two treatment options: a modified shoe or surgery. Surgical referral should be to an experienced foot orthopedist.

Suggested Reading

Mann RA. Disorders of the first metatarsophalangeal joint. J Am Acad Orthop Surg 3:34–43, 1995.

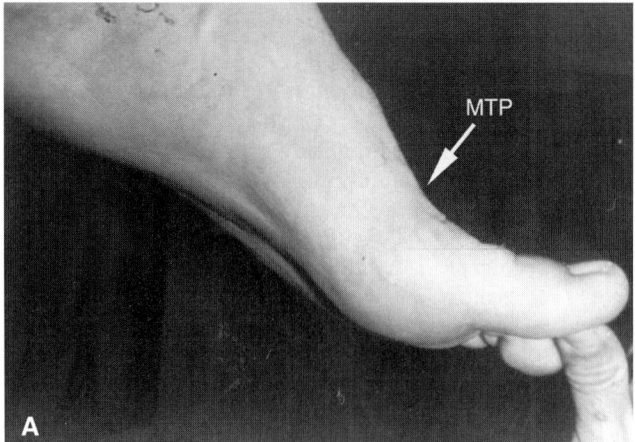 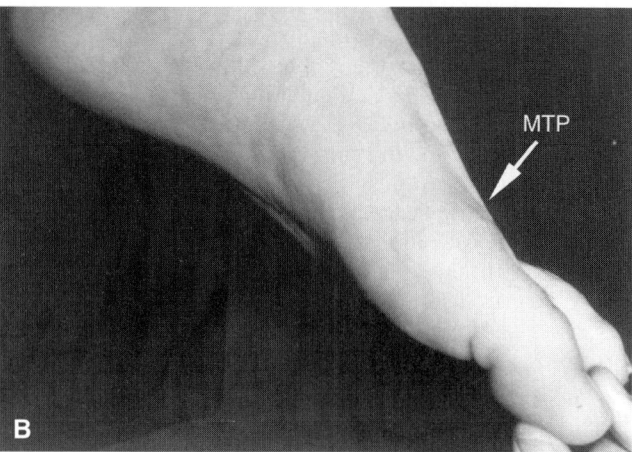

FIGURE 29–4. *Hallux rigidus.* The patient depicted had been treated for gout for 6 years. He was 32 years of age and had a history of multiple episodes of podagra, which had affected either foot, treated with indomethacin or other NSAID. Attacks had been regularly triggered by athletic efforts. Rather than in the early morning hours or during the night, as seen in gout, pain routinely appeared 1 to 2 hours after excessive activity. Examined during an asymptomatic period, both first MTPs were bulky and exhibited limited dorsal and plantar flexion (A and B). X-rays showed overgrown bone in the superior margin of the joint. There were no erosions. The left first MTP (the most frequently involved joint) was aspirated, and no crystals were seen in a small amount of fluid withdrawn. The patient was prescribed a rigid insole and was referred to the orthopedic department for possible resection of the superior osteophytes. *A,* Left foot. Minimal MTP motion in dorsiflexion. *B,* Left foot. Minimal MTP motion in plantar flexion.

Morton's Neuroma

Presentation and Progression

Morton's neuroma (Figure 29–5) is a tender nerve tissue lump formed as a result of entrapment of the digital nerve between the metatarsal heads 3 and 4, and less commonly 2 and 3. The condition is more frequent in women and is often attributed to the use of pointy, high-heel shoes that squeeze the metatarsal heads together. Contributory mechanisms include shear forces applied on the nerve (cuneiform-related metatarsals 1–3 moving en bloc alongside the cuboid-related metatarsals 4,5, which also move en bloc), nerve stretching against the overlying transverse metatarsal ligament during the terminal stance phase, and pressure by enlarged intermetatarsal bursae or ganglia.

Pain in Morton's neuroma is experienced plantarly in the forefoot while standing or walking. Some patients describe nocturnal pain. Tenderness can be elicited from the plantar side only, and an actual lump may be palpable under the examiner's fingers. Toe paresthesias and a positive Tinel's sign are rare.

Diagnosis

Summary of Diagnosis

> **MORTON'S NEUROMA**
>
> - Diagnosis is clinical based on the characteristics of pain and location of tenderness.
> - X-rays and laboratory studies are normal; they are important to rule out synovitis and stress fracture.
> - MRI may reveal the mass but should not be requested unless a tumoral lesion needs to be ruled out.

Natural History

Untreated Morton's neuroma causes chronic forefoot pain and significant gait disability.

Treatment

Methods

Morton's neuroma may be treated conservatively or surgically. Conservative therapy consists of the use of wide soft shoes with a low heel and metatarsal support to splay the toes and decrease pressure on the mass. Persistence of symptoms is an indication for the use of intralesional corticosteroids, a procedure that should be performed by a rheumatologist, an orthopedic surgeon, or a podiatrist. The technique of injection is described in the appendix. Critical to success is to apply the steroids quite deeply, past the transverse intermetatarsal ligament. The procedure may be repeated two to three times at 2 to 3 week intervals depending on symptom response. Unimproved patients should be offered surgical removal of the lump, which has a success rate of over 80%. Complications are exceptional, but recurrences sometimes occur. Prior to embarking on a repeat procedure it is critical to reevaluate diagnosis, since early synovitis may have led to an incorrect diagnosis of Morton's neuroma.

When to Refer

Patients with suspected Morton's neuroma should be prescribed the appropriate shoes and their symptoms followed. Lack of improvement after 2 to 3 weeks is an indication for referral. As mentioned, corticosteroid infiltrations should be performed only by skilled professionals. Resection of Mor-

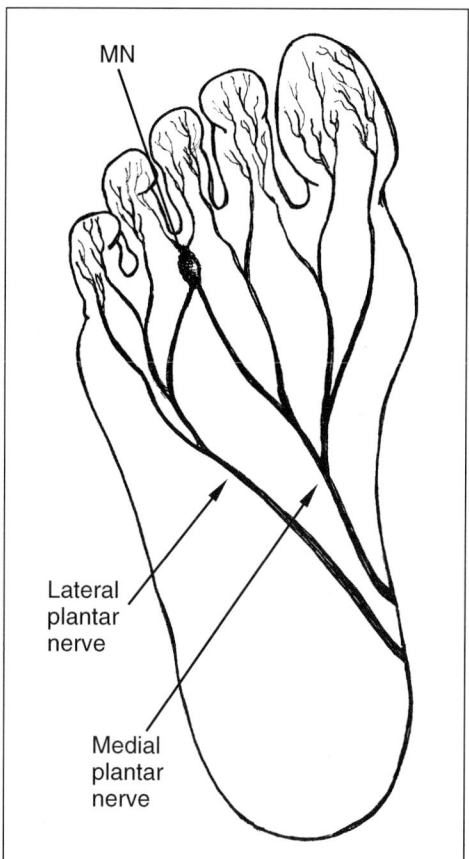

FIGURE 29–5. *Morton's neuroma.* The common digital nerve of the third space, site of most cases of Morton's neuroma, is formed by branches of the medial and lateral digital nerves. MN = Morton's neuroma.

ton's neuroma is usually done by foot orthopedists or podiatrists with surgical training.

Key Points

> **MORTON'S NEUROMA**
>
> - A frequent cause of forefoot pain, particularly in women.
> - Plantar tenderness is confined to one intermetatarsal space, usually the third.
> - A wide, soft shoe relieves pain in many patients.
> - Corticosteroid infiltrations may be very effective.
> - Surgical removal of the neuroma in refractory cases is successful in over 80% of cases.

Suggested Reading

Awerbuch MS, Shephard E, Vernon-Roberts B. Morton's metatarsalgia due to intermetatarsophalangeal bursitis as an early manifestation of rheumatoid arthritis. Clin Orthop 167:214–221, 1982.

Greenfield J, Rea J, Ilfeld FW. Morton's interdigital neuroma: Indications for treatment by local injections vs. surgery. Clin Orthop 185:142–144, 1984.

Guiloff RJ, Scadding JW, Klenerman L. Morton's metatarsalgia. Clinical, electrophysiological and histological observations. J Bone Joint Surg 66B:586–591, 1984.

Rasmussen MR, Kitaola HB, Patzer GL. Nonoperative treatment of plantar interdigital neuroma with a single corticosteroid injection. Clin Orthop 326:188–193, 1996.

Flat Foot

The clinical implications of a flat foot differ depending on the age of the patient. In neonates and infants, an appearance of flat foot is given by fat deposits that subsequently reabsorb. Even at an early age a hidden case of rigid flat foot can be detected by passive inversion of the heel. Normally, passive heel inversion elevates the longitudinal arch. In a child with a rigid flat foot, however, heel inversion fails to elevate the arch. Pediatric orthopedic consultation is in order in these patients. The discussion that follows centers on the adult flat foot.

Presentation and Progression

Cause

The vast majority of flat-footed adults are able to engage in vigorous sports activities and walk without pain or undue foot fatigue. They can hardly be considered as having a disease. Most of these patients have a flexible flat foot as a result of regional or generalized ligamentous laxity that reflects in a valgus heel, reversal of the medial contour of the foot (the apex being the head of the talus), and a fallen longitudinal arch. Patients with symptomatic flexible flat foot complain that their feet tire easily and become painful upon prolonged standing. There are also patients with a rigid flat foot caused by verticalization of the talus, tarsal coalition, an accessory navicular bone, peroneal muscle spasm (such as in some cases of RA), and posterior tibialis tendon rupture (also common in RA) with the rigidity caused in these patients by concurrent subtalar or talonavicular arthritis. These primary events, rather than the flat foot proper, cause the pain. Finally, there are acquired forms of flat foot resulting from neurologic disease.

An informed examination is essential in determining the type of flat foot present. Patients with a flexible flat foot typically develop a longitudinal arch while sitting with the feet dangling or by raising on tiptoes. Also, while the patient is sitting, simultaneous manual external rotation of the tibia and dorsiflexion of the great toe automatically correct the flat foot. A rigid flat foot is not corrected by the preceding maneuvers. Posterior tibialis rupture is suggested by a history of posterior tibialis tenosynovitis. Rupture usually results from a minor stress such as turning toward the side of the rupture. An initial snap may or not be felt, followed by acute perimalleolar pain and swelling distal and posterior to the medial malleolus. Posterior tibialis tendon rupture can be diagnosed directly by finding that the tendon is missing upon attempted inversion of the plantarly flexed foot. In addition, if the patient is viewed from the back, "too many toes" appear laterally to the patient's heel in the involved side (Figure 29–6). Finally, in the single heel rise test, whereas in the normal foot the heel goes into a stable varus position before raising (normally the posterior tibialis inverts and locks the hindfoot before the gastrocsoleus group pulls up

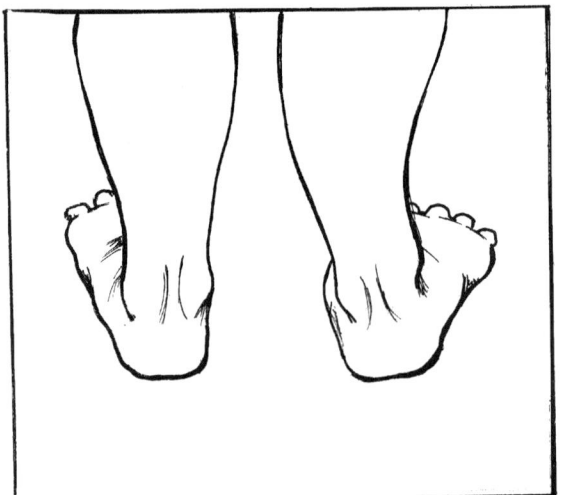

FIGURE 29–6. Characteristic of pes planus secondary to rupture of the posterior tibialis tendon is that, when viewed from the back, "too many toes" appear lateral to the patient's heel.

the heel), such a position cannot be assumed in the affected foot acutely and is both difficult and incomplete after the acute findings have subsided.

Diagnosis

Summary of Diagnosis

> **FLAT FOOT**
> - Fallen longitudinal arch.
> - Heel inversion maneuver.
> - Rising on tiptoes maneuver.
> - Tibial rotation maneuver.
> - Palpation of posterior tibialis tendon.
> - Lateral weight-bearing foot x-rays in a rigid flat foot.
> - Additional imaging procedures (oblique views, CT) to detect tarsal coalition if clinically indicated.

Natural History

Some patients with a flexible flat foot develop pain as a result of trauma or shortening of the Achilles tendon. A rigid flat foot is often a source of pain and foot tiredness. Untreated rupture of the posterior tibialis tendon leads to an irreversible valgus heel and flat foot deformity. This position is assumed in the course of one to several weeks. When a valgus heel deformity occurs, pain shifts from the medial location to the lateral ankle.

Treatment

Adult patients with a painless flexible flat foot do not require treatment beyond prophylactic stretching of the Achilles tendon. Patients with a flexible flat foot and pain should be referred to a foot orthopedist, physiatrist, or podiatrist for evaluation. The patient's level of activity may have to be decreased. It may be necessary to modify the shoe with a Thomas heel to support the talonavicular joint plus an orthotic to support the longitudinal arch and prevent hyperpronation. Very rarely, adult patients with a flexible flat foot are unable to be fitted with shoes and have pain on routine weight bearing. A wedge osteotomy of the calcaneus may be indicated in these patients.

A rigid flat foot is always an indication for orthopedic referral. Pain from traumatic posterior tibialis tendinitis (which cannot be distinguished from partial rupture) should be treated with 4 to 6 weeks of cast immobilization with the foot slightly inverted and plantar flexed. Unimproved patients may receive a single, cautious corticosteroid infiltration. Persistence of symptoms is an indication for surgical treatment, which includes tenosynovectomy plus debridement and repair as needed. Some cases need tendon augmentation prior to reattachment, the usual donor tendon being the flexor digitorum communis.

Key Points

> **FLAT FOOT**
> - A flat foot may be a result of ligament hyperlaxity, tarsal bone abnormalities, arthritis, neurologic disease, or posterior tibialis tendon rupture.
> - A painless flexible flat foot does not represent disease.
> - Excessive activity, trauma, or Achilles tendon contracture may cause pain in a flexible flat foot.
> - Pain in a rigid flat foot is usually caused by the underlying tarsal bone abnormality.
> - Posterior tibialis tendon ruptures tend to go undiagnosed; early ruptures can be repaired before irreversible changes set in.

Suggested Reading

Downey DJ, Simkin PA, Mack LA, et al. Tibialis posterior tendon rupture: A cause of rheumatoid flat foot. Arthritis Rheum 31:441–446, 1988.

Jones DC. Tendon disorders of the foot and ankle. J Am Acad Orthop Surg 1:87–94, 1993.

Myerson MS. Adult acquired flat foot deformity. J Bone Joint Surg 78A:780–792, 1996.

Pedowitz WJ, Kovatis P. Flatfoot in the adult. J Acad Orthop Surg 3:293–302, 1995.

PART V

PAIN AMPLIFICATION SYNDROMES, RELATED CONDITIONS, AND MISCELLANEA

CHAPTER 30

Pain Amplification Syndromes, Related Conditions, and Miscellanea

Benign Hypermobility Syndrome (BHS)

In addition to cases of Ehlers-Danlos syndrome in which a highly stretchable skin is present, and Marfan's syndrome in which abnormal body proportions are unmistakable, there is the benign hypermobility syndrome (BHS). Patients with BHS have lax collagenous tissues including ligaments (joint hypermobility), skin, and the support of visceral organs. As a result of increased joint excursion and faulty tendon mechanics, articular, tendinous, and fibromyalgic symptoms are quite frequent.

Presentation and Progression

Cause

BHS affects women more than men, Asians more than blacks, and blacks more than Caucasians. These findings correlate with sex and race differences in joint tightness. There is also a clear familial aggregation of BHS.

Presentation

Patients have had BHS since childhood. They all remember being able to adopt postures impossible for most. They may have excelled in gymnastics or ballet. However, as years went by, disadvantages associated with BHS outweighed the benefits. Arthralgias are common. Segments previously hypermobile may become restricted and painful. Tendinous structures such as the rotator cuff wear out. Fibromyalgic tenderness is identified in many patients. Joint hypermobility is established by using Beighton's system (Table 30–1).

Diagnosis

Summary of Diagnosis

> **BENIGN HYPERMOBILITY SYNDROME (BHS)**
>
> - BHS is a clinical diagnosis based on Beighton's criteria. (score ≥ 6).
> - Marfan's syndrome and Ehlers-Danlos syndrome must be excluded (it is not always easy).
> - Arthralgias, fibromyalgia, and later in life osteoarthritis complicate BHS.

> - Additional manifestations of collagenous hyperlaxity include skin hyperlaxity, mitral valve prolapse, recurrent joint luxations (shoulder, patella), flat feet, hernias, and prolapses.

Natural History

Expected Outcome

The condition is benign in terms of survival, but it may be quite distressing as a result of recurrent joint luxations, rotator cuff lesions, fibromyalgia, arthralgias, and secondary osteoarthritis. Mitral valve prolapse has no clinical import, but mitral regurgitation and arrhythmias may develop.

Treatment

Methods

Treatment of BHS begins with an explanation of the nature of the condition and its course. Patients may have been given multiple interpretations of their symptoms and may be quite confused and discouraged by the time they are referred to a rheumatologist. Treatment includes analgesics such as acetaminophen or mild NSAIDs such as ibuprofen or nabumetone. Patients with fibromyalgia may benefit from amitriptyline or desipramine. Physical therapy is of paramount

TABLE 30–1

BEIGHTON'S SCORING SYSTEM FOR HYPERMOBILITY SYNDROME

Score 1 point on each side of the body:
  a. Extension of fifth MCP past 90 degrees.
  b. Thumb reaches forearm on passive wrist flexion.
  c. Elbow hyperextends past 0 degrees.
  d. Knee hyperextends past 0 degrees.

Score 1 point:
Palms reach floor on anterior lumbar flexion while the knees are kept extended.

Maxium score = 9.
Hypermobility syndrome is present in patients with a score of 6 or greater.
After Beighton P, Solomon L, Soskolne C. Articular mobility in an African population. Ann Rheum Dis 32:414–418, 1973.

importance. Stretching exercises may be prescribed to treat previously hypermobile segments that are now contractured. I have often prescribed isometric and other muscle-strengthening exercises in an attempt to place a check on hypermobile joints. To my knowledge, there have been no systematic, controlled trials comparing different treatments for BHS.

Expected Response

Reassurance and analgesics work well. Little can be done for the underlying condition.

When to Refer

Patients who are hypermobile and are symptomatic should be treated with simple measures, and if there is no satisfactory improvement should be referred to a rheumatologist to check on the diagnosis and for further treatment suggestions (such as specific exercises, recommendations regarding soft tissue procedures or joint replacements, etc.).

Key Points

BENIGN HYPERMOBILITY SYNDROME (BHS)

- Patients with joint hyperlaxity are subject to articular, ligamentous, and visceral consequences of the hyperlax collagenous tissues.
- Little understood but of great concern to the patients are the arthralgias, tendinous pain, and fibromyalgic features of the condition.
- Flat feet are usually asymptomatic, but patellar and shoulder luxations produce severe recurrent disability.
- Reassurance, simple analgesics, and physical therapy work well in these patients. Associated musculoskeletal syndromes should be treated on their merits.

Suggested Reading

Beighton P, Solomon L, Soskolne C. Articular mobility in an African population. Ann Rheum Dis 32:413–418, 1973.
Grahame R. Hypermobility syndrome. In: Klippel JH, Dieppe PA (eds) Rheumatology. Mosby-Year Book, London, 5.18.1–6, 1994.

Marfan's Syndrome

In Marfan's syndrome there are striking somatic, ocular, and cardiovascular manifestations. Diagnosis is imperative because dreaded aortic complications may now be largely prevented.

Presentation and Progression

Cause

Marfan's syndrome is an autosomal dominant disorder in which there is an abnormality in fibrillin, the main component of extracellular microfibrils. As a result there is progressive dilatation of the aortic root and the ascending aorta, which results in aortic insufficiency and aortic dissection.

Presentation

Patients with Marfan's syndrome may be recognized by a positive family history plus abnormal body proportions. Patients have long limbs, an arm span 8 cm or more longer than height, arachnodactyly, thumb protrusion from the clenched fists, loose joints, kyphoscoliosis, and pectus excavatum. Additional findings include subluxed lenses (ectopia lentis) and an arched palate. Last but not least, there may be evidence of aortic dilatation that is progressive and has life-threatening complications.

Diagnosis

Summary of Diagnosis

MARFAN'S SYNDROME

- Long, thin extremities.
- Arachnodactyly.
- A positive "thumb sign" (thumbs protrude from the clenched fists).
- Kyphoscoliosis.
- Reduced vision from subluxed lenses (ectopia lentis).
- Aortic dilatation that begins at the aortic root.

Natural History

Prognosis in Marfan's syndrome depends on the time and rate of aortic dilatation. Patients may go on to develop chronic aortic regurgitation and aortic dissection, reducing life expectancy by one-third in untreated patients. Aortic enlargement may be monitored by serial echoes.

Treatment

Propranolol, in a controlled trial, has been shown to reduce the rate of aortic dilatation in patients with Marfan's syndrome. A typical treatment includes propranolol given four times daily in a dose that reduces heart rate below 100 beats during exercise. Because aortic dilatation begins early in life, a beta-adrenergic blocker should be instituted as soon as the condition is diagnosed.

When to Refer

Marfan's patients must be followed with a structured program. Compliance with beta-adrenergic blockers is vital. The aorta must be monitored by echo once a year until the size exceeds 50% of normal and every 6 months thereafter. A cardiologist must be involved in this program. Periodic orthopedic evaluation in patients with kyphoscoliosis is also essential.

Key Points

MARFAN'S SYNDROME

- Marfan's syndrome is an autosomal dominant disorder of fibrillin, a protein widely distributed in skin,

- blood vessels, perichondrium, periosteum, and suspensory ligament for the lens.
- Patients with Marfan's syndrome must be closely followed by a cardiologist working in close association with the primary care physician.
- Prognosis in Marfan's depends on the rate of aortic dilatation.
- The rate of aortic dilatation may be slowed down with the use of beta-adrenergic blockers.
- Surgical replacement of the aorta, aortic valve, and mitral valve has been successful in some patients.
- Mimicking conditions include homocystinuria, congenital contractural arachnodactyly, and the Marfanoid hypermobility syndrome.

Suggested Reading

Pyeritz RE, McKusick VA. The Marfan syndrome: Diagnosis and management. N Engl J Med 300:772–777, 1979.

Shores J, Berger KR, Murphy EA, et al. Progression of aortic dilatation and the benefit of long-term beta-adrenergic blockade in Marfan's syndrome. N Engl J Med 330:1335–1341, 1994.

Ordinary Leg Cramps

It may appear strange to discuss leg cramps separate from muscle conditions. Indeed, ordinary leg cramps are as remote to systemic myopathies as they are close to other common but bothersome syndromes affecting the lower extremities.

Presentation and Progression

Cause

The underlying mechanism of ordinary leg cramps is unknown. The condition affects with predilection people with well-developed muscles. In addition to an association with old age, ordinary cramps are frequent in the late months of pregnancy and in cirrhosis. By electromyography, ordinary cramps begin with fasciculations, followed by high-frequency muscle action potentials.

Typical patients are older individuals who report that their sleep is disrupted by cramps. The gastrocsoleus is the most frequently involved muscle. Cramps occur when an already shortened muscle is contracted. In bed, the weight of the bedclothes brings the foot into passive plantar flexion (position in which the gastrocsoleus is shortened). If the patient stretches, the active contraction of the passively shortened gastrocsoleus results in a cramp.

Diagnosis

Summary of Diagnosis

> **ORDINARY LEG CRAMPS**
> - Typically they occur at night.
> - The gastrocsoleus muscle is typically involved.
> - Diagnosis is clinical.

> - Laboratory studies, which are not required, would be normal.

Natural History

If frequent enough, nocturnal leg cramps may severely disrupt sleep.

Treatment

Patients should be reassured and instructed on the proper positioning in bed and stretching. Patients who sleep in the supine position should have the bedcovers loose and use a pillow at the end of the bed to prevent foot drop. Stretching should be done with the feet in dorsiflexion. If a cramp occurs, the foot should be forcibly dorsiflexed, which terminates the cramp within seconds. If cramps are frequent and disruptive, the patient should be started on quinine sulfate 240 to 300 mg taken at night. Randomized, placebo-controlled trials have shown that quinine is effective in reducing the frequency of nocturnal cramps. Untoward effects of quinine at this low dose are most unusual. The rare patient may develop immune thrombocytopenia.

Key Points

> **ORDINARY LEG CRAMPS**
> - Cramps occur by contraction of an already shortened muscle.
> - The shortened position should be discouraged by using loose bedclothes and by stretching while holding the feet in dorsiflexion.
> - Quinine taken at night is useful to decrease the frequency of ordinary leg cramps.

Suggested Reading

Hing M-S, Wells G. Metaanalysis of efficacy of quinine for treatment of nocturnal leg cramps in elderly people. BMJ 310:13–17, 1995.

McGee SR. Muscle cramps. Arch Intern Med 150:511–518, 1990.

Weiner IH, Weiner HL. Nocturnal leg muscle cramps. JAMA 244:2332–2333, 1980.

Reflex Sympathetic Dystrophy (RSD)

Reflex sympathetic dystrophy and causalgia, formerly considered different entities, probably represent subsets of the same condition. Although algodystrophy, a widely used designation in Europe, more appropriately conveys the clinical findings, the prevailing American designation RSD is used in this discussion.

Presentation and Progression

RSD usually follows tissue injury (often traumatic) or nerve damage (Table 30–2). Examples of the former include a minor ankle sprain, a fall on the knee, a minor surgical procedure such as carpal tunnel release, a burn, frostbite, myocardial infarction, and lung cancer. These cases are usually designated

TABLE 30–2
CAUSES OF REFLEX SYMPATHETIC DYSTROPHY

Trauma (fracture, especially Colles' fracture, minor surgery, lacerations, infections, frostbite, burns, aortic surgery)
Parkinsonism
Hemiplegia
Lumbar disc prolapse
Amyotrophic lateral sclerosis
Cervical radiculopathy
Plexus and peripheral nerve injuries
Carpal tunnel and tarsal tunnel syndromes
Myocardial infarction
Cancer
Diabetes
Hyperthyroidism
Isoniazid therapy
Uncertain

RSD. Nerve injury is the second major culprit. The injured structure may be a plexus, a main trunk, a minor sensory nerve, or the posterior tibialis nerve within the tarsal tunnel. Cases following peripheral nerve injury have traditionally been designated causalgia. Finally, there are cases in which a medication such as isoniazid appears to be involved, and others in which no explanation for RSD is found. Although the very designation of RSD suggests that the sympathetic system somehow causes these patients' symptoms, no direct evidence supports the sympathetic system involvement in causing chronic pain. Disuse atrophy, a chronic disease-type behavior, and an undiagnosed painful lesion that feeds on disuse are more plausible explanations of this syndrome.

Irrespective of its cause, RSD presents a rather stereotyped clinical picture. Several days usually elapse between the initial insult and the onset of pain. Pain is aching and burning in quality, appears out of proportion to the findings of the physical examination, spreads beyond the local area of injury, fluctuates widely, is aggravated by warmth and partially relieved by cold, and location (except in cases due to overt nerve injury) does not conform to a known nerve or vascular territory. Additional findings include *hyperpathia,* which means a delayed onset of pain after a stimulus is applied, pain persistence after the stimulus has been removed, and an emotional overreaction; and *allodynia,* which is a painful response to nonnoxious stimuli. Three stages of RSD are recognized: the acute, the dystrophic, and the atrophic. The acute phase lasts several weeks. Skin is red and warm or cold and cyanotic, and there may be persisting local edema (Figure 30–1). In the dystrophic phase pain becomes continuous; there is proximal and distal pain radiation, hyperpathia, and allodynia; and edema turns brawny. The atrophic phase begins 6 or more months after the initial injury. The affected part, for example, a hand or a foot, becomes clearly atrophic. Skin is pale, cyanotic, and glossy; fingers taper; joints become contractured. Palmar or plantar fibrosis similar to Dupuytren's contracture often develops. There is patchy osteopenia on x-rays.

Presentations may be atypical regarding location and severity of the condition. Knee RSD is a well-known variant. The majority of cases follow trauma to the patella or knee surgery, including total knee replacement. Arthroscopy seems to be the trigger in many cases. This syndrome gives protracted symptoms and often goes unrecognized. Transient osteoporosis of the hip and transient painful osteoporosis of the lower extremities are additional variants of RSD. Lesser forms of RSD are, in the experience of the author, more common than the classic forms just described. Findings include persisting burning pain, hyperpathia, cyanosis, and cold edema without dystrophic tissue changes.

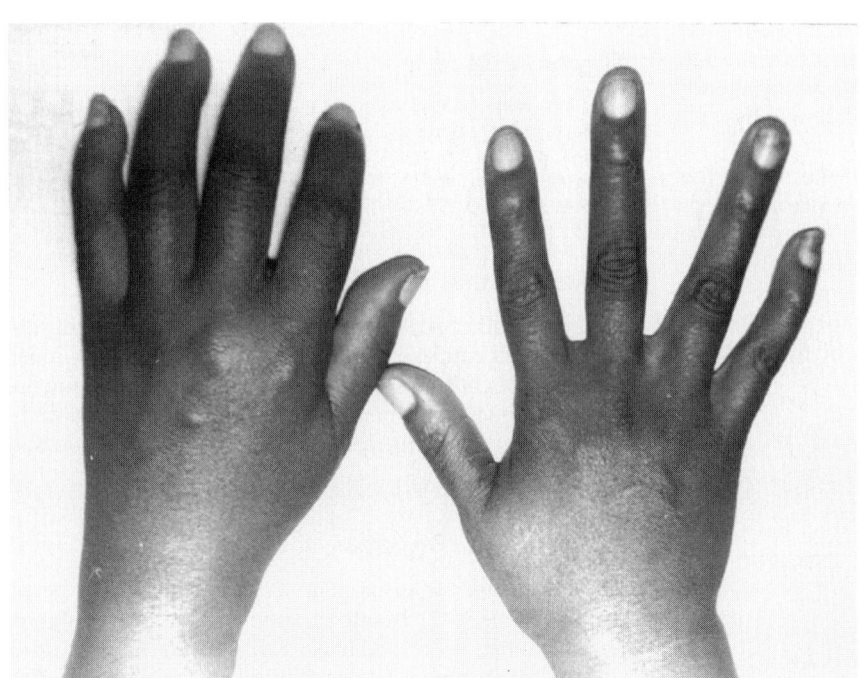

FIGURE 30–1. *Sympathetic dystrophy.* Swollen, painful left hand after carpal tunnel release. This patient, a 40-year-old woman, had open release of the left carpal tunnel for idiopathic carpal tunnel syndrome 1 month prior. She was treated with several stellate ganglion blocks and intensive physiotherapy. Three months later she was well.

Diagnosis

Summary of Diagnosis

> **REFLEX SYMPATHETIC DYSTROPHY (RSD)**
> - Follows minor soft tissue, nerve, or bone trauma.
> - Pain out of proportion to the findings.
> - Pain exacerbation with emotion and environmental warmth.
> - Burning pain, hyperpathia, allodynia, local edema.
> - Increased early uptake on bone scan.
> - Progression to tissue atrophy.
> - Patchy osteopenia on x-rays.

Natural History

Expected Outcome

Mild cases undergo spontaneous resolution after several weeks or months. Cases with persisting symptoms and dystrophy have a protracted course with progression to pronounced tissue atrophy, joint contracture, and disability. In long-term follow-up studies, at 3 years of initiation of aggressive therapy, 60% of patients still experience symptoms. Identification and correction of a pain-sustaining lesion dramatically improves prognosis.

Treatment

Methods

Because disuse atrophy is of paramount importance in RSD, the mainstay of therapy is physical therapy emphasizing passive, active, and resisted motion in the upper extremity and weight-bearing exercises and ambulation in the lower extremities. However, a meaningful physical therapy program cannot be implemented unless pain is brought under control.

To this end several treatment modalities may be used depending on the stage of the disease and availability: (1) As proposed by Kozin et al., prednisone 60 to 80 mg per day in divided doses for 2 weeks and then tapered over 1 to 2 weeks to a maintenance dose of 5 mg daily or 5 to 10 mg every other day, which is continued for 2 to 3 months, is helpful in controlling early disease. (2) Epidural blockade may be used every 1 to 2 weeks for 3 to 4 weeks in lower extremity RSD. (3) The widely used stellate ganglion or lumbar sympathetic blocks relieve pain in many patients. The effectiveness of sympathetic blocks (vs. a placebo effect) has recently been challenged. (4) A tricyclic agent such as amitriptyline or desipramine 25 to 75 mg at night, a calcium channel blocker such as nifedipine in extended release tablets 30 mg once daily or twice a day, a beta-adrenergic blocker such as propranolol in doses up to 320 mg per day, and calcitonin (especially in late cases) may be added for pain control. The author favors a short course of prednisone in upper extremity RSD and epidural blocks in lower extremity RSD, *plus* a tricyclic agent, *plus* intensive PT, which is the mainstay of therapy in all patients with RSD. At the same time, the presence of a persisting lesion that could be feeding on the RSD must be looked for fastidiously.

Expected Response

Response to corticosteroids is rapid, usually within 1 week. Epidural blocks rapidly improve pain. Delayed effects include decreased edema, a persistent rise in skin temperature, and an improved function.

Complications

Corticosteroid treatment may result in one or more of the complications of protracted glucocorticoid administration. Stellate ganglion infiltrations should be discouraged because they are not more effective than placebo, plus present an inherent risk of paresthesias, intraarterial (vertebral artery) administration leading to seizures, recurrent laryngeal nerve block, and rarely pneumothorax. The author no longer recommends stellate ganglion infiltrations in the treatment of upper extremity RSD.

When to Refer

RSD is relatively rare in a primary care setting. Because diagnosis may be difficult and the consequences of the condition severe in terms of disability, most cases of suspected RSD should be referred to a rheumatologist, neurologist, hand or foot orthopedist, physiatrist, or pain unit depending on presumed triggering mechanism, location of the syndrome, and degree of atrophy and function loss.

Key Points

> **REFLEX SYMPATHETIC DYSTROPHY (RSD)**
> - The telltale finding in RSD is pain out of proportion to physical findings.
> - Disuse atrophy appears to be central in pathogenesis.
> - Treatment includes symptomatic relief, physical measures to counteract atrophy, and a thorough search for a lesion that may be acting as a trigger.
> - Oral glucocorticoids and epidural blockade are useful in early disease.
> - Late cases may be helped by calcitonin.
> - RSD is best handled by physicians with special training.

Suggested Reading

Christensen K, Jensen EM, Noer I. The reflex sympathetic dystrophy syndrome. Response to treatment with systemic corticosteroids. Acta Chir Scand 148:653–655, 1982.

Kozin F, McCarty DJ, Sims J, et al. The reflex sympathetic dystrophy syndrome. I. Clinical and histologic studies: Evidence for bilaterality, response to corticosteroids and articular involvement. Am J Med 60:321–331, 1976.

O'Brien SJ, Ngeow J, Gibney MA, et al. Reflex sympathetic dystrophy of the knee. Causes, diagnosis, and treatment. Am J Sports Med 23:655–659, 1995.

Ochoa JL, Verdugo RJ. Reflex sympathetic dystrophy. A common clinical avenue for somatoform expression. Neurol Clin 13:351–363, 1995.

Payne R. Neuropathic pain syndromes, with special reference to causalgia and reflex sympathetic dystrophy. Clin J Pain 2:59–73, 1986.

Erythermalgia/Erythromelalgia (ETA)

These paroxysmal conditions of the extremities, believed to be part of the same pathophysiologic spectrum, are discussed under a single heading: erythermalgia/erythromelalgia, or ETA.

Presentation and Progression

Cause

Adult ETA, idiopathic or secondary, as well as early ETA are recognized. Thrombocythemia is involved in many of the adult cases. Some cases, such as those associated with SLE, are due to vasculitis. Nerve injury and microvascular disease may be involved in diabetic ETA (Table 30–3).

The involved limbs become paroxysmically red, painful, and swollen in response to dependency and environmental heat. Cold and limb elevation relieve these findings. Adult idiopathic ETA affects predominantly males between the fifth and seventh decades of life. The less frequent secondary adult ETA occurs in a variety of conditions including myeloproliferative disorders associated with thrombocythemia, SLE, RA, diabetes, pregnancy, certain viral conditions, and the use of several medications. Early ETA, which occurs in children, sometimes runs in families. There are no disease associations in early ETA.

Diagnosis

Summary of Diagnosis

> **ERYTHERMALGIA/ERYTHROMELALGIA (ETA)**
> - Paroxysmal redness, swelling, and warmth in the limbs.
> - Triggered by dependency and warmth; relieved by limb elevation and cold.
> - Rule out vascular insufficiency.
> - Determine platelet count. If elevated, seek a myelodysplastic syndrome.
> - Check for SLE, RA, and other associated conditions.

Natural History

Expected Outcome

The condition is chronic in the adult and early idiopathic forms, and parallels disease activity or exposure in secondary disease. There are no complications of ETA per se, but any of the complications of the underlying disease may occur in secondary cases.

Treatment

Methods

Adult cases associated with thrombocythemia usually respond to low-dose aspirin, which is consistent with the notion that platelet aggregation is involved in pathogenesis.

TABLE 30–3

CAUSES OF ERYTHERMALGIA/ERYTHROMELALGIA (ETA)

1. Adult, idiopathic
2. Adult, secondary
   Thrombocythemia: essential thrombocythemia, polycythemia vera, myelofibrosis, chronic myelogenous leukemia
   Vasculitis, SLE, RA
   Diabetes mellitus
   Pregnancy
   Infections: respiratory poxvirus infection
   Medications: nicardipine, nifedipine, bromocriptine
   Miscellaneous conditions: pernicious anemia, lichen sclerosus et atrophicus, arterial hypertension, etc.
3. Early forms (may be familial)

After Kraus A, Alarcón-Segovia D. Erythermalgia, erythromelalgia, or both? Conditions neglected by rheumatologists. J Rheumatol 20:1–3, 1993.

Other cases should be treated for the underlying condition, if any.

When to Refer

Cases with thrombocythemia should be referred to a hematologist. Suspected cases of connective tissue disease should be referred to a rheumatologist for evaluation.

Key Points

> **ERYTHERMALGIA/ERYTHROMELALGIA (ETA)**
> - The condition should be distinguished from vaso-occlusive disease such as thromboangiitis obliterans and arteriosclerosis obliterans and sympathetic dystrophy.
> - Underlying conditions, in particular myeloproliferative conditions and connective tissue diseases, should be ruled out.
> - Cases associated with thrombocytosis usually respond to low-dose aspirin.

Suggested Reading

Kraus A, Alarcón-Segovia D. Erythermalgia, erythromelalgia, or both? Conditions neglected by rheumatologists. J Rheumatol 20:1–3, 1993.

Fibromyalgia

Fibromyalgia, formerly known as fibrositis, is a most prevalent condition that accounts for 5% of consultations in general medical offices and 20% in rheumatology offices. In a study performed in Wichita, Kansas, the frequency of fibromyalgia in the general population was 3.4% in women and 0.5% in men. Women aged 60 to 79 had the highest prevalence, more than 7%. Patients with fibromyalgia have chronic, generalized, fluctuating pain; an inefficient sleep;

chronic fatigue; and multiple subjective dysfunctions that speak of an unusual sensitivity in target organs.

Presentation and Progression

Fibromyalgia may occur in isolation or may associate with other musculoskeletal disorders. In the past, associated cases were known as secondary fibromyalgia. However, treatment of the "primary" disease has no effect on "secondary" fibromyalgia, suggesting a chance rather than causal association. The American College of Rheumatology discourages the use of the term *secondary*.

There are also instances in which fibromyalgia develops in the context of metabolic or infectious diseases such as hypothyroidism, opiate withdrawal, corticosteroid withdrawal, bacteremia, and viremia (HIV, infectious mononucleosis). It is likely that these patients had subclinical fibromyalgia that became symptomatic as the pain threshold was further decreased by the intercurrent condition.

Patients with fibromyalgia complain of generalized pain in areas near joints, neck, and back. Pain is achy, persistent, and may have a burning quality to it. Very frequently patients describe pressure pain, such as leaning on the elbows, lying on one side, or crossing one leg over the other. Fatigue is profound and characteristically worse on arising in the morning than when retiring at night. A feeling of stiffness is characteristic; indeed, prolonged morning stiffness may be taken as an indication of RA or other inflammatory condition. Physical examination is normal, except for the unusual soft tissue tenderness. Indeed, the diagnosis may be missed if the latter is not purposefully sought.

Central to a diagnosis of fibromyalgia is the presence of a sufficient number of tender points (Figure 2–7). These points, when firmly pressed, are not only tender but also elicit an emotional response (grimace, sometimes tears) or withdrawal of the part.

It is always difficult for the uninitiated clinician to determine how much pressure to apply. Too much pressure would make anyone hurt; too little pressure might be painless even to fibromyalgia patients. A standarized amount of pressure used in research studies of fibromyalgia (5 lbs/cm^2), which is equivalent to the pressure required to produce blanching in the nail bed of the examining thumb, has been found useful in the clinical setting. The seasoned clinician has a better tool: By searching for fibromyalgic point tenderness in normals as well as in patients with fibromyalgia and other disease states, the right amount of pressure to trigger fibromyalgic pain is subconsciously learned. Fibromyalgia patients may or not experience spontaneous pain at the tender points. More often than not tender points are clinically silent with the unusual sensitivity being brought up by a directed physical examination. As a corollary, to diagnose fibromyalgia the physician must be aware of the syndrome, have a basic knowledge of tender point location, and know how much pressure to apply. Failure of detection explains the myriad patients with fibromyalgia that are considered cases of refractory "tennis elbow," "neck pain," "trochanteric bursitis," "Tietze's syndrome," and so on. Associated findings on physical examination may include crepitus on motion of the temporomandibular joint, joint hyperlaxity (benign joint hypermobility and fibromyalgia exhibit more than a chance overlap), and clinical and echocardiographic signs of mitral valve prolapse (probably an association of the joint hyperlaxity).

It is believed that an integral part of fibromyalgia is a disturbed sleep. Typically, patients wake up in the morning feeling more tired than when they retired at night. Patients may have difficulties falling asleep, or they may wake up repeatedly. The number of hours a patient sleeps is of lesser significance. Indeed, the author has seen fibromyalgia patients who slept over 24 hours straight on weekends and still felt exhausted on waking up. Researchers have studied the sleep EEGs in patients with fibromyalgia as well as in normal and diseased controls. A disturbance in the third stage of the non-REM sleep was described as characteristic of fibromyalgia. Normally, EEGs in this phase show slow delta waves. In patients with fibromyalgia the delta waves are still present but they are ragged by intrusion of fast alpha waves as if the patients were subject to auditory or other stimuli.

Interestingly, normal volunteers, who had the delta-wave sleep disturbed by auditory stimuli, after a few nights developed fatigue, achiness, and fibromyalgic tenderness. Indeed, an alpha-delta EEG pattern is seen in only a minority of patients with fibromyalgia, and a similar EEG disturbance has been documented in normal individuals as well as in patients with RA and osteoarthritis. Many features of fibromyalgia, including the sleep disturbance, are shared by the chronic fatigue syndrome. Indeed, if one could remove the tender points from the former, patients would be classified as suffering the latter. The overlap between these conditions is further underscored by the fibromyalgic tenderness that may be elicited, on directed examination, in the majority of patients with chronic fatigue syndrome.

Depression, migraine, TMJ syndrome, irritable colon, and irritable bladder (interstitial cystitis) are frequent associations of fibromyalgia. A well-known association with depression has raised the possibility that fibromyalgia is an equivalent or a somatic correlate of depression. Interestingly, although roughly 60% of fibromyalgia patients have a history of major depression prior to the onset of symptoms, less than 30% have depression concurrent with the fibromyalgic symptoms. Supporting an association between both conditions, CSF neurochemical findings in fibromyalgia are identical to those in depression. Whether depression is present is extremely important in treatment planning.

Pseudoneurologic symptoms mimicking carpal tunnel syndrome or other neuropathies are common in fibromyalgia. The bizarre and recurrent pattern of pseudoneurologic symptoms led, in several instances known by the author, to a wrong diagnosis of multiple sclerosis. Patients may complain of dry mouth and dry eyes even in the absence of tricyclic antidepressants, raising the possibility of Sjögren's syndrome. The Schirmer's test (tear production measured by placing a strip of filter paper under the lower lid for 5 minutes) is normal in fibromyalgia patients, however. Rheumatoid arthritis may be suggested by the generalized achiness and prolonged morning stiffness of fibromyalgia patients.

Diagnosis

The American College of Rheumatology classification criteria for fibromyalgia are shown in Figure 2–7. The use of these criteria can be simplified: A patient who has had generalized pain for more than 3 months and has on examination 9 or more of the 18 described tender points has fibromyalgia. Laboratory studies in fibromyalgia are normal. To exclude early inflammatory conditions that may feature generalized aches and fatigue, such as RA and SLE, it is prudent to request a CBC and ESR. Another condition that may closely resemble fibromyalgia is hypothyroidism. To rule out this condition the author routinely includes a thyroid-stimulating hormone (TSH) determination in the initial evaluation of fibromyalgia patients.

Summary of Diagnosis

> **FIBROMYALGIA**
>
> - Most prevalent in women (female/male ratio is 3.4 to 0.5).
> - Highest prevalence (> 7%) in women aged 60 to 79.
> - Pronounced fatigability.
> - Generalized pain.
> - Tenderness at 9 or more of 18 typical points.
> - Sleep disturbance in most patients.
> - Normal CBC, ESR, and TSH.

Natural History

The condition is chronic. A minority of patients have such a severe disease that they become disabled. In the remaining patients there appears to be some amelioration of the condition as years go by. This is not to say that the condition cannot be severe in some older women.

Treatment

Treatment of fibromyalgia rests on reassurance, advice on sleep hygiene, the use of tricyclic antidepressant agents, physical medicine measures, and psychiatric advice if required. Needless to say, treatment should be tailored to the severity of the condition. Patients who are minimally symptomatic and those in whom fibromyalgia was accidentally diagnosed (such as during a demonstration physical examination done on a student) should be reassured and at the most offered sleep hygiene advice. Reassurance should be based on the unusual progression to a symptomatic form of the disease and the lack of joint or muscle damage in fibromyalgia. Sleep advice includes the use of relaxation methods, techniques of stress reduction, and instruction on the deleterious effects of smoking, alcoholic beverages, and also xanthine-containing beverages such as tea or coffee past 5 p.m.

Symptomatic cases should be offered, in addition, a tricyclic agent such as amitriptyline or cyclobenzaprine, or if these agents produced unacceptable side effects or proved ineffective, doxepin or desipramine. Tricyclic agents should be started in minute doses, such as amitriptyline 10 mg, cyclobenzaprine 10 mg, doxepin 25 mg, or desipramine 10 mg 1 hour before sleep. Dose increments should be every 2 weeks aiming at reaching amitriptyline 50 mg, cyclobenzaprine 30 mg, doxepin 75 mg, or desipramine 50 mg before sleep.

It is important for primary care physicians to realize that fibromyalgia is not helped by low-dose corticosteroids such as prednisone 15 mg per day. Indeed, in a blind, randomized trial, steroids if anything showed a trend toward increasing pain. NSAIDs are also ineffective.

Physical measures include warm baths, massage in particularly painful areas, and stretching and endurance-building exercises. It has been shown that fibromyalgia patients improve when their aerobic capacity improves, for instance, by joining a cardiovascular fitness program. Help from an interested physiatrist or physiotherapist is essential in handling fibromyalgia patients.

Finally, there are a few patients, perhaps 5% of cases, who are headed toward disability (from pain and deconditioning) or have a major psychiatric component. These patients should be evaluated psychiatrically and followed accordingly.

Expected Response

Unfortunately, about 50% of patients will not be able to take one of the tricyclic medications, and about 20% will find that all of the tricyclic agents are unacceptable due to sedation or anticholinergic effects. Of patients able to take the amitriptyline, approximately one-third improve. The improvement is unrelated to changes in the sleep EEG pattern. Tachycardia may be a distressing finding in older patients taking cyclobenzaprine.

When to Refer

Although most cases of fibromyalgia can be handled by a general physician, about 30% are very difficult to cope with mainly because of patients' built-in inability to tolerate medications. These patients should be referred to a rheumatologist or, if available locally, to a fibromyalgia center or pain control unit for reevaluation and treatment. What should *not* be done is to close the door on these "bothersome" patients. A plea: Whoever treats fibromyalgia patients should have knowledge of the condition, feel empathy for chronic pain sufferers, and be willing to refer "failures of treatment" to a higher level of expertise.

Key Points

> **FIBROMYALGIA**
>
> - A chronic painful condition that predominantly affects women.
> - The characteristic feature is symmetrically placed tender points.
> - Morning stiffness and fatigue often lead to a wrong diagnosis of RA.
> - Pseudoneurologic symptoms are frequent and may be prominent, suggesting, for instance, MS.
> - Treatment of fibromyalgia rests on an understanding of the condition, tricyclic agents, and aerobic exercise.
> - Unfortunately, many patients do not tolerate medications, and of those who do, only 30% improve.
> - Treatment of fibromyalgia in specialized centers has a success rate of approximately 60%.

> • Given the information just listed, it appears prudent to advise exercising, living life as normally as possible, and avoiding a dependent life.

Suggested Reading

Carette S. Chronic pain syndromes. Ann Rheum Dis 55:497–501, 1996.

Carette S, Bell MJ, Reynolds WJ, et al. Comparison of amitriptyline, cyclobenzaprine, and placebo in the treatment of fibromyalgia: A randomized, double-blind clinical trial. Arthritis Rheum 37:32–40, 1994.

Carette S, Oakson G, Guimont C, et al. Sleep electroencephalography and the clinical response to amitriptyline in patients with fibromyalgia. Arthritis Rheum 38:1211–1217, 1995.

Clark S, Tindall E, Bennett RM. A double blind crossover trial of prednisone versus placebo in the treatment of fibrositis. J Rheumatol 12:980–983, 1985.

Wolfe F, Ross K, Anderson J, et al. The prevalence and characteristics of fibromyalgia in the general population. Arthritis Rheum 38:19–28, 1995.

Wolfe F, Smythe HA, Yunus MB, et al. The American College of Rheumatology classification criteria for fibromyalgia. Arthritis Rheum 33:160–172, 1990.

Myofascial Pain (MFP) Syndromes

Myofascial pain syndrome designates regional pain that is reproducible by palpating a tender trigger point. Additional characteristics of trigger points include an identifiable band of taut muscle fibers and a twitch response. A "latent" trigger point does not cause pain but is palpable as a taut muscle band and upon compression has a twitch response and causes referred pain. There are proponents of the MFP syndrome who believe the condition is common and explains many of the regional pains, and there are skeptics (like the author) who consider the syndrome rare even when a simplified version of the condition is accepted, that is, removing the taut bundle and the twitch response from the trigger point definition.

Presentation and Progression

Cause

Myofascial pain results in most instances from occupational factors or trauma. There are similarities among the chronic upper limb syndrome (repetitive strain injury), MFP, and fibromyalgia. Indeed, in a landmark study in which MFP patients were examined by fibromyalgia experts, most of the patients had features of fibromyalgia. In the same study, when patients with MFP, fibromyalgia, and normal controls were intermixed, an equal number of trigger points was found in the three groups. Finally, there was little reproducibility in trigger point assessment among MFP experts.

Presentation

Myofascial pain syndromes may occur everywhere but are most frequent in the upper body, involving an upper quadrant of the body or the head. They may also involve the lower hemibody, affecting predominantly the lower back. In most instances further inquiry will disclose a sleep disturbance, protracted fatigue, and multiple tender points diagnostic of fibromyalgia. Some patients, however, will only have regional pain and a true trigger point indicative of actual MFP syndrome.

Diagnosis

Summary of Diagnosis

> **MYOFASCIAL PAIN (MFP) SYNDROMES**
> • Regional pain.
> • Presence of a trigger point (reproduces the entire pain, a taut muscle band is felt, and there is a local twitch response).
> • Many patients exhibit additional findings of fibromyalgia.
> • There are no laboratory or imaging findings useful to diagnose the condition.

Natural History

Expected Outcome

The condition has a protracted course and is often recurrent.

Treatment

Methods

Proponents of the MFP syndrome believe that cold spraying of the painful area and needling or xylocaine infiltration of the trigger point relieves the syndrome. Also, in patients with headache or neckache and a trigger point at a masseter, relief may be derived from the use of a dental plate. The author has no experience with the latter. There is no indication for the use of corticosteroid infiltrations. On the other hand, if the patient has additional features that suggest fibromyalgia, the same treatment regime as for fibromyalgia applies.

Expected Response

In the author's experience, infiltration treatment of nonfibromyalgia cases works temporarily. If an occupational or recreational factor is identified that results in overuse and local pain, modification of the activity often results in pain relief.

Complications

There are no known complications of MFP treatment.

When to Refer

Patients with possible MFP syndrome should be referred to a rheumatologist for diagnostic confirmation or to identify an alternative diagnosis. Once diagnosis is clarified, whether the patient has either MFP syndrome or fibromyalgia, subsequent treatment and follow-up should be by the primary care physician.

Key Points

> **MYOFASCIAL PAIN (MFP) SYNDROMES**
> • A controversial condition; many of the patients have additional characteristics that are diagnostic of fibromyalgia.

- Another subgroup of patients has occupational disease.
- Patients with a typical trigger point and no evidence of fibromyalgia improve temporarily by xylocaine infiltration or the use of a cooling spray.
- Patients with fibromyalgia should be treated for this condition.
- When occupational factors are identified, work environment modification may afford lasting relief.

Suggested Reading

Carette S. Chronic pain syndromes. Ann Rheum Dis 55:497–501, 1996.

Smythe H. Links between fibromyalgia and myofascial pain syndromes. J Rheumatol 19:842–843, 1992.

Travell JG, Simons DG. Myofascial Pain and Dysfunction. Williams and Wilkins, Baltimore, 1983.

Tunks E, McCain GA, Hart LE, et al. The reliability of examination for tenderness in patients with myofascial pain, chronic fibromyalgia, and controls. J Rheumatol 22:944–952, 1995.

Wolfe F, Simons DG, Fricton J, et al. The fibromyalgia and myofascial pain syndromes: A preliminary study of tender points and trigger points in persons with fibromyalgia, myofascial pain syndrome and no disease. J Rheumatol 19:944–951, 1992.

Repetitive Strain Injury

Beginning in the 1980s, an epidemic of musculoskeletal symptoms, collectively known as "repetitive strain injury," appeared in Australia and some other industrialized countries among factory and office workers. Review of published data indicates that rather than being a separate entity, the condition encompasses a miscellany of syndromes that need to be diagnosed accurately to be dealt with efficiently.

Presentation and Progression

Cause

Repetitive wrist motion may result, for instance, in carpal tunnel syndrome and lateral epicondylitis. Certain occupations that imply repeated overhead lifting may cause arm, shoulder, and neck pain with typical myofascial pain (MFP) features, and so on. Not only mechanical factors are involved but also regional muscle fatigue. In addition, in certain locations, such as in Australia, a liberal compensation system, work dissatisfaction, and eager lawyers caused many instances of abuse until the law changed. However, this has not been the author's experience working either in the United States or in Mexico.

Presentation

Symptoms and findings on examination depend on the musculoskeletal syndrome at hand, and the most frequent regional pain syndromes have already been discussed. Of particular interest is occupation-related carpal tunnel syndrome in which nerve conduction studies may be normal. It is believed that the repetitive use of the wrist causes carpal tunnel edema leading to intermittent compression of the median nerve.

Diagnosis

Summary of Diagnosis

REPETITIVE STRAIN INJURY

- In most cases there is a well-defined soft tissue syndrome that needs to be accurately diagnosed if it is to be effectively treated.
- There are also instances of myofascial pain and cases of fibromyalgia that surface clinically in mechanically stressed areas.
- A minority of cases are compensation related.
- Nerve conduction studies may be normal in work-related carpal tunnel syndrome.

Natural History

Expected Outcome

Outcome depends on the specific regional pain syndrome and whether or not work-related determining factors can be modified.

Treatment

Methods

Regional pain caused by work-related repetitive strain should be treated with simple measures while an attempt is made to correct the working conditions that are responsible for the syndrome. Appropriate treatment includes splintage, capsaicin, NSAIDs, ultrasound, occasional steroid infiltrations, and most importantly therapeutic exercises for the upper extremities, shoulders, neck, and upper back. Espousing the view that work-related pain is irreversible and sooner or later will cause disability is a disservice to the worker and to society. Rather than embarking on futile major local therapies or pursuing the legal path, more effort should be made to improve the ergonomics at the workplace and a more flexible use of human resources.

When to Refer

It is important, in analyzing a patient with work-related regional pain, to enlist an occupational therapist to inspect the patient's workplace and suggest changes if these are feasible. If not, a change in job description should be attempted.

Key Points

REPETITIVE STRAIN INJURY

- Make an effort to establish an accurate diagnosis.
- If the case appears to be work related, obtain a detailed work history and enlist an occupational therapist to inspect the work environment.
- Work environment modification or a change in job description is the physiologic way of dealing with work-related regional pain.

> • Tackling the problem from the end result, that is, local or systemic treatments for the regional syndrome, at the exclusion of its cause, can be expected to fail in the majority of patients.

Suggested Reading

Johnson SJ. Therapy of the occupationally injured hand and upper extremity. Hand Clinics 9:289–298, 1993.

Littlejohn GO. Repetitive strain syndrome: An Australian experience. J Rheumatol 13:1004–1006, 1986.

Miller MH, Topliss DJ. Chronic upper limb pain syndrome (repetitive strain injury) in the Australian workforce: A systematic cross sectional rheumatologic study of 229 patients. J Rheumatol 15:1705–1712, 1988.

Rempel DM, Harrison RJ, Barnhart S. Work-related cumulative trauma disorders of the upper extremity. JAMA 267:838–842, 1992.

Chronic Fatigue Syndrome

Presentation and Progression

Cause

Patients who feel physically and mentally exhausted and in whom the most thorough evaluation fails to disclose what is wrong are encountered in any practice. Indeed, the reported frequency of fatigue lasting at least 1 month in general medical clinics in the United States was 24%. A duration of symptoms of at least 6 months is required to consider chronic fatigue, however. In the past, clinicians spoke of neurasthenia, epidemic neuromyasthenia, and so on, to describe the condition, but little effort was made to identify its cause or mechanism or to evaluate treatment methods. As recently as 1988, renewed interest in chronically fatigued patients resulted in the CDC case definition criteria that were used in epidemiologic, pathogenetic, and treatment studies. Researchers in other parts of the world were using other criteria, however, and disagreements grew.

Fortunately, the various research groups that are part of the International Chronic Fatigue Syndrome Study Group joined efforts and as a result much easier to use guidelines to evaluate and classify these patients were published in 1994. To date, the cause of chronic fatigue syndrome (CFS) is unknown. A role of viral infection has been considered by several research groups. EBV, retroviruses, enteroviruses, and human herpesvirus 6 have all been investigated without convincing results. Indeed, when physical or mental abnormalities are deemed to be the cause of fatigue (e.g., hepatitis B or C, HIV infection, or major depression), patients are excluded from the CFS category.

Presentation

Patients with CFS complain of severe fatigue, continuously or intermittently, for at least 6 months. During this period, because of exhaustion, previous levels of personal, educational, or occupational activities have declined (severe fatigue). They also complain of at least four of the following eight symptoms: (1) impaired memory or concentration; (2) sore throat; (3) tender cervical or axillary lymph nodes; (4) muscle pain; (5) multijoint pain; (6) new headaches; (7) unrefreshing sleep; (8) postexertion malaise. Along the line, investigations for a medical or psychiatric explanation of symptoms have been negative. Physical findings are normal with the exception of fibromyalgia, which is present in up to 80% of cases.

Less Typical Presentations

Patients with CFS may present predominantly neurologic symptoms suggesting, as an example, multiple sclerosis. Other patients believe they have a chronic infectious disease, such as HIV infection or "chronic infectious mononucleosis." Another form of presentation is rheumatologic; SLE is often a consideration. However, only fibromyalgic tender points are found.

Diagnosis

Summary of Diagnosis

If little thought is put into it, patients complaining of fatigue may receive excessive testing or they may be dismissed, only for the clinician to regret at a later date not having done, for instance, a TSH test. A meaningful evaluation should include tests that are likely to help and exclude others that are irrelevant.

> **ITEMS TO INCLUDE IN THE CLINICAL EVALUATION OF PROLONGED OR CHRONIC FATIGUE***
>
> • A thorough history.
> • A thorough physical examination.
> • A mental status examination.
> • CBC with differential; ESR; serum alanine aminotransferase, total protein, albumin, globulin, alkaline phosphatase, Ca, P, glucose, BUN, electrolytes, and creatinine; TSH determination; and urinalysis.

> **TESTS NOT RECOMMENDED IN THE CLINICAL EVALUATION OF PROLONGED OR CHRONIC FATIGUE***
>
> • Serologic tests for EBV, retrovirus, human herpesvirus 6, enteroviruses, and *Candida albicans*.
> • Tests of immunologic function.
> • Brain imaging studies.
>
> *Additional testing may be required in individual cases.
> International Chronic Fatigue Syndrome Study Group; see Fukuda K, Straus SE, Hickie I, et al. The chronic fatigue syndrome: A comprehensive approach to its definition and study. Ann Intern Med 121:953–959, 1994.

Natural History

Chronic fatigue syndrome is a recently described condition and little data are available on long-term outcome. It has been observed, however, that some patients appear to improve.

Treatment

Methods

There is no known effective treatment for CFS. In general, the treatment of CFS is similar to the treatment of the closely related fibromyalgia. Patients should be treated with sympathy. They should be reassured that an immunologic, infectious, or malignant condition is not present. Mainstays of therapy are tricyclic antidepressant agents, in particular amitriptyline, and physical therapy. Patients with CFS are typically profoundly deconditioned, and any sudden change in physical activities is poorly tolerated. Treatment should stress stretching exercises and a programmed buildup of strength and endurance. Psychologic support is frequently required. Because a viral etiology of the condition has often been suggested, researchers have considered the use of antiviral agents. Acyclovir has been tested double blind with negative results. Trials with other antiviral agents are underway.

When to Refer

Because no effective treatment is available and provided that the diagnostic evaluation has been complete, there is little to gain by referring chronic fatigue patients to a specialist. If a research group is available locally, however, the team work that is usually available, plus the prospect of joining therapeutic trials, makes the referral of these patients highly advisable.

Suggested Reading

Fukuda K, Straus SE, Hickie I, et al. The chronic fatigue syndrome: A comprehensive approach to its definition and study. Ann Intern Med 121:953–959, 1994.

Holmes GP, Kaplan JE, Gantz NM, et al. Chronic fatigue syndrome: A working case definition. Arch Intern Med 108:387–389, 1988.

Joints That Rub, Squeak, Crack, or Snap

For 15 years the author has taught a course in the pathophysiology of the musculoskeletal system for second-year medical students, and the most frequently asked question has been, "Doctor, my joints crack; what does it mean? What should I do?" Also, many patients have complained that their joints crack, sometimes with pain, or have discomfort that was relieved after the joint was made to crack or snap. Finally, few signs in clinical medicine are as striking as the soft tissue friction rubs that occur in scleroderma.

Presentation and Progression

Cause

Fingers: The well-known finger cracking is caused by synovial fluid fracture (cavitation) when the MCP joint is pulled with a load of 10 to 16 k. About 20 minutes must elapse before the joint can be made to crack again, which is the time required for a radiographically demonstrable gas bubble to return into solution. Purposeful finger cracking is both a pathognomonic sign of poor manners and a nuisance when silence is required. Snaps, often audible at a distance, are a classic finding in trigger finger. They may also occur at the base of the thumb in patients with joint hyperlaxity.

Wrists, Distal Forearms, Ankles, and Distal Legs: A leathery rub felt on palpation and sometimes heard at a distance may be a dramatic finding in patients with diffuse scleroderma. A stethoscope magnifies the rub, but the observer must be aware of the normal auscultatory findings around tendon sheaths and joints. Scleroderma rubs originate within tendon sheaths, joints, and superficial bursae.

Elbows: Snapping at the elbow may occur due to dislocation of the ulnar nerve in and out of the groove (often associated with ulnar paresthesias), the triceps over the medial epicondyle, and the brachialis over the medial rim of the trochlea. The latter may cause a median nerve neuropathy.

Neck: Some individuals, usually over the age of 50, complain of painless neck cracking that is viewed (rightfully so) as a sign of aging. Of the many potential sources for these cracks, which are perceived by osseous transmission, none can be blamed with certainty.

Shoulders: Subacromial cracks are common in elderly individuals from fraying in the rotator cuff tendons. Gross cracking is a common accompaniment of subacromial impingement. In the Milwaukee shoulder, excruciatingly painful squeaks occur between the eburneated and irregular humeral head and the contacting acromion or glenoid.

Scapula: Scapular snaps are relatively frequent and may occur from bursitis affecting normal or adventitious bursae, an excessive forward curvature of the medial angle of the scapula, or an osteochondroma projecting from the chest wall or the anterior scapula (Luschka's tubercle in the superomedial angle). There are cases that indicate occupational disease and others that are voluntary, attained by excessive tightening of the scapulothoracic muscles during elevation of the arm. Compulsive scapular snapping does occur. In an extreme case seen by the author, the patient was totally concentrated and pale as he repeatedly rotated the scapula until an unbelievably loud, compound snap occurred. This was immediately followed by a calmed countenance and total relaxation, resembling an orgasm.

Hips: Hip snaps are generally asymptomatic and harmless. Lateral snaps occur as the fascia lata or gluteus maximus jump over the greater trochanter. Anterior snaps occur when the femur is moved from a flexed position to extension corresponding to a displacement of the iliopsoas tendon (from a lateral to a medial position) over the femoral head or, less frequently, the iliopectineal eminence. Painful clicks are more likely to be intraarticular such as in labral detachments, small fracture fragments, and osteochondromas.

Knees: Squeaks may normally occur at the patella as individuals rise from a sitting position. Painful patellofemoral squeaks and cracks are common in chondromalacia patella and patellofemoral osteoarthritis. A loud snap, usually painful, may be produced in the lateral knee in patients with a tense iliotibial tract. This sound indicates a jump of the taut tendon over the lateral epicondyle in the femoral condyle. A similar sound in the medial knee may result from a hypertrophic plica. A snap, usually painful, followed by normalization of joint motion is an unequivocal indication of internal derangement of the joint.

Diagnosis

Summary of Diagnosis

> **JOINTS THAT RUB, SQUEAK, CRACK, OR SNAP**
>
> - In most instances diagnosis is clinical.
> - Tendon sheath rubs are elicited by finger motion, bursal rubs by skin displacement, and joint rubs by angular motion.
> - Squeaks are brought about by the motion of contacting bare bone.
> - Joint cracks and snaps, when associated with sudden changes of range of motion, are unequivocal evidence of an internal derangement of the joint and an indication for arthroscopy.
> - Scapular snaps should be investigated with oblique or profile scapular x-rays, and possibly CT.
> - Hip snaps are located by palpation during flexion/extension movements. Knee snaps are located by palpation during flexion-extension movements.

Natural History

Expected Outcome

Outcome depends on the structure at fault and the use of the part. Thus, although occasional finger cracking is harmless, compulsive cracking may result, over the years, in accelerated osteoarthritis. Loose bodies, revealed by the catching phenomenon, should be removed to alleviate symptoms and prevent wearing of the joint.

Treatment

Methods

Treatment of trigger finger and subacromial decompression in the impingement syndrome have been described. Arthroscopy is the preferred method to remove loose bodies in shoulder and knee. Scapular osteochondromas and chronically inflamed subscapular bursae may be treated by open or arthroscopic surgery. Symptomatic hip snaps may be treated by a corticosteroid infiltration plus lengthening exercises for the involved structure: fascia lata in lateral snaps, and iliopsoas tendon in anterior snaps. Unrelieved anterior hip snaps may be treated by surgical release of the iliopsoas tendon.

When to Refer

From the preceding discussion it should be clear that most abnormal sounds are inconsequential and only require reassurance of the patient. Soft tissue rubs in scleroderma associate with disseminated disease that, given its course and prognosis, falls within the realm of rheumatology. Painful snaps and clicks dictate orthopedic consultation.

Key Points

> **JOINTS THAT RUB, SQUEAK, CRACK, OR SNAP**
>
> - Soft tissue rubs in scleroderma indicate severe disease.
> - Articular squeaks usually reveal denuded contacting bone.
> - Finger cracking, which is normally harmless, if abused may lead to mechanical deterioration of the joint.
> - Painful clicks, cracks, and snaps indicate internal derangement in joints or inflammation at a prominent site or hole in extraarticular snaps.

Suggested Reading

Allen WC, Cope R. Coxa saltans: The snapping hip revisited. J Acad Orthop Surg 3:303–308, 1995.
Cardinal E, Buckwalter KA, Capello WN, et al. US of the snapping iliopsoas tendon. Radiology 198:521–522, 1996.
Coonrad RW, Spinner RJ. Snapping brachialis tendon associated with median neuropathy. J Bone Joint Surg 77A:1891–1893, 1995.
Lyons JC. The snapping iliopsoas tendon. Mayo Clin Proc 59:327–329, 1984.
Milch H. Snapping scapula. Clin Orthop 20:139–150, 1961.
Taylor GR, Clarke MNP. Surgical release of the "snapping iliopsoas tendon." J Bone Joint Surg 77B:881–883, 1995.
Unsworth A, Dowson D, Wright V. "Cracking joints." A bioengineering study of cavitation in the metacarpophalangeal joint. Ann Rheum Dis 30:348–358, 1971.

Soft Tissue Pain and Fever: Pyomyositis, Necrotizing Fasciitis, and Spontaneous Gas Gangrene

Serious infections may mimic a musculoskeletal pain syndrome. This is particularly true in pyomyositis, necrotizing fasciitis, and spontaneous gas gangrene. An early diagnosis may be life saving in these conditions. The location of common soft tissue infection is shown in Figure 30–2.

Presentation and Progression

Cause

Pyomyositis in the tropics (tropical pyomyositis) often has no identifiable portal of entry or risk factor. In nontropical countries, and certainly in the United States, pyomyositis is largely confined to intravenous drug users, patients with AIDS, diabetics, and patients with hematopoietic and other debilitating disorders. The most prevalent agent (over 90%) in tropical pyomyositis is *S. aureus;* in nontropical cases a variety of agents are involved including *S. aureus* (about 60%), streptococci (about 20%), and other agents including gram negative bacteria, anaerobes, and even fungi.

Necrotizing fasciitis is more common in diabetics, alcoholics, drug users, and postoperatively in pelvic and abdominal surgery. The prevailing agent in limb necrotizing fasciitis is group A streptococcus (GAS). As is well known from the media, over the past 10 years there has been an epidemic of deep GAS soft tissue infections, particularly of the M-1 and M-3 serotype. These agents frequently produce the pyrogenic

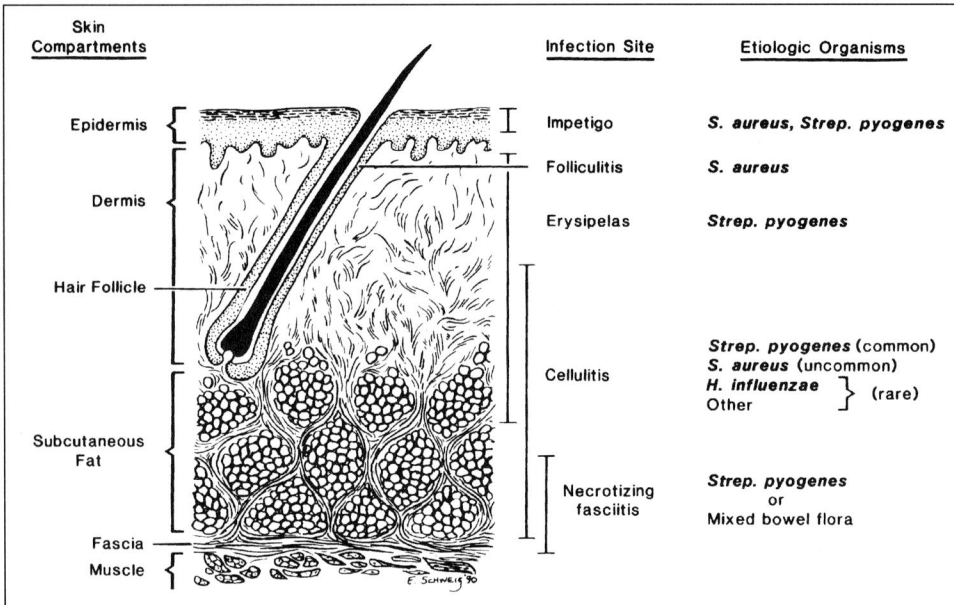

FIGURE 30–2. *Anatomy of soft tissue infections.* Depth and prevailing bacteriology of various infections are shown. For the purpose of this discussion, attention should be paid to subcutaneous fat, deep fascia, and muscle. (After Feingold DS, Hirschmann JV. Skin and soft tissue infections. In: Gorbach SL, Bartlett JG, Blacklow NR [eds] Infectious Diseases. W. B. Saunders, Philadelphia, 1065, 1992.)

exotoxin A (the scarlet fever exotoxin), which appears to be involved in the pathogenesis of the streptococcal toxic shock syndrome. Postoperative cases may be caused by GAS or a mixed flora that comprises anaerobic bacteria such as *Bacteroides* or *Peptostreptococcus* plus facultative bacteria such as streptococci (not group A) or *Enterobacteriaceae*.

Spontaneous gas gangrene occurs in older individuals with an often unrecognized ulcerated neoplasm in the GI tract, usually in the colon. Agents include *C. septicum* and *C. histoliticum.*

Presentation

Pyomyositis causes focal muscle induration and tenderness and later a fluctuant mass. Most frequently involved regions include the thighs, buttocks, paraspinal muscles, upper arms, and shoulders (Figure 4–2). Fever need not be prominent and may be absent at onset. Only one muscle or muscle group is usually involved, but other muscle abscesses as well as suppurative infection elsewhere may surface on follow-up.

In necrotizing fasciitis events occur at an astonishing speed, and sometimes the only external indication of infection is severe focal soft tissue tenderness. Skin necrosis is present in a minority of patients at initial evaluation. Indeed, pain out of proportion to local signs of infection in a toxic individual should raise the suspicion of necrotizing fasciitis. It has been stressed by Bisno and Stevens that renal failure in streptococcal toxic shock may precede hypotension and that catastrophic toxic shock may occur without cutaneous evidence of necrotizing fasciitis. Premorbid risk factors include age older than 50, diabetes mellitus, malnutrition, intravenous drug use, and renal failure. Clues suggesting necrotizing fasciitis include fever, restlessness, obtundation, diffuse limb edema, severe soft tissue pain, hypotension, and renal failure. Blisters, bullae, and diffuse cutaneous necrosis soon follow. Similar systemic findings, plus local crepitus, occur in spontaneous gas gangrene.

Diagnosis

Summary of Diagnosis

SOFT TISSUE PAIN AND FEVER

Pyomyositis
- Tropical pyomyositis occurs in seemingly normal individuals. Local trauma may precede muscle infection.
- Nontropical pyomyositis affects drug users, patients with AIDS, diabetics, and patients with other debilitating conditions.
- Focal induration and tenderness in muscle; fluctuation later in the course.
- Thighs, buttocks, paraspinal muscles, upper arms, shoulders.
- Fever.
- Leukocytosis (with eosinophilia in tropical cases).
- Documentation by ECHO, CT with contrast, or MRI.
- Bacteriologic diagnosis by needle or catheter aspiration, or surgical drainage.

Necrotizing Fasciitis
- Type I (mixed infections) frequently postoperative and in diabetics; predilection for abdomen or perineum.
- Type II (group A streptococcus, or GAS) usually in alcoholics or intravenous drug users; predominant limb involvement.
- Severe local pain; patch of cellulitis that evolves to bulla formation and necrosis; local anesthesia; there may be crepitus.
- Hypertermia, less often hypotermia; systemic toxicity.
- Systemic toxicity and hypotension in a patient with

severe localized soft tissue pain should suggest streptococcal necrotizing fasciitis.
- Surgical debridement is both diagnostic and therapeutic.

Spontaneous Gas Gangrene
- Abrupt onset of pain, swelling, and tenderness.
- Patient appears gravely ill; pale, sweaty, delirious, manic, or apathetic.
- Crepitation.
- Rapid evolution to full thickness necrosis with bullae and blebs.
- Diagnosis proven at surgery: pale or brick-colored muscle that is not contractile and does not bleed.
- Gram stain of exudate: gram positive rods.

Natural History

Expected Outcome

Tropical pyomyositis has an excellent prognosis. Prognosis in nontropical pyomyositis is guarded mainly because of the debilitated condition of the host. Involvement of additional muscles may surface on follow-up in both forms of pyomyositis. Metastatic infection to internal structures, such as the pericardium, sometimes occurs. Untreated, both necrotizing fasciitis and gas gangrene are uniformly lethal.

Treatment

Methods

Treatment of pyomyositis varies with the stage of the condition. Early disease may be diagnosed prior to suppuration. These cases respond to systemic antibiotics. Later in the course catheter or surgical drainage becomes necessary. Mortality of pyomyositis is 2% to 3% in the tropics, and higher, around 10%, in temperate areas of the world probably as a result of debilitating comorbid conditions.

Treatment of necrotizing fasciitis is with immediate surgical debridement with removal of all necrotic tissue plus systemic antibiotics. Discriminating cellulitis from necrotizing fasciitis is the critical step. Symptoms that far outweigh physical signs, lack of response to antibiotics, and a toxic appearance of the patient all indicate that the patient has necrotizing fasciitis rather than cellulitis and that prompt surgical exploration is warranted. Initial antibiotics should include a combination of ampicillin (or penicillin G), gentamycin, and clindamycin. Overall mortality is about 50% but is less in drug addicts, GAS etiology, and cases with debridement within 12 hours of admission.

Gas gangrene is treated with surgical removal of all infected muscle and systemic antibiotics, usually penicillin plus clindamycin. Hyperbaric oxygen, if available, may be used as an addition to the outlined treatment.

When to Refer

Suspicion of pyomyositis, necrotizing fasciitis, or gas gangrene calls for immediate surgical referral and an infectious disease consult.

Key Points

SOFT TISSUE PAIN AND FEVER: PYOMYOSITIS, NECROTIZING FASCIITIS, AND GAS GANGRENE

- Serious infection should be considered any time a patient with local pain and tenderness has fever or systemic toxicity.
- Intravenous drug use, AIDS, malignancy, diabetes, and other debilitating illnesses are often in the background.
- Muscle induration and tenderness suggests pyomyositis.
- Severe toxemia with mental changes suggests necrotizing fasciitis and gangrene.
- Crepitation may occur in necrotizing fasciitis and is the rule in gangrene.
- Suspected fasciitis and gangrene call for immediate surgical exploration.
- Prognosis is good in pyomyositis, poor in fasciitis, and dismal in gas gangrene.

Suggested Reading

Bisno AL, Stevens DL. Streptococcal infections of skin and soft tissues. N Engl J Med 334:240–245, 1996.
Canoso JJ, Barza M. Soft tissue infections. Clin Rheum Dis 19:293–309, 1993.
Falasca GF, Reginato AJ. The spectrum of myositis and rhabdomyolysis associated with bacterial infection. J Rheumatol 21:1932–1937, 1994.
Gómez-Reino JJ, Aznar JJ, Pablos JL, et al. Nontropical pyomyositis in adults. Sem Arthritis Rheum 23:396–405, 1994.
Lille ST, Sato TT, Engrav LH, et al. Necrotizing soft tissue infections: Obstacles in diagnosis. J Am Coll Surg 182:7–11, 1996.
Shbeeb MI, Cockerill FR, Gabriel SE. Musculoskeletal manifestations of invasive group A streptococcal infection. Arthritis Rheum 39:1260–1261, 1996.

The Patient with a Soft Tissue Mass

It may seem odd to have a section on soft tissue masses in a book devoted to rheumatic conditions. However, every once in a while a patient believed to have bursitis or joint swelling will in fact have a tumoral mass. Most of these lesions will be benign but others will be a sarcoma. Confronted with a suspicious situation, a plan of action should be available to take the right preliminary steps and, more importantly, to make early and appropriate referral.

Presentation and Progression

Cause

A deep lump at the root of a limb, for example, in the buttock or proximal thigh, has a high likelihood of being a sarcoma. Other possibilities include a benign soft tissue tumor such as a lipoma and, rarely, a distended iliopsoas or trochanteric bursa. Conversely, a lump around the knee may represent synovial effusion, a tumoral synovial condition such as synovial chondromatosis or pigmented villonodular synovitis (PVNS), a meniscal cyst, a Baker's cyst, a ganglion, a popliteal artery aneurysm, or a sarcoma. Somewhere in between fall lumps in the foot, shoulder, elbow, and hand. Superficial lipomas can be readily recognized and dismissed, unless they pose a cosmetic problem, if additional lesions are found elsewhere in the subcutaneous tissue.

In superficial bursitis the lump is clearly within the confines of a bursa except when bursal rupture has occurred, in which case the differential is not with a tumor but with diffuse infection. Articular effusions can be typically displaced around the joint and its recesses. Because synovial effusions occur in damaged joints, evidence of degenerative or inflammatory disease will be present: In the former, joint excursion will be irregular; in the latter, all endpoints of motion will be painful. Meniscal cysts are peculiar in that they become prominent in semiflexion of the knee and disappear in full flexion and full extension. Conversely, Baker's cysts harden in knee extension and soften in flexion (Foucher's sign). Other soft tissue masses are unaffected by joint position. Soft or fluctuant masses may represent distended bursae, ganglia, or lipomas. Soft tissue sarcomas are fleshy, firm, or hard and are firmly lodged within muscle or in a fascial plane; they may or may not be tender.

Although pain is not a main feature of soft tissue sarcomas, bone malignancies, whether primary (such as osteosarcoma, chondrosarcoma, multiple myeloma, or lymphoma) or metastatic are typically painful. Pain from bone tumors is relentless and becomes worse at night. Both intramedullary and surface bone tumors may grow into the soft tissues, mimicking a primary soft tissue mass. Plain x-rays, although seldom informative in soft tissue tumors, are always important in the assessment of bone malignancy. There may be pleasant surprises: A painful bone lesion may end up being osteomyelitis or an osteoid osteoma.

Diagnosis

Summary of Diagnosis

THE PATIENT WITH A SOFT TISSUE MASS

- Obtain a detailed history (trauma, pain, growth rate).
- Rule out an articular or bursal origin of the mass.
- Determine by palpation the structure in which the mass is lodged: subcutaneous tissue, muscle/fascia, bone.
- Obtain plain x-rays. Phleboliths are characteristic of hemangiomas. Soft tissue osteochondromas exhibit stippled calcification. Other focal calcifications are nonspecific and occur frequently in certain neoplasms (e.g., synovial sarcoma).
- Obtain an ECHO to determine the internal structure of the mass.
- If the mass is not cystic, enlist a musculoskeletal oncologist to conduct further evaluation.
- The next step is likely to be an MRI followed by an incisional (rarely excisional), fine-needle, or Tru-cut needle biopsy.

Natural History

Outcome of course depends on the nature of the soft tissue lesion. Two tumoral conditions of joints, both of them benign and monoarticular, have a synovial derivation: PVNS and synovial chondromatosis. PVNS is a chronic condition that owes its name to chocolate-colored, hemosiderin-laden synovium that projects in irregular masses. Enzymes produced by this lesion are capable of eroding adjacent bone. The true nature of PVNS, whether inflammatory or neoplasic, is still under debate. Clinically, PVNS behaves as a chronic monoarthritis with episodic tense effusions. Synovial fluid is characteristically blood tinged or chocolate in color, and noninflammatory.

In *synovial chondromatosis*, multiple intrasynovial metaplastic cartilaginous nodules develop within a joint. These nodules pedunculate and are subsequently delivered free into the joint space where they may ossify (synovial osteochondromatosis). Synovial chondromatosis causes chronic enlargement of a single joint. The free play of the joint is interfered with and pressure erosions may develop, particularly in the hip. Synovial effusions are clear and noninflammatory.

Paraarticular myxoma is a benign, ganglionlike tumoral condition that develops adjacent to the knee and sometimes in the vicinity of the acromioclavicular joint. Resection is often followed by recurrence.

Lipomas are the prevailing soft tissue tumors. Three main types of soft tissue lipomas are recognized: (1) solitary subcutaneous lipomas, which are the most frequent; (2) multiple subcutaneous lipomatosis, which has approximately one-tenth of the frequency of solitary subcutaneous lipomas; and (3) subfascial lipomas, which are rare. Most soft tissue lipomas occur in the trunk, shoulder, upper arm, and neck. Lipomas involving the supraclavicular fossa and the shoulders that frequently associate with peripheral neuropathy have already been described. Over 80% of lipomas are less than 5 cm in diameter. Thigh lipomas are rare.

On the other hand, *soft tissue sarcomas* occur most frequently proximally in the lower extremity followed by the distal lower extremity, the upper extremity, and the trunk. Deep-seated lesions, which are the most frequent, tend to be larger than 5 cm in diameter by the time of diagnosis. The most frequent histologic types include malignant fibrous histiocytoma, which accounts for 40% of sarcomas, followed by leiomyosarcoma, liposarcoma, synovial sarcoma (which despite its name only exceptionally grows intraarticularly), and several rarer lesions. At diagnosis about 8% of sarcomas have already metastasized, principally to the lung. Prognosis in soft tissue sarcoma relates to tumor size (worse in tumors larger than 5 cm in diameter), malignancy grade, presence of necrosis, and vascular invasion. A sizable proportion of sarcomas of the extremities, perhaps 30%, have a subcutaneous location. Prognosis of these lesions is better than in deep-seated sarcomas. The difference is accounted for by the smaller size of superficial lesions.

Thus, distinguishing lipomas from small subcutaneous sarcomas clinically may be impossible, and only when multiple lesions are present can a clinical diagnosis of lipoma be made with certainty.

Treatment

Treatment of PVNS is with surgical or arthroscopic synovectomy. Recurrences are frequent. In synovial chondromatosis, synovectomy is required in active disease, but removal of the free bodies may be all that is needed in late stages of the disease after the synovial lining of the joint has once again become normal. Recurrences are rare. Lipomas may be removed or, if they are small (as multiple lipomas usually are), they may be left alone. Treatment of soft tissue sarcomas is beyond the scope of this book. However, it needs to be stressed that a correctly planned, placed, and executed biopsy is definitely a part of the treatment plan. Preferably, the biopsy should be performed by the same surgeon who will be responsible for the definitive operative procedure.

When to Refer

Any patient with a soft tissue mass that is not bursal or synovial, a superficial lipoma in the context of lipomatosis, or a ganglion should be referred to a musculoskeletal oncologist for further imaging studies and biopsy.

Key Points

THE PATIENT WITH A SOFT TISSUE MASS

- Soft tissue malignancy should be suspected in patients with a soft tissue mass that is not synovial or bursal.
- Superficial lipomas can be confidently diagnosed if more than one lesion is present.
- Ganglia can be confirmed or ruled out by ultrasound.
- All other patients should be suspected of having soft tissue malignancy and should be expediently referred to a musculoskeletal oncologist.
- Ideally, the biopsy should be performed by the same surgeon who will be in charge of the definitive surgical treatment.
- Open biopsies allow an accurate diagnosis of soft tissue sarcomas. Of the closed biopsy techniques, Tru-cut needle biopsies are best because they provide tissue with the original architecture preserved. Fine-needle biopsies are helpful to diagnose local recurrences as well as to sample enlarged lymph nodes.

Suggested Reading

Canoso JJ. Soft tissue tumors. In: Koopman WN (ed) Arthritis and Allied Conditions, 13th ed. Williams and Wilkins, Baltimore, 1867–1886, 1996.

Gustafson P. Soft tissue sarcoma. Epidemiology and prognosis in 508 patients. Acta Orthop Scand 65:1–31, 1994.

Rydholm A, Berg NO. Size, site and clinical incidence of lipoma. Factors in the differential diagnosis of lipoma and sarcoma. Acta Orthop Scand 54:929–934, 1983.

Sim FH, Frassica FJ, Frassica DA. Soft-tissue tumors: Diagnosis, evaluation, and management. J Am Acad Orthop Surg 2:202–211, 1994.

Simon MA, Bierman JS. Biopsy of bone and soft-tissue lesions. J Bone Joint Surg 75A:616–621, 1993.

Simon MA, Finn HA. Diagnostic strategy for bone and soft-tissue tumors. J Bone Joint Surg 75A:622–631, 1993.

Springfield DS, Rosenberg A. Biopsy: Complicated and risky. J Bone Joint Surg 78A:639–643, 1996.

APPENDIX

Injection and Aspiration Techniques

Primary care physicians should learn (they probably did during training) how to aspirate superficial bursae, such as the olecranon and prepatellar, and certain joints, such as the knee and the wrist. The technique is simple, and the frequency of involvement is high. There are also corticosteroid infiltrations that are easy to perform and that provide satisfactory results. These include infiltrations for trigger finger, carpal tunnel syndrome, rotator cuff tendinitis, trochanteric bursitis, and anserine bursitis. However, because primary care physicians may work in areas without rapid or convenient access to a rheumatologist or an orthopedist, a description of procedures is provided here.

Corticosteroid Infiltrations

Indications

> ARTHRITIS: Sterile arthritis not controlled with systemic medications (RA, spondyloarthropathy, some cases of gout and pseudogout).
> BURSITIS: Olecranon and prepatellar (traumatic*); retrocalcaneal (spondyloarthropathy, RA); trochanteric; anserine.
> TENOSYNOVITIS: Trigger finger; RA; de Quervain's; carpal tunnel syndrome; tarsal tunnel syndrome.
> FASCIITIS: Plantar fasciitis (spondyloarthropathy).
> ELBOW PAIN: Tennis elbow.[†]
> SHOULDER PAIN: Structural impingement; frozen shoulder; acromioclavicular arthritis.
> FOREFOOT PAIN: Morton's neuroma.
> TRIGGER POINTS in the myofascial syndromes.[‡]

---

*Seldom an indication.
[†]In my opinion, seldom an indication.
[‡]Only xylocaine 1%–2% should be used; there is no rationale for the use of corticosteroids.

Complications

a. *Facial flushing.* Very common, perhaps 40% of intraarticular injections. Transient and inconsequential but may worry unwarned patients.
b. *Postinjection flare.* Uncommon, perhaps 5% of intraarticular injections. Pain appears hours after the procedure and lasts several hours to 1 day. Protracted pain, lasting days or weeks, may follow tennis elbow infiltrations.
c. *Skin atrophy.* Very common following superficial infiltrations and olecranon bursa injections. May lead to chronic pressure pain.
d. *Hipopigmentation.* A very frequent complication of superficial infiltrations (i.e., de Quervain's tenosynovitis). The hypopigmented patch, which may be very disfiguring in blacks, persists up to 2 years.
e. *Infection.* Possible but extremely rare, except in injections in the olecranon bursa.
f. *Tendon rupture.* Usually indicates abuse of the procedure or intratendinous injection. Prevalent in athletes who received multiple infiltrations around the Achilles tendon.
g. *Steroid arthropathy.* Abuse of intraarticular injections may result in a Charcot's-type arthropathy similar to the one reported in CPPD crystal deposition disease.
h. *Systemic complications.* It must be remembered that corticosteroid esters are absorbed and have systemic effects, including transient hipophyseal inhibition. Serial infiltrations may cause adrenal suppression. Rare cases of osteonecrosis have been reported.

Techniques (by Anatomic Regions)

All procedures must be done according to the rules of universal precautions. The techniques that follow may be used for diagnostic aspiration or corticosteroid infiltration. For diagnosis, #20 needles (or #18 if bacterial infection is suspected) should be used. Narrower needles are used for infiltration. Needles should be of sufficient length. Long needles may be needed in the shoulder (GH) and the trochanteric bursa in obese patients. The skin is sterilized with povidone-iodine solution for 2 minutes or 70%–90% alcohol for 1 minute. The corticosteroid doses recommended are based on the use of methylprednisolone acetate (Depomedrol). When triamcinolone hexacetonide (Aristospan) is used the lower dose of the range should be chosen. In general, I prefer to immobilize the injected site for at least 48 hours following the procedure. Longer immobility may lead to better results (albeit with more muscle atrophy) and should be considered in special circumstances.

Finger and metacarpophalangeal joints

a. *Indications.* RA, psoriatic arthritis, etc.
b. *Dose.* 10–15 mg (#25 needle).
c. *Entry.* Dorsolateral, digit in semiflexion. Multiple joints may be injected in one session.

d. *Precautions.* Do not hyperdistend joint; fluid tends to back up.
e. *Complications.* Joint hyperlaxity, capsular calcification (frequent but inconsequential).

Flexor tendon sheaths

a. *Indications.* Trigger finger, RA, psoriatic arthritis, etc.
b. *Dose.* 15–20 mg mixed with 1–2 ml xylocaine (#25 needle or #23 butterfly).
c. *Entry.* Palmar crease of thumb, proximal palmar crease (index), distal palmar crease (long and ring fingers) with needle held at a 45 degree inclination.
d. *Precautions.* Avoid intratendinous injection. Tendon engagement is present if the needle moves reciprocally upon gentle finger motion.
e. *Complications.* Superficial extravasation may produce focal palmar atrophy.

Dorsal wrist tenosynovitis

I seldom inject these structures. Persistent (months) tenosynovitis should be evaluated by a hand surgeon, since a tenosynovectomy may be necessary to prevent tendon rupture.

Wrist extensor (ECU, ECR) and flexor (FCU, FCR) tendon sheaths

Inflammation in these structures is common in RA and psoriatic arthritis. Considerations similar to those for flexor tendon sheath injections apply.

Carpal Tunnel Syndrome (CTS)

a. *Indications.* All etiologies of CTS except acute cases due to fracture, hemorrhage or infection, and the CTS of late pregnancy.
b. *Dose.* 20–30 mg mixed with 2–3 ml xylocaine (#22 needle or #23 butterfly).
c. *Entry.* Distal wrist crease medial to the palmaris longus (PL) tendon. If the PL tendon is absent (in 25% of people), use the midline. The needle should be inserted 1 cm with a 45 degree distal inclination and a 45 degree radial inclination.
d. *Precautions.* Paresthesias indicate median nerve engagement; reposition the needle. Reciprocal needle motion upon gentle finger motion indicates tendon engagement; reposition the needle.
e. *Complications.* Transient increase of paresthesias.
NOTE: A resting splint in neutral position (lowest intra CT pressures) should be used continuously for 48 hours and as a night splint for the ensuing 12 days.

Elbow

a. *Indications.* RA, psoriatic arthritis, etc.
b. *Dose.* 30–40 mg (#22 needle).
c. *Entry.* Midpoint between the olecranon tip and the lateral epicondyle. Aim the needle to the center of the joint. Alternatively, the radiocapitular joint may be entered from the side just proximal to the radial head.

d. *Precautions.* None.
e. *Complications.* None.

Olecranon bursa

a. *Indications.* Aseptic bursitis (traumatic). A negative bursal fluid culture is required for the procedure to be performed.
b. *Dose.* 20 mg (#22 needle). Use methylprednisolone acetate only.
c. *Entry.* Lateral through normal skin toward the center of the bursa.
d. *Precautions.* Taps at the tip of the bursa may create a chronic leak. Medial entries may damage the ulnar nerve.
e. *Complications.* Skin atrophy, pain on leaning, septic bursitis.
NOTE: I recommend conservative initial treatment, namely, avoidance of leaning on the elbow for 3 months. Intrabursal corticosteroids may be tried in cases that fail to resolve during that period.

Tennis elbow

a. *Indications* (arguable). Failures of conservative treatment; to speed up recovery in high-performance athletes (I dislike this indication).
b. *Dose.* 20–30 mg (#22 needle).
c. *Entry.* At the most tender point. Use xylocaine alone. Failure to eradicate pain on resisted wrist dorsiflexion indicates the wrong injection site; reposition the needle and reinfiltrate with xylocaine. The steroid should be injected at the successful site.
d. *Precautions.* Avoid injecting too superficially.
e. *Complications.* Transient increase in pain in 40% of patients. Repeated corticosteroid infiltrations may result in chronic pain.
NOTE: The current trend is to be conservative and shy away from infiltrations. Failure to improve with xylocaine suggests compressive neuropathy of the deep branch of the radial nerve at Frohse's arcade.

Shoulder (GH joint)

a. *Indications.* RA, spondyloarthropathy, Stages I and II frozen shoulder.
b. *Dose.* 40–60 mg (#22 or #25 needle).
c. *Entry.* Two entries will be described, an anterior entry, which is the one I use, and a posterior entry, which is preferred by several authorities because it causes less apprehension and pain. *Anterior:* The patient sits (landmarks are lost in recumbency) with the arm hanging at the side of the body, the elbow flexed 90 degrees, the forearm in the sagittal plane. The needle is entered anteroposteriorly 1 cm distal and 1 cm lateral to the coracoid process (prior to any movement of the needle some xylocaine is injected so as to move through an anesthesized front). Once bone is touched (which happens soon after the capsular toughness is felt), the forearm is passively brought into internal rotation as the needle is gently pushed into the articular space. *Posterior:* The patient sits. The needle is inserted posteroanteriorly 1 cm below and 1 cm medial to the posterior

corner of the acromion, aimed at the coracoid process anteriorly until bone is touched at the articular space.
  d. *Precautions.* Use a chair with armrests; have an assistant; watch for fainting.
  e. *Complications.* Vasovagal syndrome. Misplaced anterior injections may encounter neurovascular structures.

Subacromial bursa

  a. *Indications.* Subacromial impingement; occasional cases of calcific tendinitis.
  b. *Dose.* 30–40 mg (#22 or #25 needle).
  c. *Entry.* Here again two entries will be described, the anterior, which I use, and the posterolateral, which is preferred by others. *Anterior:* The needle is aimed anteroposteriorly flush with the inferior surface of the acromion, 1 cm lateral to the acromioclavicular joint. Once a tough structure is passed (the coracoacromial ligament) tissue resistance ceases. Easy flow indicates the bursal location of the needle. *Posterolateral:* The needle is aimed anteromedially under the acromion with the tip directed to the undersurface of the acromion. Easy flow indicates a bursal injection.
  d. *Precautions.* None.
  e. *Complications.* None.
  NOTE: Subacromial bursa injections, similar to glenohumeral joint injections, are technically difficult. Only about 50% of injections are on target.

Acromioclavicular (AC) joint

  a. *Indications.* OA, RA, spondyloarthropathy.
  b. *Dose.* 15–20 mg (#22 needle or #23 butterfly).
  c. *Entry.* Vertically at articular cleft; advance the needle 0.5 cm; inject to distend joint.
  d. *Precautions.* Difficult tap; very narrow joint plus partial meniscus.
  e. *Complications.* None.

Interspinous ligaments

  a. *Indications.* Reactive arthritis, ankylosing spondylitis.
  b. *Dose.* 10–20 mg (#22 needle).
  c. *Entry.* Posteroanterior at midline; infiltrate the ligament and its attachments.
  d. *Precautions.* None.
  e. *Complications.* None.

Trigger points in the myofascial syndromes

  a. *Indications.* Acute cases if pressure on the point or the nodule reproduces regional pain.
  b. *Dose.* 3–5 ml xylocaine (do not use corticosteroids) (#22 needle).
  c. *Entry.* Aim at the tender point or the center of the nodule, which should be infiltrated radially throughout the indurated area.
  d. *Precautions.* None.
  e. *Complications.* None.
  NOTE: "Dry needling," rubbing pressure on the nodule, or gentle stretching of the contractured muscle under a hot shower is frequently effective.

Hip

I do not inject or aspirate hips. These procedures belong in the realm of orthopedics and radiology. Because the usual concern leading to aspiration is pyogenic infection, the procedure should be done to maximize the likelihood of yield—i.e., under fluoroscopic, ultrasound, or CT guidance.

  a. *Indications.* Diagnosis of septic arthritis of the hip, including presumed septic arthritis in a prosthetic hip.
  b. *Dose. None; the procedure is done strictly for diagnosis.*
  c. *Entry.* The femoral neck projection follows a bisecting line of the angle formed by the inguinal ligament and the femoral artery. The needle is inserted anteroposteriorly with some cephalic and medial inclination 1 finger breadth lateral to the femoral artery and 2 finger breadths distal to the inguinal ligament.
  d. *Precautions.* The danger of injuring the femoral neurovascular bundle is averted by using an imaging procedure as a control.
  e. *Complications.* None.

Trochanteric "bursa"

  a. *Indications.* Trochanteric "bursitis."
  b. *Dose.* 30–40 mg mixed with 3 ml of 1% xylocaine (#22 1½ inch needle; use a spinal tap needle with obese patients).
  c. *Entry.* With the patient lying on the opposite side, the greater trochanter is identified by ascending palpation along the femur. Maximal tenderness is usually at the posterior corner of the greater trochanter. The needle is inserted vertically to the periosteum. Xylocaine infiltration should cover the base of a cone 3 cm in diameter, half on bone and half on soft tissue. Next, the mixture of the steroid and xylocaine is infiltrated in the same area.
  d. *Precautions.* The needle should be of sufficient length.
  e. *Complications.* None.
  NOTE: Rather than bursitis, this process represents a stress enthesopathy at the gluteus medium and minimus insertion. The cause of the excessive pull should be sought (foot, knee, hip, or back disorder; discrepant leg length) and addressed to achieve sustained relief.

Knee

  a. *Indications.* RA, spondyloarthropathies, OA. Occasionally crystal-induced synovitis.
  b. *Dose.* 40–60 mg (#20 or #22 needle).
  c. *Entry.* Medial, with the needle aimed at the patellar undersurface, midway between the upper and lower poles of the patella (the lateral patellofemoral cleft is narrower than the medial, and the joint capsule is tougher laterally than medially).
  d. *Precautions.* Beware of superimposed septic arthritis in RA patients. Postpone injection of an acutely inflamed joint until a negative SF culture result becomes available.
  NOTE: If SF analysis has not been performed, any fluid removed during the procedure should be studied with cell count, differential, crystal search, and culture. Because corticosteroid crystals remain in joints for weeks and even months, an erroneous diagnosis of

gout or pseudogout can be made in a previously injected patient.
e. *Complications.* None.

Baker's cyst

Aspiration or injection of the cyst is unnecessary. In adults, Baker's cysts develop in connecting gastrocnemius-semimembranosus bursae and depend for their persistence and growth on excessive synovial fluid produced by the knee. Baker's cysts are best treated by correcting the causative knee disorder by systemic treatment, corticosteroid injection, or surgery.

Anserine "bursitis"

a. *Indications.* The syndrome of anserine bursitis.
b. *Dose.* 20–30 mg mixed with 2–3 ml of xylocaine (#22 needle).
c. *Entry.* Medial upper tibia about 5 cm distal to the medial articular line. The injection site is best determined following the medial tendinous border of the thigh, with the knee in semiflexion, to the tibia, where a mark is placed. The knee is then brought to extension, and the needle is entered perpendicular to the skin to tibial contact. An area 3 cm in diameter is infiltrated adjacent to the periosteum.
d. *Precautions.* None.
e. *Complications.* None.
NOTE: Because anserine bursitis is almost always secondary (genu valgum, patellofemoral osteoarthritis, etc.), the condition may be expected to recur unless the primary process has been addressed. A vigorous program of isometric quadriceps exercises should be initiated.

Ankle

a. *Indications.* Same as in knee.
b. *Dose.* 20–30 mg (#22 needle).
c. *Entry.* With the patient supine on the examining table, seek the cleft between the tibia and talus by gently moving the foot. Insert the needle vertically, medial to the posterior tibialis tendon.
d. *Precautions.* None.
e. *Complications.* None.

Subtalar joint

a. *Indications.* Same as in knee.
b. *Dose.* 20–30 mg (#22 needle).
c. *Entry.* By gently inverting and everting the foot, find a soft cleft (sinus tarsi) anterior to the lateral malleolus. Enter the needle obliquely toward the tip of the medial malleolus. Aspiration of fluid proves articular insertion. Inject under low pressure.
d. *Precautions.* None.
e. *Complications.* None.

Posterior tibialis tendon sheath

a. *Indications.* Posterior tibialis tenosynovitis; tarsal tunnel syndrome. Only one, cautious injection allowed.
b. *Dose.* 20–30 mg (#22 needle).
c. *Entry.* The patient lies supine with the injected leg resting on the contralateral knee. The needle is entered toward the posterior surface of the tibia 3 finger breadths proximal to the tip of the medial malleolus. Inject under low pressure. Fluid may be felt distending the sheath.
d. *Precautions.* Avoid injection within tendon substance.
e. *Complications.* Intratendinous injection may lead to rupture.

Retrocalcaneal bursa

a. *Indications.* Refractory Achilles tendon enthesitis in the spondyloarthropathies; RA.
b. *Dose.* 10–15 mg (#22 needle or butterfly).
c. *Entry.* The patient is prone on the examining table. The foot is outside the mattress. Allow calf relaxation. The needle is advanced vertically (PA), transtendinously aiming to the posterior superior calcaneal angle. Touch bone and back up 1 mm. Aspiration of fluid (usually a trace) proves the intrabursal location. Do not inject large volumes; high pressures produce back flow as the needle is removed. Bursal pressures may be decreased by keeping the foot in slight plantar flexion.
d. *Precautions. This procedure should be performed only by rheumatologists, orthopedists, or podiatrists.* The distal leg and foot should be casted for 10 days to achieve maximum antiinflammatory effect.
e. *Complications.* I have not observed tendon rupture or other complications but would discourage more than one reinjection after 2–3 weeks.

Plantar fascia attachment

a. *Indications.* Refractory plantar fasciitis in the spondyloarthropathies.
b. *Dose.* 20–30 mg diluted with 2 ml of xylocaine (#22 needle).
c. *Entry.* Medial, with the needle parallel to the plantar skin, 2 cm deep to the plantar surface. Aim the needle to the medial plantar tubercle of the calcaneus. Resilience indicates a fascial location. Relocate the needle and inject deep and superficial to the fibrous fascia.
d. *Precautions. This procedure should be performed only by rheumatologists, orthopedists, or podiatrists.*
e. *Complications.* Repeated infiltrations may result in fat atrophy and pressure plantar heel pain. Discourage more than one reinjection after an interval of 2–3 weeks.

Morton's neuroma

a. *Indications.* Morton's neuroma.
b. *Dose.* 20–30 mg mixed with 1 ml xylocaine.
c. *Entry.* Dorsal between the metatarsal heads; the needle must be advanced about 2 cm and passed through tough fibrous resistance (the transverse metatarsal ligament).
d. *Precautions.* Inject under low pressure.
e. *Complications.* None; up to two reinjections 2–3 weeks apart are allowed.

Metatarsophalangeal joints

  a. *Indications.* RA, spondyloarthropathies.
  b. *Dose.* 10–20 mg (#22 needle).
  c. *Entry.* Dorsal, lateral, or medial to the extensor tendon.
  d. *Precautions.* None.
  e. *Complications.* None.

Suggested Reading

Blyth T, Hunter JA, Stirling A. Pain relief in the rheumatoid knee after steroid injection. A single-blind comparison of hydrocortisone succinate and triamcinolone acetonide or hexacetonide. Brit J Rheumatol 33:461–463, 1994.

Carette S, Marcoux S, Truchon R, Grondin C, Gagnon J, Allard Y, Latulippe M. Facet joint injection of corticosteroids in chronic low back pain: A randomized double-blind placebo controlled trial. N Engl J Med 325:1002–1007, 1991.

Emkey RD, Lindsay R, Lyssy J, Weisberg JS, Dempster DW, Shen V. The systemic effect of intraarticular administration of corticosteroids on markers of bone formation and bone resorption in patients with rheumatoid arthritis. Arthritis Rheum 39:277–282, 1996.

Gatter RA. Arthrocentesis technique and intrasynovial therapy. In: McCarty DJ, Koopman WJ (eds). Arthritis and Allied Conditions, 12th ed. Lea & Febiger, Philadelphia, 711–720, 1993.

Neustadt DH. Local corticosteroid injection therapy in soft tisssue rheumatic conditions of the hand and wrist. Arthritis Rheum 34:923–926, 1991.

Price R, Sinclair H, Heinrich I, Gibson T. Local injection of tennis elbow. Hydrocortisone, triamcinolone and lignocaine compared. Brit J Rhumatol 30:39–44, 1991.

Smith DL, McAfee JH, Lucas LM, Kumar KL, Romney DM. Treatment of nonspecific olecranon bursitis. A controlled, blinded prospective trial. Arch Intern Med 149:2527–2530, 1989.

Weinstein PS, Canoso JJ, Wohlgethan JR. Long-term follow-up of corticosteroid injection for traumatic olecranon bursitis. Ann Rheum Dis 43:44–46, 1984.

Physical Therapy Instructions

Fitness Program

Patients with regional and systemic rheumatic diseases derive measurable benefit from a fitness program. A fitness program may be implemented in most patients by tailoring one of several possible programs to existing limitations. Aerobic exercise may take a variety of forms, including jogging, fast walking, using a stationary bike, swimming, floating, and walking across water. Fast walking may be the choice in patients with a painful back or shoulder, whereas floating and walking across water may be best for rheumatoid arthritis patients with multiple painful joints. Exercises need not be carried out forcefully. They should be performed for 30 minutes, including a warm-up period (fast walking for 5 minutes followed by general stretching) and a cool-down period (5 minutes of slower walking and then general stretching).

Isometric Exercises (Quadriceps, Gluteus Maximus, Abdominal)

Isometric exercises play a major role in the treatment of joint and tendon conditions. They are effective in the prophylaxis of muscle atrophy in patients with acute arthritis involving the hip or knee. Prime examples of knee conditions helped by quadriceps setting exercises include septic arthritis, flares of RA, gout, and pseudogout. Isometric exercises are also essential in the treatment of arthritis patients who first consult after muscle atrophy has set in. Another important use of isometric exercises is in painful anterior knee conditions such as chondromalacia patella, in which dysfunction of the quadriceps-patella-patellar tendon unit is intimately involved in pathogenesis. Gluteus maximus exercises are an important adjunct in the treatment of hip joint arthritis and low back pain. Quadriceps, gluteus, and abdominal wall isometric exercises should be included in the daily exercise routine of older patients in an attempt to prevent the loss of muscle mass associated with aging. To prevent the cardiovascular risk of an inadvertently performed Valsalva maneuver, it has been suggested that patients count backward from 6 out loud while doing the isometric exercise.

Quadriceps Setting Exercises

Goal: To strengthen anterior thigh muscles for stair climbing, rising from a chair, and squatting.

This exercise is done with the patient lying in bed face up. If the condition affects only one knee, the exercise is done on the healthy side first.

1. With the knee extended, the patient concentrates on the anterior thigh and contracts the quadriceps (front thigh muscle) maximally. The contraction is held 6 seconds (counted with a watch), and then the muscle is allowed to relax. The exercise is then attempted on the affected side. It is important, in the beginning, to have an assistant (child, spouse) in charge of ascertaining that muscle contraction actually occurs. This may be difficult at first, particularly when the knee is inflamed. Also, the knee may not be able to extend fully as a result of knee effusion or synovitis. This should not be an obstacle to performing the exercise as long as there is no pain. A modest twitch or contraction may be all that can be achieved at first, but fuller contractions will appear sooner or later.
2. The isometric contraction is repeated _____ times on each leg, always on alternating sides.
3. These exercises are done twice a day.
   NOTE: In patients who are not bedridden (such as for restoration of thigh strength in patients with longstanding knee problems, i.e., chondromalacia patella) it may be found convenient to perform the exercises before getting up in the morning and upon retiring at night.

Gluteus Maximus Setting Exercises

Goal: To strengthen the hip extensor muscles and to decrease pelvic obliquity (thus decreasing lumbar lordosis).

This exercise may be performed with the patient standing or lying in bed face up.

1. The buttock muscles are contracted against each other as if one were holding a sheet of paper between the buttocks. The contraction is held 6 seconds, and then the muscles are relaxed.
2. The contraction is repeated _____ times.
3. These exercises are performed twice a day after the quadriceps isometric exercises.

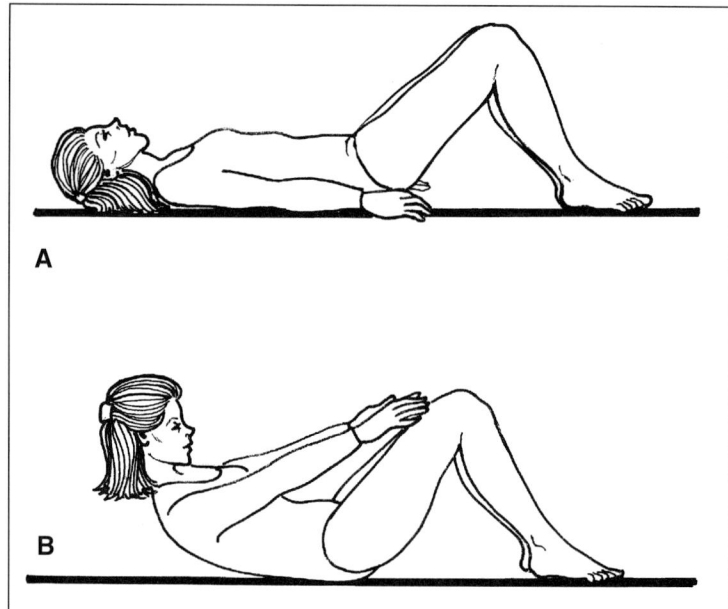

FIGURE A–1. *Abdominal wall strengthening exercises. A,* Patient lies flat on floor. *B,* Patient reaches with hands toward knees while slightly raising head and shoulders and flattening lumbar spine. (See text for details).

Abdominal Wall Strengthening Exercises (Figure A–1)

Goal: To strengthen the abdominal wall muscles to decrease lumbar lordosis. This exercise is used for the treatment of back pain as well as to improve general conditioning.

1. Lie flat on the floor or on a firm bed with both knees bent, your feet on the floor, and your arms by your sides.
2. Reach your hands toward your knees, slightly raising your head and shoulders while flattening the lumbar curvature (partial sit-up). Hold this position while counting backward from 6, one count per second.
3. Return to the initial position. The exercise is repeated _____ times.

To Begin Loosening Up

General stretching may be started with two exercises that are performed on the floor.

Longitudinal Stretch (Figure A–2)

Goal: To achieve the maximum possible longitudinal stretching.

1. Lying flat on the floor with the arms straight up and the feet pointing down, stretch as much as you can, holding the stretched position 4 seconds.
2. From the previous position, without allowing the knees to flex, bend your feet up with the toes pointing to your head. You'll feel the calf muscles being stretched. Hold this position 4 additional seconds.
3. Now relax.
   Repeat the general stretching _____ times.

Knee to Chest Stretch (Figure A–3)

Goal: To extend the benefit from the previous loosening exercise.

1. Lying flat on the floor, raise one leg and with both hands clasp the upper leg, or the thigh if the knee hurts.
2. Pull the leg toward your chest (keeping the opposite knee extended) gently but firmly, feeling a stretch in the hip and buttock muscles. Hold this position 4–6 seconds.
3. Return to the initial position.
   Repeat the stretching _____ times.

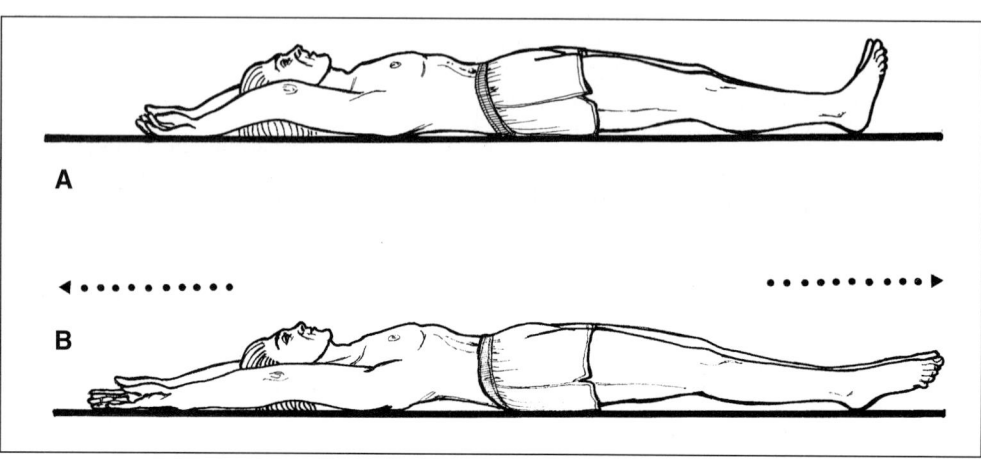

FIGURE A–2. *Longitudinal stretch. A,* Patient flat on floor. *B,* Stretched position. (See text for details.)

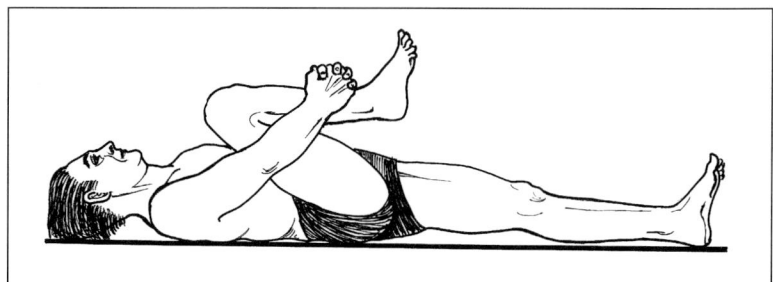

FIGURE A–3. *Knee to chest stretch exercise. (See text for details.)*

Neck Exercises

Neck motion becomes progressively limited during aging, but much of the loss is due to less demanding use (leading to restriction) rather than to disease. Restricted soft tissues make injuries more likely upon unprepared-for motions or minor trauma. Neck motions include flexion and extension movements, lateral bendings, and lateral turnings.

Neck Flexibility Exercises

Goal: To stretch joints, muscles, and ligaments, allowing for a freer neck. These exercises may be performed lying in bed, sitting, or standing. It is recommended that older people perform these exercises sitting in a chair. Different muscles will be active whether these exercises are performed in bed or in the sitting/erect position. Neck exercises are illustrated in Figures A–4 through A–6.

Flexion-extension exercise (Figure A–4)

1. Bend the neck forward, allowing the weight of the head to stretch the posterior neck structures, for 4–6 seconds.
2. Bend the neck backward, holding the fully extended position for 4–6 seconds.
3. The full (forward-backward) motion is repeated _____ times.

Right-left turning (Figure A–5)

1. Turn the head fully to the right, holding the position for 4–6 seconds.
2. Turn the head fully to the left, holding the position for 4–6 seconds.
3. The full (right-left) motion is performed _____ times.

Right-left bending (Figure A–6)

1. Bend the neck to the left, bringing the left ear close to the left shoulder (which should not be raised); hold the position 4–6 seconds.
2. Bend the neck to the right, bringing the right ear close to the right shoulder (which should not be raised); hold the position 4–6 seconds.
3. The full (left-right) motion is performed _____ times.

FIGURES A–4, A–5, A–6. *Neck flexibility exercises. (See text for details.)*

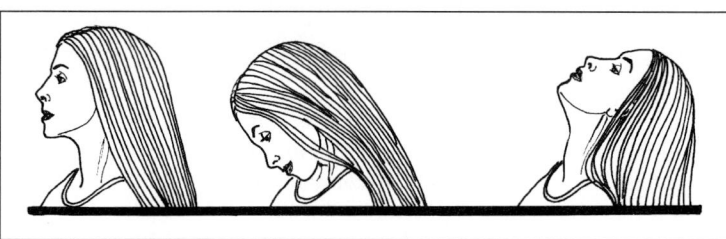

A–4

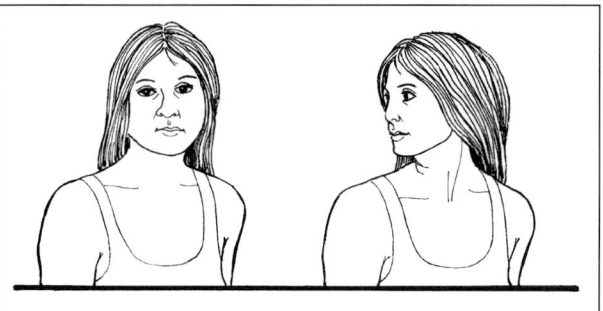

A–5

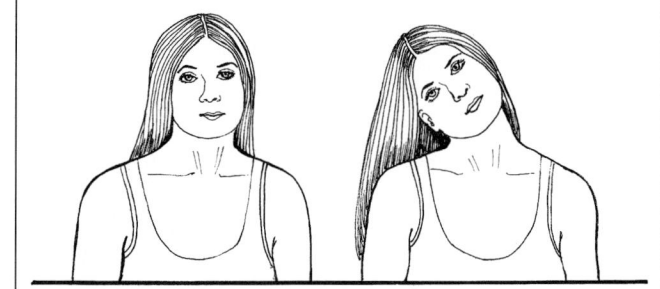

A–6

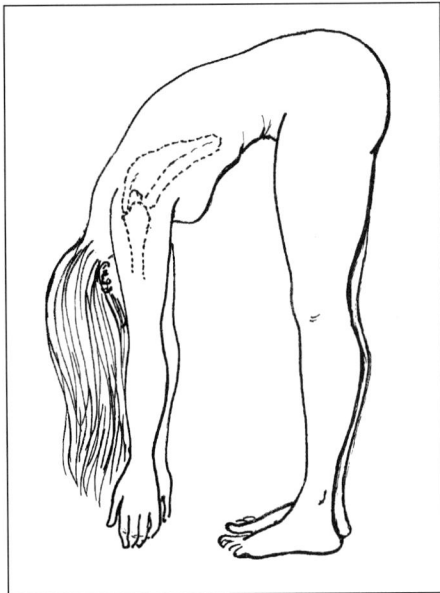

FIGURE A–7. *Rationale for Codman's pendular exercises.* In the stooping position the gravity of the arm allows abduction without the need of a fulcrum. In addition, the shoulder muscles, which have various directions of pull with the arms at the sides of the body, all arrange in concentric cones in the stooping position.

Shoulder Exercises

Before approaching shoulder exercises, a word must be said about shoulder immobilization. The shoulder takes immobility very poorly. However, short-term immobilization is important in the treatment of acute rotator cuff tendinitis. Shoulder immobilization is conveniently achieved with the use of a sling. Once pain begins to lessen, which usually occurs within 8 to 24 hours, the sling is removed, and a program of Codman's pendular exercises is initiated.

Codman's Pendular Exercises

Codman's exercises are extremely useful to maintain shoulder motion in subacute shoulder conditions and to relieve pain and regain motion in obstructive impingements and the frozen shoulder. In the stooped forward position the upper arm painlessly abducts (Figure A–7), and the weight of the extremity applies gentle traction on capsular and tendinous structures.

Goal: To decrease shoulder pain, to discourage limitation, and to regain glenohumeral motion.

1. If your right shoulder is involved, stand behind a chair and stoop forward, resting your left hand on the back of the chair. Bring the right shoulder to a dependent position so that the extremity may act as a pendulum. Make sure your back feels comfortable.
2. With little force, start pendular motions: clockwise and counterclockwise circles, back and forth motions, and side to side motions, always within a cone of painless motion. Initially, have someone check that your shoulder muscles are relaxed as you perform the exercise.
3. Perform the pendular motion for 3 minutes.
4. Pendular exercises should be carried out every _____ hours while awake.

Shoulder Stretching*

Overhead reach of the arm (Figure A–8)

Goal: To stretch a restricted shoulder.

1. Lie flat on your back with your arms at your sides.
2. Grasp with the opposite hand the involved arm and bring it up as far as it goes comfortably.
3. Keep a firm pressure on the tissues to a count of 10 initially, progressing slowly to a count of 100.
4. Return the arm to the initial side position. Repeat the stretch 3 times.
   This exercise is performed _____ times a day.
   NOTE: An alternative technique for the overhead stretch is shown in Figure A–9. With the patient sitting next to a table, the involved arm is rested flat on the table. Stretching is achieved by bending the trunk forward.

External rotation of the arm (Figure A–10)

Goal: To stretch a restricted shoulder.

1. Lie flat on your back with your elbows at your sides.
2. Bend both elbows to a right angle.
3. With the opposite hand, using a stick, push the involved extremity away from your body while keeping your elbow at your side. Maintain a gentle stress to a count of 10 initially, and then work up to a count of 100.
4. Return the hands to the starting position. Repeat the exercise 3 times.
   The exercise is performed _____ times a day.

*Data from Matsen FA, Lippitt SB, Sidles JA, Harryman DT II. Practical Evaluation and Management of the Shoulder. WB Saunders, Philadelphia, 167–175, 1994.

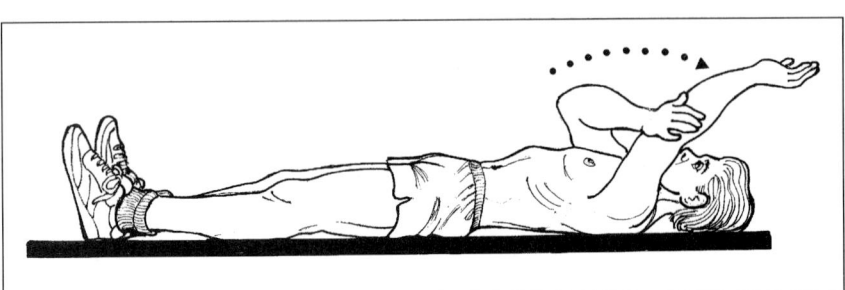

FIGURE A–8. *Shoulder stretching: overhead reach of the arm.* (See text for details.)

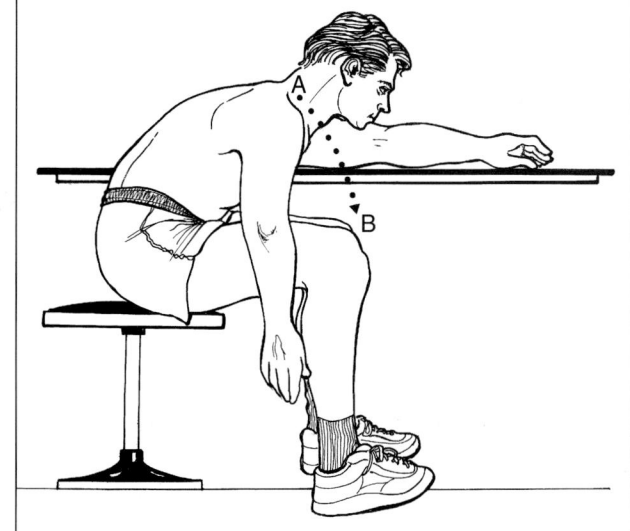

FIGURE A–9. *Shoulder stretching: alternative position for overhead reach.* As the trunk is bent forward (*A* to *B*) the shoulder is stretched. (See text for details.)

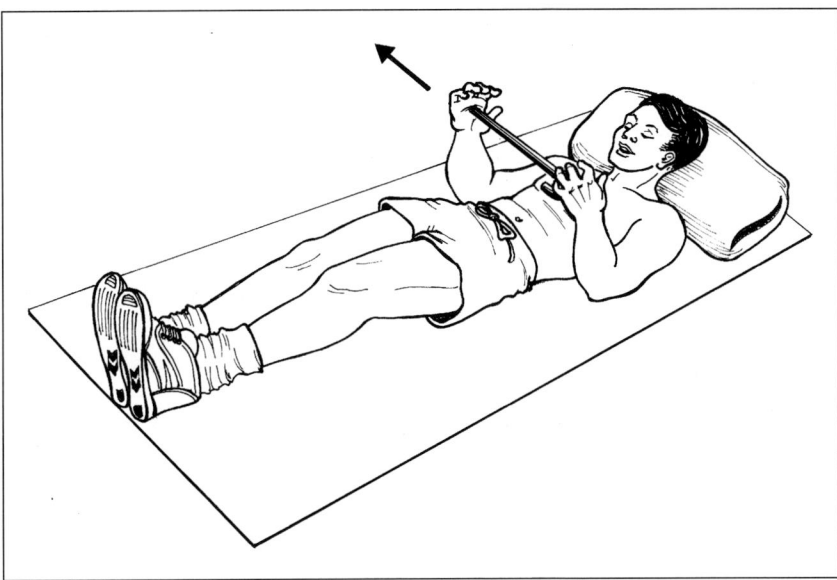

FIGURE A–10. *Shoulder stretching: external rotation of the arm.* (See text for details.)

Reaching up the back (Figure A–11)

Goal: To stretch a restricted shoulder.

1. This exercise is performed standing. Grasp a towel with the hand of the diseased shoulder behind your back and the opposite hand behind your neck.
2. Pull up the towel, which makes the involved shoulder go into internal rotation.
3. Keep the pull to a count of 10 initially, and progress gradually to a count of 100.
4. Repeat the exercise 3 times.
   The exercise is performed _____ times a day.

Shoulder Strengthening Exercises*

Two groups of muscles must be exercised: the external and internal rotators of the shoulder and the muscles that move the scapula up and forward.

*Data from Matsen FA, Lippitt SB, Sidles JA, Harryman DT II. Practical Evaluation and Management of the Shoulder. WB Saunders, Philadelphia, 167–175, 1994.

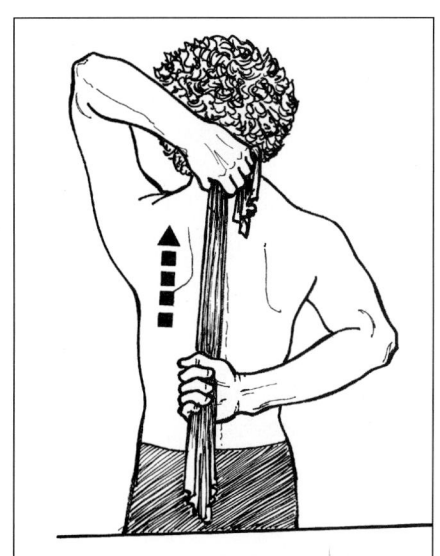

FIGURE A–11. *Shoulder stretching: reaching up the back.* (See text for details.)

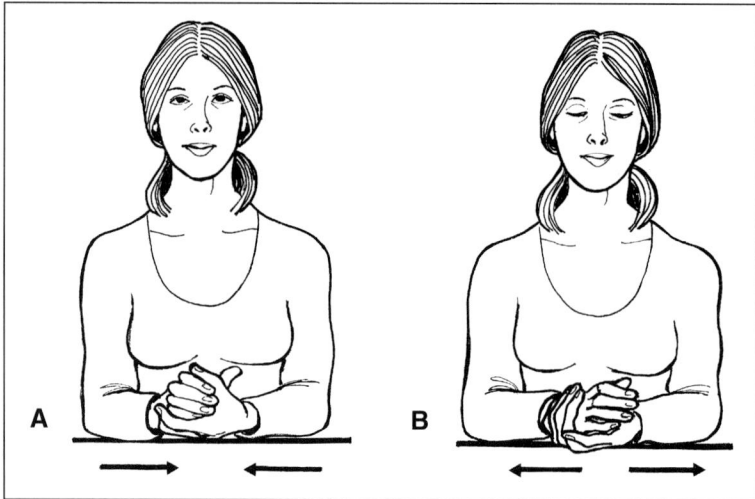

FIGURE A-12. Shoulder strengthening exercises. A, Internal rotation strengthening. B, External rotation strengthening. (See text for details.)

Internal rotators strengthening (Figure A-12A)

These exercises are performed sitting or standing.

1. Keep the arm of the painful shoulder at the side of your body with the elbow flexed 90 degrees.
2. Try to rotate the arm inward against the opposite hand, holding the pressure for 3 seconds. Repeat the movement 20 times.
   The exercise is performed _____ times a day.

External rotators strengthening (Figure A-12B)

1. Keep the arm of the painful shoulder at the side of your body with the elbow flexed 90 degrees.
2. Try to rotate the arm outward against the opposite hand, holding the traction 3 seconds. Repeat the movement 20 times.
   The exercise is performed _____ times a day.

Strengthening the muscles that lift your shoulder blade (the trapezius, levator scapulae, and rhomboids)

This exercise may be performed standing or sitting.

1. With your arms at your sides, shrug and hold the shoulders up for 3 seconds.
2. Return to the initial position.
3. Repeat the movement 20 times.
   Progressive weights may be subsequently added, building to a maximum 20% of your body weight. Don't add weights that you can't lift 20 times.

Strengthening the muscles that move your shoulder blade forward (the serratus and the pectoralis)

This exercise is performed by a bench press-type exercise (Figure A-13) while you lie on your back holding a small weight.

1. Lift your shoulder blade off the bed or floor.
2. Return to the previous position. Once you can control the weight for 20 movements, it is time to add weights, progressing to a maximum of 10% of your body weight. This exercise can also be done without using weights by forcibly holding the shoulder in the forward position for 3 seconds and repeating the motion 20 times.

Back Exercises

In addition to the actual performance of back exercises, patients should receive specific instructions on proper posture for bed rest and techniques for safe bending and lifting.

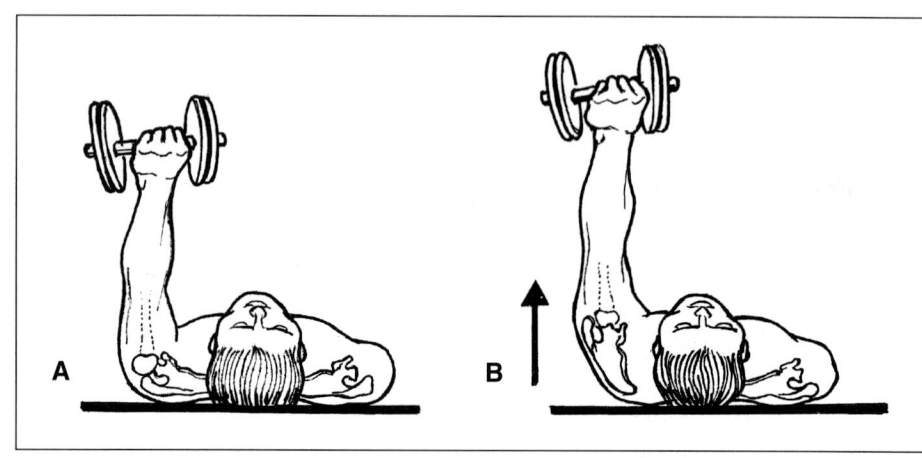

FIGURE A-13. Strengthening of muscles that move the shoulder blade forward. A, lie on your back holding weight. B, Lift your shoulder blade off the bed or floor.

Bed Rest

In general, bed rest should be discouraged in low back pain. Even a few days of bed rest tend to prolong symptoms in patients with acute low back pain. An exception should be made in some patients with particularly severe sciatica, but even in these cases bed rest should be used for less than 4 days. The preferred position for bed rest in sciatica is to lie supine on a firm mattress with the knees slightly bent on a pillow. Lateral decubitus with the legs drawn up, also known as the fetal position, is also well tolerated. To get up from bed to go to the bathroom, the patient should turn to the side near the edge of the bed and then sit upright with the help of the arms. Progressive ambulation should be encouraged as soon as symptoms improve. Bed rest should be avoided altogether in chronic low back pain.

Safe Lifting

The following recommendations are important for avoiding injury to the spine while lifting:

1. Avoid stooping and bending forward.
2. Face the object to be lifted and stand close to it.
3. Have a firm footing and a wide stance.
4. Bend at the hips and knees, and keep your back straight.
5. Avoid objects that are awkward or heavier than arm strength.
6. Divide the object into smaller parts if possible.
7. Lift the object by straightening the knees.
8. Lift steadily; do not jerk.
9. Do not lift objects above waist level.
10. If you have to turn, shift your feet; do not twist your back.

To Counteract a Tendency to Kyphosis in Ankylosing Spondylitis

Patients with ankylosing spondylitis have a tendency to develop a flexion deformity of the dorsal spine. To prevent this deformity it is recommended that patients lie flat on the floor 20 minutes each day (the time may be used to read the newspaper).

Abdominal wall strengthening exercises (Figure A–1)

Goal: To strengthen the abdominal wall muscles, thereby decreasing lumbar lordosis. This exercise is used to treat back pain as well as to improve general conditioning.

1. Lie flat on the floor or on a firm bed with the knees bent, your feet on the floor, and your arms by your sides.
2. Reach your hands toward your knees, slightly raising your head and shoulders while flattening the lumbar curvature (partial sit-up). Stay in this position while counting backward from 6, one count per second.
3. Return to the initial position. The exercise is repeated _____ times.

Hamstring muscles stretch (Figure A–14)

Goal: To lengthen the hamstring muscles. These muscles get tight in individuals with back ailments and further reduce flexibility.

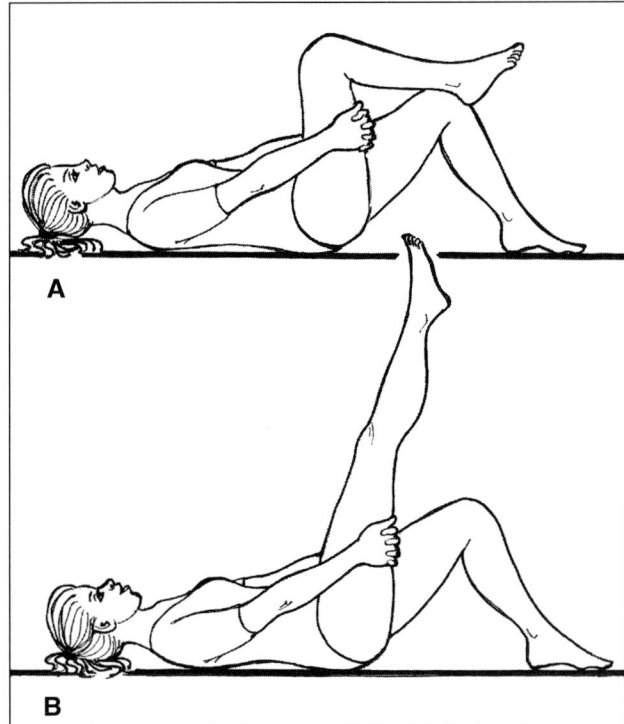

FIGURE A–14. *Hamstring muscles stretch. A, Grasp the back of one thigh with both hands. B, Straighten the knee and then pull the thigh up. (See text for details.)*

1. Lie flat on the floor with the knees bent and your feet flat on the floor.
2. Grasp the back of one thigh with both hands.
3. Straighten the knees.
4. Pull the thigh up as high as it can go, keeping the knees straight. Hold for 6 seconds.
5. Go back to the starting position and relax. Repeat the exercise _____ times.

Hamstring muscles stretch (alternative exercise) (Figure A–15)

This exercise may be better suited to older patients than the previous one.

1. Sit in a chair with a stool in front of you.
2. Raise one leg and rest your heel on the stool. Keep the knee fully extended.
3. Bend the body forward; keep the tension in the back of the extended knee 3–6 seconds.
4. Go back to the starting position. Then repeat the cycle with the opposite leg. Repeat the entire set _____ times.

Back rotation (Figure A–16)

Goal: To improve spinal and pelvic rotation.

1. Lie flat on the floor or on a hard bed with your hands resting on your abdomen.
2. Without moving your shoulders or neck, turn your pelvis (and legs) to one side. Hold for 3–6 seconds. Now turn your pelvis (and legs) to the other side. Hold for 3–6 seconds.

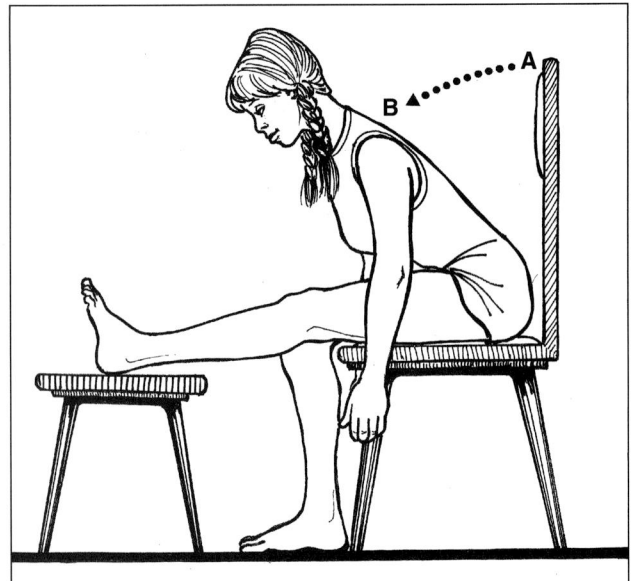

FIGURE A–15. *Hamstring muscles stretch* (alternative posture). (See text for details.) The hamstring muscles are stretched as the body is bent forward from *A* to *B*.

3. Return to the starting position.
   Repeat the entire exercise _____ times.

Back rotation alternative (Figure A–17)

This exercise is done with the patient sitting on a stool.
Goal: To improve back and pelvic rotation.

1. Sit straight on a stool with your arms crossed in front of you.
2. Turn to the right, holding the position to a count of 3.
3. Now turn to the left, holding the position 3 seconds.
   Repeat the full exercise (right plus left turn) _____ times before ending in the starting position.

Back extension exercise

Goal: To strengthen the paraspinal muscles and increase dorsal spine flexibility.

1. Lie flat on your abdomen on the floor or on a hard mattress, your arms at your sides, having placed a pillow under your abdomen at the thoracolumbar junction.
2. Lift your head and shoulders, holding the position while you count down 3 seconds.
3. Return to the previous position.
   Repeat _____ times. Now relax.
4. Now bring your arms up.
5. Lift your arms, shoulders, and head, holding the position while you count down 3 seconds.
6. Return to the previous position.
   Repeat _____ times.

Pectoral stretch (Figure A–18)

This is a very important exercise in ankylosing spondylitis patients.
Goals: To assist in correcting the stooping of the shoulders and in strengthening the pectoral muscles.

1. Stand facing a corner of the room.
2. Place one hand on each wall at shoulder level.
3. Lean forward slowly, feeling a stretch at the front of your chest, to a count down from 6.
4. Return to the starting position.
   Repeat _____ times.

Lateral bending exercises (Figure A–19)

This exercise is begun after a week or two of performing flexion and/or extension back exercises.
Goal: To stretch the contralateral quadratus lumborum and latissimus dorsi muscles.

1. Stand straight with your arms at your sides.
2. Raise one arm, placing the forearm on your head. Keep the contralateral arm extended at your side.
3. Bend your body to the side of the extended arm, which makes your hand slide down along your leg. You'll feel a stretch on your convex side. Hold this position while you count down from 6.
4. Return to the standing position.

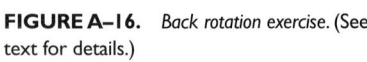

FIGURE A–16. *Back rotation exercise.* (See text for details.)

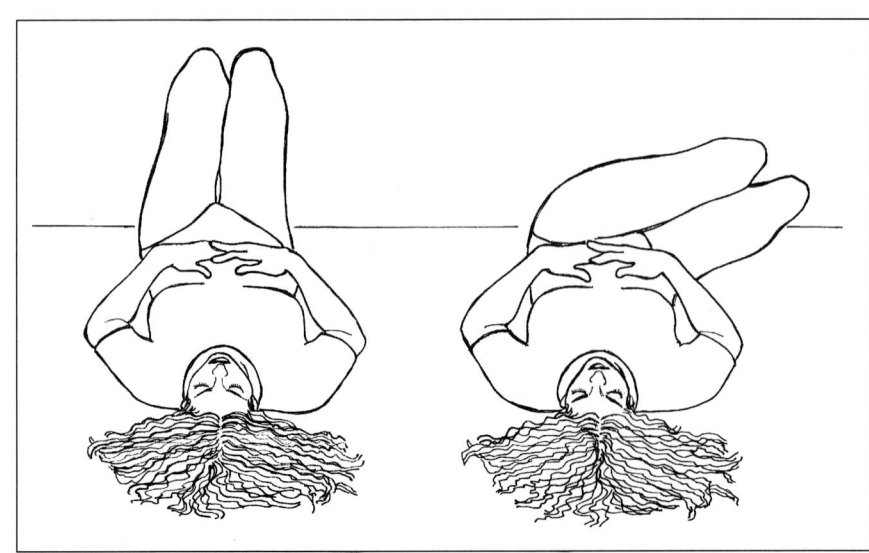

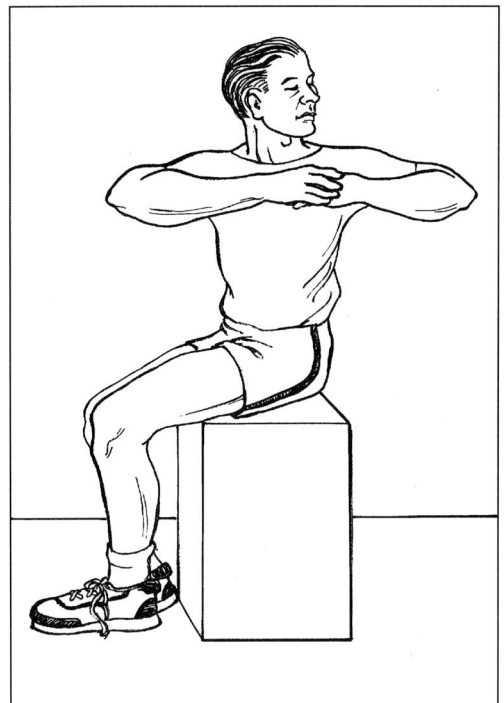

FIGURE A–17. *Back rotation alternative.* (See text for details.)

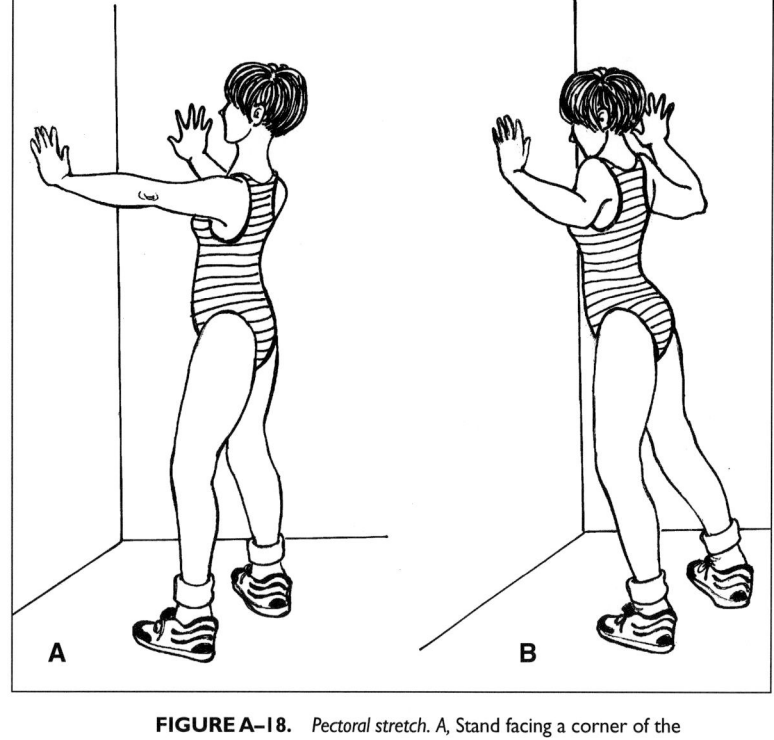

FIGURE A–18. *Pectoral stretch.* A, Stand facing a corner of the room. B, Lean forward slowly. (See text for details.)

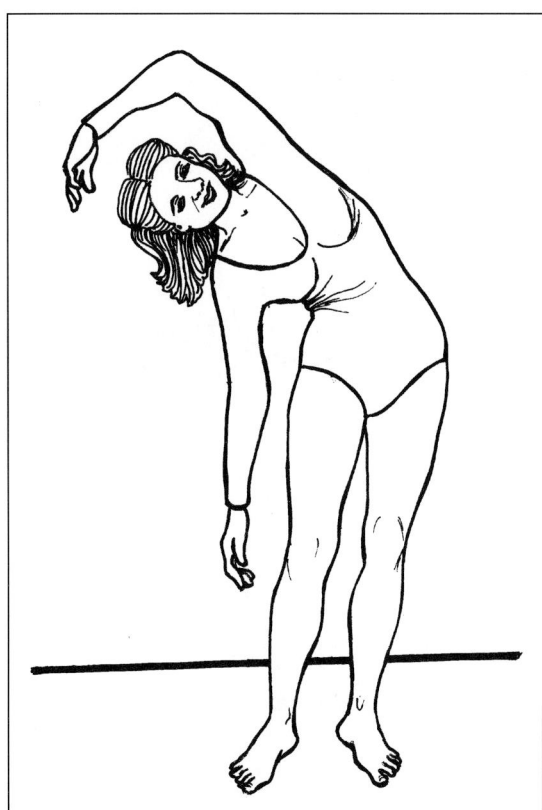

FIGURE A–19. *Lateral bending.* (See text for details.)

Now do the exercise on the opposite side.
Repeat the exercise _____ times on each side.

Hip Exercises

Hip Extension Exercise (Figure A–20)

Goal: To strengthen the hip extensor muscles and correct flexor deformity of the hip.

1. Lie flat on your abdomen on the floor or on a hard mattress, your arms at your sides, having placed a pillow under your abdomen at the thoracolumbar junction.
2. Raise one leg 4–6 inches off the floor.
3. Hold this position while you count down from 6.
4. Return to the starting position.
   Repeat this exercise _____ times with each leg.

Quadriceps Stretch (Knee and Hip Stretch) (Figure A–21)

Goal: To stretch the front thigh muscles (quadriceps) and the hip and knee joints to improve posture and discourage flexor deformity of the hip.

1. Stand in front of a wall.
2. Place one hand on the wall for support, and flex the opposite knee.
3. Grasp your ankle and start a steady pull of the flexed leg. You should feel a stretch in the anterior thigh.
4. Hold this position while you count down from 6.
5. Return to the standing position.
   Repeat this exercise _____ times with each leg.

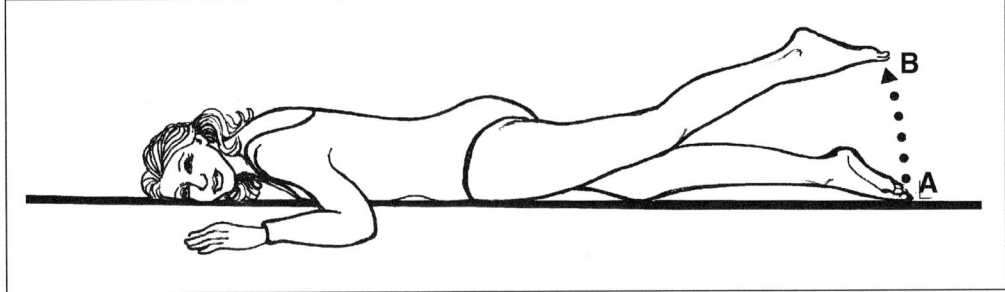

FIGURE A–20. Hip extension exercise. Raise one leg 4–6 inches off the floor. (See text for details.)

Iliotibial Tract Stretch

The iliotibial tract is often contractured in people with back and hip problems, leading to the syndrome of trochanteric bursitis. Running athletes may develop iliotibial tract tendinitis in the outer aspect of the knee. Both groups of patients benefit from iliotibial tract stretch.
Goal: To lengthen the iliotibial tract when it is contractured.

1. To stretch the right iliotibial band, lie near the side of the bed on the left side, with the left leg slightly bent at the hip and knee and the right leg straight on top.
2. Slide back the extended right leg just enough to clear its support, and let it descend on its weight, stretching the iliotibial band to a count down of 6 seconds.
3. Return the right leg to the starting position.
   The exercise is repeated _____ times.
   Now do the exercise to stretch the opposite iliotibial tract, following the same guidelines.

Hand Exercises

Hand Protection

1. Use as many electrical appliances as possible.
2. Use lightweight utensils (aluminum, plastic) rather than heavy ones made of glass or metal.
3. Large handles are easier to hold than small ones.
4. Zippers may be hard to handle. Use a ring on the zipper tab, and place a finger through the loop.
5. Replace buttons with Velcro fasteners.
6. Use a single-lever-type faucet rather than one that requires turning and twisting.
7. Use a wall-mounted jar opener that allows you to hold the can with both hands. If a jar opener is not available, place a rubber sheath on the jar lid, and open it with the palm rather than the fingers.
8. Replace small metal drawer handles by large, wooden handles to spread the stress.
9. To lift a heavy object, get under the object and lift it with the palms of both hands.

Hand Exercises

Goals: Hand exercises are aimed at maintaining and enhancing function in the intrinsic muscles and the muscles of the thenar and hypothenar eminences. It is recommended that the patient soak both hands in warm (not hot) water for 5–8 minutes prior to exercising. Patients with any degree of neuropathy in whom thermal sensation may be decreased should not soak in warm water except under supervision. Both hands are exercised simultaneously. All exercises start with the fully extended hand.

1. Flex the stretched fingers (index through small) at the metacarpophalangeal joint while keeping the fingers straight (Figure A–22).
2. Return the fingers to the initial position.
   Repeat this movement _____ times.
3. Move the thumb toward each fingertip, returning to the stretched hand position in between (Figure A–23).
   Repeat this movement _____ times.
4. Now bring the stretched fingers in side contact with each other and separate them (Figure A–24).
   Repeat this movement _____ times.

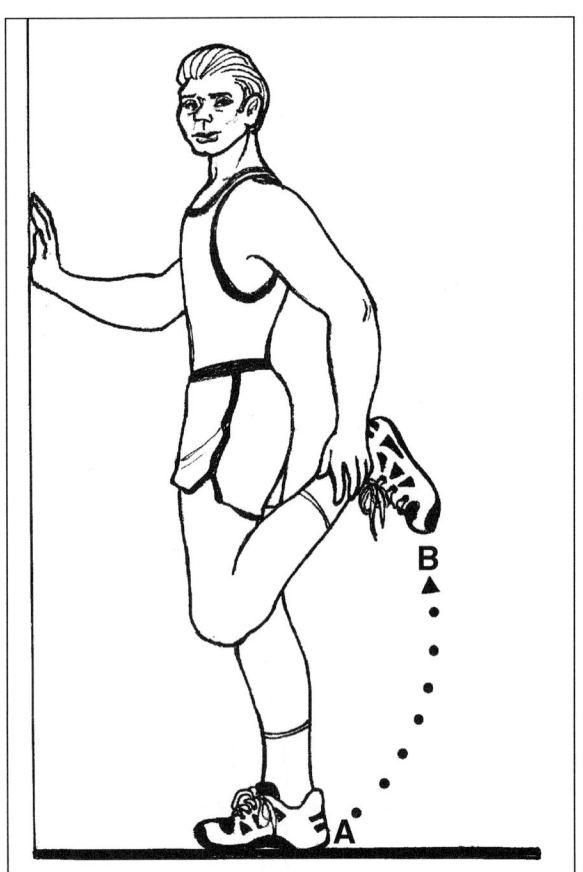

FIGURE A–21. *Quadriceps stretch.* Pull the flexed leg from A to B. (See text for details.)

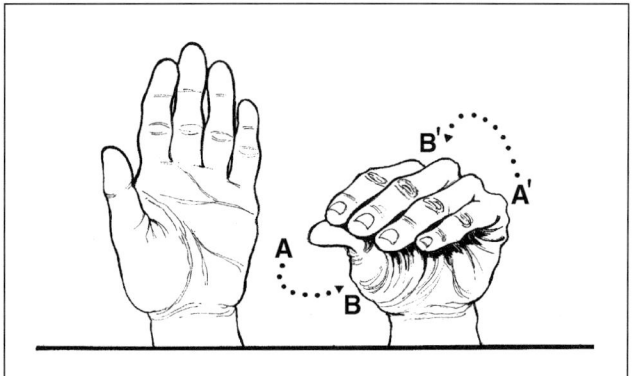

FIGURE A–22. Hand exercises. (See text for details.)

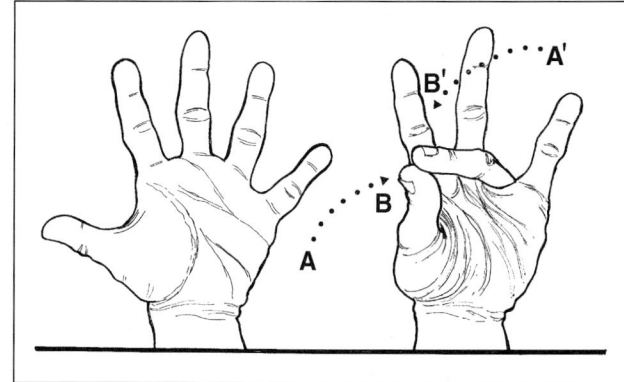

FIGURE A–23. Hand exercises. (See text for details.)

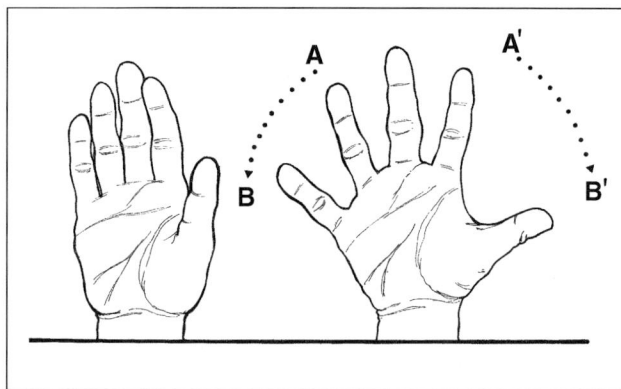

FIGURES A–24. Hand exercises. (See text for details.)

Respiratory Exercises

Goal: To maintain motion of the costovertebral joints and to strengthen the diaphragm. These exercises are very important in ankylosing spondylitis.

Abdominal-Diaphragmatic Breathing Exercises

1. Inspire by using the diaphragm. This is achieved if the abdomen inflates like a balloon, with minimal movement of the chest wall.
2. Purse your lips and exhale, using the strength of your abdominal muscles.
   Repeat the exercise _____ times.

Maximal Breathings

1. Inspire maximally. Feel your chest wall motion with your hand.
2. Purse your lips and exhale forcibly.
   Repeat the exercise _____ times.

Heat Application

It is common knowledge that heat (and cold) relieves musculoskeletal pain. Everyone has had the opportunity of ascertaining this when afflicted with neck, low back, or other pain. The point cannot be argued. On the other hand, there are indications that collagenase, an enzyme involved in cartilage and fibrous tissue degradation, is more active when temperatures are raised, for instance, from the normal 32–32.5° C to 36–37° C. For this reason there is concern that increasing intraarticular temperature may result in additional joint damage when deep heat modalities are used in the treatment of rheumatoid arthritis.

Significant intraarticular temperature elevations have been noted when warm packs and short-wave diathermy were used in the knee. Maximal temperatures were reached 20–25 minutes after completion of a 10–15-minute heat application, and return to baseline took almost 3 hours. Similar changes could be expected from the use of ultrasound. In contrast, with cool applications intraarticular temperatures fell by as much as 10° C. The lowest temperatures were obtained with ice compresses applications.

Given these findings, there is a theoretical advantage in using ice compresses rather than heat in the treatment of inflammatory conditions. In general, the following broad recommendations can be made:

1. In acute trauma (such as an ankle sprain) cold packs should be used in the initial 24 hours and warm packs thereafter.
2. In acute arthritis (such as in gout) the joint should be temporarily immobilized. Warm packs may dramatically *increase* pain. Cold applications have a theoretical advantage and should be used whenever a splint plus appropriate antiinflammatory medications do not afford prompt relief, as well as patients who are unable to take the latter.
3. Prior to ligamentous stretching in a restricted shoul-

der, a painful back, or a contractured knee, heat should be used in the form of a warm shower, an immersion bath, ultrasound, or shortwave diathermy. Heat is beneficial because collagen fibers stretch more at higher temperatures.

4. In chronic inflammatory conditions such as RA there is a theoretical advantage in using cold packs. However, to relieve muscle contracture and in postinflammatory fibrosis (a residually restricted shoulder or elbow) heat application prior to stretching works best.
5. Heat applications with a paraffin tank are useful in the treatment of painful Heberden's and Bouchard's nodes. The commercially available tanks (Parabath, obtained from Talcott Laboratories Inc., 301 E. Barr Street, McDonald, Pennsylvania 15057 (412)926-3011) operate on regular home current and are permanently kept on with the melted paraffin thermostatically controlled at 126–130° F. The affected hand is dipped 5–7 times into the melted paraffin to establish a proper glove thickness. The hand is then wrapped in cellophane or Saran Wrap. Paraffin gloves keep the warmth for approximately 20 minutes. The paraffin glove is then peeled off and thrown back into the tank.

Suggested Reading

Burkhardt CS, Mannerkorpi K, Hedenberg L, Bjelle A. A randomized, controlled clinical trial of education and physical training for women with fibromyalgia. J Rheumatol 21:714–720, 1994.
Gerber LH. Exercise and arthritis. Bull Rheum Dis 39(6):1–6, 1990.
Hicks JE, Nicholas JJ, Swezey RL (eds). Handbook of Rehabilitative Rheumatology. American Rheumatism Association, Atlanta, 1988.
Oosterveld FGJ, Rasker JJ, Jacobs JWG, Overmars HJA. The effect of local heat and cold therapy on the intra-articular and skin surface temperature of the knee. Arthritis Rheum 35:146–151, 1992.
Stenström CH. Home exercise in rheumatoid arthritis functional class II: Goal setting versus pain attention. J Rheumatol 21:627–634, 1994.
Swezey RL (ed). Straight Talk on Spondylitis, 2nd ed. Spondylitis Association of America, Sherman Oaks, CA, 1992.

Choosing Shoes

Choosing adequate shoes is both an art and a science. Unfortunately, fashion and esthetics often conflict with foot mechanics, particularly in women's footwear. The choice should be simple; but then, what constitutes an adequate shoe? The truth is that no shoe is the best shoe. It all depends on the foot. Basic principles will be reviewed first, and advice about specific foot problems will follow. It is interesting that until the 18th century shoes were symmetrically shaped and could be worn indifferently on either foot.

Anatomy of a Shoe (Figure A–25)

Primary care physicians need to become acquainted with pedorthic terminology:

1. *Upper:* everything but the sole.
2. *Toe box:* the forepart of the shoe that covers the toe area.
3. *Vamp:* the part of the shoe that covers the instep.
4. *Quarter:* the back half of the shoe's upper.
5. *Counter:* the part of the quarter behind the heel.

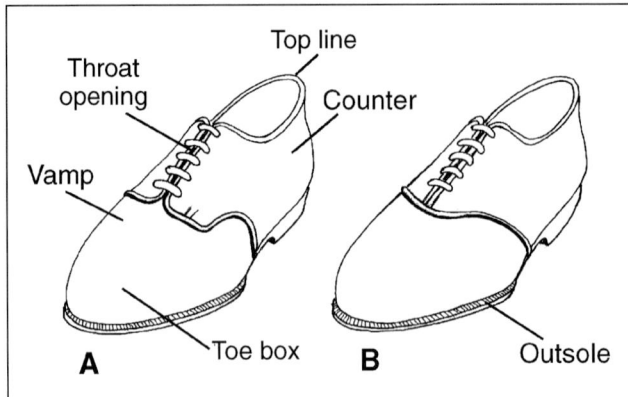

FIGURE A–25. Anatomy of a shoe. A, Blucher. B, Balmoral. (See text for details.)

6. *Sole:* the insole (the inside surface for the foot) and the outsole, which provides traction, insulation, and shock absorption and helps in maintaining the shape of the shoe.

Which elements should be taken into consideration when choosing a shoe?

Shoe shape: In principle, a shoe's shape should match the foot's shape. This is usually the case in men's shoes but it seldom is in women's shoes, which accounts for the high prevalence of hallux valgus and other deformities in women. A high toe-box shoe and a rounded toe provide the best fit for the toes. In contrast, a tapered toe box and a pointed toe force the toes, cause calluses, and result in deformity. The vamp should be high enough so that pressure is not put on the instep. There are two types of throat openings, the Blucher and the Balmoral (Figure A–25). The Blucher allows for greater adjustability and should be preferred, all other things being equal.
Shoe size: The foot should be measured for overall length, arch length, and width. A proper shoe accommodates the first MTP joint at its widest point. Both feet should be measured.
Proper fit: Since the foot stretches during gait, the shoe should have ⅜ to ½ inch toe room between the end of the shoe and the longest toe. Make sure that the shoe is wide enough. There should be a snug fit around the heel. Fit shoes on both feet while bearing weight. Check that the first MTP is at the widest point.
Extra-depth shoes: Shoe retailers that specialize in orthopedic shoes carry extra-depth shoes that can accommodate swollen and deformed toes. Extra-depth shoes include pumps in a broad range of sizes and widths.
Low-heel shoes: These are preferable to high-heel shoes. With a low heel, weight is more evenly distributed on the sole, rather than concentrated over the ball of the foot.
Running shoes: Nike Air Craft (Nike, Beaverton, Oregon) have a thick insole with an excellent cushioning property. New Balance (Boston, Massachusetts) provides running shoes with a variety of widths. *Running shoes are an excellent alternative to orthopedic shoes.*

The use of padded socks and the removal of calluses add significantly to reduce plantar pressures.

To find out which shoe stores in your area are staffed by certified pedorthics, call 1-800-673-8447. The stores listed will carry a selection of off-the-shelf wide or extra-depth shoes and will be able to fill prescriptions for specialized orthoses.

American Orthopaedic Foot and Ankle Society* Guidelines for Proper Footware

1. Sizes vary among shoe brands and styles. Don't select shoes based on the size marked inside the shoe. Pick the shoe by how it fits your foot.
2. Select a shoe that conforms as nearly as possible to the shape of your forefoot.
3. Have your feet measured regularly. The size of your feet may change as you grow older.
4. Have both feet measured (often one foot is larger than the other). The shoe should be fitted to the larger foot.
5. Have your shoes fitted at the end of the day when your feet are the largest.
6. Stand during the fitting process because the foot lengthens as you are standing. There should be one finger breadth (½ inch or 1.3 cm) between your longest toe and the end of the shoe.
7. The ball of your foot should fit snugly into the widest part of the shoe, but the shoe should not be too tight.
8. If the shoes don't fit, don't purchase them. Don't expect them to "stretch to fit."
9. Your heel should fit comfortably in the shoe with a minimum amount of pistoning.
10. While you are still in the shoe store, walk to make sure that the fit feels correct.

Suggested Reading

Coughlin MJ, Thompson FM. The high price of high-fashion footware. Instructional course lectures, DW Jackson (ed). Amer Acad Orthopedic Surgeons 44:371–377, 1995.

Janisse DJ. The art and science of fitting shoes. Foot Ankle 13:257–262, 1992.

Assistive Devices for Walking

Proper Use of a Cane

A cane, properly used, removes the center of gravity from the affected hip, knee, or foot and thus partially removes the pain associated with ambulation.

1. *Fitting a cane.* For proper fit a cane must reach the waist when the patient is upright. In an obese man cane length should equal the height of the greater trochanter. The cane should reach 8 inches lateral to the front of the foot in the unaffected side as the elbow is flexed 15–30 degrees. A rubber tip will prevent dangerous slipping. The cane should be held with the hand opposite the painful hip or knee.

*Brochures are available from the American Orthopaedic Foot and Ankle Society, 701 16th Avenue, Seattle, Washington 98122.

2. *Use of the cane.* To initiate walking, the good leg should be advanced first, and then the "bad" leg, which is applied on the ground synchronous with the cane. The patient should exert force on the cane as if the ground were pushing up on the cane. This allows removing part of the weight from the painful structure. As an example, by applying 20 pounds of force on the cane, the affected (contralateral) hip is relieved of more than 150 pounds of force.
3. *Stairs.* In negotiating stairs, the adage "up with the good, down with the bad" should be followed.

Proper Use of a Walker

Walkers are light, movable devices made of metal tubing. A walker is superior to a cane when there is bilateral lower-extremity disease and when extra safety is required. There are several problem with walkers: They are difficult to transport, they are bulky appliances that are difficult to handle indoors, the speed of ambulation with them is quite slow, and a normal gait pattern is difficult to perform.

1. *Fitting a walker.* As with canes, walkers should be waist or greater trochanter high.
2. *Using a walker.* The patient holds the hand grips on the upper bars and advances the walker and the protected extremity. Then the good limb steps up to the walker.

Proper Use of Crutches

There are two types of crutches, the double adjustable Lofstrand or forearm crutches and the axillary crutches. Use of the latter is described here. Axillary crutches require good standing balance; functional strength in the trunk and upper extremities is required for most gait patterns; they may cause damage to axillary vessels; and elderly patients often feel insecure with their use. Patients with shoulder or elbow arthritis find the use of forearm crutches more comfortable.

1. *Fitting crutches.* To fit axillary crutches the following steps must be taken: (a) the length should be 3–4 finger breadths below the axilla to a point 15 cm (6 inches) lateral to the patient's heel; (b) hand grips are positioned such that while supporting weight the elbows should be flexed 20–25 degrees; (c) to decrease risk of accidental damage to the brachial plexus, once crutch length and hand grip position have been determined, the 3–4 finger-breadth distance between the crutch pad and the axilla should be verified.
2. *Using crutches.* The basic crutch stance is the tripod position in which the crutches are placed 15 cm in front and lateral to each foot. If one limb should be protected, the tripod position includes the good foot plus the crutches. A commonly used crutch gait is the three-point gait in which the painful or otherwise protected leg does not bear weight. In this gait weight is borne in the uninvolved leg and then on both crutches, then repeating the sequence. In the modified three-point gait ("touch-down" gait) the patient is permitted full weight bearing on one leg but only partial weight bearing on the other. Here the crutches and the partial

weight-bearing extremity are advanced simultaneously. Then the full weight-bearing extremity is advanced while weight is distributed between the crutches and the protected limb in the desired proportion. In the touch-down gait, patients should be encouraged to use a heel-strike gait or to place the foot with minimal weight, rather than the toe.

3. *Stairs.* To ascend stairs (a) the patient transfers weight to the crutches; (b) the unaffected leg is advanced to the stairs; and (c) the patient aligns both crutches on the stairs, and so on with the next step. To descend stairs the patient (a) transfers body weight to the good leg; (b) the crutches are placed on the step, and the patient begins to transfer weight to the crutches; and (c) the good leg is moved to the stairs with the crutches, and so on.
4. *Sitting with crutches.* (a) The patient first stands in front of the center of the chair with the back side of the good leg touching the chair; (b) the patient transfers the involved side crutch to the opposite hand, which now holds both crutches by the handle; (c) the affected-side hand grasps the arm of the chair; and (d) the patient lowers himself or herself into the chair. The opposite sequence is used to stand. The fully erect patient assumes the tripod position before walking.

Suggested Reading

Blount WP. Don't throw away the cane. J Bone Joint Surg 38A:695–708, 1956.

Pierson FM. Ambulation aids, patterns, and activities. In: Principles and Techniques of Patient Care. WB Saunders, Philadelphia, 99–148, 1994.

1. Community Resources and Government Agencies

National Arthritis and Musculoskeletal and Skin Diseases Information Clearinghouse (NAMSIC). C/o JBS, Inc. 8630 Fenton Street, Suite 1200, Silver Springs, MD 20910.

NAMSIC is a program of the National Institute of Arthritis and Musculoskeletal and Skin Diseases, National Institutes of Health. It is a national resource center for health professionals seeking information about arthritis and other rheumatic conditions, musculoskeletal diseases (including sports injuries), and skin diseases. NAMSIC collects and disseminates publications, patient education brochures, and bibliographies. NAMSIC also maintains a subfile on the Combined Health Information Database.

The Arthritis Foundation (AF). Patient Services Department, Professional Education Department, 1324 Spring Street, N.W., Atlanta, GA 30309.

The AF has educational materials for physicians and health professionals about the various rheumatic diseases. There are self-study videotapes, publications, medications briefs, and patient education literature for a clinician's office. Some materials are available free or on loan from local chapters of the AF. Others may be ordered in quantity from the national office.

Ankylosing spondylitis. Spondylitis Association of America (SAA), 14827 Ventura Boulevard, #119, P.O. Box 5872, Sherman Oaks, CA 91413. Tel. (818)981-1616, (800)777-8189.

The SAA provides educational books, exercise videotapes, and pamphlets on ankylosing spondylitis and related spondyloarthropathies. Spanish language booklets are available, and there is a physician referral service.

Behçet's syndrome. The American Behçet's Disease Association (ABDA), P.O. Box 27494, Temple, AZ 85285-7494. Tel. (602)917-9603, (800)723-4238.

The ABDA is a nonprofit organization formed to offer support to Behçet's patients, their families, and their physicians. Services include a telephone hotline, a quarterly newsletter, patient/family conferences, and literature. The ABDA also serves as a source for patients for medical research and referrals to physicians knowledgeable about Behçet's.

Fibromyalgia. National Fibromyalgia Research Association (NFRA), P.O. Box 500, Salem, OR 97308. Tel. (503)588-1411.

The NFRA is a nonprofit organization dedicated to education, treatment, and the finding of a cure for fibromyalgia.

Fibromyalgia. Fibromyalgia Network (incorporated as Health Information Network, Inc.), P.O. Box 31750, Tucson, AZ 85751. Tel. (602)290-5508, fax (520)290-5505.

The network offers information on symptom management, patient coping techniques, conference updates, advances in research, and fibromyalgia in children. There is a newsletter, *Fibromyalgia Network,* and patient education handouts on fibromyalgia, chronic fatigue syndrome, and related conditions are available.

Osteoporosis. National Osteoporosis Foundation (NOF), 1150 17th Street, N.W., Suite 500, Washington, D.C. 20036-4603. Tel. (202)223-2226, 1-800-464-6700.

The NOF provides useful brochures on osteoporosis and densitometry tests.

Psoriatic arthritis. National Psoriasis Foundation, 6600 S.W. 92nd, Suite 300, Portland, OR 97223. Tel. (503)244-7404, 1(800)723-9166 ext. 11 for publications; fax (503)245-0626.

The foundation publishes useful information for both patients and their physicians. Notable publications include the *Bulletin* and the *Pharmacy News,* aimed at patients, and *Psoriasis Forum,* which is directed to medical professionals. It also offers many pamphlets, some translated into Spanish, audiocassettes, and videotapes.

Scleroderma. Scleroderma Federation (SF), Peabody Office Building, One Newbury Street, Peabody, MA 01960. Tel. (508)535-6600, fax (508)535-6696.

The SF is a network of affiliated groups emphasizing patient service and research funding. It administers a broad-based collaborative research program. A physician referral database is maintained and is provided to patients; educational literature is also available to physicians for patient dissemination.

Scleroderma. United Scleroderma Foundation, PO Box 399, Watsonville, CA 95077. Tel. (408)728-2202, fax (408)728-3328.

This nonprofit health foundation has strived to bring hope and knowledge to scleroderma patients worldwide. It offers a scleroderma handbook, specialized brochures, quarterly newsletters, and a fact sheet. There are patient support groups throughout the United States and Canada. Physician referrals are offered.

Sjögren's syndrome. National Sjögren's Syndrome Association (NSSA), 3201 West Evans Drive, Phoenix, AZ 85023-5632. Tel. (602)516-0787, (800)395-NSSA; fax (602)516-0111.
The NSSA is a clearinghouse for information about Sjögren's syndrome. It publishes the *Sjögren's Digest;* a patient education series; and an educational video, *Living Well with Sjögren's Syndrome*. The NSSA is devoted to research and educational efforts.

Sjögren's syndrome. Sjögren's Syndrome Foundation (SSF), 333 North Broadway, Jericho, NY 11753. Tel. (516)933-6365, fax (516)933-6368.
The purposes of the SSF are to increase medical and public awareness about Sjögren's syndrome and to provide opportunities for patients to share ways of coping with a chronic illness. The SSF is the publisher of *The Moisture Seekers Newsletter* and *The Sjögren's Syndrome Handbook: An Authoritative Guide for Patients.*

Systemic lupus erythematosus. Lupus Foundation of America (LFA), 4 Research Place, Suite 180, Rockville, MD 20850-3226. Tel. (301)670-9292, fax (301)670-9486.
Patient education is a key factor in managing patients with lupus. The LFA provides an extensive array of brochures and fact sheets, including: *Living Well with Lupus, Laboratory Tests, Joint and Muscle Pain, Nervous System Involvement, Steroids, Antimalarials,* and *NSAIDs*. Brochure packets, Rolodex cards, Social Security disability information, and other help are also available.

Sun Protection

The ill effects of excessive sun exposure are well known. An increased incidence of basal cell and squamous cell carcinoma and possibly melanoma, premature and deep wrinkling of the skin, leathery skin, and possibly an increased rate of cataracts represent the unfortunate cost of keeping up a suntan. In addition, discoid lupus, systemic lupus erythematosus (SLE), dermatomyositis, polymorph light eruption, and porphyria cutanea tarda, among other conditions, may flare up following sun exposure. Finally, patients taking a multiplicity of drugs (Table A–1) may become sun sensitive and should therefore be advised to use a sunscreen when sun exposure cannot be avoided. Thus, a discussion of practical aspects of ultraviolet light protection needs little apology.

Ultraviolet (UV) radiation—of which there are three types: ultraviolet light A (UVA), ultraviolet light B (UVB), and ultraviolet light C (UVC)—is part of the solar electromagnetic spectrum (Table A–2). Whereas stratospheric ozone absorbs large amounts of UVC, and to a lesser extent UVB, little UVA radiation is absorbed by the atmosphere. As a result, 10 to 100 times more UVA than UVB radiation reaches the earth. Because 1,000 times more UVA than UVB energy is required to cause erythema in human skin, sunburns are caused mostly by UVB and to a lesser extent by UVA (90% and 10%, respectively).

Guidelines for Sun Protection

1. *Minimal erythema dose (MED)* is the exposure time required to develop erythema. Because the thickness of the ozone layer varies with the angulation of the sun in reference to the zenith, at 4 p.m. standard time there is a fourfold increase in the time required to induce erythema as compared with noon. This consideration underlies the recommendation we give our patients: Avoid sun exposure from 10 a.m. to 4 p.m. (11 a.m. to 5 p.m. during daylight saving time).

2. *Sun protection factor (SPF),* the label used to rate the strength of sunscreens, is a ratio obtained by dividing the MED of protected skin (with the product being rated) by the MED of unprotected skin. Thus, a sunscreen with an SPF of 6 delays erythema 6-fold; i.e., from the 35–40 minutes that it takes to get a sunburn at noon in June in Boston, Massachusetts, to 3.5 to 4 hours. An important consideration is that

TABLE A–1

SOME OF THE MEDICATIONS THAT PRODUCE SYSTEMIC PHOTOSENSITIZATION

Phototoxic reactions (erythematous, nonimmune reaction)
  Doxycycline
  Tetracyclines (especially demethylchlortetracycline)
  Nalidixic acid
  Sulfonamides
  Sulfonylureas
  Amiodarone
  Furosemide
  Thiazides
  Phenothiazines
  5-Fluorouracil
  Vinblastine
  Retinoids
  Psoralens

Photoallergic reactions (pruritic, eczematous dermatitis due to a delayed hypersensitivity response)
  Sulfonamides
  Thiazides
  Piroxicam
  Naproxen (pseudoporphyria)
  Phenothiazines

TABLE A–2

ELECTROMAGNETIC RADIATION SPECTRUM

Gamma rays	
X-rays	
Ultraviolet	
C (10–290 nm)	Does not reach earth (absorbed in stratospheric ozone)
B (290–320 nm)	Causes sunburn and cancer (partially absorbed by stratospheric ozone; absorbed by window glass)
A (320–400 nm)	Causes wrinkles and contributes to sunburns and cancer (passes window glass)
Visible (400–800 nm)	White light used for vision
Infrared (800–1,700 nm)	Supplies heat
Microwave	
Radiowave	

TABLE A–3
A PARTIAL LIST OF AVAILABLE SUNSCREENS ARRANGED BY PERFORMANCE*

	Wet Time Claim
SPF 15–18, extended water resistance	
Bullfrog Sunblock, the Body Gel	6 hours
Neutrogena Sunblock	6 hours
Vaseline Intensive Care Moisturizing	6 hours
Bain de Soleil All Day Waterproof	6 hours
SPF 15, 80-minute waterproof	
Shade Sunblock Oil-free Gel	80 minutes
Presun Sensitive Skin Sunscreen	80 minutes
Avon Sunseekers	80 minutes
Mary Kay Sun Essentials Sensible Protection	80 minutes
SPF 29–35, extended water resistance†	
Bain de Soleil All Day for Kids	8 hours
Hawaiian Tropic Just for Kids	8 hours
Coppertone Kids Sunblock	8 hours
Hawaiian Tropic Baby Faces	8 hours
SPF 30, 80-minute waterproof†	
Johnson's Baby Sunblock	80 minutes
Waterbabies by Coppertone	80 minutes
Vaseline Intensive Care Baby Moisturizing	80 minutes
Eckerd Children's Sunblock	80 minutes

*Modified from Consumer Reports, "Putting Sunscreens to the Test." May 1995, pp. 338–339.
†Children's products may be used by adults.

increasing SPFs deliver decreasing returns. For example, a sunscreen with an SPF of 15 excludes more than 93% of UV light in sunlight, whereas another with an SPF of 30 removes 97%, which is a marginal difference.

Although sunscreens were formulated on the basis of UVB protection, sunscreens with an SPF of 8 or higher have a protective effect of at least 66% on UVA as well. To exert their action sunscreens must remain on the skin. This opens the issue of water and sweat resistance (the wet time claim). For different products, wet time ranges from 1 hour to about 8 hours. In general, SPFs decrease with length of immersion, so that by the end of the time claim some SPF 30 sunscreens may rate a humble 15 to 20. Because para-amino benzoic acid (PABA) may irritate the skin, products containing this chemical should be avoided. A partial list of sunscreens available on the market is given in Table A–3.

From the foregoing discussion, the use of SPF 15 sunscreens is more than adequate for most purposes. However, there are specific indications to use SPF 30 filters: (1) in children, since 50%–80% of lifetime sun exposure occurs before the age of 18; (2) in photosensitive conditions, as listed above; (3) in people with light-colored skin; (4) when full-day protection from both direct and reflected light (such as at the beach) is required; (5) in sojourns to high altitudes; and (6) when vacationing at southerly locations such as in Florida or Cancun.

Suggested Reading

Consumer Reports. Putting sunscreens to the test. 334–339, May 1995.
Lowe NJ, Shaath NA (eds). Sunscreens. Developments, Evaluation, and Regulatory Aspects. Marcel Dekker, New York, 1–624, 1990.

Guidelines for the Prevention of Corticosteroid-Induced Osteoporosis*

Long-term glucocorticoid use is a major cause of osteoporosis and osteoporosis-related fractures. While daily prednisone doses of >7.5 mg per day are known to adversely affect bone mass, particularly within the initial 6 months of therapy, the safety of lower corticosteroid doses has not been shown. Alternate-day dosing also reduces bone mass. Guidelines recently published by the American College of Rheumatology (ACR) give specific recommendations to minimize the effect of glucocorticoids on bone.

As reviewed in Chapter 22, individuals whose bone mineral density (BMD) is more than 1 standard deviation below mean peak bone mass (T-score) have low a BMD, and those with a T-score >−2.5 are considered to have osteoporosis. Because bone mass cannot be predicted clinically, it is recommended that all patients facing corticosteroid treatment for more than 6 months undergo baseline bone densitometry. Dual-energy x-ray absorptiometry (DEXA) provides highly accurate BMD measurements with a minimal amount of radiation.

General recommendations to prevent glucocorticoid-induced bone loss include (a) use of the lowest effective oral and parenteral doses; (b) a preferential use (if applicable) of topical and inhaled preparations, (c) life-style modifications, including cessation of smoking, reduction of alcohol intake, and increased levels of weight-bearing exercises; and (d) an optimal calcium intake (1,500 mg per day) through either diet or supplements, plus vitamin D supplementation (either 800 IU per day or 50,000 IU 3 times per week) or calcitriol 0.5 µg per day. If high-dose vitamin D or calcitriol is used, serum and urine calcium levels should be monitored. The following clinical scenarios are contemplated in the ACR guidelines.

Scenario I

Patients on long-term corticosteroids seen *after they have sustained an osteoporotic fracture* (usually hip, rib(s), vertebra(e), ankle, or foot). These patients should be evaluated as shown in Table A–4. A follow-up visit should be scheduled within 2 weeks for discussion of results. Follow-up testing should be done as indicated in Table A–5. There should be implementation of prophylaxis and treatment based on DEXA findings plus the results of laboratory evaluation:

*From American College of Rheumatology Task Force on Osteoporosis Guidelines. Recommendations for the prevention and treatment of glucocorticoid-induced osteoporosis. Arthritis Rheum 39:1791–1801, 1996.

1. T-Score <–1; Normal Laboratory Results

   a. Calcium plus vitamin D supplementation.
   b. Referral to physical therapy (PT).
   c. Hormone replacement therapy (HRT).
      Postmenopausal women: estrogen replacement therapy; add progestine if uterus is intact. If estrogen is refused or contraindicated, prescribe calcitonin or bisphosphonates.

      Premenopausal women with intact ovarian function (ages 13–50): estrogen-containing oral contraceptives with 50 µg of estradiol or equivalent. If refused or contraindicated, prescribe calcitonin.

2. T-Score <–1; Abnormal Laboratory Results

   a. Ca plus vitamin D supplementation.
   b. Referral to PT.
   c. Treat underlying condition (Table A–5).

3. T-Score ≥–1; Normal Laboratory Results

   a. Calcium plus vitamin D supplementation.
   b. Referral to PT.
   c. HRT as in (1). In men, adjust testosterone levels if abnormally low. If testosterone is refused or contraindicated, prescribe calcitonin or bisphosphonates.

4. T-Score ≥–1; Abnormal Laboratory Results

   a. Calcium and vitamin D supplementation.
   b. Referral to PT.
   c. HRT as in (1). In men, treat as in (3).
   d. Treat underlying causes (Table A–5).

A follow-up DEXA measurement should be obtained after 6–12 months. If BMD has declined less than 5% over 12 months, treatment should be continued. A greater decline calls for alternative or additional therapy. If the patient has been receiving HRT, the addition or substitution of either calcitonin or a bisphosphonate should be considered.

TABLE A–4

INITIAL EVALUATION OF A PATIENT TAKING GLUCOCORTICOIDS WHO HAS A NONTRAUMATIC FRACTURE*

HISTORY AND PHYSICAL MEASURES

Documentation of height, weight in bare feet, lower-extremity muscle strength, balance, vision
Documentation of medical history
Documentation of menstrual history in menstruating women and impotence or infertility in men
Family history (mother and father) of fractures

LIFE-STYLE MODIFICATION: DOCUMENTATION OF MODIFIABLE INFLUENCES

Calcium and vitamin D intake
Smoking
Medications (thyroid hormone, diphenylhydantoine, coumadin, heparin, cyclosporin A, antigonadotrophins)
Alcohol intake

PATIENT EDUCATION

Prevention of falling
Physical therapy
  Back extension exercises (see p. 330 in this appendix)
  Posture training
  Balance
  Gait evaluation
  Assistive devices
  Kypho-orthosis (as needed)

PAIN CONTROL

Nonpharmacologic therapies
Calcitonin (injectable or intranasal†)
Muscle relaxants
Analgesics; narcotics when necessary

LABORATORY

Complete blood cell count
Erythrocyte sedimentation rate
Serum creatinine, calcium, phosphorus, alkaline phosphatase, liver enzymes, albumin, and electrolytes
24-hour urinary calcium
Serum 25-hydroxyvitamin D
Serum testosterone (male)
Serum luteinizing hormone (female)

DUAL-ENERGY X-RAYS ABSORPTIOMETRY

Hip (all patients)
Spine (patients under 60; anterior osteophytes may falsely increase lumbar spine BMD in elderly patients)

*Modified from American College of Rheumatology Task Force on Osteoporosis Guidelines. Recommendations for the prevention and treatment of glucocorticoid-induced osteoporosis. Arthritis Rheum 39:1791-1801, 1996. © American College of Rheumatology.
†The lesser bioavailability of intranasal calcitonin makes subcutaneous administration preferable when an analgesic effect is desired.

TABLE A–5

FOLLOW-UP FOR ABNORMAL LABORATORY FINDINGS IN PATIENTS TAKING GLUCOCORTICOIDS WHO HAVE A NONTRAUMATIC FRACTURE*

Abnormal Findings	Follow-up Evaluation
High serum Ca, low serum P, high urinary Ca	Measure intact PTH
Low serum Ca, low serum P, low urinary Ca	Measure 25-hydroxyvitamin D
Taking thyroid replacement	Measure TSH
High serum creatinine	Evaluate for renal osteodystrophy
Elevated 24-hour urinary Ca	Add thiazide diuretic with potassium supplement
Elevated total protein or serum globulin	Obtain serum protein electrophoresis and serum and urine immunoelectrophoresis

*From American College of Rheumatology Task Force on Osteoporosis Guidelines. Recommendations for the prevention and treatment of glucocorticoid-induced osteoporosis. Arthritis Rheum 39:1791–1801, 1996.

Scenario II

Patients on long-term corticosteroid therapy *who have not had an osteoporotic fracture* should be evaluated as outlined above. All patients should be started on Ca and vitamin D supplementation. If the BMD is normal, calcium supplementation should be adjusted in a follow-up visit 1 month later. A thiazide should be added for patients with hypercalciuria (urinary Ca >300 mg/day). HRT is recommended in postmenopausal women. Patients with abnormal BMD and/or laboratory tests should be evaluated and treated like patients who have already sustained a fracture. Follow-up is in 12 months, as in Scenario I.

Scenario III

Patients *who are beginning long-term corticosteroid therapy* should be evaluated as indicated in Table A–4. All patients should be started on Ca and vitamin D supplementation and have BMD determination by DEXA. Postmenopausal patients with normal BMD should be encouraged, unless there is contraindication, to start HRT. Patients with low BMD should be started on HRT, or if there is contraindication, a bisphosphonate or calcitonin. One month later, if 24-hour urine Ca is >300 mg per day and the patient is not taking calcitriol, a thiazide diuretic should be added. Follow-up is in 12 months, as in Scenario I.

Clinical Practice Guidelines

TABLE A–6
DIAGNOSTICALLY USEFUL CLINICAL FEATURES IN THE INITIAL EVALUATION OF THE PATIENT WITH ACUTE MUSCULOSKELETAL SYMPTOMS*

	Tendinitis/Bursitis	Noninflammatory Problems†	Systemic Rheumatic Disease
SYMPTOMS			
A.M. stiffness	Focal, brief	Focal, brief	Significant, prolonged
Constitutional symptoms	Absent	Absent	Present
Peak period of discomfort	With use	After prolonged use	After prolonged inactivity
Locking or instability	Unusual, except rotator cuff tear, trigger finger	Implies loose body, internal derangement or weakness	Uncommon
SIGNS			
Symmetry	Uncommon	Occasional	Common
Tenderness	Focal, periarticular, or tender points	Unusual	Common
Inflammation (fluid, pain, warmth, erythema)	Over tendon or bursa	Unusual	Common
Instability	Uncommon	Occasional	Uncommon
Multisystem disease	No	No	Often

*American College of Rheumatology Ad Hoc Committee on Clinical Guidelines. Guidelines for acute musculoskeletal symptoms. Arthritis Rheum 39:1–8, 1996.
†For example, osteoarthritis or internal derangement.

TABLE A–7
"RED FLAGS" SUGGESTING THE NEED FOR URGENT EVALUATION AND MANAGEMENT OF THE PATIENT WITH MUSCULOSKELETAL SYMPTOMS*

Feature	Differential Diagnosis
History of significant trauma	Soft tissue injury, internal derangement, or fracture
Hot, swollen joint	Infection, systemic rheumatic disease, gout, pseudogout
Constitutional signs and symptoms (e.g., fever, weight loss, malaise)	Infection, sepsis, systemic rheumatic disease
Weakness	
Focal	Focal nerve lesion (compartment syndrome, entrapment neuropathy, mononeuritis multiplex, motor neuron disease, radiculopathy†)
Diffuse	Myositis, metabolic myopathy, paraneoplastic syndrome, degenerative neuromuscular disorder, toxin, myelopathy,† transverse myelitis
Neurogenic pain (burning, numbness, paresthesia)	
Asymmetric	Radiculopathy,† reflex sympathetic dystrophy, entrapment neuropathy
Symmetric	Myelopathy,† peripheral neuropathy
Claudication pain pattern	Peripheral vascular disease, giant cell arteritis (jaw pain), lumbar spinal stenosis

*American College of Rheumatology Ad Hoc Committee on Clinical Guidelines. Guidelines for acute musculoskeletal symptoms. Arthritis Rheum 39:1–8, 1996.
†Radiculopathy and myelopathy may be due to infectious, neoplastic, or mechanical processes.

TABLE A–8
RECOMMENDATIONS FOR THE DIAGNOSTIC USE OF THE ERYTHROCYTE SEDIMENTATION RATE (ESR)*

1. The ESR should not be used to screen asymptomatic persons for disease.
2. The ESR should be used selectively and interpreted with caution when the history and physical examination fail to provide any evidence for a specific diagnostic hypothesis in a symptomatic person.

    Significant infectious, inflammatory, or neoplastic disease is unlikely in such patients, and the ESR must be markedly elevated to be diagnostically useful. Extreme elevation of the ESR seldom occurs in patients with no evidence of serious disease.

3. If there is no immediate explanation for an increased ESR, the physician should repeat the test in several months rather than search for occult disease.

    A careful history and physical examination will generally disclose the cause of an elevated ESR. An increased ESR in the setting of a normal examination is usually transitory and is infrequently the harbinger of serious occult disease.

4. The ESR is indicated for diagnosis and monitoring of temporal arteritis and polymyalgia rheumatica.

    A normal ESR excludes the diagnosis of temporal arteritis in most patients who are suspected of having the disease. However, when the ESR is normal, despite other strong clinical evidence of temporal arteritis, aggressive diagnostic or therapeutic intervention is still indicated.

    Although the ESR is an indicator of disease activity in temporal arteritis and polymyalgia rheumatica, the patient's clinical status must be taken into account in adjusting the dosage of corticosteroids.

5. In diagnosing and monitoring patients with rheumatoid arthritis, the ESR should be used principally to help resolve conflicting clinical evidence. The role of the ESR in other rheumatic diseases has not been studied.
6. The ESR may be helpful in monitoring patients with treated Hodgkin's disease.

*From Sox HC, Liang MH. The erythrocyte sedimentation rate. Guidelines for rational use. Ann Intern Med 104:515–523, 1986.

Author's note: I would add unequivocally that the ESR is useful to distinguish aseptic loosening of a prosthesis from loosening due to infection and also in the follow-up of patients with osteomyelitis.

TABLE A–9

CENTERS FOR DISEASE CONTROL RECOMMENDATIONS FOR THE SEROLOGIC DIAGNOSIS OF LYME DISEASE*

Test Performance and Interpretation

RECOMMENDATION 1.1. TWO-TEST PROTOCOL

All serum specimens submitted for Lyme disease testing should be evaluated in a two-step process. First is a sensitive serological test, such as an enzyme immunoassay (EIA) or immunofluorescent assay (IFA). Second, all specimens found to be positive or equivocal by a sensitive EIA or IFA should then be tested by a standardized Western blot (WB) procedure. Specimens found to be negative by a sensitive EIA or IFA need not be tested further.

RECOMMENDATION 1.2. WB CONTROLS

Immunoblotting should be performed using a negative control, a weakly reactive positive control, and a high-titered positive control.

RECOMMENDATION 1.3. TESTING AND STAGE OF THE DISEASE

When WB is used in the first 4 weeks after disease onset (early Lyme disease), both IgM and IgG procedures should be performed. Most Lyme disease patients will seroconvert within this 4-week period. In the event that a patient with suspected early disease has a negative serology, serologic evidence is best obtained by testing paired acute- and convalescent-phase samples. In late Lyme disease the predominant antibody is usually IgG. It is highly unusual for a patient with active disease to have only an IgM response to *Borrelia burgdorferi* after 1 month of infection. A positive IgM test result alone is not recommended for determining active disease in persons with illness of longer than 1 month duration because the likelihood of a false positive result is high for these individuals.

RECOMMENDATION 1.4. WB CRITERIA

An IgM blot is considered positive if two of the following three bands are present: 24 (OspC), 39 kDa, and 41 kDa. An IgG blot is considered positive if five of the following ten bands are present: 18, 21 (OspC), 28, 30, 39, 41, 45, 58, 66, and 93 kDa.

RECOMMENDATION 1.5. REPORTING OF RESULTS

An equivocal or positive EIA or IFA result followed by a negative immunoblot result should be reported as negative. An equivocal or positive EIA or IFA result followed by a positive immunoblot result should be reported as positive. An explanation and interpretation of test results should accompany all reports.

*Centers for Disease Control. Proceedings of the Second National Conference on Serologic Diagnosis of Lyme Disease, 1st ed. Association of State and Territorial Public Health Laboratory Directors, Washington, DC, 1–111, 1994.

TABLE A-10

Antirheumatic Therapy in Pregnancy and Lactation and Effects on Fertility*

	FDA Use in Pregnancy Rating†	Crosses Placenta	Major Maternal Toxicities	Fetal Toxicities	Breast-feeding	Fertility
Aspirin	C; D in 3rd trimester	Yes	Anemia, peripartum hemorrhage, prolonged labor	Premature closure of ductus, ICH, pulmonary hypertension	Use cautiously; excreted at low concentration; doses greater than one (325 mg) tablet result in high infant plasma concentrations	No data
NSAIDs	B; D in 3rd trimester	Yes	As for aspirin	As for aspirin	Compatible according to AAP	No data
Corticosteroids Prednisone / Dexamethasone	B / C	Dexamethasone and betamethasone	Exacerbation of diabetes and hypertension; PROM	IUGR	5–20% of maternal dose excreted in breast milk; compatible but wait 4 hours if dose > 20 mg	No data
Hydroxychloroquine	C	Yes; fetal concentration 50% of maternal	Few	Few	Contraindicated (slow elimination rate, potential for accumulation)	No data
Gold	C	Yes	No data	One reported cleft palate and severe CNS abnormalities	Excreted into breast milk (20% of maternal dose); rash, hepatitis, and hematologic abnormalities reported but AAP considers compatible	
D-penicillamine	D	Yes	No data	Cutis laxa; connective tissue abnormalities	No data	No data
Sulfasalazine	B, D if near term	Yes	No data	No increase in congenital malformations, kernicterus if administered near term	Excreted into breast milk (40–60% of maternal dose); bloody diarrhea in one infant; AAP recommends caution	Females: no effect; males: significant decrease in sperm counts; 2 months to return to normal
Azathioprine	D	Yes	No data	IUGR (up to 40% rate) and prematurity; transient immunosuppression in neonate; effect on germlines of offspring	No data; hypothetical risk of immunosuppression outweighs benefit	Not studied; can interfere with effectiveness of IUD
Chlorambucil	D	Teratogenic effect potentiated by caffeine	No data	Renal agenesis	Contraindicated	No data
Methotrexate	X	No data	Spontaneous abortion	Fetal abnormalities (including cleft palate and hydrocephalus)	Contraindicated; small amounts excreted with potential to accumulate in fetal tissues	Females: infrequent long-term effect; males: reversible oligospermia
Cyclophosphamide	D	Yes, 25% of maternal level	No data	Severe abnormalities; case report male twin developed thyroid papillary cancer at 11 years and neuroblastoma at 14 years	Contraindicated; has caused bone marrow depression	Females: age > 25 years, concurrent radiation, prolonged exposure increase the risk of infertility; males: dose dependent, oligo- and azoospermia regardless of age or exposure
Cyclosporine A	C	Yes	No data	IUGR and prematurity; one case report: hypoplasia of right leg; not an animal teratogen and unlikely to be a human one	Contraindicated due to potential for immunosuppression	No data

*From American College of Rheumatology Ad Hoc Committee on Clinical Guidelines. American College of Rheumatology Guidelines for Monitoring Drug Therapy in Rheumatoid Arthritis. Arthritis Rheum 39:723–731, 1996.

†Key to FDA use-in-pregnancy ratings:

A = Controlled studies show no risk. Adequate, well-controlled studies in pregnant women have failed to demonstrate risk to the fetus.

B = No evidence of risk in humans. Either animal findings show risk but human findings do not, or, if no adequate human studies have been done, animal findings are negative.

C = Risk cannot be ruled out. Human studies are lacking, and animal studies are either positive for fetal risk or lacking as well. However, potential benefits may justify the potential risk.

D = Positive evidence of risk. Investigational or postmarketing data show risk to the fetus. Nevertheless, potential benefits may outweigh the potential risk.

X = Contraindicated in pregnancy. Studies in animals and humans, or as investigational or postmarketing reports, have shown fetal risk that clearly outweighs any possible benefit to the patient.

Abbreviations: AAP = American Academy of Pediatrics; ICH = intracranial hemorrhage; IUGR = intrauterine growth retardation; PROM = premature rupture of membranes; CNS = central nervous system; IUD = intrauterine device.

TABLE A-11
AMERICAN COLLEGE OF RHEUMATOLOGY GUIDELINES FOR THE MANAGEMENT OF RHEUMATOID ARTHRITIS*

I. BASELINE EVALUATION

Subjective

Degree of pain in specific symptomatic joints
Duration of morning stiffness
Presence or absence of fatigue
Functional status

Physical Examination

Documentation of actively inflamed joints
Documentation of mechanical joint problems or loss of motion, crepitus, instability, alignment abnormalities, and deformity

Laboratory

ESR/CRP, rheumatoid factor, ANA
CBC and chemistry profile as baseline for medications, search for systemic and concurrent disease
Synovial fluid analysis if necessary to rule out other diseases†

Radiographs

Radiographs of limited diagnostic value early in disease, but radiographs of selected involved joints establish baseline for monitoring disease progression and response to treatment

Parameters for Response to Treatment (Outcomes)

Patient and physician global assessment
Tender and swollen joints
Pain assessment
Functional status assessment

II. NSAIDS FOR RHEUMATOID ARTHRITIS

Goals

Symptomatic relief of pain and swelling

Limitations

Probably unable to prevent damage

Factors for Selecting Drugs

Dosing regimen
Efficacy
Tolerance
Costs
Patient's age
Presence of co-morbid disease(s)
Concurrent drugs
Patient preferences

Monitoring Efficacy

Symptoms and signs of active synovitis

III. DISEASE-MODIFYING ANTIRHEUMATIC DRUGS (DMARDS) FOR RHEUMATOID ARTHRITIS

Goals

Remission or optimal control of inflammatory joint disease

Limitations

May or may not prevent damage in spite of apparent clinical control
May or may not have lasting efficacy
May or may not be tolerated due to toxicity

Factors for Selecting Drugs

Convenience and cost of medication and monitoring for toxicity
Risk of adverse reactions, including frequency and seriousness
Physician's estimate of efficacy and prognosis

Monitoring Efficacy

Is disease in remission or optimally controlled?

Monitoring Toxicity‡

---

*American College of Rheumatology Guidelines for the Management of Rheumatoid Arthritis. I–VI. Arthritis and Rheumatism. Kwoch CK, Simms RW, co-chairmen. 1996, in press. © American College of Rheumatology.

†*Author's note:* Gout and calcium pyrophosphate dihydrate (CPPD) crystal deposition disease may mimic RA to perfection. Joint aspiration is essential to rule out these conditions.

‡For more detailed information on monitoring the symptoms and signs of toxicity, see American College of Rheumatology Guidelines for Monitoring Drug Therapy in Rheumatoid Arthritis page 347.

(Continued)

TABLE A-11 *(Continued)*

IV. DMARDS FOR RHEUMATOID ARTHRITIS

Drugs	Time Delay to Benefit	Usual Maintenance Dosing	Toxicity
Hydroxychloroquine	2–4 months	200 mg bid	Infrequent rash, diarrhea, rare retinal toxicity
Sulfasalazine	1–2 months	1,000 mg bid or tid	Rash, infrequent myelosuppression, liver toxicity
Methotrexate	1–2 months	7.5–15 mg once weekly	GI, stomatitis, rash, infrequent myelosuppression, hepatotoxicity. Rare but serious (and even life threatening) pulmonary toxicity.
Injectable gold salts	3–6 months	IM injection 25–50mg q 1–4 weeks	Rash, stomatitis, myelosuppression, thrombocytopenia, proteinuria
Oral gold	4–6 months	3 mg qd or bid	Same as injectable gold plus frequent diarrhea
Azathioprine	2–3 months	50–150 mg qd	Myelosuppression, infrequent hepatotoxicity. Early flulike illness with fever, GI symptoms, elevated LFTs
Penicillamine	3–6 months	250–750 qd	Rash, stomatitis, dysgeusia, proteinuria, myelosuppression. Infrequent but serious autoimmune disease

V. GLUCOCORTICOID THERAPY

Local Injection

Goals

Early local treatment of most involved joints
Flare of one or a few joints during treatment program
Attempt to recover lost joint motion

Limitations

Local joint treatment but systemic process. Temporary benefit if disease is not systemically controlled

Factors for Selecting Drugs

Need for long-acting preparation; concentration varies with size of joint being injected

Monitoring Efficacy

Improvement in synovitis, restoration of range of motion

Monitoring Toxicity

Avoid repetitive injections in the same joint more than once every 3 months

Systemic, Low-dose Oral (≤ 10 mg prednisone daily)

Goals

Bridging treatment awaiting DMARD response
Short course for flares or special life events
Disease not adequately controlled (unacceptable discomfort or limitations of function) in spite of optimal NSAID, DMARD trials

Limitations

Damage may progress; probably no disease-modifying properties§

Factors for Selecting Drugs

Initial and maintenance dose selection critical

Monitoring Efficacy

Improvement in symptoms and signs of synovitis; improvement in function

Monitoring Toxicity

VI. MONITORING RA ACTIVITY

Each visit: Evaluate for evidence of active disease
- Degree of joint pain
- Duration of morning stiffness
- Severity of fatigue
- Synovitis on examination
- Limitation of function

Periodically: Evaluate for disease activity or progression on physical examination (loss of motion, instability, malalignment, and/or deformity)
- Erythrocyte sedimentation rate or C-reactive protein (CRP) elevation
- Progression of radiographic damage of involved joints

Outcomes
- Patient and physician global assessment of disease activity
- Pain, function
- Joint counts (tenderness and swelling)
- Functional status assessment

---

§*Author's note:* A recent study by Kirwan JR, et al. N Engl J Med 333:142–146, 1995, p. 44, (Glucocorticoids) has shown a lesser rate of erosions in low-dose corticosteroid-treated patients.

TABLE A-12

RECOMMENDATIONS FOR MONITORING FOR HEPATIC SAFETY IN RHEUMATOID ARTHRITIS (RA) PATIENTS RECEIVING METHOTREXATE*

A. Baseline
 1. Tests for all patients
    a. Liver blood tests (aspartate aminotransferase [AST], alanine aminotransferase [ALT], alkaline phosphatase, albumin, bilirubin), hepatitis B and C serologic studies
    b. Other standard tests, including complete blood cell count and serum creatinine
 2. Pretreatment liver biopsy (Menghini suction-type needle) only for patients with:
    a. Prior excessive alcohol consumption
    b. Persistently abnormal baseline AST values
    c. Chronic hepatitis B or C infection
B. Monitor AST, ALT, albumin at 4–8-week intervals
C. Perform liver biopsy if:
 1. Five of 9 determinations of AST within a given 12-month interval (6 of 12 if tests are performed monthly) are abnormal (defined as an elevation above the upper limit of normal)
 2. There is a decrease in serum albumin below the normal range (in the setting of well-controlled RA)
D. If results of liver biopsy are:
 1. Roenigk grade I, II, or IIIA, resume MTX and monitor as in B, C1, and C2 above
 2. Roenigk grade IIIB or IV, discontinue MTX
E. Discontinue MTX in patient with persistent liver test abnormalities, as defined in C1 and C2 above, who refuses liver biopsy

*From Kremer JM, et al. Methotrexate for rheumatoid arthritis. Suggested guidelines for monitoring liver toxicity. Arthritis Rheum 37:316–328, 1994.

Roenigk grade I = normal findings; possibly mild fatty changes, anisonucleosis, and mild portal inflammation.

Roenigk grade II = above plus spotty hepatocellular necrosis.

Roenigk grade IIIA = mild portal fibrosis, with or without fibrotic septae extending into the lobe.

Roenigk grade IIIB = piecemeal necrosis or portal-portal fibrosis or portal triad to central vein bridging.

Roenigk grade IV = frank cirrhosis.

TABLE A-13
RECOMMENDED MONITORING STRATEGY FOR DRUG TREATMENT OF RHEUMATOID ARTHRITIS*†

Drug	Toxicities Requiring Monitoring	Baseline Evaluation	Monitoring System Review/Examination	Laboratory
Salicylates, nonsteroidal anti-inflammatory	Gastrointestinal bleeding and ulceration	CBC, creatinine, ALT, AST	Dark/black stool, dyspepsia, nausea, vomiting, abdominal pain, dyspnea, edema	Yearly CBC, LFTs, creatinine testing may be required‡
Glucocorticoids (oral, ≤10 mg of prednisone or equivalent)	Hypertension, hyperglycemia, osteoporosis	BP, chemistry panel; bone densitometry in high-risk patients	Polyuria, polydipsia, dyspnea, edema, BP at each visit; visual changes, weight gain	—
Hydroxychloroquine	Macular damage	None, unless patient is over 40 or has previous eye disease	Visual changes; fundoscopy and visual fields every 6–12 months	—
Sulfasalazine	Myelosuppression	CBC and AST or ALT in patients at risk; G6PD	Symptoms of myelosuppression,§ photosensitivity, rash	CBC q 2–4 weeks for first 3 months, then q 3 months
Methotrexate	Myelosuppression, hepatic fibrosis, cirrhosis, pulmonary infiltrates, pulmonary fibrosis	CBC, chest radiography within past year, hepatitis B, C serology in high-risk patients, AST or ALT, albumin, bilirubin, alkaline phosphatase, and creatinine	Symptoms of myelosuppression,§ dyspnea, nausea/vomiting, oral ulceration, lymph node swelling	CBC, AST, or ALT, albumin, creatinine q 4–8 weeks
Gold, intramuscular	Myelosuppression, proteinuria	CBC, creatinine, and urine dipstick for protein	Symptoms of myelosuppression,§ edema, rash, oral ulcers, diarrhea	CBC and urine dipstick before each injection
Gold, oral	Myelosuppression, proteinuria	CBC, urine dipstick for protein	Symptoms of myelosuppression,§ edema, rash, diarrhea	CBC and urine dipstick for protein every 4–12 weeks
D-penicillamine	Myelosuppression, proteinuria	CBC, urine dipstick for protein, creatinine	Symptoms of myelosuppression,§ edema, rash	CBC and urine dipstick every 2 weeks until dose stable, then q 1–3 months
Azathioprine	Myelosuppression, hepatotoxicity, lymphoproliferative disorders	CBC, creatinine, ALT, or AST	Symptoms of myelosuppression§	CBC q 1–2 weeks with changes in dose every 1–3 months thereafter
Agents for Refractory RA or Severe Extraarticular Complications				
Cyclophosphamide	Myelosuppression, myeloproliferative disorders, malignancy, hemorrhagic cystitis	CBC, urinalysis, creatinine, AST, or ALT	Symptoms of myelosuppression	CBC and platelet count every 1–2 weeks with changes in dose every 1–3 months thereafter; urinalysis and urine cytology every 6–12 months after cessation
Chlorambucil	Myelosuppression, myeloproliferative disorders, malignancy	CBC, urinalysis, creatinine, AST, or ALT	Symptoms of myelosuppression	CBC every 1–2 weeks with changes in dose every 1–3 months thereafter
Cyclosporine A	Renal insufficiency, anemia, hypertension	CBC, creatinine, uric acid, BP	Edema	Creatinine monthly and BP

*From American College of Rheumatology Ad Hoc Committee on Clinical Guidelines. Guidelines for monitoring drug therapy. Arthritis Rheum 39:723–731, 1996.
†Potential serious toxicities that may be detected by monitoring before clinically apparent or harmful to patient. This list mentions toxicities that occur enough to justify monitoring. Patients with co-morbidity, concurrent medications, and other specific risk factors may need further studies to monitor for specific toxicity.
‡Package insert for diclofenac (Voltaren) recommends that AST and ALT be monitored within the first 8 weeks of treatment and periodically thereafter. Monitoring of serum creatinine should be performed weekly for at least 3 weeks in patients receiving concomitant angiotensin-converting enzyme inhibitors or diuretics.
§Symptoms of myelosuppression include fever, symptoms of infection, easy bruisability, and bleeding.
ALT = alanine aminotransferase; AST = aspartate aminotransferase; BP = blood pressure; CBC = complete blood count (hematocrit, hemoglobin, white blood cell count), including differential and platelet count.

TABLE A-14

DEFINITION OF IMPROVEMENT IN RHEUMATOID ARTHRITIS*

Required: >20% improvement in tender joint count
>20% improvement in swollen joint count
plus
>20% improvement in 3 of following 5:
  Patient pain assessment
  Patient global assessment
  Physician global assessment
  Patient self-assessed disability
  Acute phase reactant (ESR or CRP)

1. Tender joint count: ACR tender joint count,[†] an assessment of 28 or more joints. The joint count should be done by scoring several aspects of tenderness, as assessed by pressure and joint manipulation on physical examination. The information on various types of tenderness should then be collapsed into a single tender-versus-nontender dichotomy.
2. Swollen joint count: ACR swollen joint count, an assessment of 28 or more joints. Joints are classified as either swollen or not swollen.
3. Patient's assessment of pain: a horizontal visual analog scale (usually 10 cm).
4. Patient's global assessment of disease activity: the patient's overall assessment of how the arthritis is doing. One acceptable method for this is the question from the AIMS instrument: "Considering all the ways your arthritis affects you, mark 'X' on the scale for how well you are doing."
5. Physician's global assessment of disease activity: a horizontal visual analog scale (usually 10 cm).
6. Patient's assessment of physical function (HAQ, AIMS).
7. Acute phase reactant value: A Westergren erythro sedimentation rate or a C-reactive protein level.

*After Felson DT, Anderson JJ, Boers M, et al. American College of Rheumatology preliminary definition of improvement in rheumatoid arthritis. Arthritis Rheum 38:727–735, 1995.

[†]Arthritis Rheum 21:28–32, 1994; Arthritis Rheum 37:463–464, 1994.

Author's note: This guideline is for use in clinical trials; however, it shows well the clinical criteria that experienced clinicians use to determine improvement in patients with RA.

TABLE A-15

GUIDELINES FOR THE MEDICAL TREATMENT OF OSTEOARTHRITIS. PART I. OSTEOARTHRITIS OF THE HIP*

A. Goals of treatment
  1. Control of pain and other symptoms
  2. Patient and family education
B. Make certain that pain is due to osteoarthritis; consider bursitis (trochanteric, anserine syndrome) and pain radiation from a spinal condition (see Chapter 27)
C. Use the American College of Rheumatology classification criteria to determine that a patient indeed has hip osteoarthritis (see Chapter 20 on osteoarthritis)
D. Medical management of patients with osteoarthritis of the hip:
  1. Nonpharmacologic therapy
    a. Patient education; self-management programs (such as the Arthritis Self-Help Course)
    b. Health professional social support via telephone contact
    c. Weight loss if overweight
    d. Physical therapy
      1) Range of motion exercises
      2) Strengthening exercises
      3) Assistive devices for ambulation (e.g., a cane)
    e. Occupational therapy
      1) Joint protection and energy conservation
      2) Assistive devices for activities of daily living (bathing, dressing, toileting, performing household chores)
      3) Aerobic aquatic exercise programs (such as the Aquatic Program sponsored by the Arthritis Foundation)
  2. Pharmacologic therapy
    a. Nonopioid analgesics (e.g., acetaminophen up to 1 g qid); if no response:
    b. Nonsteroidal anti-inflammatory drugs in low dose such as ibuprofen (up to 400 mg qid) or nonacetylated salicylates; if no response:
    c. Nonsteroidal anti-inflammatory drugs in full dose (with misoprostol in patients with risk factors for UGI bleeding or ulcer disease[†])
    d. If response is inadequate, consider referral for joint surgery (osteotomy, total joint arthroplasty)
    e. Opioid analgesics (e.g., propoxyphene, codeine, oxycodone)

*Modified from Hochberg, MC, Altman RD, Brandt KD, et al. Guidelines for the medical management of osteoarthritis. Part I. Osteoarthritis of the hip. Arthritis Rheum 38:1535–1540, 1995.

[†]Risk factors for UGI bleeding: age 65 or older, history of peptic ulcer disease or upper GI bleeding, concomitant use of corticosteroids and anticoagulants, and possibly smoking and alcohol consumption.

TABLE A-16

GUIDELINES FOR THE MEDICAL MANAGEMENT OF OSTEOARTHRITIS. PART II. OSTEOARTHRITIS OF THE KNEE*

A. Goals of treatment
   1. Control of pain and other symptoms
   2. Patient and family education
B. Make certain that pain is due to osteoarthritis; consider anserine, infrapatellar, or prepatellar bursitis (as well as other soft tissue causes of knee area pain in Chapter 28). Rule out referred pain from the hip or spine.
C. Use the American College of Rheumatology classification criteria to determine that a patient indeed has knee osteoarthritis (see Chapter 20).
D. Medical management of patients with osteoarthritis of the knee:
   1. Nonpharmacologic therapy
      a. Patient education; self-management programs (such as the Arthritis Self-Help Course)
      b. Health professional social support via telephone contact
      c. Weight loss if there is overweight
      d. Physical therapy
         1) Range of motion exercises
         2) Quadriceps strengthening exercises
         3) Assistive devices for ambulation (a cane, etc.)
      e. Occupational therapy
         1) Joint protection and energy conservation
         2) Assistive devices for activities of daily living (bathing, dressing, toileting, performing household chores)
      f. Aerobic exercise programs (such as the Aquatic Program sponsored by the Arthritis Foundation)
   2. Pharmacologic therapy
      a. If effusion is present, consider aspiration (which will serve to rule out crystal-induced disease) and injection of intraarticular steroids (see "Injections and Infiltrations" in this appendix)
      b. Nonopioid analgesics (e.g., acetaminophen up to 1 g qid). If necessary, add:
      c. Topical analgesics (e.g., capsaicin and methylsalicylate creams); if no reasponse:
      d. Nonsteroidal anti-inflammatory drugs in low dose such as ibuprofen (up to 400 mg qid) or nonacetylated salicylates; if response is inadequate:
      e. Nonsteroidal anti-inflammatory drugs in full dose (with misoprostol in patients with risk factors for UGI bleeding or ulcer disease†)
      f. Opioid analgesics (e.g., propoxyphene, codeine, oxycodone)
      g. If response is inadequate, and surgery is contraindicated, consider referral for joint lavage and/or arthroscopic debridement
      h. If response is inadequate, consider referral for joint surgery (osteotomy, total joint arthroplasty)

*Modified from Hochberg MC, Altman RD, Brandt KD, et al. Guidelines for the medical management of osteoarthritis. Part II. Osteoarthritis of the knee. Arthritis Rheum 38:1541–1546, 1995.

†Risk factors for UGI bleeding: age 65 or older, history of peptic ulcer disease or upper GI bleeding, concomitant use of corticosteroids and anticoagulants, and possibly smoking and alcohol consumption.

TABLE A-17

CLINICAL PRACTICE GUIDELINES FOR ACUTE LOW BACK PAIN*

PATIENT EDUCATION
1. Recommendation: about expectations, methods of symptom control, activities modifications, prevention of recurrences, instruction about red flags for infection and neoplasia, and actions to take should symptoms persist (B); "back school" in workplaces (C)
2. Option: "back school" in nonoccupational setting (C)
3. Recommended against: none

MEDICATION
1. Recommendation: acetaminophen (C), NSAIDs explaining potential side effects (B)
2. Option: muscle relaxants (C); short course of opioids (C)
3. Recommended against: opioids >2 weeks (C); oral steroids (C); antidepressants (C)

PHYSICAL TREATMENT
1. Recommendation: manipulation in the first month if no radiculopathy since neurologic deterioration may follow manipulation (B)
2. Option: manipulation after 1 month or if radiculopathy (C); self-application of heat and cold (C); corset at work for prevention (C)
3. Recommended against: prolonged manipulation (D); traction (B); TENS (C); biofeedback (C); corset for treatment (D)

INJECTIONS
1. Recommendation: none
2. Option: epidural steroids for radicular pain
3. Recommended against: epidural steroids for back pain (D); trigger facet, ligamentous (C); acupuncture (D)

BED REST
1. Recommendation: none
2. Option: 2–4 days for severe radiculopathy (D)
3. Recommended against: >4 days may lead to debilitation and is not recommended (B)

EXERCISE
1. Recommendation: aerobic (C); trunk conditioning (C); resume normal activities (B)
2. Option: none
3. Recommended against: therapeutic back stretching (D)

A = Multiple randomized clinical trials. B = One high-quality (randomized, controlled) study or multiple adequate (but not randomized) studies. C = At least one adequate study. D = No adequate studies.

*After Bigos SJ, Bowyer OR, Braen GR, et al. Acute low back problems in adults. Agency for Health Care Policy and Research, Rockville, MD, publication No. 95-0642. Clinical Practice Guideline No. 14. Public Health Service, US Department of Human Services, December 1994.

Author's note: Manipulation in the first month has the highest patient satisfaction, but the outcome is no different (see Carey, Garrett, Jackman, et al., 1995; cited in "Acute Nonspecific Low Back Pain," Chapter 26); also, a recommendation to resume ordinary activities as promptly as possible produced more rapid return to work and better clinical outcomes than did 2 days of bed rest or a formal back-mobilizing exercise program (see Malmivaara, Häkkinen, Aro, et al., 1995; cited in "Acute Nonspecific Low Back Pain," Chapter 26).

TABLE A–18
GUIDELINES FOR THE CLINICAL UTILIZATION OF BONE MASS MEASUREMENTS IN THE ADULT POPULATION*

1. Bone mass measurements (BMMs) predict a patient's future risk of fracture. The ability of bone mass to predict future fracture risk is as valuable as cholesterol testing or blood pressure measurements for the prediction of heart attack or stroke and should be used more widely to identify at-risk patients.
2. Osteoporosis can be diagnosed on the basis of BMMS even in the absence of prevalent fractures. Diagnosing osteoporosis before a fracture occurs is an important concept advancement. It is justified on the recognized inverse and exponential relationship between low bone mass and future fracture risk and the exceedingly high risk observed for a second fracture once the first fracture has occurred.
3. BMMs provide information that can affect the management of patients. A BMM should be performed in any patient of any age or sex when the result will influence a clinical decision. The clinical decision(s) that may follow BMM results are diverse, but include whether to initiate hormonal replacement therapy, to diagnose osteoporosis in a young fracturing amenorrheic athlete, or to monitor longitudinal changes in a patient receiving pharmacological therapy to prevent or treat osteoporosis. There are, therefore, a wide variety of clinical decisions that can be made more objectively with knowledge of BMM results.
4. The choice of the appropriate site(s) for the assessment of bone mass or fracture risk may vary depending on the specific circumstances of the patient. Different skeletal sites can be measured in order to diagnose osteoporosis and predict fracture risk. Since bone mass is discordant in the younger, perimenopausal population, if the first skeletal site measured is normal, it may be necessary to measure a second skeletal site in order to make an accurate diagnosis. Measuring more than one skeletal site may also be necessary if artifacts invalidate a particular site. Decisions about which site to measure and how many sites to measure should be the clinician's choice. In general, since cancellous bone changes more rapidly than cortical bone over time or with therapeutic intervention(s), cancellous bone sites (axial skeleton, calcaneus, or distal radius) may be the preferred site(s) to measure, though cortical bone sites (midradius, femoral neck) may also provide valuable and independent data. Additionally, when performing serial measurements in patients to monitor the natural course of bone loss (or gain) or the response to pharmacologic intervention, clinicians must know if the changes are real or within the precision error of a particular measurement and if they are the result of a particular technique.
5. The choice of the appropriate technique for BMMs in any given clinical circumstance should be based on an understanding of the strengths and limitations of the different techniques. All BMM techniques are valuable for making the diagnosis of osteoporosis and predicting fracture risk. The choice of which technique(s) to use for any individual patient should be at the discretion of the physician. In most countries, dual energy x-ray absorptiometry (DXA) is the most widely used technique because of its low precision error, low radiation exposure, and capacity to measure multiple skeletal sites. However, other techniques such as quantitative computerized tomography (QCT), ultrasound, single x-ray absorptiometry of the wrist or calcaneus, peripheral quantitative computerized tomography (PQCT), or hand radiogrammetry are valuable and may offer information not assessed by DXA. Some of these lower-cost techniques may be used as screening techniques to detect a larger percentage of the high-risk population at potentially lower health care costs. Whatever technique is used, quality control and quality assurance are paramount for providing competent patient assessment.
6. BMMs should be accompanied by a clinical interpretation. The computer printout data provided by the bone mass manufacturers do not fully provide the clinical information that the primary care physician needs to have in order to direct patient care. BMM results have wide implications for clinical decisions in the care of patients with low bone mass and may lead to broader diagnostic and therapeutic interventions that can be provided by blood pressure measurements or blood chemistry results. A brief narrative report correlating the BMM to a technician-obtained patient questionnaire database can allow the clinician interpreting the BMM to suggest to the primary care physician wider diagnostic and intervention possibilities. In this way the value of the BMM result is enhanced for the patient and physician alike.

*From Miller PD, Bonnick S, Rosen C. Guidelines for the clinical utilization of bone mass measurement in the adult population. For a Panel of the Society for Clinical Densitometry. Calcif Tissue Int 57:251–252, 1995.

TABLE A-19
NAMES AND DEFINITIONS OF VASCULITIDES ADOPTED BY THE CHAPEL HILL CONSENSUS CONFERENCE ON THE NOMENCLATURE OF SYSTEMIC VASCULITIS*

LARGE VESSEL VASCULITIS[†]

Giant cell (temporal) arteritis	Granulomatous arteritis of the aorta and its major branches, with a predilection for the extracranial branches of the carotid artery. (Often involves the temporal artery. Usually occurs in patients older than 50 and is often associated with polymyalgia rheumatica.)
Takayasu arteritis	Granulomatous inflammation of the aorta and its major branches. (Usually occurs in patients younger than 50.)

MEDIUM-SIZED VESSEL VASCULITIS

Polyarteritis nodosa (classic)	Necrotizing inflammation of medium-sized or small arteries without glomerulonephritis or vasculitis in arterioles, capillaries, or venules.
Kawasaki disease	Arteritis involving large, medium-sized, and small arteries and associated with mucocutaneous lymph node syndrome. (Coronary arteries are often involved. Aorta and veins may be involved. Usually occurs in children.)

SMALL VESSEL VASCULITIS

Wegener's granulomatosis[‡]	Granulomatous inflammation involving the respiratory tract and necrotizing vasculitis affecting small to medium-sized vessels (e.g., capillaries, venules, arterioles, and arteries). (Necrotizing glomerulonephritis is common.)
Churg-Strauss syndrome[‡]	Eosinophil-rich and granulomatous inflammation involving the respiratory tract and necrotizing vasculitis affecting small to medium-sized vessels. (Associated with asthma and eosinophilia.)
Microscopic polyangiitis[§] (microscopic polyarteritis)[†]	Necrotizing vasculitis, with few or no immune deposits, affecting small vessels (i.e., capillaries, venules, or arterioles). (Necrotizing arteritis involving small and medium-sized arteries may be present. Necrotizing glomerulonephritis is very common. Pulmonary capillaritis often occurs.)
Henoch-Schönlein purpura	Vasculitis, with IgA-dominant immune deposits, affecting small vessels (i.e., capillaries, venules, or arterioles). (Typically involves the skin, gut, and glomeruli and is associated with arthralgias or arthritis.)
Essential cryoglobulinemic vasculitis	Vasculitis, with cryoglobulin immune deposits, affecting small vessels (i.e., capillaries, venules, or arterioles) and associated with cryoglobulins in serum. (Skin and glomeruli are often involved.)
Cutaneous leukocytoclastic angiitis	Isolated cutaneous leukocytoclastic angiitis without systemic vasculitis or glomerulonephritis.

*From Jennette JC, Falk RJ, Andrassy K, et al. Nomenclature of systemic vasculitis. Proposal of an International Consensus Conference. Arthritis Rheum 37:187–192, 1994.
[†]Large vessel refers to the aorta and the largest branches directed toward major body regions (e.g., to the extremities and the head and neck); medium-sized vessel refers to the main visceral arteries (e.g., renal, hepatic, coronary, and mesenteric arteries); small vessel refers to venules, capillaries, arterioles, and the intraparenchymal distal arterial radicals that connect with arterioles. Some small and large vessel vasculitides may involve medium-sized arteries, but large and medium-sized vessel vasculitides do not involve vessels smaller than arteries. Essential components are represented by material not in parentheses; material in parentheses represents usual, but not essential, components.
[‡]Strongly associated with antineutrophil cytoplasmic autoantibodies.
[§]Preferred term.

INDEX

Abdominal muscles, isometric exercises for, 323
Abdominal wall, strengthening exercises for, 324, *324*, 329
Abscess, intramuscular, computed tomography of, 23, *23*
    metaphyseal (Brodie's), 206
    renal, low back pain in, 262
Acetaminophen, 43
    for hand osteoarthritis, 177, 178
    for knee osteoarthritis, 180
Achilles tendinitis, in reactive arthritis, 136, 137
    in spondyloarthropathy, 288
    posterior calcaneal pain in, 288
Acquired immunodeficiency syndrome (AIDS), rheumatic conditions with, 162t, 162–164
Acrodermatitis chronica atrophicans, in Lyme borreliosis, 172
Acromegaly, in endocrine disorders, 52
Acromioclavicular joint, 238
    arthritis of, pain in, 238–239, *239*, 240, *241*
    corticosteroid infiltration in, 321
    osteoarthritis of, 248
    osteophytes of, impingement from, 241
    pain in, 248
    pseudogout of, 248
    septic arthritis of, 165, 248
Adiposis dolorosa, 251
Adjuvant disease, breast implants and, 112–114
B-Adrenergic blockers, for reflex sympathetic dystrophy, 303
Adrenocorticotropic hormone, for gout, 44, 155
Aging, bone mass in, 191
    regional pain syndromes in, 50–51
    rheumatic disease in, 50–51
    rotator cuff degeneration in, 244–245
    systemic conditions in, 51
Alanine aminotransferase, 27
Aldolase, 27
Alkaline phosphatase, 27
    serum levels of, in ankylosing spondylitis, 134
        in Paget's disease, 190
Alkylating agents, 47
Allergy, to nonsteroidal anti-inflammatory drugs, 42
Allodynia, in reflex sympathetic dystrophy, 302
Allopurinol, uric acid reduction with, 44, 156

Aluminum, in renal osteodystrophy, 199
Amitriptyline, 43
    for fibromyalgia, 306
    for reflex sympathetic dystrophy, 303
Amyloidosis, 184–186
    hemodialysis-related, 185, 186
    in rheumatoid arthritis, 65
    light chain, 185, *185*
        joint pain in, 19–20
        subcutaneous nodules in, 15
    presentation of, 185, *185*
    secondary, weight loss in, 17
    serum protein A in, 185
Amyotrophy, diabetic, 101
Analgesics, vs. nonsteroidal anti-inflammatory drugs, 43
Anemia, 27
    in rheumatoid arthritis, 65
Aneurysm, abdominal, low back pain in, 259, 261
Angiitis, cutaneous leukocytoclastic, 351t
Angioedema, 118
Angioma, radiography of, 21
Ankle, arthritis of, vs. subtalar arthritis, 285
    corticosteroid infiltration of, 322
    extension at, 285
    flexion at, 285
    pain in, 286
    rub in, 310
Ankle sprain, 286
    cause of, 286–287
    complications of, 287
    diagnosis of, 287
    persistent pain after, 288t
    presentation of, 287
    radiography in, 287, *287*
    treatment of, 287–288
Ankylosing spondylitis, 133–135
    aortic regurgitation in, 18
    cause of, 133
    criteria for, 133t
    diagnosis of, 134
    enteric infection in, 16

Ankylosing spondylitis *(Continued)*
    enthesitis in, 17
    flexion deformity in, prevention of, 329
    in pregnancy, 50
    joint pain in, 20
    mechanical vs. inflammatory findings in, 10
    methotrexate for, 45
    natural history of, 134
    neck pain in, 255
    physical examination in, 5
    presentation of, 133–134
    radiography of, 22
    referral in, 135
    sacroiliitis in, 16
    treatment of, 134–135
    urogenital infection in, 16
    vs. polymyalgia rheumatica, 20
Anserine bursitis, 278, 279–280
    corticosteroid injection for, 322
Anterior drawer sign, in anterior cruciate ligament tear, 281, *282*
Anti-B^{-2} glycoprotein 1, 32t
Antibiotics, for septic arthritis, 167
    in orthopedic surgery, 49
Anticardiolipin antibody, 32t
Anticoagulation, for antiphospholipid syndrome, 92, 92t
    for systemic lupus erythematosus, 83
    in orthopedic surgery, 49
Anti-DNA antibody, 32t
Anti-double-stranded DNA antibody, 32t, 33
Antihistone antibody, 32t
Antihypertensive agents, in systemic sclerosis, 107
Anti-La antibody, 32t, 33
Anti-neutrophil-cytoplasmic antibody, 34
Antinuclear antibodies, 32, 32t, *33*
    in adjuvant disease, 113
    in systemic lupus erythematosus, 74
Anti-P antibody, 32t
Antiphospholipid antibody, 34
Antiphospholipid syndrome, in pregnant patient, 87, 88, 92
    primary, 91–92
        treatment of, 92, 92t
Anti-RA33, 32t
Antirheumatic therapy, during lactation, 343t
    during pregnancy, 343t
Antiribonucleoprotein antibody, 32t, 33–34
Anti-RNP antibody, 32t, 33–34
Anti-Ro antibody, 32t, 33
Antisignal recognition particle syndrome, 97, 98
Anti-Sm antibody, 32t, 33
Antisynthetase syndrome, 97, 98
Aortic regurgitation, in arthritis, 18
Arc of motion, shoulder, in acromioclavicular arthritis, *241*
    in rotator cuff impingement, *241*
Arcade of Frohse, 230
Arcuate ligament, in medial elbow, 227, *228*
Arteritis, giant cell. See *Giant cell arteritis.*
    Takayasu. See *Takayasu arteritis.*
    vessel caliber in, 115
Arthralgia, in human immunodeficiency virus infection, 162
    in systemic sclerosis, 105
Arthritis, acromioclavicular, pain in, 238–239, *239*, *240*, *241*
    acute, joint aspiration in, 12–13
        joint positions in, 5, 5t, *6*
        musculoskeletal examination in, 5, 5t, *6*

Arthritis *(Continued)*
    pattern recognition in, 12–13
    vs. acute bursitis, 6, 235
  axial, in inflammatory bowel disease, 141
  cancer and, 54
  chronic, peripheral neuropathy in, 19
  chronic gouty, 153, *154*
  corticosteroids for, 319
  crystal-induced, 150–161. See also specific type, e.g., *Gout.*
    in endocrine disorders, 53
  degenerative. See *Osteoarthritis.*
  distal interphalangeal, 16, 143, 145
  elbow motion in, 228
  fever with, 13–14
  fungal, 170–171
  gonococcal, 13, 168–170
  heart murmur in, 17–18
  in inflammatory bowel disease, 140–141
  in Lyme borreliosis, 172, 173, 174
  in secondary syphilis, 174–175
  in systemic sclerosis, 105
  infectious. See *Septic arthritis.*
  meningoccocal, 165, 166t
  muscle weakness in, 19
  mycobacterial, 170–171
  peripheral, in inflammatory bowel disease, 141
  pseudoseptic, 65
  psoriatic. See *Psoriatic arthritis.*
  rash in, pattern recognition in, 13–14, 18–19
  reactive. See *Reactive arthritis.*
  rheumatoid. See *Rheumatoid arthritis.*
  rubella, 13, 164
  septic. See *Septic arthritis.*
  subacute, peripheral neuropathy in, 19
  subcutaneous nodules in, 60, *60*, 65–66, *66*
    pattern recognition in, 15–16
    vs. pulmonary neoplasms, 66
  subtalar, 285–286
  viral, 164
  vs. tenosynovitis, 7
  weight loss in, 17
Arthritis mutilans, 143, 145
Arthropathy, corticosteroids and, 319
  neuropathic, in endocrine disorders, 53
Arthroplasty, 48–49
  septic arthritis after, 166
Arthroscopy, 48
Articular (paraarticular) mass, imaging of, 22–23
Aspartate aminotransferase, 27
Aspiration, 319–323
Aspirin, 41, 41t
  in pregnancy, 343t
Assessment, 37–40
Atlantoaxial subluxation, in rheumatoid arthritis, 65
Atrophy, in rheumatoid arthritis, 65
  of plantar fat pad, 285, *285*
Autoantibodies, in myositis, 97
  in systemic lupus erythematosus, 74
Axial joint disease, mechanical vs. inflammatory findings in, 10
Azathioprine, for polymyositis, 98
  for rheumatoid arthritis, 46, 63
  in pregnancy, 343t
  methotrexate plus, 47
Azithromycin, for gonococcal arthritis, 169

Baastrup's disease, 262
Back exercises, 328–330, *329–331*
Back pain. See also *Low back pain.*
  in endocrine disorders, 53
Back rotation, 329–330, *330, 331*
Back strain, 262–264
  presentation of, 262–263, 263t
Bacterial arthritis, 165–168
Bacterial endocarditis, 34–35
  back pain in, 89
  peripheral arthritis in, 18
  vs. systemic lupus erythematosus, 89
Baker's cyst, 282, 314
  anatomy of, 274
  aspiration/injection of, 322
  diagnosis of, 283–284
  imaging of, 22
  in children, 283
  natural history of, 284
  pathophysiology of, *283*
  presentation of, 283
  referral in, 284
  rupture of, pseudothrombophlebitis from, 283, 283t
  thrombophlebitis with, 283, 284
  treatment of, 284
Basic calcium phosphate crystal deposition disease, 158–161
  tendinitis in, 159
Bed rest, 329
Behçet's disease, 146–147
  presentation of, 146, *146*
Beighton's scoring system, for benign hypermobility syndrome, 299t
Benign hypermobility syndrome, 299t, 299–300
Biceps brachii tendon, 227, 238
  in rotator cuff impingement, 240
  tear of, 242
Biceps femoris tendon, 274
Bisphosphonate, for osteoporosis, 193
  for Paget's disease, 202
Bladder, toxic effects of cyclophosphamide on, 47
Blindness, in giant cell arteritis, 127
Bone, avascular necrosis of, in endocrine disorders, 53
  cortical, 189
  cyst of, 215
  formation of, 190
  infection of. See *Osteomyelitis.*
  lysis of, in systemic sclerosis, 106, *106*
  malignancy of, 314
  metabolism in, 189
  necrosis of. See *Osteonecrosis.*
  radiography of, 21, 24, *25*
  remodeling of, 189
  resorption of, 190
  sclerotic, 24, *25*
  trabecular, 189
  turnover of, at menopause, 190
Bone densitometry, 24–25
Bone disease, 189–208. See also specific type, e.g., *Osteoporosis.*
  assessment of, 189–190, 190t
  dual x-ray absorptiometry in, 189, 190t
  quantitative computed tomography of, 189
  radiography of, 189
Bone mass, aging and, 191
  in osteoporosis, 191
Bone mass measurements, 350t

Bone matrix, 189
Bone mineral density, appendicular, 190, 190t
  axial, 190, 190t
  in fracture risk, 191
  measurement of, 190t
Borrelia burgdorferi, 171
Borreliosis, Lyme. See *Lyme borreliosis.*
Bouchard's nodes, in hand osteoarthritis, 177
Brachial plexus, compromise of, in thoracic outlet syndrome, 250
Brachialis, 227
Brachioradialis, 227
  ganglia of, 214
Breast implants, connective tissue disease from, 112–114
Breathing exercises, 333
Brodie's abscess, 206
Bronchiolitis obliterans, in systemic lupus erythematosus, 84t, 85
Brown tumor, in osteitis fibrosa cystica, 198
Brucellosis, polyarthritis in, 15
  spondyloarthropathy from, 16
Buerger's disease, 120–121
Bursa, aspiration of, 28–29
Bursa anserina, 279
Bursitic edema, 235
Bursitis, 209
  acute, vs. acute arthritis, 6, 235
  anserine, 278, 279–280
    steroid injection for, 322
  corticosteroids for, 319
  iliopsoas, 272–273, 273t
  infrapatellar, 278
  olecranon, 234–237. See also *Olecranon bursitis.*
  prepatellar, 276–277
    septic, vs. acute arthritis, 5, *6*
  radiography of, 21
  septic, olecranon bursitis from, 234
  shoe-related, 289
  subcutaneous, synovial fluid analysis in, 29t
  superficial, 314
  trochanteric, 270–271
    in hip osteoarthritis, 181
    lateral hip pain in, 270, *271*

Calcaneal plantar fat pad, atrophy of, 285, *285*
Calcaneus, plantar, pain in, 286, 288t, 290
  posterior, pain in, 286, 288t, 288–289
Calcific tendinitis, 243–244
Calcification, ectopic, in renal osteodystrophy, 199
Calcinosis, in systemic sclerosis, 106, *106*
Calcitonin, for osteoporosis, 193
  for Paget's disease, 201–202
Calcitriol, for renal osteodystrophy, 199
  in bone metabolism, 189
Calcium, serum levels of, bone metabolism and, 189
  in renal osteodystrophy, 199
  supplemental, for osteoporosis, 193
  urinary levels of, bone resorption and, 190
Calcium channel blockers, for reflex sympathetic dystrophy, 303
  for systemic sclerosis, 106
Calcium crystals, tendinitis from, 243–244
Calcium oxalate stones, in gout, 153–154
Calcium phosphate deposition disease, radiography of, 22
Calcium pyrophosphate (dihydrate crystal) deposition disease, *157*, 157–159
  conditions associated with, 157t

Calcium pyrophosphate *(Continued)*
   in synovial fluid, 29, *30*
   pseudospondylitic, 158
   radiography of, 22
Calciuria, in osteitis fibrosa cystica, 197
Camptocormia, 101
Cancer, rheumatic manifestations of, 54
Cane, use of, 335
Capsaicin, 43
   for knee osteoarthritis, 180
Capsulitis, adhesive, 245. See also *Frozen shoulder.*
Carisoprodol, 43
Carpal tunnel, 223
   decompression of, for amyloidosis, 186
Carpal tunnel syndrome, 223–226
   and repetitive strain injury, 308
   cause of, 223, 223t
   cervical spondylosis with, 257
   corticosteroid infiltration in, 320
   diagnosis of, 224
   electrodiagnostic tests in, 225, 225t
   in endocrine disorders, 52, 53
   in pregnancy, 50
   in rheumatoid arthritis, 65
   maneuvers for, 219, 224
   nerve conduction studies of, 25–26
   nonresolving, 225, 225t
   outcome of, 224
   patient evaluation in, 224t
   presentation of, 223–224
   recurrent, 225, 225t
   referral in, 225
   surgery for, 225
   treatment of, 224–225
Carpometacarpal osteoarthritis, torque test for, 219
Cauda equina syndrome, low back pain in, 260
   sciatica in, 264, 265
Ceftriaxone, for gonococcal arthritis, 169
Cellulitis, vs. acute digital tenosynovitis, 220
Cervical myelopathy, 23
Cervical spine, pain in, 254–258
Cervical spondylosis, 257–258
Charcot's joint, chronic monoarthritis in, 15
Chemonucleolysis, for sciatica, 266
Chest expansion, in spondyloarthropathy, 10–11
   test for, 10–11
Chest wall, anterior, pain in, 252–253
Children, Baker's cyst in, 283
Chiropractic manipulation, 48
Chlorambucil, in pregnancy, 343t
Chloroquine, side effects of, 46, 46t
Choline magnesium trisalicylate, for systemic lupus erythematosus, 77
Chondrocalcinosis, in calcium pyrophosphate deposition disease, 157, *157*
   radiography of, 22
Chondrocostal joint, swelling of, 252
Chondromalacia patellae, 277
Chondromatosis, synovial, 15, 314
Chondrosternal joint, swelling of, 252
Chopart's joint, motion at, 286
Chorea, in acute rheumatic fever, 148, 149
Chronic fatigue syndrome, 309
   testing in, 309
   treatment of, 309–310
   vs. fibromyalgia, 305

Churg-Strauss syndrome, 123–124, 351t
   classification of, 123, 123t
   peripheral neuropathy in, 19
Ciprofloxacin, Achilles tendinitis from, 136–137
   for gonococcal arthritis, 169
Cirrhosis, methotrexate and, 45–46
Claudication, neurogenic, in spinal stenosis, 266, 267, *268*
Clavicle, osteolysis of, 248
Clear cell sarcoma, vs. tennis elbow, 230
Coccygodynia, 262
Codman's pendular exercises, 326, *326*
Coffee cup sign, 228
Cognitive disturbance, in systemic lupus erythematosus, 83
Colchicine, for Behçet's ulcers, 147
   for calcium pyrophosphate deposition disease, 158
   for gout, 44, 155
Collagen, type 1, in bone, 189
Collateral ligament of knee, 274
   medial, 274
Community resources, 336–337
Complement, levels of, 34
Complete blood count (CBC), 27
Computed tomography, 23–24
Connective tissue disease, breast implants and, 112–114
   mixed. See *Mixed connective tissue.*
   vs. idiopathic inflammatory myopathy, 101, 102t
Coracoacromial arch, anomalies of, rotator cuff impingement from, 240
Coronary artery disease, gout in, 154
Corticosteroids, bone mineral loss from, 44
   crystals of, vs. gout, 29
   for amyloidosis, 186
   for Behçet's ulcers, 147
   for chronic low back pain, 269
   for de Quervain's tenosynovitis, 219, *220*
   for digital stenosing tenosynovitis, 217, 218t
   for giant cell arteritis, 128
   for gout, 155
   for knee osteoarthritis, 180
   for lupus pleuritis, 85
   for neuropsychiatric systemic lupus erythematosus, 83
   for olecranon bursitis, 236
   for polymyositis, 98
   for pregnancy-associated lupus, 88
   for reflex sympathetic dystrophy, 303
   for renal systemic lupus erythematosus, 80
   for rheumatoid arthritis, 63, 345t
   for sarcoidosis, 184
   for sciatica, 265–266
   for systemic lupus erythematosus, 78
   for systemic sclerosis, 107
   for Takayasu arteritis, 130
   for tennis elbow, 229
   for Wegener's granulomatosis, 126
   in pregnancy, 343t
   infiltration of, 319–323
      complications of, 319
      indications for, 319
   osteoporosis from, 194–195
Costochondritis, 252–253
Costovertebral joint, motion of, chest expansion in, 10–11
Cotton sponge test, in Sjögren's syndrome, 93
Coumadin, for antiphospholipid syndrome, 92, 92t
Cracking, joint, 310
Cramps, leg, 301

C-reactive protein, 27–28
Creatine phosphokinase, 27
Creatinine, 27
    excretion of, bone resorption and, 190
CREST (calcinosis, Raynaud's phenomenon, esophageal dysmotility, sclerodactyly, telangiectasis), 104. See also *Scleroderma*.
Crohn's disease, arthritis in, 140
    extraintestinal manifestations of, 141t
Cruciate ligament of knee, anterior, 274
    tear of, anterior drawer sign in, 281, *282*
        meniscal tear with, 281, *282*
    posterior, 274
Crutches, use of, 335–336
Cryofibrinogen, determination of, 35, 132
Cryofibrinogenemia, 35, 131–132
    classification of, 35, 35t
Cryoglobulin, determination of, 34–35, 132
Cryoglobulinemia, 131–132
Crystals, polarizing set for, 31
Cubital tunnel syndrome, 233–234
    cause of, 233, *233*
    provocative test for, 227, 233
Cutaneous lupus erythematosus, subacute, *86*, 86–87
Cyclobenzaprine, 43
Cyclophosphamide, 47
    for Takayasu arteritis, 130
    for Wegener's granulomatosis, 126
    in pregnancy, 343t
Cyclosporine, for rheumatoid arthritis, 47
    in pregnancy, 343t
    methotrexate plus, 47
Cytomegalovirus, arthritis from, 164
Cytotoxic agents, 47

Dactylitis, in reactive arthritis, 136, *137*
    psoriatic, 143
Dapsone, for Behçet's ulcers, 147
De Quervain's tenosynovitis, 218–220
    child care and, 50
    differential diagnosis of, 219t
    Finkelstein's test for, 218, *219*
    treatment of, 219, *220*
Deep breathing test, and diaphragmatic shoulder pain, 239
Degenerative arthritis. See *Osteoarthritis*.
Degenerative spondylolisthesis, 254
Deltoid, 238
Denervation, vs. idiopathic inflammatory myopathy, 101, 102t
Dental caries, in Sjögren's syndrome, 94
Deoxypyridinoline, in bone matrix, 189
Depression, and fibromyalgia, 305
Dercum's disease, 251–252
Dermatitis/arthritis syndrome, gonococcal, 168, 169
Dermatomyositis, 99–101
    presentation of, *99*, 99–100
    rash in, 18
Dermatosis, acute febrile, 18–19
Desipramine, 43
    for reflex sympathetic dystrophy, 303
Diabetes mellitus, carpal tunnel syndrome in, 225
    foot osteomyelitis in, 205
    frozen shoulder in, 245
    in septic prepatellar bursitis, 276
Diclofenac, for calcific tendinitis, 244
Diffuse idiopathic skeletal hyperostosis, in endocrine disorders, 53
    spondylitis mimicker in, 16

Digital extensor tendon, 212
Digital flexor tendon sheath, 211, *212*
Disability, 55–56
    criteria for, 55t
Discectomy, for sciatica, 266
Discoid lupus erythematosus, 86–87
Disseminated idiopathic skeletal hyperostosis, neck pain in, 255
Diuretics, thiazide, for osteoporosis, 193
Dorsal spine pain, 254, 258–259
Double-crush syndromes, 224, 257
Doxepin, 43
Doxycycline, for gonococcal arthritis, 169
    for reactive arthritis, 139
Drawer sign, anterior, in anterior cruciate ligament tear, 281, *282*
Drug abuse, intravenous, joint infection in, 165, 165t
Drugs, muscle weakness from, vs. idiopathic inflammatory myopathy, 101, 102t
    photosensitization from, 337, 337t
    systemic lupus erythematosus from, 90t, 90–91
Dupuytren's contracture, 213–214
Dupuytren's diathesis, 213

Edema, bursitic, 235
    hand, 12
    leg, in Baker's cyst, 283
        in iliopsoas bursitis, 273
    pitting, remitting seronegative synovitis with, 72–73
Effusion, 276
    sympathetic, vs. septic arthritis, 276
Elbow, anatomy of, *227*, 227–228, *228*
    carrying angle of, 227
    chronic hygroma of, 235
    corticosteroid infiltration in, 320
    impingement of, vs. arthritis, 228
    lateral pain in, 228, 228t
    microtrauma to, olecranon bursitis from, 234, 236
    motions of, 227, 228
    pain in, 227–237
        corticosteroids for, 319
    physical examination of, 228
    snapping of, 310
    ulnar nerve compression at, 233
Elderly, hip fracture in, physiologic factors in, 190
    recurrent hemorrhagic shoulder of, 242
Elderly-onset rheumatoid arthritis, 51, 68-70, 69t
Electrodiagnosis, 25
Electromagnetic radiation, spectrum of, 337, 337t
Electromyography, 25
Encephalitis, rheumatic, 148
Encephalopathy, in Lyme borreliosis, 172
Endarteritis, *Salmonella typhi* and, in Takayasu arteritis, 130
Endocarditis, bacterial, 34–35
    back pain in, 89
    peripheral arthritis in, 18
    vs. systemic lupus erythematosus, 89
Endocrine disorders, rheumatic manifestations of, 52t, 52–53
Endometriosis, low back pain from, 262
Enthesitis, 17
    patellar, 278
    psoriatic, 143, 145
Enthesopathy, 209
    pattern recognition in, 17
Eosinophilia-myalgia syndrome, 111–112
    L-tryptophan in, 111

Eosinophilic fasciitis, 111–112
    groove sign in, 111, *112*
Epicondyle, lateral, 274
Epicondylitis, lateral, 228–230. See also *Tennis elbow.*
    medial, 232–233
Episcleritis, in rheumatoid arthritis, 66
Epstein-Barr virus, arthritis from, 164
Ergotamine tartrate, pseudovasculitis from, 116, *116*
Erysipelas, in systemic lupus erythematosus, 89, *89*
Erythema, in dermatomyositis, 99, *99*
Erythema marginatum, in acute rheumatic fever, 13, 148
Erythema migrans, in Lyme borreliosis, 13, 171–172
Erythermalgia, 304, 304t
Erythrocyte sedimentation rate, 27, 27t
    diagnostic use of, 341t
    in giant cell arteritis, 128
Erythromelalgia, 304, 304t
Esophagitis, reflux, in systemic sclerosis, 107
Estrogen, for osteoporosis, 193
Exercise, 323–333
    for ankylosing spondylitis, 134
Extensor digiti minimi tendon, assessment of, 212
Extensor indicis tendon, assessment of, 212
Extensor pollicis longus tendon, assessment of, 212
Eye(s), in rheumatoid arthritis, 66, 67t
    in Sjögren's syndrome, 93, 93t, 94t

Facet joint, osteoarthritis of, hyperextension maneuver for, 262
    low back pain from, 262, *263*
Facial flushing, corticosteroids and, 319
Familial Mediterranean fever, 14
Fasciitis, 209
    corticosteroids for, 319
    eosinophilic, 111–112, *112*
    necrotizing, 311–313
        radiography of, 21
Fasciitis-panniculitis syndromes, 111, 111t
Fatigue, chronic, 305, 309–310
Felty's syndrome, in rheumatoid arthritis, 65
Femoral condyles, lateral, 274
    medial, 274
Fever, familial Mediterranean, 14
    in arthritis, 13–14
    in septic arthritis, 165
    in soft tissue pain, 311–313
    systemic lupus erythematosus and, 88–90
        erysipelas in, 89, *89*
Fibromyalgia, 304–307
    diagnosis of, 305–306
    dorsal, 259
    frequency of, 304
    in endocrine disorders, 52
    in Sjögren's syndrome, 93
    neck pain in, 255
    patient interview in, 4
    pattern recognition in, 20
    presentation of, 305
    tender points in, 7, *10*, 305
    tricyclic antidepressants for, 43
    vs. systemic lupus erythematosus, 32–33
    vs. tennis elbow, 229
Fibrosis, retroperitoneal, low back pain in, 261
    systemic, in endocrine disorders, 53
Fibrositis. See *Fibromyalgia.*
Fibula, distal, stress fracture of, 286

Finger(s), acute tenosynovitis of, 220–221
    corticosteroid infiltration in, 319–320
    intrinsic muscles of, 212
    joint cracking in, 310
    telescoping, in psoriatic arthritis, 143
    trigger, 216–218
        frequency of, 217, *217*
        treatment of, 217–218, 218t
Finkelstein's test, for de Quervain's tenosynovitis, 218, *219*
Fitness program, 323
Flare, postinjection, corticosteroids and, 319
Flat foot, 295
    cause of, 295–296, *296*
    rigid, posterior tibialis tendon rupture and, 295, *296*
Flat foot heel inversion maneuver, 295
Flexor carpi radialis, ganglia of, 214
Flexor digitorum profundus tendon, assessment of, 212
Flexor retinaculum of hand, 211
Flexor tendons of fingers, corticosteroid infiltration in, 320
Fluorescent light, ultraviolet B radiation in, 77
Fluoride, for osteoporosis, 193
Fluoroquinolones, Achilles tendinitis from, vs. reactive arthritis, 136–137
    response of tendons to, 17
Fluoxetine, 43
Flushing, facial, corticosteroids and, 319
    for rheumatoid arthritis, 46
Folate, supplemental, for elderly-onset rheumatoid arthritis, 70
Foot, flat, 295–296, *296*
    function of, 285
    pain in, 285–296
    weight distribution in, 285
Forearm, distal, rub in, 310
Forefoot, pain in, 286
    corticosteroids for, 319
    plantar pain in, 288t
    plantar tenderness of, in Morton's neuroma, 294
Forefoot pain maneuvers, 286
Foreign body synovitis, 15
Forestier's disease, spondylitis mimicker in, 16
Foucher's test, for Baker's cyst, 283
Fracture, in Paget's disease, 201
    in renal osteodystrophy, 199
    osteoporotic, treatment of, 194
Friction rubs, in scleroderma, 106
Frohse's arcade, 131, 230
Frozen shoulder, 245–247
    motion restriction in, 240
    radiography of, 23
Fungal arthritis, 170–171

Ganglia, 214–216
    cause of, 214, *215*
    intraosseous, 215
Gangrene, radiography of, 21
Gas gangrene, spontaneous, 311–313
Gastrocnemius, 274
Gastrocnemius-soleus cramping, 301
Gastrointestinal tract, in systemic sclerosis, 105
    ulcer of, nonsteroidal anti-inflammatory drugs and, 42, 42t
Genitals, ulcer of, in Behçet's disease, 146, *146*
Giant cell arteritis, 126–128, 351t
    classification of, 126, 127t

Giant cell arteritis *(Continued)*
  in elderly, 51
  in polymyalgia rheumatica, 70
Glenohumeral joint, 238
  disorders of, motion restriction in, 240
    pain in, 240
Glomerulonephritis, in systemic lupus erythematosus, 79
  poststreptococcal, 148
Glucocorticoids, 44–45. See also *Corticosteroids*.
  complications from, 44–45, 45t
  for eosinophilic fasciitis, 112
  in fibromyalgia, 52
Gluteus maximus, exercises for, 323
Gold therapy, for rheumatoid arthritis, 46, 63
  in pregnancy, 343t
Golfer's elbow, 232–233
Gonococcal arthritis, 13, 168–170
Gottron's sign, in dermatomyositis, 99
Gout, 150–157
  acute, 153
    treatment of, 154–155
  after orthopedic surgery, 49
  cardiovascular risk in, 154
  cause of, 150
  characteristics of, 157
  chronic tophaceous, vs. rheumatoid arthritis, 153, *154*
  colchicine for, 44
  diagnosis of, 153
  early-onset, 152
  forefoot pain in, 286
  hemarthrosis in, 13
  hyperuricemia in, treatment of, 155t, 155–156
  in myeloproliferative disorders, 54
  interval, treatment of, 155t
  joint aspiration in, 152
  joint involvement in, 151
  laboratory studies in, 152
  marginal erosion in, 153, *154*
  medications for, 44
  monosodium urate crystals in, 44
  nephropathy in, 44, 154
  nodal, 16, 151
  nodule aspiration in, 152, *152*
  olecranon bursitis in, 234, 236
  oligoarthritis in, 16
  outcome of, 153–154, *154*
  painful swollen hands in, 12
  patient interview in, 4
  polyarticular, 151–152
    synovial fluid analysis in, 30–31
  prepatellar bursitis in, 276
  presentation of, 150–152, 151t, *152*
  pseudorheumatoid arthritis in, 15
  pseudorheumatoid deformities in, 153, *154*
  radiography of, 21–22
  referral in, 156
  spinal, 152
  stages of, 150
  tophaceous, 44, 153
  treatment of, 154–156
  uric acid excretion in, 152
  uric acid levels in, 150, 150t, 151
  urinary stones in, 153–154
  vs. pseudopodagra, 151, 151t
Government agencies, 336–337

Granuloma, sarcoid, 183
  vs. Wegener's granulomatosis, 125, 125t
Groove sign, in eosinophilic fasciitis, 111, *112*

Haglund's deformity, 288, *289*
Hallux rigidus, 293, *294*
  pain in, 286
Hallux valgus, 292–293
  pain in, 286
Hallux valgus angle, 292
Hamstring muscles, stretching of, 329, *329*
  tightness of, in sciatica differentiation, 263
Hand(s), pain in, 211–226
  pattern recognition in, 12
  painful swollen, 12
  palmar side of, 211, *211*
Hand exercises, 332, *333*
Hand protection, 332
Health Assessment Questionnaire, 37–38, 39t–40t
Heart, in acute rheumatic fever, 148
  in Lyme borreliosis, 172
  in systemic sclerosis, 105
  myxoma of, peripheral arthritis in, 18
  valvular disease of, arthritis in, 17–18
Heart murmur, in arthritis, 17–18
Heat application, 333–334
Heberden's nodes, in hand osteoarthritis, 177
  urate deposits in, 16
Heel. See also *Calcaneus*.
  plantar, pain in, 290
Heel rise test, single, in posterior tibialis tendon rupture, 295
Heel spur, 290
Hemarthrosis, 13
Hematologic disease, rheumatic manifestations of, 53–54
Hematoma, low back pain in, 261
Hemochromatosis, subcutaneous nodules in, 16
Hemophilia, hemarthrosis in, 13
  rheumatic manifestations of, 53–54
Henoch-Schönlein purpura, 119–120, 351t
  classification of, 119, 119t
  vs. hypersensitivity vasculitis, 117
Hepatitis A virus, arthritis from, 164
Hepatitis B virus, arthritis from, 164
  in polyarteritis nodosa, 121
Hepatitis C virus, in polyarteritis nodosa, 121
Hepatoxicity, nonsteroidal anti-inflammatory drugs and, 42
Herpes simplex virus, arthritis from, 164
Herpes zoster, dorsal spine pain in, 258
  sciatica in, 265
Hip, corticosteroid infiltration in, 321
  disease of, vs. iliopsoas bursitis, 273t
  osteoarthritis of, medical therapy for, 347t
    trochanteric bursitis in, 181
  pain in, 5, *7*, 270–273
    differential diagnosis of, 270, 270t
    in trochanteric bursitis, 270, *271*
  snapping of, 310
Hip exercises, 331, *332*
HLA. See *Human leukocyte antigen*.
Hoffa's fat body, inflammation of, 278
Human immunodeficiency virus (HIV) infection, musculoskeletal disease in, 162–164
  myositis in, 101
  osteomyelitis in, 206
  reactive arthritis in, 136

Human immunodeficiency virus (HIV) infection (Continued)
  weakness in, 19
  weight loss in, 17
Human leukocyte antigen B27, determination of, 35–36
  in ankylosing spondylitis, 133
  in inflammatory bowel disease arthritis, 140
Human leukocyte antigen DR3, in Sjögren's syndrome, 93
Human leukocyte antigen DR4, determination of, 35
Humerus, distal, 227
Hydrochlorothiazide, for corticosteroid-induced osteoporosis, 195
Hydroxyapatite crystal, in synovial fluid, 29, 30
Hydroxychloroquine, for rheumatoid arthritis, 46, 63
  for systemic lupus erythematosus, 77
  in pregnancy, 77–78, 343t
  methotrexate plus, 47
  ocular toxicity of, 46
  side effects of, 46, 46t
Hydroxyproline, urinary levels of, bone resorption and, 190
Hygroma, of elbow, 235
Hyperextension maneuver, for facet joint syndrome, 262
  thigh, for referred low back pain, 261
Hyperglobulinemic purpura, in cryoglobulinemia, 131
Hyperimmunoglobulin D syndrome, 14
Hypermobility syndrome, benign, 299–300
    Beighton's scoring system for, 299t
Hyperostosis, diffuse idiopathic skeletal, in endocrine disorders, 53
    spondylitis in, 16
Hyperparathyroidism, 197
  musculoskeletal findings in, 197–198
  osteitis fibrosa cystica in, 197
Hyperpathia, in reflex sympathetic dystrophy, 302
Hypersensitivity vasculitis, 117–118
  classification of, 117, 117t
Hypertrophic osteoarthropathy, 207–208
Hyperuricemia, classification of, 150, 150t, 151
  treatment of, 155t, 155–156
Hyperviscosity syndrome, in cryoglobulinemia, 131
Hypopigmentation, corticosteroids and, 319
Hypothenar eminence, 211, 211
Hypothyroidism, in Sjögren's syndrome, 94
  vs. fibromyalgia, 20
Hypoxanthine-guanine phosphoribosyltransferase, deficiency of, 152

Ibuprofen, for elderly-onset rheumatoid arthritis, 70
  for hand osteoarthritis, 178
Iliohypogastric nerve, compressive neuropathy maneuver for, 270
Iliopsoas bursitis, 272–273
  and leg edema, 273
  vs. hip disease, 273t
  vs. iliopsoas tendinitis, 273t
Iliopsoas tendinitis, vs. iliopsoas bursitis, 273t
Iliotibial tract, 274
Iliotibial tract stretch, 332
Iliotibial tract syndrome, 274–275
Imaging studies, 21–26
Immune complexes, 34
Immunoglobulin D, elevated serum levels of, and arthritis or arthropathy, 14
Immunoglobulin G antibodies, in Lyme borreliosis, 172
Immunoglobulin M antibodies, in Lyme borreliosis, 172
Immunoglobulins, intravenous, 47
Immunologic studies, 32–36
Immunosuppressive agents, for polymyositis, 98

Impingement, elbow, vs. arthritis, 228
  of posterior tibial nerve, 290
  rotator cuff, 240–243. See also *Rotator cuff impingement.*
Indomethacin, for ankylosing spondylitis, 135
Infection, corticosteroids and, 319
  fibromyalgia in, 305
  hematogenous, in osteomyelitis, 204–205
  low back pain in, 259–260
  methotrexate and, 45
  patient interview in, 4
Infectious arthritis, 162–175. See also *Septic arthritis.*
Inflammation, enthesial, radiography of, 21
  patient interview in, 3
Inflammatory bowel disease, arthritis in, 140–141
    axial, 140, 141
    peripheral, 140, 141
    presentation of, 140, 141t
  spondyloarthropathy in, radiography of, 22
  weight loss in, 17
Infrapatellar bursitis, 278
Infraspinatus tendon, calcium-induced inflammation of, 243
  in rotator cuff impingement, 240
Infraspinatus tendon tear, 242
Injection, techniques for, 319–323
Interleukin-1, in rheumatoid arthritis, 65
Intermetatarsal angle, 292
Interphalangeal joint, distal, 212
  arthritis of, 16
  in Swan-neck deformity, 212
  proximal, 212
Interspinous ligaments, corticosteroid infiltration in, 321
Interstitial lung disease, in systemic lupus erythematosus, 84t, 85
Intervertebral disc, herniation of, 264
  sciatica from, 254
Intravenous drug use, musculoskeletal infection in, 165, 165t
Isometric exercises, 323

Jaccoud's arthritis, 148
Joint(s), bleeding into, 13
  cracking of, 310–311
  drainage of, in septic arthritis, 167
  expansion of, in ganglion formation, 214, 215
  infiltrative conditions of, 183–186
  magnetic resonance imaging of, 24t
  pain in, stiffness and, 19
  radiography of, 21
  rubbing of, 310–311
  snapping of, 310–311
  splintage of, for septic arthritis, 167
  squeaking of, 310–311
Joint prosthesis, infection of, 166, 167–168
Jumper's knee, 278

Kawasaki disease, 13–14, 351t
Keratoconjunctivitis sicca, in Sjögren's syndrome, 93, 93t–95t, 95
  treatment of, 95, 95t
Keratoderma blennorrhagica, in reactive arthritis, 137, 137
Kidney(s), abscess in, low back pain in, 262
  diseases of, nonsteroidal anti-inflammatory drugs in, 42
  in systemic lupus erythematosus, 79t, 79–81
Knee, anatomy of, 274
  anterior pain in, 277–279
    shrug sign in, 277
    sustained flexion test for, 277, 277
  aspiration of, 28–29

Knee (Continued)
   corticosteroid infiltration in, 321–322
   disorders of, 275t
      magnetic resonance imaging of, 22
   effusions of, prepatellar bursitis with, 276
   masses around, 313–314
   medial, bursae in, 281
      bursitis of, 280–281
   osteoarthritis of, medical therapy for, 348t
   pain in, 274–284
   reflex sympathetic dystrophy of, 302
   squeaking of, 310
   synovium of, 274
   unstable, 274
Knee flexion test, in patellar pain, 277
Knee to chest stretch, 324, 325

Laboratory studies, 27–31
Lachman test, in anterior cruciate ligament tear, 281, 282
Lactation, antirheumatic therapy in, 343t
Lasègue's maneuver, in sciatica, 263, 264
Lateral bending exercises, 330–331, 331
Latissimus dorsi, 238
LE cells, 74. See also Systemic lupus erythematosus.
Leg(s), distal, rub in, 310
   edema of, and iliopsoas bursitis, 273
Leg cramps, 301
Leg length discrepancy, low back pain from, 262, 263
Leprosy, 19
   lepromatous, arthritis in, 19
      painful swollen hands in, 12
Leukemia, rheumatic manifestations of, 54
Leukopenia, 27
Lifting, injury avoidance in, 329
Light chain amyloidosis, 15, 19–20, 185, 185
Lip(s), ulcer of, in Behçet's disease, 146, 146
Lipoma, 313, 314
Lipomatosis, multiple symmetric, 251–252
   shoulder girdle, 251–252
Livedo reticularis, in inflammatory bowel disease, 140
Liver, methotrexate effects on, in rheumatoid arthritis, 346t
Longitudinal stretch, 324, 324
Low back pain, 254
   acute nonspecific, 262–263
   cause of, 259
   chronic, 268–269
   clinical practice guidelines for, 349t
   diagnosis of, 260
   inflammatory vs. mechanical, 260, 260t
   outcome of, 261
   presentation of, 259–260
   prevalence of, 259, 260t
   radiography of, 23
   referral in, 261
   referred, 260, 261–262
   treatment of, 261
Lumbago, 262–264
Lumbosacral pain, 254
Lung(s), hemorrhage of, in systemic lupus erythematosus, 84t, 85
Lupus anticoagulant, in thrombophilia, 34, 34t
Lupus autoantibodies, clinical correlates of, 32, 32t, 33
Lupus erythematosus. See Systemic lupus erythematosus.
Lupus-like illness, in cancer, 54
Lyme borreliosis, 171–174
   erythema migrans in, 13

Lyme borreliosis (Continued)
   laboratory studies in, 172–173, 173t
   neurologic findings in, 172
   oligoarthritis in, 16
   presentation of, 171–172, 172t
   prevention of, 173t
   serologic diagnosis of, 342t
   stages of, 171–172
   treatment of, 173t, 173–174
   vs. secondary syphilis, 174
Lyme borreliosis antibody test, 35
Lymphokines, in rheumatoid arthritis, 65
Lymphoma, in Sjögren's syndrome, 94–95
   low back pain in, 261
   rheumatic manifestations of, 54
Lymphopenia, 27

Magnetic resonance imaging, 24, 24t, 25
Major histocompatibility complex, in polymyositis, 97
Malignancy, low back pain in, 260
   rheumatic manifestations of, 54
Marfan's syndrome, 300–301
McMurthy's sign, in carpal tunnel syndrome, 224
Medsger's syndrome, 213, 213
   painful swollen hands in, 12
Melphalan, for amyloidosis, 186
Meningismus, nonsteroidal anti-inflammatory drugs and, 42
Meningitis, in Lyme borreliosis, 172
Meningococcemia, 13
   septic arthritis in, 165–166, 166t
Meniscus (menisci), 274
   tear of, 281
      anterior cruciate ligament tear with, 281, 282
Menopause, bone turnover at, 190
Mental changes, nonsteroidal anti-inflammatory drugs and, 42
Meralgia paresthetica, 272
Metabolism, disorders of, enthesitis in, 17
   fibromyalgia in, 305
Metacarpophalangeal joint, corticosteroid infiltration in, 319–320
   cracking of, 310
   in Swan-neck deformity, 212
   palmar crease and, 211, 211
Metatarsophalangeal joint, congruency of, 292
   corticosteroid infiltration of, 322
   pain in, 286
   rigidity of, 293, 294
   valgus deformity of, 292–293
Methocarbamol, 43
Methotrexate, combination therapy with, 47
   for elderly-onset rheumatoid arthritis, 70
   for polymyositis, 98
   for rheumatoid arthritis, 45, 62–63
   for systemic lupus erythematosus, 78
   for Wegener's granulomatosis, 126
   hepatic effects of, in rheumatoid arthritis, 346t
   in pregnancy, 343t
   side effects of, 45t, 45–46
Microdiscectomy, for sciatica, 266
B_2-Microglobulin, accumulation of, in renal insufficiency, 184, 199
Microscopy, compensated polarizing, 31
Milwaukee shoulder, 242
   arthroplasty for, 49
   squeaks in, 310
Minimal erythema dose, 337
Minocycline, for rheumatoid arthritis, 47

Misoprostol, for stomach ulcer, 42
Mitral regurgitation, in acute rheumatic fever, 18
Mitral stenosis, in acute rheumatic fever, 18
Mixed connective tissue disease, 107–109
    antiribonucleoprotein antibodies in, 33–34
    diagnosis of, 108, 108t
    painful swollen hands in, 12
    weakness in, 19
Monoarthritis, chronic, 14–15
    purulent gonococcal, 168, 169
Monoclonal antibodies, for rheumatoid arthritis, 47
Mononeuritis multiplex, nerve conduction studies of, 26
Monosodium urate crystal, deposition of, 150
    in gout, 44
    in synovial fluid, 29, 30
Morphea, 104, 105t
Morton's neuroma, 294–295, 295
    corticosteroid infiltration of, 322
    forefoot pain in, 286
Mouth, in Sjögren's syndrome, 93, 93t, 94t
Multiple myeloma, back pain in, 260
    joint pain in, 19
Mumps, arthritis from, 164
Muscle, atrophy of, in rheumatoid arthritis, 65
    biopsy of, 25
    inflammation of, 97–103. See also *Myositis* and specific conditions, e.g., *Polymyositis*.
Muscle dystrophy, vs. idiopathic inflammatory myopathy, 101, 102t
Muscle relaxants, 43
Muscle weakness, in arthritis, 19
    in polymyositis, 97
Musculocutaneous nerve, compressive neuropathy of, 229–230
Musculoskeletal disease, 209
    clinical features in, 341t
    in human immunodeficiency virus infection, 162–164
    treatment of, 41–49
Musculoskeletal examination, 5–11
    brief, 7, 8t–9t
    detailed, 7
    in acute arthritis, 5, 5t, 6
Musculoskeletal infection, fungal, 170–171
    mycobacterial, 170–171
Mutilans arthritis, 143, 145
Myalgia, in human immunodeficiency virus infection, 162
Mycobacterial arthritis, 170–171
Myelopathy, cervical, 23
    compressive, 257
Myofascial pain syndromes, 307–308
    dorsal, 259
    neck, 255
    trigger points in, 255, 259, 307, 321
        corticosteroid infiltration of, 321
Myopathy, idiopathic inflammatory, 101–103
    conditions mimicking, 101, 102t
    in endocrine disorders, 53
Myositis, 97–103
    autoantibodies in, 97
    human immunodeficiency virus and, 101
    inclusion body, 101–103
    patient interview in, 4
    zidovudine and, 163
Myxoma, cardiac, peripheral arthritis in, 18
    paraarticular, 314

Nabumetone, for elderly-onset rheumatoid arthritis, 70

Nabumetone *(Continued)*
    for hand osteoarthritis, 178
Nail fold, capillaries of, in Raynaud's disease, 110
    inspection of, 104, 110
Naproxen, for calcific tendinitis, 244
Neck, cracking of, 310
    exercises for, 325, *325*
    motion of, shoulder pain from, 239–240
Neck pain, 254–258
    acute nonspecific, 254–255
    myofascial, 255
    radiography of, 23
Necrotizing fasciitis, 311–313
    radiography of, 21
Neisseria gonorrhoeae, arthritis from, 168–169
Neonatal lupus syndrome, 50
Neoplasms, dermatomyositis with, 99, 100
    weight loss in, 17
Nephritis, lupus. See also *Systemic lupus erythematosus, renal.*
    classification of, 79t, 79–80
Nephropathy, gouty, 154
Nerve conduction studies, 25–26
Neurogenic claudication, in spinal stenosis, 266, 267, *268*
Neuroma, Morton's, 236, 294–295, *295*, 322
Neuromuscular junction disease, nerve conduction studies of, 26
    vs. idiopathic inflammatory myopathy, 101, 102t
Neuropathy, compressive, 209, 223–226, 230–231, 233, 240
    ganglia and, 215
    peripheral, in arthritis, 19
        in Lyme borreliosis, 172
    proximal, vs. idiopathic inflammatory myopathy, 101, 102t
No name–no fame bursitis, 280
Nonsteroidal anti-inflammatory drugs, 41t, 41–42
    allergic reactions to, 42
    combination therapy with, 47
    for acute rheumatic fever, 149
    for ankylosing spondylitis, 134–135
    for calcific tendinitis, 244
    for chronic low back pain, 269
    for elderly-onset rheumatoid arthritis, 70
    for gout, 155
    for polymyalgia rheumatica, 71
    for remitting seronegative symmetrical synovitis with pitting edema, 72
    for rheumatoid arthritis, 62, 344t
    for systemic lupus erythematosus, 77
    gastrointestinal ulcer from, 42, 42t
    hepatoxicity of, 42
    in pregnancy, 343t
    meningismus from, 42
    mental changes from, 42
    renal disease from, 42
    vs. analgesics, 43
Nucleus pulposus, herniation of, 254
    sciatica from, 264

Ober test, in iliotibial tract syndrome, 275
Obesity, in knee osteoarthritis, 178
    plantar heel pain with, 290
Occupational therapy, 47–48
Ofloxacin, Achilles tendinitis from, 136–137
Olecranon bursa, 227–228
    corticosteroid infiltration in, 320
Olecranon bursitis, 234–237
    in gout, 234, 236

Olecranon bursitis (Continued)
  presentation of, 234–235, 235, 236
  rheumatoid, 234, 236
  septic, 234, 235, 235, 236, 236
Oligoarthritis, pattern recognition in, 16
  psoriatic, 143, 144, 145
Ophthalmoscope, in nail fold assessment, 104, 110
Orthopedic surgery, 48–49
  antibiotics in, 49
  anticoagulation in, 49
  clearance for, 49
  gout after, 49
  indications for, 49
  rehabilitation after, 49
Os peroneum syndrome, pain in, 286
Osgood-Schlatter disease, vs. spondyloarthropathy, 278
Osteitis, sternoclavicular, 249
Osteitis condensans ilii, in pregnancy, 50
Osteitis fibrosa cystica, 197–198
  hyperparathyroidism and, 197
Osteoarthritis, 176–182
  acetaminophen for, 43
  acromioclavicular, 248
  aging in, 50–51, 176
  carpometacarpal, torque test for, 219
  diagnosis of, 38, 40
  distal interphalangeal joint in, 16
  erosive, 61, 61
  facet joint, low back pain from, 262, 263
  hand, 176–178
    classification of, 176t
    radiography of, 177
  hip, 181–182
    classification of, 181t
    medical therapy for, 347t
    trochanteric bursitis in, 181
  history in, 176
  in calcium pyrophosphate deposition disease, 158
  in hallux valgus, 292
  in old age, 50–51
  knee, 178–180
    classification of, 179t
    medical therapy for, 349t
    pain in, 178–179
  mechanical vs. inflammatory findings in, 9
  patellofemoral, 278
  radiography of, 21
  vs. rheumatoid arthritis, 61, 61
Osteoarthropathy, hypertrophic, 207
  cause of, 207, 207t
  presentation of, 207, 207
Osteoblasts, in bone remodeling, 189
Osteocalcin, in bone formation, 189
  serum levels of, bone turnover and, 190
Osteodystrophy, renal, 198–200
Osteomalacia, 196–197
  biochemical determinations in, 196t
  in old age, 51
  joint pain in, 19
  rickets and, 195–197
  spondylitis in, 16–17
  vitamin D deficiency and, 195–196
  vs. fibromyalgia, 20
Osteomyelitis, 204–207
  bone pain in, 205

Osteomyelitis (Continued)
  dorsal spine pain in, 258
  imaging studies in, 205t, 205–206
  sickle cell disease and, 53
  spinal, 260
    Mycobacterium tuberculosis and, 170
Osteonecrosis, 202–204
  cause of, 203, 203t
  corticosteroid use and, 78
  hemarthrosis in, 13
  in polymyositis, 98
  pain in, 203
  passive motion restriction in, 203
  spontaneous, magnetic resonance imaging of, 24, 25
Osteopenia, bone mineral density and, 191
  in endocrine disorders, 53
  in renal osteodystrophy, 199
  in spinal fracture, 191, 192
Osteoporosis, 191–195
  bone mass in, 191
  bone mineral density in, 191
  cause of, 191, 191t
  corticosteroid-induced, 194–195
  diagnosis of, 192
  fracture treatment in, 194
  involutional, 191
  laboratory findings in, 192
  outcome of, 192
  prophylaxis for, 194
  radiography in, 191, 192
  referral in, 194
  treatment of, 192–193
  vertebral fractures in, 191–192, 192
Ottawa Ankle Rules, 287, 287
Oxalate crystal, in synovial fluid, 29, 30

Paget's disease, 200–202
  radiography of, 200
  treatment of, 201–202, 202t
Pain, distal radiation of, physical examination in, 5, 7
  regional, in old age, 50–51
    in pregnancy, 50
Pain amplification syndromes, 299–315
Palindromic rheumatism, patient interview in, 4
  pattern recognition in, 14
Palmar fascia, 212
Paraarticular mass, imaging of, 22–23
Paraspinal muscles, contracture of, in low back pain, 262
Parathormone, in bone metabolism, 189
  in osteitis fibrosa cystica, 197
Parathyroidectomy, for renal osteodystrophy, 199
Parotid gland, enlargement of, in Sjögren's syndrome, 93
Parvovirus infection, arthralgia in, 15
  arthritis in, 164
  rash in, 13
Patella, 274
  instability of, 277
  pain in, 277
Patellar ligament, 274
Patellar retinaculum, lateral, 274
Patellar tendon, 274
  acute calcium-induced inflammation of, 278
Patellofemoral joint, osteoarthritis of, 278
Pectoral stretch, 330, 331
Pectoralis major, 238

D-Penicillamine, for systemic sclerosis, 106–107
  in pregnancy, 343t
Penicillin, for Whipple's disease, 142
  prophylactic, in acute rheumatic fever, 149
Pericarditis, in rheumatoid arthritis, 66
Perinephric abscess, low back pain in, 262
Periodontitis, in Sjögren's syndrome, 94
Periostosis, in hypertrophic osteoarthropathy, 207, *207*
Peripheral joint disease, mechanical vs. inflammatory findings in, 9–10
Peripheral nerve, in cryoglobulinemia, 131
  injury to, reflex sympathetic dystrophy from, 302
Peripheral neuropathy, in arthritis, 19
  in Lyme borreliosis, 172
Peroneal tenosynovitis, pain in, 286
Pes anserinus, 274
Pes planus, 295–296, *296*
Phalen's test, in carpal tunnel syndrome, 224
Pharyngitis, streptococcal, in acute rheumatic fever, 149
Phosphate, serum levels of, in renal osteodystrophy, 199
Phosphoribosylpyrophosphate synthetase hyperactivity, 152
Photosensitization, drugs and, 337, 337t
Physical examination, 5–11
  brief, 7, 8t–9t
  detailed, 7
  in acute arthritis, 5, 5t, 6
Physical medicine, 47–48
Physical therapy, 47–48, 323–333
  for elderly-onset rheumatoid arthritis, 70
  for rheumatoid arthritis, 62–64
  for systemic sclerosis, 106
Pigmented villonodular synovitis, 15, 314
  hemarthrosis in, 13
  synovial fluid characteristics of, 15
Piriformis muscle syndrome, sciatica in, 265
Placebo effect, 43–44
Plantar fascia, corticosteroid infiltration of, 322
Plantar fasciitis, in reactive arthritis, 136, 137
  insertional tenderness in, 290
Plantar fat pad deficiency maneuver, 290
Plantar heel pain, 290–291
Plantar tenderness maneuver, 294
Pleural effusion, in rheumatoid arthritis, 66
  in systemic lupus erythematosus, 84–85
Pleuritis, in rheumatoid arthritis, 66
  in systemic lupus erythematosus, 84t, 84–85
Plica syndrome, 278
Pneumonitis, acute lupus, 84t, 85
  interstitial, methotrexate and, 45
  rheumatic, 148
Podagra, in gout, 151
Polarizing set, 31
Polyangiitis, microscopic, 351t
Polyarteritis nodosa, 121–123, 351t
  classification of, 121, 122t
  vs. rheumatoid arthritis, 19
Polyarthralgia, in secondary syphilis, 174
Polyarthritis, distal chronic, in calcium pyrophosphate deposition disease, 158
  in rheumatoid arthritis, 15
  in secondary syphilis, 174
  protracted distal symmetric, 15
  seronegative, in endocrine disorders, 52
Polychondritis, relapsing, aortic regurgitation in, 18

Polymyalgia rheumatica, 70–72
  corticosteroid complications in, 71
  giant cell arteritis in, 70
  glucocorticoids for, 44
  in elderly, 51
  in giant cell arteritis, 127
  joint pain in, 19
  painful swollen hands in, 12
  vs. ankylosing spondylitis, 20
  vs. elderly-onset rheumatoid arthritis, 69t
Polymyositis, 97–99
  osteonecrosis in, 98
  rash in, 18
Popliteal artery, 274
Popliteal fossa (popliteal space), 274
  cyst in. See *Baker's cyst.*
  ganglia at, 215
Posterior tibialis tendon, corticosteroid infiltration of, 322
  rupture of, in rigid flat foot, 295, *296*
  tenosynovitis of, 286
Postinjection flare, corticosteroids and, 319
Pregnancy, ankylosing spondylitis in, 50
  antiphospholipid syndrome in, 87, 88, 92
  antirheumatic therapy in, 343t
  carpal tunnel syndrome in, 50
  complications of, in systemic lupus erythematosus, 50, 87–88
  hydroxychloroquine in, 77–78
  low back pain in, 50
  osteitis condensans ilii in, 50
  regional pain syndromes in, 50
  rheumatic disease in, 50
  rheumatoid arthritis in, 50
  scleroderma in, 50
Prepatellar bursa, 274
  sepsis of, vs. acute arthritis, 5, 6
Prepatellar bursitis, 276–277
  gouty, 276
  septic, 276
  traumatic, 276
Pretendinous bursa, 274
Probenecid, and uric acid excretion, 44, 152, 156
Pronator syndrome, 224
Propranolol, for reflex sympathetic dystrophy, 303
  in Marfan's syndrome, 300
Prostate, carcinoma of, low back pain from, 262
Proteinuria, in rheumatoid arthritis, 65
Pseudocyst, mucinous, in hand osteoarthritis, 177
Pseudogout, acromioclavicular, 248
  hemarthrosis in, 13
  in calcium pyrophosphate deposition disease, 158
  oligoarthritis in, 16
  painful swollen hands in, 12
Pseudolymphoma, in Sjögren's syndrome, 94–95
Pseudoneurologic symptoms, in fibromyalgia, 305
Pseudopodagra, vs. gout, 151, 151t
Pseudothrombophlebitis, ruptured and Baker's cyst, 283, 283t
Pseudovasculitis, 115–116, *116*, 116t
Psoriasis, in human immunodeficiency virus infection, 163
Psoriatic arthritis, 18, 142–146
  asymmetric oligoarthritis in, 143, *144*
  cause of, 143
  diagnosis of, 144
  distal interphalangeal joint, 16
  enthesitis in, 17

Psoriatic arthritis *(Continued)*
   intertriginous lesion in, 144, *144*
   methotrexate for, 45
   oligoarthritis in, 16
   outcome of, 144–145
   presentation of, *143*, 143–144, *144*
   pseudorheumatoid type, 143, *143*, 144–145
   referral in, 145
   telescoping fingers in, 143
   treatment of, 145
Psoriatic dactylitis, 143
Psoriatic oligoarthritis, 143, *144*, 145
Psoriatic spondylitis, 143, 145
Psoriatic spondyloarthropathy, 16
   radiography of, 22
Psychosis, corticosteroids and, 83
   lupus, 82
Purpura, Henoch-Schönlein, 117, 119t, 119–120, 351t
   hyperglobulinemic, 131
Pyelonephritis, low back pain in, 262
Pyoderma gangrenosum, in inflammatory bowel disease, 140
Pyomyositis, 311–313
   in acquired immunodeficiency syndrome, 162
   in human immunodeficiency virus infection, 163
   tropical, 311
Pyridinoline, in bone matrix, 189
   urinary levels of, bone resorption and, 190

Quadriceps, isometric exercises for, 323
   tightness maneuver for, 278
Quadriceps setting exercises, 323
Quadriceps stretch, 331, *332*
Questionnaires, 37–40
Quinidine, systemic lupus erythematosus from, 90–91
Quinine sulfate, for leg cramps, 301

Radial artery, aneurysm of, vs. ganglia, 215
Radial nerve, 227, *227*
   deep branch, compression of, 230–231
Radial tunnel release, 231t
Radial tunnel syndrome, 230–231
   treatment of, 231, 231t
   vs. tennis elbow, 229, 230
Radiation, spectrum of, 337, 337t
Radiculopathy, in cervical spondylosis, 257
Radiography, 21–23, *22*
Radionuclide bone scan, 24
Rash, in arthritis, 13–14, 18–19
Raynaud's disease, 109–111
   vs. secondary Raynaud's phenomenon, 109, 109t
Raynaud's phenomenon, in systemic sclerosis, 104
   secondary, 109–111
      conditions associated with, 109, 109t
      vs. Raynaud's disease, 109, 109t
   treatment of, 106
Reactive arthritis, 135–139
   aortic regurgitation in, 18
   cause of, 136
   dactylitis in, 136, *137*
   diagnosis of, 138
   enteric, 136, 136t
   enthesitis in, 17
   in human immunodeficiency virus infection, 162–163
   keratoderma blennorrhagica in, 137, *137*

Reactive arthritis *(Continued)*
   methotrexate for, 45
   oligoarthritis in, 16
   outcome of, 139
   postdysenteric, 16
   postvenereal, 16
   presentation of, 136–138, *137*, *138*
   radiography of, 22, *22*, 138
   rash in, 18
   sacroiliitis in, 138, *138*
   "sausage toe" in, 136, *137*
   syndesmophytes in, 138, *138*
   treatment of, 139
Recurrent hemorrhagic shoulder of elderly, 242
Reflex sympathetic dystrophy, 301–303
   cause of, 301–302, 302t
   frozen shoulder and, 245
   painful swollen hands in, 12
   presentation of, 302, *302*
   stages of, 302
   treatment of, 303
   vs. thoracic outlet syndrome, 250
Reflux esophagitis, in systemic sclerosis, 107
Rehabilitation, after orthopedic surgery, 49
   vocational, 55t, 55–56
Reiter's syndrome, 137, *137*
Remitting seronegative synovitis with pitting edema, 72–73
   painful swollen hands in, 12
   vs. elderly-onset rheumatoid arthritis, 69t
Renal failure, in systemic sclerosis, 105
   osteodystrophy in, 198–200
   systemic lupus erythematosus and, 80
Renal osteodystrophy, 198–200
Repetitive strain injury, 308–309
Repetitive stress syndrome, neck pain in, 254–255
Respiratory exercises, 333
Respiratory infection, upper, in Sjögren's syndrome, 94
Reticulohistiocytosis, multicentric, subcutaneous nodules in, 16
Retinaculum, lateral patellar, tightness of, 277
Retrocalcaneal bursa, corticosteroid infiltration of, 322
Retroperitoneal fibrosis, low back pain in, 261
Retroperitoneal tumors, low back pain in, 261
Rhabdomyolysis syndrome, 97
Rheumatic disease, hand in, 211–226
   in old age, 50–51
   in pregnancy, 50
   regional, 209
   treatment of, 41–49
   wrist in, 211–226
Rheumatic encephalitis, 148
Rheumatic fever, acute, 147–149
   diagnosis of, 148t, 148–149
   mitral disease in, 18
   subcutaneous nodules in, 15–16
Rheumatism, palindromic, patient interview in, 4
   pattern recognition in, 14
Rheumatoid arthritis, 59–73
   acromioclavicular, 248
   age onset in, 59
   amyloidosis in, 65
   anemia in, 65
   articular aspects of, 59–64
   atlantoaxial subluxation in, 65

Rheumatoid arthritis (Continued)
   azathioprine for, 46
   carpal tunnel syndrome in, 65
   cause of, 59, 65
   classification of, 59t
   corticosteroids for, 44
   cricoarytenoid arthritis in, 65
   diagnosis of, 38, 40, 61
   differential diagnosis of, 60
   drug therapy for, 61–62, 347t
   elderly-onset, 51, 68–70, 69t
      vs. polymyalgia rheumatica, 69t
      vs. remitting seronegative symmetrical synovitis with pitting edema, 69t
   experimental treatment of, 47
   Felty's syndrome in, 65
   forefoot pain in, 286
   functional classification of, 38, 40t
   glucocorticoids for, 44
   gold therapy for, 46, 63
   guidelines for, 64
   hydroxychloroquine for, 46
   improvement in, 347t
   in pregnancy, 50
   laboratory studies in, 60
   late, 61
   lymphokines in, 65
   malignant, 61
   marginal erosion in, 61, *61*
   methotrexate for, 45t, 45–56
      hepatic effects of, 346t
   muscle atrophy in, 65
   natural history of, 61, 61t
   neck pain in, 255
   nonsteroidal anti-inflammatory drugs for, 41
   ocular involvement in, 66, 67t
   olecranon bursitis in, 234, 236
   orthopedic surgery in, 48–49
   osteonecrosis in, 203
   outcome in, 61
   painful swollen hands in, 12
   palindromic, 61
   parenchymal pulmonary involvement in, 66
   patient interview in, 4
   pericarditis in, 66
   physical examination in, 60
   physical therapy for, 62–64
   pleuritis in, 66
   polyarthritis in, 15
   presentation of, 59–61, *60*, *61*, 65
   proteinuria in, 65
   radiography of, 21, 60–61, *61*
   referral in, 64
   remission of, 61, 61t
   seronegative, vs. ankylosing spondylitis, 133
   slow-acting agents for, 45–46
   sternoclavicular, 249
   subcutaneous nodules in, 60, *60*, 65–66, *66*
   sulfasalazine for, 46
   systemic manifestations of, 64–68, 65t
   tendon rupture in, 60, *60*
   treatment of, 61–64, 344t–345t
      response to, 64
   vasculitis in, 66–67

Rheumatoid arthritis (Continued)
   vs. chronic tophaceous gout, 153, *154*
   vs. osteoarthritis, 61, *61*
   vs. polyarteritis nodosa, 19
   weakness in, 19
   weight loss in, 65
Rheumatoid factor, 32
Rheumatology, pattern recognition in, 12–20
   practice of, 3–4
"Rhupus" (rheumatoid arthritis/lupus), 107–109
Rickets, biochemical determinations in, 196t
   clinical manifestations of, 196t
   osteomalacia and, 195–197
   vitamin D deficiency and, 195–196
Romberg's test, 267
Rose bengal test, in Sjögren's syndrome, 94
Rotator cuff, 238
   age-related degeneration of, 244–245
   arthropathy of, 242
   exercises for, 328, *328*
   tendinitis of, 240
Rotator cuff arthropathy, arthroplasty for, 49
Rotator cuff impingement, 240–243
   cause of, 240, 240t
   presentation of, 240–241, *241*
   shoulder arc of motion maneuver in, *241*
   tendon rupture in, 242
Rotator cuff tendons, disorders of, pain in, 240
   humeral insertion of, 238
Rubella arthritis, 13, 164
Rubs, 106, 310
Running, iliotibial tract syndrome from, 274–275

Sacroiliac joint, abnormalities of, 11t
   physical examination of, 11
   septic arthritis of, 165
Sacroiliitis, 11
   in ankylosing spondylitis, 16
   in reactive arthritis, 138, *138*
   low back pain in, 260
Salicylates, 41, 41t
   nonacetylated, for systemic lupus erythematosus, 77
Salmonella typhi, in Takayasu arteritis, 129–130
Salsalate, for systemic lupus erythematosus, 77
SAPHO (synovitis, acne, pustulosis, hyperostosis, osteomyelitis) syndrome, 249, 252
Sarcoidosis, 183–184
   rash in, 18
   skin lesion in, 14
   subcutaneous nodules in, 15
Sarcoma, 313
   clear cell, vs. tennis elbow, 230
   soft tissue, 314
   synovial, radiography of, 21
      vs. proliferative tenosynovitis, 221, *222*
"Sausage toe," in reactive arthritis, 136, *137*
Scapholunate joint, ganglia of, 214
Scapula, snapping of, 310
Scapulothoracic joint, 238
Schirmer test, in Sjögren's syndrome, 93, 94
Schober test, 10
Sciatica, 264–266
   disc herniation and, 254
   prevalence of, 260t

Sciatica (Continued)
   pyriformis muscle maneuver in, 265
Scleroderma, 104–107
   acral calcification in, 106, *106*
   breast implants and, 113
   cause of, 104
   classification of, 104, 104t
   diagnosis of, 105
   diffuse, 104, 104t, 106
   disorders confused with, 111, 111t
   gastrointestinal tract in, 105
   in pregnancy, 50
   in Sjögren's syndrome, 105
   limited, 104t, 104–105
   linear, 104, 105t
   localized, 104, 105t
   outcome of, 105–106, *106*
   patient interview in, 4
   presentation of, 104–105
   Raynaud's phenomenon in, 104
   referral in, 107
   renal failure in, 106
   skin hardening in, 104–105
   treatment of, 106–107
   weakness in, 19
   weight loss in, 17
Sclerosis, radiography of, 24, *25*
Scotoma, in systemic lupus erythematosus, 82
Seizure, in systemic lupus erythematosus, 82
Sepsis, prepatellar bursitis in, 276
Septic arthritis, 165–168
   acromioclavicular, 248
   after arthroplasty, 166
   antibiotics for, 167
   cause of, 165
   diagnosis of, 166
   infected prosthesis and, 166, 167–168
   joint drainage for, 167
   outcome of, 167
   physical measures for, 167
   presentation of, 165t, 165–166
   referral in, 168
   sternoclavicular, 249
   treatment of, 167–168
   vs. osteomyelitis, 205
   vs. septic prepatellar bursitis, 5, *6*
   vs. sympathetic effusion, 276
Shock, toxic, in olecranon bursitis, 234, *235*
Shoes, anatomy of, 334, *334*
   selection of, 334–335
Shoulder. See also specific joint, e.g., *Glenohumeral joint.*
   anatomy of, 238
   corticosteroid infiltration in, 320–321
   cracking of, 310
   frozen, 23, 240, 245–247
   lipomatosis of, 251–252
   motion in, 238
   pain in, 5, *7*, 238–253
      causes of, 238t
      corticosteroids for, 319
      diaphragmatic, 239
      patterns of, 238–239, *239*
   recurrent hemorrhagic, of elderly, 242
   rheumatic disease of, in old age, 50–51

Shoulder (Continued)
   tendinitis of, vs. arthritis, 240
Shoulder arc of motion maneuver, in acromioclavicular arthritis, 240, *241*
   in rotator cuff impingement, 241, *241*
Shoulder exercises, 326–328, *326–328*
   strengthening, 327–328, *328*
   stretching, *326*, 326–327, *327*
Shoulder force-couple, 238
Shoulder impingement syndrome, radiography of, 23
Shrinking lung syndrome, in systemic lupus erythematosus, 84t, 85
Shrug sign, in anterior knee pain, 277
Shulman's disease, 111–112, *112*
Sickle-cell disease, bone infection in, management of, 53, 53t
   rheumatic manifestations of, 53
Silicone breast implants, connective tissue disease from, 112–114
Silicone gel, connective tissue disease from, 113
Single heel rise test, in posterior tibialis tendon rupture, 295
Sjögren's syndrome, 93–96
   anti-La antibodies in, 33
   cause of, 93
   complications of, 94–95
   in human immunodeficiency virus infection, 162
   in systemic sclerosis, 105
   keratoconjunctivitis sicca in, 93, 93t, 94t
      treatment of, 95, 95t
   laboratory findings in, 93–94
   ocular dryness in, 93, 93t, 94t
   oral dryness in, 93, 93t, 94t
   outcome of, 94
   patient interview in, 4
   presentation of, 93t, 93–94, 94t
   referral in, 95
   slow-acting agents for, 45–46
   tests for, 93
   treatment of, 95, 95t
   vaginal dryness in, 93
Skin, effects of corticosteroids on, 319
   in acute rheumatic fever, 148
   in cryoglobulinemia, 131
   in lupus erythematosus, *86*, 86–87
   in systemic sclerosis, 104–105
SLE. See *Systemic lupus erythematosus.*
Sleep, in fibromyalgia, 305
Slipping rib syndrome, 252–253
Snaps, joint, 310, 311
Social Security Administration, disability guidelines of, 55t, 56
Soft tissue, infection of, 311, *312*
   magnetic resonance imaging of, 24t
   mass in, 313–315
   pain in, fever and, 311–313
   radiography of, 21
   sarcoma of, 314
Spinal canal, trefoil, 266, *267*
Spinal disease, mechanical vs. inflammatory findings in, 10
Spinal stenosis, 265–268
   cause of, 266, *267*, 267t
   neurogenic claudication in, 266, *267*, *268*
   radiography of, 23
Spine, cervical, pain in, 254–258. See also *Neck pain.*
   dorsal, pain in, 254, 258–259
   fracture of, in ankylosing spondylitis, 134
      low back pain in, 260
   lumbar, motion of, 10

Spine *(Continued)*
    nerve root irritation of, 264
      pain in, 254. See also *Low back pain.*
      sympathetic blockade of, for reflex sympathetic dystrophy, 303
    metastasis to, radiography of, 23
    osteomyelitis of, *Mycobacterium tuberculosis* and, 170
Spinous processes, kissing, low back pain from, 262, 263
    tenderness in, in spinal disease, 259
Spondylitis, pattern recognition in, 16–17
    psoriatic, 143, 145
Spondyloarthropathy, 133–149. See also specific type, e.g., *Ankylosing spondylitis.*
    Achilles tendinitis in, 288
    acromioclavicular pain in, 248
    brucellosis and, 16
    chest expansion in, 10–11
    diagnosis of, 38, 40
    dorsal pain in, 259
    forefoot pain in, 286
    human leukocyte antigen B27 in, 35–36
    low back pain in, 260
    mechanical vs. inflammatory findings in, 10
    patient interview in, 4
    physical maneuvers in, 10, 11
    plantar heel pain in, 290
    psoriatic, 16
    radiography of, 21, 22, *22*
    slow-acting agents for, 45–46
    sternoclavicular pain in, 249
    undifferentiated, 135–140
      diagnosis of, 138
    Whipple's disease and, 16
Spondylolisthesis, degenerative, 254
Spondylosis, 254
    cervical, 257–258
      pain in, 255, 257
Squeaks, in bone-on-bone contact, 311
Staphylococcus aureus, in acute digital tenosynovitis, 220
    in osteomyelitis, 205
Stellate ganglion, blockade of, for reflex sympathetic dystrophy, 303
Stenosing tenosynovitis, 216
Sternoclavicular joint, 238
    arthritis of, 238–239, *239*
      pain in, 249
      septic arthritis of, 165
      swelling of, 252
Steroids. See *Corticosteroids.*
Stiffness, proximal joint pain and, 19–20
Still's disease, 14
Straight leg raising test, 263
    in sciatica, 264, 265
Streptococcal antibodies, in acute rheumatic fever, 148
Streptococcus, group A, in necrotizing fasciitis, 311–312
Streptococcus pyogenes, acute rheumatic fever from, 147
    in acute digital tenosynovitis, 220
Streptomycin, for Whipple's disease, 142
Stretching exercises, 324, *324*
Subacromial bursa, 238
    corticosteroid infiltration in, 321
Subacromial cracking, 310
Subacromial impingement, anatomy of, *239*
    pain in, 241, *241*
    treatment of, 242
Subacute cutaneous lupus erythematosus, *86,* 86–87
Subclavian artery, in Takayasu arteritis, 129, *130*

Subcostal nerve, compressive neuropathy maneuver for, 270
Subcutaneous nodules, in acute rheumatic fever, 148
    in sarcoidosis, 15
    rheumatoid, 60, *60,* 65–66, *66*
      pattern recognition in, 15–16
      vs. pulmonary neoplasms, 66
Subtalar joint, arthritis of, 285–286
    corticosteroid infiltration of, 322
    eversion at, 285
    inversion at, 285
Sulfasalazine, for ankylosing spondylitis, 135
    for rheumatoid arthritis, 46, 63
    in pregnancy, 343t
    methotrexate plus, 47
Sulfinpyrazone, uric acid reduction with, 44, 156
Sun protection, 337t, 337–338, 338t
Sun protection factor, 337–338
Sunscreens, 338, 338t
Supraclavicular pain, assessment of, 239–240
Suprascapular nerve, compression or entrapment of, 240, 247–248
Supraspinatus, in rotator cuff impingement, 240
Supraspinatus tendon, calcium-induced inflammation of, 243
    in rotator cuff impingement, 240
    tear of, 242
Swan-neck deformity, 212
Sweet's syndrome, rash in, 18–19
Sydenham's chorea, in acute rheumatic fever, 148, 149
Syndesmophytes, in reactive arthritis, 138, *138*
Synovial chondromatosis, 15
Synovial fluid analysis, 28t, 28–31
    bloody, 13
    crystal identification in, 29, *30*
    errors in, 28–29
    in subcutaneous bursitis, 29t
    technique of, 29–31, *30*
Synovial fluid fracture, in joint cracking, 310
Synovitis, foreign body, 15
    in secondary syphilis, 174–175
    osteonecrosis in, 203
    pigmented villonodular, 13, 15, 314
    remitting seronegative, pitting edema with, 12, 72–73
    tuberculous, 170–171
Syphilis, secondary, 13
    polyarthritis in, 15
    synovitis in, 174–175
Systemic lupus erythematosus, 74–86
    anti-La antibodies in, 33
    antinuclear antibodies in, 32, 32t, *33,* 74
    antiphospholipid syndrome in, 87, 88
    anti-Ro antibodies in, 33
    autoantibodies in, 74
    bronchiolitis obliterans in, 84t, 85
    chronic interstitial lung disease in, 84t, 85
    classification of, 74, 75t
    diagnosis of, 38, 40, 74
    differential diagnosis of, 74
    drug-induced, 90t, 90–91
    environmental factors in, 74
    fever in, 88–90
      erysipelas in, 89, *89*
    genetic predisposition to, 74
    glucocorticoids for, 44
    heart murmurs in, 18
    immune complex mediation of, 74
    immunologic findings in, 74

Systemic lupus erythematosus *(Continued)*
   infection in, 88–90
   late-onset, 51
   LE cells in, 74
   mild, 75–79
      autoimmune disease in, 77
      cause of, 75
      corticosteroids for, 78
      diagnosis of, 76
      hydroxychloroquine for, 77
      laboratory studies in, 76
      methotrexate for, 78
      nonsteroidal anti-inflammatory drugs for, 77, 337–338
      outcome of, 76
      presentation of, 75–76, *76*
      referral in, 78
      support groups for, 78
      treatment of, 76–78
      ultraviolet light protection in, 77
      urinalysis in, 76
      vasculitis in, 75, *76*
   mortality in, 75
   neuropsychiatric, 81–83
      manifestations of, 81, 81t
      pathogenesis of, 82t
   osteonecrosis in, 203
   outcome of, 75
   patient interview in, 4
   pericarditis in, 84, 89
   pleuritis in, 84t, 84–85
   pleuropulmonary, 82–86
      presentation of, 84t, 84–85
   pneumonitis in, 84t, 85
   polyarthritis in, 15
   pregnancy in, 50, 87–88
   pulmonary hemorrhage in, 84t, 85
   quinidine and, 90–91
   rash in, 18
   renal, 79–81
      acute changes in, 79, 79t
      chronic changes in, 79, 79t
      classification of, 79t, 79–80
   severity of, 37, 38t
   shrinking lung syndrome in, 84t, 85
   vs. infective endocarditis, 89
   weakness in, 19
Systemic Lupus Erythematosus Damage Index, 37, 39t
Systemic Lupus Erythematosus Disease Activity Index, 37, 37t–38t
Systemic Lupus International Cooperating Clinics SLE Damage Index, 39t
Systemic sclerosis, 104–107. See also *Scleroderma.*

Takayasu arteritis, 129, 351t
   classification of, 129, 129t
   presentation of, 129–130, *130*
Tarsal joint, transverse, motion at, 286
Tarsal tunnel, 291, *291*
Tarsal tunnel syndrome, 291–292
   cause of, 291, 291t
   nerve conduction studies of, 26
Tartrate-resistant acid phosphatase, bone resorption and, 190
Tender points, in fibromyalgia, 305
Tendinitis, 209
   Achilles, in reactive arthritis, 136, 137
      in spondyloarthropathy, 288

Tendinitis *(Continued)*
      posterior calcaneal pain in, 288
   calcific, 243–244
      patellar, 278
   iliopsoas, vs. iliopsoas bursitis, 273t
   in basic calcium phosphate crystal deposition disease, 21, 159
   radiography of, 21
   rotator cuff, 240
   shoulder, vs. arthritis, 240
Tendon(s), fluoroquinolone effect on, 17
   rupture of, corticosteroids and, 319
      in rheumatoid arthritis, 60, *60*
      rotator cuff impingement and, 242
      vs. paralysis, 212
Tennis elbow, 228–230
   cause of, 228, 228t
   corticosteroid infiltration in, 320
   treatment of, 229, 229t
   vs. clear cell sarcoma, 230
   vs. radial tunnel syndrome, 230
Tenodesis effect, differential diagnosis of ruptured tendon, 212
Tenosynovitis, 209
   acute digital, 220–221
   calcific, 220, 221
   corticosteroids for, 319
   crepitating, 218
   de Quervain's, 218–220. See also *De Quervain's tenosynovitis.*
   digital stenosing, 216–218
      frequency of, 217, *217*
      treatment of, 217–218, 218t
   dorsal wrist, corticosteroid infiltration in, 320
   in acute rheumatic fever, 148
   nodular pigmented, 221, *221*
   peroneal, pain in, 286
   proliferative, 221–223
      Mycobacterium tuberculosis and, 170–171
      vs. synovial sarcoma, 221, *222*
   suppurative, 220
   vs. arthritis, 3, 7
Teres major, 238
Thalidomide, for Behçet's ulcers, 147
Thenar eminence, 211, *211*
Thigh, hyperextension maneuver of, for referred low back pain, 261
Thomas' test, for Achilles tendon rupture, 288
Thoracic outlet syndrome, 250–251
   provocative maneuvers in, 250, 250t
Thromboangiitis obliterans, 120–121
Thrombocytosis, 27
Thromboembolism, risk for, 34t
Thrombophilia, lupus anticoagulant with, 34, 34t
Thrombophlebitis, Baker's cyst with, 283, 284
Thrombosis, in antiphospholipid syndrome, 91–92
Thumb, 211, *211*
   extension of, 211
   flexion of, 211
   opposition movement of, 211–212
Thyroid gland, disease of, frozen shoulder in, 245
Thyroiditis, autoimmune, in Sjögren's syndrome, 93–94
Tibial nerve, 274
   posterior, calcaneal branches of, impingement maneuver for, 290
Tibialis tendon, posterior. See *Posterior tibialis tendon.*
Tietze's syndrome, 252–253
Tinel sign, in carpal tunnel syndrome, 224
   in compression neuropathy, 219, 224, 291

Toe, great. See *Hallux* entries.
   "sausage," in reactive arthritis, 136, *137*
Tongue, in amyloidosis, 185, *185*
Tongue depressor test, in Sjögren's syndrome, 93
"Too many toes" sign, in posterior tibialis tendon rupture, 295
Torque test, for carpometacarpal osteoarthritis, 219
Trapezium-trapezoid joint, ganglia of, 214
Trapezius, 238
Trauma, prepatellar bursitis from, 276
Treatment, 41–49
Trendelenburg's lurch, 181
Trendelenburg's sign, 181
Triamcinolone, for Behçet's ulcers, 147
   for gout, 155
Trick knee, 281
Tricyclic antidepressants, 43
   for fibromyalgia, 306
Trigger finger, 216–218, *217*
Trigger phenomenon, in stenosing tenosynovitis, 216, 307
Trigger points, corticosteroids for, 319, 321
   in dorsal spine pain, 259
   in myofascial pain syndromes, 255, 259, 307, 321
Trimethoprim-sulfamethoxazole, for Whipple's disease, 142
Trochanteric bursa, corticosteroid infiltration in, 321
Trochanteric bursitis, 270–271
   lateral hip pain in, 270, *271*
Tropheryma whippelii, 141
L-Tryptophan, in eosinophilia-myalgia syndrome, 111
Tuberculosis, musculoskeletal, 170–171
   osteomyelitis in, 206
   synovitis from, 170–171
   vs. sarcoidosis, 183

Ulcer(s), gastrointestinal, nonsteroidal anti-inflammatory drugs and, 42, 42t
   in Behçet's disease, 146, *146*
Ulcerative colitis, arthritis in, 140
   extraintestinal manifestations of, 141t
Ulnar nerve, compression of, 233
Ultrasonography, 24
Ultraviolet B radiation, from fluorescent light, 77
Undifferentiated connective tissue disease, 107–109
Ureter(s), calculi in, low back pain from, 262
Uric acid, serum levels of, 27
   in gout, 150, 150t, 151
   reduction of, 44, 156
Uricosurics, 156
Urinalysis, 27
   in systemic lupus erythematosus, 76
Urolithiasis, in gout, 153–154
Urticaria, chronic, 18, 118–119
   vs. urticarial vasculitis, 118, 118t
   vasculitic, 14, 18
Uterus, carcinoma of, low back pain from, 262

Vagina, dryness of, in Sjögren's syndrome, 93
Valvular heart disease, arthritis in, 17–18
Varicella-zoster virus, arthritis from, 164
Vasculitis, 115–132
   classification of, 115t
   essential cryoglobulinemic, 351t
   hypersensitivity, 117–118

Vasculitis (Continued)
   classification of, 117, 117t
   in rheumatoid arthritis, 66–67
   in systemic lupus erythematosus, 75, *76*
   large vessel, 351t
   medium-sized vessel, 351t
   patient interview in, 4
   small vessel, 351t
   urticarial, 118–119
      vs. chronic urticaria, 118, 118t
   vessel caliber in, 115, *115*
Vastus lateralis, 274
Vastus medialis, 274
Vertebrae, fractures of, dorsal spine pain in, 258
   in osteoporosis, 191–192, *192*
   herniation of discs between, 264
   and sciatica, 254
Vibration white finger, 109
Viral arthritis, 164
Viruses, in chronic fatigue syndrome, 309
Vitamin D, deficiency of, 196
   osteomalacia from, 195
   rickets from, 195
   for corticosteroid-induced osteoporosis, 195
   for osteomalacia, 196
   for osteoporosis, 193
Vocational rehabilitation, 55t, 55–56

Walker, use of, 335
Walking, assistive devices for, 335–336
Weakness, in arthritis, 19
   in myositis, 97
Wegener's granulomatosis, 124–126, 351t
   arthritis in, 19
   classification of, 124, 125t
   peripheral neuropathy in, 19
   pulmonary-renal vasculitic syndromes in, 125, 125t
   vs. midline granuloma, 125, 125t
Weight loss, in arthritis, 17
   in rheumatoid arthritis, 65
Wheal, urticarial, 118
Whiplash injury, 256–257
   classification of, 256t
Whipple's disease, 141–142
   spondyloarthropathy from, 16
   subcutaneous nodules in, 16
   weakness in, 19
   weight loss in, 17
Wrist, dorsal, tenosynovitis of, 320
   dorsiflexion of, in tennis elbow, 228
   ganglia of, 214
   nerve compression at. See *Carpal tunnel syndrome*.
   pain in, 211–226
      differential diagnosis of, 219t
   palmar flexion of, in golfer's elbow, 232
   repetitive strain injury to, 308
   rub in, 310
   tendons of, corticosteroid infiltration in, 320
   volar, 211, *211*

Xiphodynia, 252–253

Zidovudine, myositis from, 163

ISBN 0-7216-6080-0

```
RC          Canoso, Juan J.
927
C323        Rheumatology in
1997         primary care.
```

$52.00   35409

DATE			

SOUTH COLLEGE
709 Mall Blvd.
Savannah, GA 31406

BAKER & TAYLOR